T0203981

Target Organ Toxicology Series

Ophthalmic Toxicology

Target Organ Toxicology Series

Series Editors
A. Wallace Hayes, John A. Thomas, and Donald E. Gardner

Target Organ Toxicology Series

Ophthalmic Toxicology

Second Edition

Editor

George C. Y. Chiou, Ph.D.

Institute of Ocular Pharmacology
Department of Medical Pharmacology and Toxicology
Texas A&M University College of Medicine
College Station, Texas

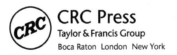

CRC Press
Taylor & Francis Group
Boca Raton London New York

CRC Press is an imprint of the
Taylor & Francis Group, an **informa** business

A TAYLOR & FRANCIS BOOK

OPHTHALMIC TOXICOLOGY, 2/E

First published 1999 by Taylor & Francis

Published 2018 by CRC Press
Taylor & Francis Group
6000 Broken Sound Parkway NW, Suite 300
Boca Raton, FL 33487-2742

© 1999 by Taylor & Francis Group, LLC
CRC Press is an imprint of Taylor & Francis Group, an Informa business

First issued in paperback 2019

No claim to original U.S. Government works

ISBN-13: 978-0-367-44756-4 (pbk)
ISBN-13: 978-1-56032-722-6 (hbk)

This book contains information obtained from authentic and highly regarded sources. Reasonable efforts have been made to publish reliable data and information, but the author and publisher cannot assume responsibility for the validity of all materials or the consequences of their use. The authors and publishers have attempted to trace the copyright holders of all material reproduced in this publication and apologize to copyright holders if permission to publish in this form has not been obtained. If any copyright material has not been acknowledged please write and let us know so we may rectify in any future reprint.

Except as permitted under U.S. Copyright Law, no part of this book may be reprinted, reproduced, transmitted, or utilized in any form by any electronic, mechanical, or other means, now known or hereafter invented, including photocopying, microfilming, and recording, or in any information storage or retrieval system, without written permission from the publishers.

For permission to photocopy or use material electronically from this work, please access www. copyright.com (http://www.copyright.com/) or contact the Copyright Clearance Center, Inc. (CCC), 222 Rosewood Drive, Danvers, MA 01923, 978-750-8400. CCC is a not-for-profit organization that provides licenses and registration for a variety of users. For organizations that have been granted a photocopy license by the CCC, a separate system of payment has been arranged.

Trademark Notice: Product or corporate names may be trademarks or registered trademarks, and are used only for identification and explanation without intent to infringe.

Visit the Taylor & Francis Web site at
http://www.taylorandfrancis.com

and the CRC Press Web site at
http://www.crcpress.com

A CIP catalog record for this book is available from the British Library.

Library of Congress Cataloging-in-Publication Data available from publisher.

Contents

Contributing Authors

Jimmy D. Bartlett, O.D.   *Department of Optometry, School of Optometry, University of Alabama at Birmingham, Birmingham, Alabama 35294*

George C.Y. Chiou, Ph.D.   *Institute of Ocular Pharmacology, Department of Medical Pharmacology and Toxicology, Texas A&M University College of Medicine, College Station, Texas 77843*

Linda C. Epner, M.D.   *Department of Ophthalmology, Cullen Eye Institute, Baylor College of Medicine, Houston, Texas 77030*

Keith Green, Ph.D., D.Sci.   *Department of Ophthalmology and Department of Physiology and Endocrinology, Medical College of Georgia, Augusta, Georgia 30912*

Nicholas J. Millichamp, D.V.M., Ph.D.   *Department of Small Animal Medicine and Surgery, College of Veterinary Medicine, Texas A&M University, College Station, Texas 77843*

Brooks H. Rohde, Ph.D.   *Institute of Ocular Pharmacology, Department of Medical Pharmacology and Toxicology, Texas A&M University College of Medicine, College Station, Texas 77843*

Zhao Hui Song, Ph.D.   *Department of Medical Pharmacology and Toxicology, Texas A&M University Health Science Center, College Station, Texas 77843*

Ann Schroeder, B.S.   *Department of Medical Pharmacology and Toxicology, Texas A&M University Health Science Center, College Station, Texas 77843*

Bo Xuan, M.D.   *Institute of Ocular Pharmacology, Department of Medical Pharmacology and Toxicology, Texas A&M University College of Medicine, College Station, Texas 77843*

Series Preface
Target Organ Toxicology Series

The concept of a Target Organ Toxicology Series began nearly two decades ago with the late Dr. Robert L. Dixon. His early vision provided the initial stimulus and the guidance for the early years of the series. The series began at a time when technical achievements in the field of toxicology were undergoing rapid growth leading to a vast accumulation of scientific information, much of which was focused on identifying the mechanisms associated with the biological action of chemicals on various physiological systems. Emerging knowledge enhanced the understanding of the hazards of environmental contaminants, and the resultant basic assessment led to the formation of a number of federal and state policies promulgating the protection of the public from exposure to chemicals in the environment. The rapid growth of toxicology created a need to address critical issues and recent advances in the assessment of the mechanism of chemically induced toxicity in various target organs. The Target Organ Toxicity Series set out to meet this challenge and has become internationally recognized as a successful series of monographs devoted to the careful and articulate review of critical areas in toxicology and environmental health and also as a major influence affecting future trends in the field of toxicology.

The objectives and goals of the series have always been to highlight a particular organ system and to present a comprehensive and critical synthesis of advances leading to a better understanding of the toxicology of that organ system.

The series is written for a broad scientific audience yet provides comprehensive coverage of specific areas of toxicology. The authors focus their presentation so that the information can be used not only to gain a general understanding of the principles of toxicology but also to be a resource guide directing readers who want a deeper understanding regarding mechanisms of response of a specific substance on a specific target organ.

Beyond being a basic reference resource, the series serves readers with more focused needs. For researchers, who are interested in comparing target organ responses between and among species, the series provides a timely source useful in guiding future research. For educators, the series is a basic reference source as well as a directory to other related toxicological literature. For regulatory scientists, it is a repository of comprehensive information useful in making and supporting regulatory decisions with a toxicological database that may not be available in other single publications.

The series is comprised of monographs edited by leading, internationally recognized scientists with expertise in toxicology and the environmental sciences. The contributors of the various monographs are drawn from a diverse multidisciplinary background and represent industrial, governmental, academic, and research establishments but are always experts on the advances, issues, and concepts of the chapter's topic area. While for each of the topic areas coverage may appear to be highly specialized, together the complete series represents an unique overview of an interdisciplinary approach to evaluate target organ toxicity.

The series editors recognize that the field of toxicology continues to change rapidly, and that new and important advances will be forthcoming. As the needs arise and new knowledge is gained in the field of toxicology, the Target Organ Toxicology Series will provide timely new topics written by international experts.

Preface to the Second Edition

Unlike most ocular toxicology books, which merely list a multitude of toxic compounds and their ophthalmic toxicities, this edition of *Ocular Toxicology* retains its uniqueness by covering specific actions and affinities of ophthalmic poisons to various eye tissues and the animal species; research methods in vivo and in vitro; ophthalmic toxicities of representative chemicals via systemic and/or local delivery; and medical treatment of chemical injuries. As a result, this book can be used by a wide variety of readers in academia, industry, clinics, research laboratories, and government agencies.

Although written by the same author, Dr. K. Green, "History of Ophthalmic Toxicity" (Chapter 1) has been extensively revised and updated, particularly in the sections Definition of Ophthalmic Toxicology, Toxicity Testing, Development of Techniques, and Future Areas for Development.

A new chapter, entitled "Molecular Basis of Ophthalmic Toxicology," by Drs. Song and Shroeder, has been added in this edition because of rapid advancement in ophthalmic toxicology at the molecular level. The chapter is presented in concise, accessible language so that it can be easily read and understood.

Chapter 5, entitled "In Vivo Eye Irritation Test Methods," was completely rewritten by the new author, Dr. K. Green. He expanded the introduction markedly to include the discussion of toxicity versus irritation; in vitro versus in vivo methods; primary test system; and eye responses. In the section regarding the Draize test, he reviewed in detail not only the method itself but also the strengths versus the weaknesses; the advantages versus the disadvantages; the easiness versus the difficulty of the methods; the albino versus the pigmented rabbit; and the systemic versus the local administration of chemicals. This is basically a brand-new chapter that includes 265 references, compared with the old chapter with only 48 references.

In Chapter 6, entitled "In Vitro Methods in Ophthalmic Toxicology," the introduction has been rewritten and newer methods, such as isolated chicken eye, have been added. The section on cell cultures has been completely revised by providing common test methods first, with various cell cultures given later as specific examples. By doing so, repetitive presentations of the same methods in different cell cultures were avoided, thereby saving space.

Major additions have been made in Chapter 8, entitled "Ophthalmic Toxicology by Local Agents," by including, in a condensed, concise form, two chapters from the first edition: "Air Pollution and Ocular Toxicity" and "Occupational Hazards and Ocular Toxicity."

The last chapter, "Treatment of Chemical Ocular Injury" has been revised and updated by Dr. L. Epner. This chapter is very practical and useful for clinicians and health-related professionals for emergency treatment of chemical eye injury. It is also useful for those using chemicals in laboratories or factories, providing commonsense, on-the-spot pretreatment for the injured eyes before the patient(s) is (are) sent to the hospital.

To accommodate the revisions and changes in the structure of the references, a heavy workload of editing, typing, and proofreading has been imposed on the secretarial staff. Without the outstanding assistance provided by Mrs. Patty Sampson, Ms. Misti Frodyma, and Mr. Payton Mayes, this book could not have been completed as planned. I am deeply grateful to all contributors and secretaries for their close cooperation and support in this difficult task.

George C. Y. Chiou
October 23, 1998

Acknowledgments

It was a delightful experience working with all of the contributors to this book. Completing the chapters on time was not an easy task, and I am grateful to all of the contributors, who understood my requests and cooperated fully in meeting the deadline. Because of the vast amount of information and the wide range of fields covered in this book, it took almost two years to develop. I am deeply grateful to the secretarial assistance provided by Mrs. Patty Sampson. Without her superb handling of the word processor and her careful proofreading, this book could not have been completed as efficiently and pleasantly as it was.

Preface to the First Edition

The uniqueness of this book is the coverage of all aspects of ophthalmic toxicology, including the history and research methods of ophthalmic toxicology: tissue specificity and species differences in ocular responses to chemical injuries, eye toxicities caused by systemic drugs, local agents, air pollutants, and occupational hazards, and medical treatment of chemical eye injuries. Although several books are available that cover one or two aspects of the aforementioned areas on an individual basis, none is available that covers all of them in one book as does *Ophthalmic Toxicology*. Therefore, this book will be useful to a broad audience, including researchers, teachers, students, ophthalmologists, optometrists, pharmacists, nurses, and general health-related professionals.

Another unique feature of this book is the concise text that provides an ample amount of reference literature. The references provide readers with useful information needed for ordinary purposes or for in-depth information and further investigation of certain aspects of ophthalmic toxicology.

Chapter 1 summarizes the historical perspective of ophthalmic toxicology. Although the history of ophthalmic toxicology originated in 1785 when Withering first noted the visual side effects of foxglove, the explosive development of ophthalmic toxicology is a relatively recent event in medical science.

Chapter 2 concisely reviews the tissue specificity in response to toxic agents. This chapter is designed to assist in the understanding of ocular toxicity caused by systemic and local agents that are presented in later chapters. Although numerous articles are available that discuss the species specificity of anatomy, physiology, and pharmacology, this is the first time that species specificity of ophthalmic toxicology has been summarized and analyzed.

Good research on ophthalmic toxicology depends very much on reliable animal models. Although the Draize test has been used since 1944 and still is used as the official test method for prediction of clinical toxicities on the eyes in humans, it has inherited numerous problems and disadvantages, as discussed in Chapter 4. For humane reasons, the Draize test should be used as a safety assurance rather than for toxicity testing and only after in vitro tests or skin irritation tests show either no irritation or only a mild irritation of the agents. In addition to the skin test, various in vitro methods have been developed recently as alternatives to the Draize test (Chapter 5). However, no single in vitro method can be used as a complete alternative to the Draize test, as the eye in vivo is a very complex structure that is capable of producing a wide variety of responses to toxic insults.

The toxic eye responses caused by representative systemic agents are presented in Chapter 6. The author lists each class of agent with pathogenesis, ocular manifestation, and patient management.

The toxic ocular responses to local contacts are presented in Chapter 7. Unlike systemic agents, tens of thousands of new chemicals are introduced into the world every year, and a large portion of these compounds are toxic to the eyes. Therefore, local agents are treated differently from the systemic drugs by mentioning the ocular toxicity of only a few representative chemicals in each class of agent based on their uses.

Chapters 8 and 9 discuss the ocular toxicity caused by air pollutants and occupational hazards, respectively. Ocular irritations caused by smog and air pollution have become a daily problem for those residents of cities and industrial towns, while ocular toxicities in chemical plants are obvious problems that are experienced by many workers.

The medical treatment of ophthalmic toxicity is presented in Chapter 10. With proper and immediate treatment of ocular toxicity, the result can be happy restoration of eyesight; without it, tragic loss of partial or total eyesight can occur. Therefore, this chapter should be read not only by ophthalmologists, optometrists, nurses, and emergency personnel but by general health-related professionals as well.

George C. Y. Chiou

Ophthalmic Toxicology
Edited by George C. Y. Chiou
Copyright © 1999 Taylor & Francis

1

History of Ophthalmic Toxicology

Keith Green

*Department of Ophthalmology and Department of Physiology and Endocrinology,
Medical College of Georgia, Augusta, Georgia, USA*

- **Definition of Ophthalmic Toxicology**
  - Evaluation
  - Rechallenge
  - Need for Assessment
  - Constituents
- **Diversity of Ocular Toxicology**
- **Observations of Ocular Toxicology**
- **Clinical Observations**
- **Need for Documentation of Toxic Responses**
- **Toxicity Testing**
  - Introduction of Draize Test
  - Modification of Draize Test
  - Other Refinements
  - Replacement of Draize Test
- **Development of Techniques**
- **Publications**
- **Future Areas for Development**
- **Acknowledgments**
- **References**

DEFINITION OF OPHTHALMIC TOXICOLOGY

Despite the occurrence of many events and observations over a period of decades concerning the influence of drugs, products, raw materials, or devices upon the eye, the science of ocular toxicology, as a recognizably separate discipline from other subspecialties, is of relatively recent origin. The majority of incidents of ocular toxicology, of either single drug effects or of drug interactions, are case reports where the use or addition of a systemic or topical medication, or exposure to certain chemicals, has led to an unexpected or unwanted reaction or adverse side effect. Ideally, any drug, agent, or device designated and specifically targeted for ocular use as a therapeutic or corrective measure should only initiate one event, namely, that which is intended. This ideal situation is rarely, if ever, achieved. Similarly, the inadvertent exposure of the eye to agents not designed for ocular use can cause unwanted effects.

Ocular toxicology, therefore, includes the unwanted response of the eye to compounds or devices designed to come into contact with the ocular surface as well as those occurrences when materials accidentally reach the eye, usually by the topical route but not excluding a systemic route. The latter approximation of tissue and material by accidental exposure comprises ocular irritancy where the responses are usually (but not always) confined to the ocular surface. The consequences of deliberate exposure usually occur in many eye tissues over a longer time period and are associated with toxicity. It is important to keep this not only semantic but also very real differentiation in mind during discussions of acute ocular irritancy versus true tissue toxicity.

Evaluation

As is evident later in this chapter, acute ocular irritation studies are only performed with evaluation of but three eye tissues, namely, the cornea, conjunctiva, and iris, for these are the only criteria included in the test paradigm. Tissues that are known to be more responsive, in many cases (and dependent upon the origin of the stimulus), such as the lens and retina, are simply not evaluated in ocular irritancy testing. This major divergence in experimental outcomes means that any attempt to assess toxicity using the standard ocular irritation test paradigm is doomed at the outset to be less than successful. The irritation test only addresses three ocular tissues in a qualitative (or, at best, semiquantitative manner) after only a single administration of test agent or product.

Clinical experience has taught us that true ocular toxicity can present in a variety of eye tissues in a multiplicity of different ways. Use of the irritation test system, therefore, for anything other than elimination of ophthalmic products for human use at an early stage of development is not a productive step. The two approaches are, in reality, mutually exclusive due to the very limited conditions under which the irritation test is conducted. Historically, they may have been thought to overlap or be part of a continuum, but this is incorrect. Even the species used primarily in the irritation test, the albino rabbit, is a poor model for toxicity studies because melanin can interplay with either the primary compound or metabolites to alter drug pharmacokinetics. Despite these shortcomings, the Draize test still has a place in the evaluation of products or chemicals. These lie in two areas: (1) that for which the test was designed, namely, to provide an index of the acute irritation potential of a variety of materials that can accidentally reach the eye; (2) the initial phases of the evaluation of products designed for ocular use in the treatment of eye diseases or disorders.

Rechallenge

Very few reports offer the results of a rechallenge with the same drug used by a patient to discern whether or not the drug, or some component of the product, was indeed the cause of the initial reaction. The latter, of course, represents the ultimate test of drug or product toxicity, namely, that a repetition of the response occurs as a result of reuse or reapplication of the same drug or product. Many of these observations, therefore, are anecdotal since they rely upon single individual observations.

Deductions, conclusions, extrapolations, or inferences are frequently drawn from a series of events or the experience of the observer(s) to discern the source of the adverse effect. Careful history taking with repetition of questions in different forms is imperative to help establish a singular cause of the undesirable response. Such questioning, together with examination of the labeling of the material under examination, may yield valuable clues that will help in the determination of the probable underlying inducer of the adverse effect. These observations are sometimes given as case reports. Individually, each report may be of relatively little importance, but when a number of similar observations are accumulated they may represent a significant finding that is indicative of a true drug-induced reaction. Reactions to drugs or agents may be idiosyncratic or reflect a true adverse ill effect that is noted in a significant number of individuals exposed to a particular drug or agent.

Need for Assessment

The expansion of medicine into a scientific and drug-based discipline rather than an empirical and herbal art, which occurred in the late 19th and early 20th centuries, gave rise to the development of specific drug products. Following World War II, the use of specific, targeted drugs exploded and gave rise to the need to assess these compounds for side effects before their exposure to man (Jackson, 1992). The philosophical change that accompanied this transition resulted in the development of many single chemical entities that were created or designed to attack specific pathophysiological conditions. This progress, in turn, led to the need for an assessment of a single variable against a background of relative constants (Jackson, 1984).

The veritable explosion of new chemicals and devices requires research protocols not only to determine their efficacy, but also to attempt to discern any side effects. This has given rise, over the past three or four decades, to the study of mechanisms of drug effects rather than solely descriptions of responses. Similarly, the recognition of toxic or irritation responses of the eye to a variety of chemicals or finished products in the marketplace has led to the development of test paradigms to evaluate toxic responses.

Constituents

Ocular irritation assessment and toxicology consists of two primary systems: First, the study of drugs, devices, or agents given prophylactically in animal trials before their use in man, to provide some prediction of any potential hazard in human use. This aspect, further, has at least two components that include assessment of the ocular toxicity of compounds designed to be administered therapeutically to the eye in topical form or drugs given systemically that will reach the eye. Another component is the evaluation of the ocular irritation potential of chemicals that may accidentally reach the ocular surface, either directly by accidental spillage or through the systemic circulation; this category includes materials such as eye cosmetics as well as those represented by office products, household chemicals, volatile organic solutes, shampoos, and raw materials used in manufacturing. Historically, the use of test systems to evaluate the ocular irritation potential of materials that would accidentally reach the eye preceded testing of ocular products (Green, 1998).

Second, the study of the effect of drugs, agents, or drug interactions that have been shown to create adverse effects following their use in, or exposure to, man. The latter include not only ocular effects of systemic drugs (e.g., chloroquine, ethambutol, etc.), but also the systemic effects of ocular drugs (Bartlett and Jaanus, 1989; Newcomb and Priest, 1989) (e.g., timolol, phenylephrine) and the obvious ocular effects of ocular drugs (e.g., echothiophate, pilocarpine gel). Such definitions must be viewed relatively conservatively, however, or many substances would be considered toxic. Most drugs or agents, for example, will cause an adverse effect if a sufficiently high concentration is reached. Even oxygen if inhaled at 100% concentration is toxic, and distilled water, if continually ingested, would ultimately lead to severe systemic problems.

The nature and time course of adverse effects depend upon many factors. These include the drug or agent per se, the route of administration or exposure, the frequency and longevity of exposure, whether or not a disease or disorder preexists (e.g., the corneal penetration of a drug may be altered during anterior segment or corneal inflammation), age and sex of the recipient, use or exposure to other drugs or agents, and idiosyncrasies. The key is to make careful observations to determine any correlation with drug intake or exposure and identify the variable. One then makes observations that explore the accuracy, or truthfulness, of the observed effects, and their precision or reproducibility. Once a causal relationship has been established, then one can indicate that a toxic effect has occurred (Havener, 1983). It then behooves the investigator to quantitate the observations in an appropriate manner using modern in vitro and in vivo technological methodologies.

Sometimes, despite appropriate establishment of apparent safety in preclinical and clinical trials, the full complement of adverse effects is not realized until a drug is widely used in the population for which it is targeted. An example of such drugs is the first-generation topical beta-adrenergic blockers for reduction of intraocular pressure. Although these drugs, especially timolol, received extensive phase II and III testing relative to drugs that preceded these compounds into the marketplace and set standards by which all new drugs are tested, most of the trial participants were not of the normally elderly population that has glaucoma. Only when the drugs were used widely in the population in which glaucoma was prevalent were a spectrum of adverse effects noted.

Some of these responses were due to poor recounting of medical history by patients or poor history taking on the part of ophthalmologists who then prescribed the beta-blocker in patients for whom their medical history should have precluded use of these drugs, and some responses were due to true adverse effects of the drugs. The ability to distinguish these responses is often clouded; thus adverse effects might be over-reported. On the other hand, such responses might be dismissed as idiosyncratic reactions and remain unreported. Whether these two mechanisms cancel each other is a matter of conjecture. It is against such a background that adverse drug effects are sometimes noted, together with more classical observations.

DIVERSITY OF OCULAR TOXICOLOGY

Given the huge number of prescription drugs (reportedly over 30,000 in the United States alone and obviously many more worldwide) and over-the-counter medications (reportedly about 300,000 in the United States) together with all of the various manufactured and natural products to which we are exposed (Meyer and Fraunfelder, 1987), it is not surprising that toxic or adverse reactions occur within the general population. Accidental exposure of man to any chemical substance in our environment is always a possibility, and precautionary measures should be known in order to treat such incidences. These occurrences may be due to a single drug, device, or agent or due to an interaction between two or more drugs.

Instances occur of accidents, such as train derailments and vehicle crashes, or occurrences, such as sick building syndrome, that are often triggered by volatile organic solvents used in paint or carpet, within the public domain, and emergency treatment procedures should be delineated to minimize the sequelae of such events. There is also an entire ocular toxicology associated with cosmetics that includes safety testing and prognostic ocular toxicology. This area includes mascaras, eyeliners, eye shadows, and eyebrow pencils, as well as devices such as eyelash curlers.

There was, and still is, a need for standardization of the observations and an appropriate means of record keeping. These standards have been set by various authorities (e.g., the European Community [Schnieders, 1987; Lehnert and Ulrich, 1990], United States [Hackett, 1990], and others) and must be met before approval for human use is permitted. Such steps are vital for the protection of human health. There is still a need for the acceptance of worldwide standards for the labeling of drugs, medications, chemicals, products, and agents, especially those with the potential for eye damage. Of particular benefit would be worldwide acceptance of standard criteria for ocular toxicity testing. Such standards would allow transference of data from one continent to another, alleviating the need for duplication of effort and expediting the utilization of medications on a wider basis. This process is under continuous review, known as international harmonization, and universally accepted standards are slowly and gradually becoming part of the criteria used worldwide.

OBSERVATIONS OF OCULAR TOXICOLOGY

Perhaps the earliest observation of ocular toxicity was in 1785 by Withering (1785), who noted that ingestion of foxglove caused confused vision in man, with objects appearing green or yellow. These observations were supported by Carroll (1945), who noted similar eye and vision changes after the use of digitalis. Grant (1974) has summarized over 100 years of observations on the effects of drugs or agents on the visual system in an elegant synopsis of what is known about substances having toxic effects on the eye. Some observations are dependent upon data from laboratory studies, but the majority of observations are case reports. This text has undergone revisions more recently (Grant and Schuman, 1993).

CLINICAL OBSERVATIONS

Bron (1979) drew attention to the remarkable diversity of ocular responses that drugs may cause, some occurring during drug intake and others showing the occurrence of a toxic response after drug withdrawal. Experience has taught us that corticosteroids may cause cataracts and/or elevated intraocular pressure and that chloroquine can induce a keratopathy and/or a retinopathy. These side effects of drugs used for the treatment of non-ocular disorders, among others, are well known. Experience has also taught us when it is prudent to monitor for toxic side effects of drugs (Bron, 1979). A variety of tests may be employed to determine whether certain parameters of ocular function fall within normal limits; these include direct and indirect ophthalmoscopy, slit-lamp biomicroscopy, intraocular pressure, near and distance visual acuity, visual fields, electroretinography, color vision, dark adaptation, and fluorescein angiography (Green, 1998). Changes that may disturb vision include corneal deposits, cataracts, glaucoma, retinal and optic nerve disease, and nystagmus (Bron, 1979). Appropriate quantitation of these effects, as they occur in vivo, can be made using different techniques (Green, 1998).

NEED FOR DOCUMENTATION OF TOXIC RESPONSES

The *Physicians' Desk Reference* (PDR) (1996) and *Physicians' Desk Reference for Ophthalmology* (1996) are frequently used as reference sources of drug side effects. Both PDRs contain the same information as supplied on the FDA-approved package insert that is made available by the drug manufacturer or supplier. The PDR began in 1946 and the PDR for Ophthalmology in 1974, indicating an early awareness of the need to provide a resource that listed the possible side effects and complications, as well as precautions to be taken with the use, of various medications. These side effects were recognized as extensions of the observed therapeutic effect, with some responses being of an allergic nature (*Physicians' Desk Reference*, 1996), and reflected the transition from descriptive to mechanistic medicine. Inorganic materials tend to cause an irritant reaction that has as its components hyperemia, edema, increased vascular permeability, and blistering. Organic compounds cause many effects on different tissues, with many of the effects being reversible upon withdrawal of the drug (Duke-Elder, 1972).

Many observations and descriptions were made dating to the late 1800s and early 1900s for cataracts and other, less evident, ocular disorders. As steroids began to be introduced and more widely used to combat either ocular or systemic inflammatory diseases, the dual secondary effects of cataract and elevated intraocular pressure became evident. Other examples of such side effects are the cataract-inducing effects of echothiophate, which may take a decade of continued use to be revealed, and the occurrence of superficial punctate keratitis due to surfactants used as preservatives in topical medications, which appears long after the primary disease has disappeared.

One of the major concerns of ocular toxicology research in the mid-1960s was the development of a meaningful and practical test of safety of many manufactured products. These products include drugs, medicines, devices, and agents in addition to the multitude of chemicals to which the consumer is exposed in the home or office, ranging from household cleaning products to cosmetics and from copy machine toners to solvents, respectively. Knowledge of the mechanisms of an injury to the eye caused by direct contact of toxic substances is, in the majority of cases, unknown. Many compounds are, rather, known only as an inducer of a response (Beckley, 1965).

As discussed below, the underlying question concerning the similarity and relationship of the response of the widely chosen test model, the rabbit, relative to the effects in man caused by the same agent, is one that remains unanswered. Similarly, the induction of like responses (i.e., corneal edema, conjunctival hyperemia) by different stimuli raises some questions concerning the common nature of the underlying biochemical changes. Furthermore, an expansion of the major test paradigm occurred from testing of products, chemicals, or agents, that normally only gain access to the eye by accidental exposure or by systemic intake, to the different perspective of irritation testing of ophthalmic products using the same test system. Any, and all, testing regimens have their inherent limitations that permit evaluation of any material only to the degree that the test model allows. Given the limitations of any model system, it is not surprising that adverse effects are noted when materials are allowed access to the general population. The mis-use, or even the correct use, of any substance may lead to adverse reactions, especially in the sensitive tissues of the eye.

TOXICITY TESTING

Introduction of Draize Test

The aim of the study of ocular toxicology is to anticipate and avoid considerable side effects of drugs or agents. This is achieved best through a series of comprehensive tests prior to human use. Testing normally occurs in animals, with the choice of the model system being very important because different species give different responses to the same stimulus (Bito, 1984). Testing is usually performed by noting the severity of injury to the eye, and the data are used as a guide to determine any precautionary labeling of the drug or agent for human use or potential human exposure (Green, 1998). Because many agents, chemicals, or drugs reach the eye by a topical route, considerable emphasis was placed originally on the assessment of ocular injury or irritation by this route.

The earliest standardized test schedule for determining external ocular toxicity was published in 1944 by Friedenwald and co-workers (Friedenwald et al., 1944). This basic grading schedule was upgraded by Draize and his co-workers (Draize et al., 1944) with a system that was modified in 1952 and 1959 (Draize and Kelley, 1952; Draize, 1959). Standard use of this scheme for testing commercial substances in the albino rabbit has occurred through its specified use by several different government agencies. The Federal Hazardous Substances Act (Consumer Product Safety Commission, 1979), as detailed in the 1979 Code of Federal Regulations (1979), provided the criteria for determining what constitutes "safe" or "hazardous" materials. The Federal Hazardous Substances Act Regulation (1982) is the most recent outline of the protocols to be employed in the United States.

No discussion of the history of ocular toxicity would be complete without an exploration of the use of the Draize test and the various other in vitro and in vivo tests that it has generated. It could be said that the other tests would have evolved anyway, and in some cases the technology has been developed because of other needs, such as the understanding of physiological, biochemical, or pathophysiological processes, but there is little question that the Draize test has acted as a stimulus for the development of many in vitro or alternative systems. More sensitive in vivo test methodologies have also been developed as the Draize test was adapted from its original role as a method for testing ocular irritancy of substances that could accidentally reach the eye, to a test used for discerning and evaluating the safety and toxicity and irritation of ophthalmic products.

The latter use of the Draize test, namely, for the determination of the ocular toxicity potential of compounds designed for ophthalmic use, represents a large philosophical change from the original use of the test, which was to evaluate chemicals or products that would not normally deliberately reach the eye. The Draize test has several limitations in terms of a one-time exposure to test material, very limited qualitative evaluation of only a few eye tissues (cornea, conjunctiva, and iris) with no evaluation of lens or retina, very limited scope of tissue examination, and limited evaluation time. Ophthalmic products are designed and made for the alleviation of some pathological occurrence in the eye, ideally without themselves inducing any adverse response. While irritation testing in early stages of drug development would be of value in eliminating those drugs that might cause undesirable side effects, final testing of ophthalmic products using a test paradigm that is as crude and restrictive as the Draize test does not provide the necessary precision and sensitivity to assess potential damage to ocular tissues from such products.

Newer, more sensitive methodologies have been developed not only to provide better conditions for the assessment of potential ophthalmic products but also for the determination of underlying physiological and biochemical tissue responses. The latter has been the primary driving force in the technological developments, namely, the desire and need to understand how the eye tissues normally function in order that pathophysiological processes can be better understood and regulated. Through such further comprehension, disease or aging processes may be better controlled or influenced. Toxicological assessments of tissue–product interaction can also be better understood by adopting the new techniques to such studies.

The so-called Draize test has been subject to analysis by a number of authors who have addressed the accuracy and reproducibility of the method, the scoring system (Weltman et al., 1965; Baldwin et al., 1973), and comparisons of rabbit data, in which the test is specified, to the human experience. The Draize eye irritation test scores the effects of drugs or agents, when delivered as 0.1 g (100 mg) of a solid or 0.1 ml (100 μl) of a liquid into the lower cul-de-sac of the eye. The effects on the cornea, conjunctiva, and iris of rinsed and unrinsed eyes are evaluated at 1, 24, 48, and 72 hours, and 4 and 7 days after administration of the test material. Because of the scoring procedures, corneal and iris lesions have greater emphasis in the accumulation of "points" for the total score (Green, 1992a). The corneal scores, because of the multiplication of the different individual subsections, tend to rank very high (80 of 110, or 72%). The observations required by the testing agencies involve only nonmicroscopic observations of the eye. To assist in the evaluation process, a series of color slides indicating different scores of the various responses are available (Federal Register, 1964; Food and Drug Administration, 1965). Many authors have stressed greater precision and sensitivity of the test by using different grading systems, slit-lamp biomicroscopy, or objective physical measurements of parameters, such as corneal thickness (Burton, 1972; Green et al., 1981, 1985, 1990; Morgan et al., 1987; Kennah et al., 1989) or corneal epithelial permeability to fluorescein (Green et al., 1985; Ramselaar et al., 1988). Several aspects of this literature have been reviewed earlier (McDonald and Shadduck, 1977; McDonald, Seabaugh et al., 1987; McDonald, Hiddeman et al., 1987; Chan and Hayes, 1988; Green et al., 1997).

The Draize test, as originally described, was designed for the evaluation of the ocular irritancy potential of products that were not designed to reach the ocular surface except by accident. The use of a one-time application was used to simulate this situation. The application of this test to determine ocular toxicity has several inherent difficulties. Not the least of the problems relates to the number of applications of the test product. Ocular toxicity frequently does not occur after a single product application but rather after a series of applications, sometimes over a long time period. This requires an adjustment in the test paradigm. Ocular toxicological changes are not necessarily confined to the ocular surface, as more often occurs with irritation responses, and requires appropriate steps for the evaluation of ocular tissues other than cornea, conjunctiva, and iris. Thus, although the chemicals may be similar, different responses would be anticipated in determining the ocular irritation potential of a finished product versus the ocular toxicity of long-term lower level exposure in the work place to various ingredients of that product, or even the final compound, during its manufacture. The ability to distinguish between these two approaches is fundamental to comprehension of irritation potential versus toxicity. Ocular toxicity cannot be evaluated by the Draize test for the reasons outlined above. Furthermore, the albino rabbit, in which the eye irritation test is normally specified to be performed, is not an ideal model for examining and predicting drug behavior in man.

The primary objections to the Draize eye irritation test are those of interlaboratory variation and the accuracy of predicting effects on man. These concerns have been expressed for quite some time, but the level of concern has increased over the past 10 years as greater accuracy and sensitivity have been sought in order to increase the predictive value of the test. Laboratory-to-laboratory variation is expected because the observations required in the Draize test are subjective, although comparisons of unknown samples to known standards often produce similar data. The greater reactivity of the rabbit eye compared to that of man has been one of the major problems with the Draize test. The development of more intense, and prolonged, responses on the rabbit eye compared to man means that the effects are overestimated relative to human responses. Similarly, the use of a large amount, or volume, of test material relative to the smaller amount that humans are estimated to receive on their ocular surface tends to maximize the response of the rabbit eye. The use of other species has been suggested as a means of overcoming this problem. Nevertheless, the rabbit remains the mainstay of the testing protocols required by regulatory agencies.

Modification of Draize Test

Primate testing, however, although providing more accurate comparisons to man than rabbit testing (Green et al., 1978) has the disadvantage of much greater cost, restricted availability, dangers associated with their handling, and the potential for loss of sight for these animals. Other alternatives (Griffith et al., 1982) suggest that making the rabbit eye irritation test less severe so as to give results consistent with the known human experience is a more practical approach. This is especially true for the lids and conjunctiva of the rabbit, which have a much more vigorous reaction than those same tissues in man. The corneal response in each species is almost equal.

Historically, a reduction in dose of applied material and an assessment of reversibility of the response were suggested by the National Research Council Committee of the National Academy of Sciences. This group was asked by the Consumer Product Safety Commission to review the criteria utilized in the Federal Hazardous Substances Act for their ability to predict human ocular responses. As a result of their deliberations the committee suggested, 20 years ago, that a smaller dose be used, to reduce the ocular responses of rabbits to a range more consistent with known responses available from the human experience (Committee for the Revision of NAS Publication 1138, 1977). The committee further suggested that the use of at least two dose levels would provide useful information, and that longer observation times would allow the factoring of reversibility of any response. Testing of a series of substances with different degrees of recognized irritation potential indicated that the Federal Hazardous Substance Act test criteria overrated the irritancy of all the moderate irritants. The National Academy of Sciences test criteria, however, when using a 0.01 ml (10 μl) dose, best predicted the human experience (Green, 1998). The latter, of course, are based on anecdotal information, reports to companies from consumers, and occupational incidents and, in many cases, form only an incomplete series of reports.

Other Refinements

Subsequent studies, during the intervening years, on the interrelationship between animal experimental data and the human experience after exposure to the same materials has only supported the notion that ocular irritation responses after low dose applications of materials in rabbits is equivalent to human responses. This result has been substantiated in several studies (Griffith et al., 1982; Freeberg et al., 1984; Arthur et al., 1986; Freeberg, Hooker et al., 1986; Freeberg, Nixon et al., 1986; Allgood, 1989). It is evident, therefore, that a further modification of the Draize test that incorporates dilute solutions or smaller quantities or volumes of material needs to be accepted by the appropriate authorities to allow more appropriate use of this test for predication of human responses. Not only does this maneuver provide a more valid test model, but it also allows a more accurate determination of the underlying tissue events. With a more restricted response that does not produce maximal responses in all aspects of the test, it is possible, using more sophisticated methods, to discern the underlying mechanisms of action of the test agent.

Fewer numbers of animals have also been advocated for in vivo irritancy testing, and this has been demonstrated to provide equally adequate data for eye irritancy potential (Talsma et al., 1988). Regulatory agencies have responded to these recommendations, and decreases in the number of animals from the usual six to one or three, depending upon the observed response, is acceptable. Use of fewer animals, together with decreased amounts of applied test materials, allows a greater number of more quantitative observations to be made in the same time period. More subtle changes can be more readily detected using more sophisticated techniques.

Replacement of Draize Test

Several in vitro tests have been developed that complement the Draize test and allow initial screening of drugs, products, chemicals, or agents prior to final testing in an in vivo animal-model system. In vitro tests, such as the isolated bovine cornea (Muir, 1985), isolated eyes (Burton et al., 1981; Himber et al., 1985; Price and Andrews, 1985; Maurice and Singh, 1986), isolated rabbit ileum (Muir, 1983), tissue cultured cells of ocular and nonocular origin (Bracher et al., 1987/8; North-Root et al., 1982, 1985; Kemp et al., 1983, 1985; Nardone and Bradlaw, 1983; Scaife, 1985; Rink and Hockwin, 1987; Simmons et al., 1987; Ward et al., 1997), chick chorioallantoic membrane (CAM) (Leighton et al., 1985; Luepke, 1985; Parish, 1985), and nonliving systems (Gordon and Bergman, 1987, 1988; Wallin et al., 1987; Gordon et al., 1990) have been employed.

Each of these alternative testing methods has drawbacks compared with the response of the in vivo eye. The isolated cornea represents but one facet of the ocular response by eliminating the vasoactive and chemotic components of the conjunctival response; tissue cultured cells have no blood supply, thus no vascular response can be observed; the CAM offers an elegant alternative for the ocular vascular response but does not include the membranes and connective tissue similar to the cornea and, in addition, an assumption is made concerning a relationship between angiogenesis and inflammation; the totally synthetic system (Eyetex) offers no vascular response, although apparently showing clouding similar to the corneal stroma (Gordon and Bergman, 1987, 1988; Gordon et al., 1990). The latter, however, uses the response of jackbean protein to simulate the complex stromal environment of glycosamino-glycans and collagen where it is the collagen fibril arrangement pattern that acutely governs clarity or opacity of the stroma. Alterations in the glycosaminoglycans of the stroma change the spatial distribution and arrangement of the collagen fibrils; thus the synthetic model uses totally different physical and chemical bases to simulate the cornea.

Initial testing using these in vitro systems has a valuable role in the assessment of potential toxicity of materials that we use or are exposed to either accidentally or deliberately. These methodologies, despite their limitations and lack of relationship to integrated ocular responses, provide a means of screening products or chemicals in order that irritants can be either excluded from in vivo testing or used in dilute form in in vivo test systems. All roads for the present, however, lead to use of the final in vivo assessment (albeit modified in scope and numbers of animals) as the ultimate test procedure. Further testing of in vitro methodologies may yield a system, or a combination of systems, that may predict the behavior of chemicals, drugs, and agents in man. At present, however, this notion appears quite remote.

Can one, with sufficient accuracy, predict the human experience from rabbit or even in vitro data? The present evidence, if the correct low dosage in vivo test is used in rabbit, is that it is possible to obtain a valid comparison that would be predictive of and reflect human eye behavior to ocular irritants. Known experience after exposure to specific chemicals is most often less drastic in man than equivalent exposure in other test species. The predictive experience, thus far, with entirely in vitro test methods appears somewhat promising, although it is probably very unlikely that a single test will replace the Draize, and conclusive agreement upon valid tests may take several years to achieve.

As Beckley (1965) points out, however, we would condemn the placement of unknown substances into the human eye without first testing it for safety in animal eyes. This does not imply that one treats the in vivo test with impunity, but approaches the test in a compassionate and thoughtful manner with use of a lower initial concentration of the material in only a few test cases before proceeding to the test of the full-strength material if that is justified on the basis of lack of response to low doses. The final stage of testing in animals follows in vitro tests that eliminate harmful irritants and restrict animal testing only to compounds that are not likely to induce severe effects.

In 1981, the cosmetics industry took the lead in expanding studies on alternative approaches to assessment of in vivo irritancy by establishing the Center for Alternatives to Animal Testing (CAAT) based in the School of Hygiene and Public Health at the Johns Hopkins University Medical Institutions. The aim of this center is to serve as a focal point for the utilization of industry funds for the study of cellular and molecular events occurring with inflammatory processes in cell and tissue culture systems. The results of the studies supported by the center have been published (Goldberg, 1983, 1984, 1985, 1987a,b, 1988, 1989). In the in vitro agarose diffusion organic test system, a high correlation has been obtained with the in vivo Draize test (Wallin et al., 1987; Jackson et al., 1988). Indeed, the relatively high success rate and predictability of this test have already caused some cosmetic companies to adopt this method as an in vitro alternative for ocular irritancy testing (Jackson, 1992). There has been a marked transition over the last 50 years, therefore, from the introduction of the Draize test to a spectrum of alternative tests that allow the use of fewer animals and, in some cases, possible total replacement of animals by batteries of other test systems.

A similar arrangement exists in Europe with the formation of the European Centre for the Validation of Alternative Methods (ECVAM). The express founding of this group is to offer a means of testing the validity, sensitivity, and predictability of in vitro tests as alternatives to the Draize (Balls and Fentem, 1997). Tests by this group, and many others, have revealed that no one test has the ability to accurately predict all phases of the eye irritation response to a specific stimulus. Indeed, some groups differ widely in their assessment of the usefulness and validity of individual test systems (Bruner et al., 1991, 1996; Spielmann et al., 1991, 1997; Bagley et al., 1992; O'Brien et al., 1992; Christian and Diener, 1996; Bradlaw and Wilcox, 1997; Chamberlain et al., 1997). The only factor that has been clearly demonstrated is that compounds may be initially evaluated by physicochemical information and structure–activity relationships that seem to contribute to the ability to reduce test procedures. In vitro test systems can be effectively used as a further progression in the test system as a screen to categorize materials and products into broad species of compounds that may be used to eliminate certain chemicals from further testing. This constitutes the so-called three-tier system that involves the initial use of physicochemical data (Leahy et al., 1997), followed by in vitro testing, and, finally, limited in vivo testing as dictated by previous information and initial testing protocols (Avalos et al., 1997; de Silva et al., 1997).

DEVELOPMENT OF TECHNIQUES

While there has been an emphasis on the Draize test and its modification or possible replacement with alternative in vitro test systems over the years, there has also been a vast expansion in oculotoxicity methods for all eye tissues, including the cornea, lens, and retina (Hockwin et al., 1992). These techniques have developed out of a need for better quantitation and greater understanding of changes that occur in tissues as a result of a variety of applied perturbations. The appropriation, adaptation, and use of the new technologies to toxicity and irritation testing have been a logical step as more subtle tissue changes were found during physiological studies. These developments have permitted the identification of not only the effects of lower doses of products, but also the changes induced by pharmacological agents or other external influences during exploration of normal tissue behavior where overt irritation is not necessarily noted.

These more sensitive in vivo techniques have been developed out of a need to evaluate the response of ocular tissues in finer detail in order to understand how to regulate these tissues to prevent, arrest, or reverse pathophysiological events in the eye (Hockwin et al., 1992). Use of these methods has permitted a much greater understanding of the basic mechanisms that govern the behavior of different eye tissues and their interrelationships. In addition, new drug development, with the associated toxicity testing and establishment of a better safety profile, has been enhanced through a greater comprehension of underlying physiology and biochemistry. The incorporation of these tests into toxicological studies has been a logical expansion that includes the use of pigmented animals, examination of the response of other ocular tissues (e.g., trabecular meshwork, retina, lens, ciliary body, extraocular tissues), and the use of quantitative techniques to document tissue changes. This allows the study of ocular toxicology rather than ocular irritation.

The simple addition of slit-lamp biomicroscopy, direct or indirect ophthalmoscopy, or magnification loupes has enabled another layer of objectivity to be introduced into the test system. These provisions allow further details to be revealed, especially at lower test-agent concentrations. The use of a slit-lamp enables details to be revealed that would normally be overlooked with a simple illumination system (Green et al., 1981).

Specifically for the cornea, the use of specular microscopy (with or without simultaneous pachymetry [Santoul et al., 1990]) has allowed the assessment of corneal endothelial changes in the living eye by permitting measurement of cell density and shape. Sophisticated analytical software methods exist that allow one to distinguish the various changes in corneal endothelial cell morphology, such as polymegathism or pleomorphism, that may occur in the endothelium (Edelhauser and Ubels, 1992). These morphological changes may well reflect underlying alterations in physiology that initiate the structural rearrangements that occur to compensate for changes in passive permeability, enzyme activity, other cellular biochemical processes, and so on (Green, 1991).

Similarly, new technologies have allowed assessment of lens changes in the formation of cataracts. These technologies arose due to a need for more accurate and quantitative measures of lens changes in aging, diabetes, and radiation as well as after drug influence. As in vitro techniques provided more precise information concerning cataract formation, so newer in vivo techniques were required to assess the subtle changes occurring in the in situ eye. Equipment developed to allow slit-image photography of the lens using Scheimpflug's principle has permitted quantitative analysis of lens toxicity (Dragomirescu et al., 1978; Eckerskorn et al., 1987; Lehnert et al., 1987; Lerman, 1987; Wegener and Hockwin, 1987; Wegener et al., 1987).

Evaluations have been made of a whole range of environmental and drug influences upon the development of cataracts in different animal models, allowing a differentiation to be made between drug-induced effects, aging changes, and alterations induced in diabetes or by radiation (Wegener and Hockwin, 1987; Kojima et al., 1990; Schmitt et al., 1990). In addition, more recent analytical techniques, such as nuclear magnetic resonance, have been used in vivo and in vitro to examine lens changes (Lerman, 1990). In vitro examination methods for analyzing changes in lenses after experimental study have also become available. These techniques allow the use of smaller portions of tissue such that thin sections can now be analyzed, instead of whole lenses, to provide information on regional lens changes (Bours et al., 1990). Use has also been made of chemical structures and known phototoxicity of chemicals in predicting their behavior in lenses (Roberts and Dillon, 1990).

Other studies on eye tissues, such as those in the anterior segment or relative to intraocular pressure control and aqueous humor formation, have also profited from the application of new techniques and equipment (Green, 1992b,c). Electrophysiological studies of the retina (Blain et al., 1990; Brown et al., 1990), combined with morphological studies, have enabled toxicity tests to be performed on a variety of inorganic (Hennekes et al., 1987; Paylor et al., 1987; Green et al., 1993) and organic compounds (D'Amico et al., 1985; Baldinger et al., 1986; Small et al., 1987; Fiscella et al., 1988; Zlioba et al., 1988). Detailed examinations have also outlined age-related tissue changes (Weisse et al., 1990) as well as the toxicological response differences between pigmented and albino animals (Rubin, 1990).

The response of an eye to a foreign agent or chemical is determined, in part, by the longevity of the agent or chemical residence on the corneal surface. Experimentally, however, it has been found that irrigation of eyes is of little benefit if delayed for more than 20 to 30 seconds after exposure to a test agent (Davies et al., 1976; Swantson, 1983). This may be related to the production of prostaglandins and other eicosanoids during arachidonic acid metabolism and release of other mediators (such as histamine or kinins) in eye tissues following exposure to chemicals or agents that contact the eye. While the degree of susceptibility of different tissues from different species is highly variable in terms of the quantities of metabolites produced (Kulkarni et al., 1984; Yousufzai et al., 1988), there is a common underlying release of prostaglandins and other eicosanoids in response to a physical or chemical insult. It has been well documented, however, that different species respond in quite different ways to the same stimulus (Bito, 1984), thus the impact of prostaglandin metabolism differs between species.

In vitro tests have demonstrated a variety of responses depending upon the type of cells used and the chemical under test. Good correlations, or even inverse correlations, have been reported with different cell systems used in a variety of different techniques (Swantson, 1983). The data obtained with surfactants suggests that the mechanism of surfactant irritation to the eye is not straightforward, being complicated by the degree of hydrophobicity of the cornea. Thus, data obtained would be considered as a guide for the test compounds, but not a result that could be slavishly followed. The in vitro tests might be used to exclude certain chemicals, drugs, or agents that would be extremely harmful in the living eye.

Toxicity testing has undergone an evolution during the past 40 years or so on at least two fronts. In one, there has been a shift from anecdotal reports based upon single observations of drug-induced side effects in recipients to a more sophisticated reporting system exemplified in the United States by the National Registry of Drug-Induced Ocular Side Effects. On the second front, there has been a revolution in the assessment of toxicity. These changes range from the subjective Draize type of test to ones including the use of quantitative measures of different parameters, whether this be the specular microscope to permit corneal endothelial cell counts to be performed, Scheimpflug photography of the lens with subsequent quantitative densitometric analysis, or electroretinographic determinations.

Each of these, and other, technological advances has allowed a more precise and quantitative analysis to be performed on the effects of drugs, whether they be primary or secondary. The adaptation of these advanced, quantitative techniques to ocular toxicity studies has resulted in a quantum leap of knowledge that has allowed mechanistic interpretation of responses rather than only descriptive results. This alone has led to the dramatic increase in ocular toxicity as a science and as an acceptable analytic method. Furthermore, the original limited focus of the Draize test to cornea, conjunctiva, and iris has been expanded to include all ocular tissues. This philosophical change has altered the scenery of ophthalmic toxicology and transformed it into a 20th-century science.

Despite these advances, and the publication of drug-induced side effects either from laboratory or from clinical experience, it must be remembered that, by far, the largest proportion of all the data in ocular toxicology studies (as with all toxicology) is held within the proprietary interests of drug companies. Much of what has been published has come from the public sector when scientists or physicians have had access to materials for testing before or after public release, and this data has resulted in publications. Although there has been a considerable increase in the quantity and quality of data published in the area of toxicology, the validation of the data concerning drug-induced side effects or drug-induced ocular toxicology occurs primarily through epidemiological studies. Studies of this type are not only rare but also tremendously expensive; voluntary reporting of side effects and suspected ocular toxicology through a system such as the National Registry of Drug-Induced Ocular Side Effects in the United States or the Clinical Toxicology Center, Marseilles, France is a cost-effective means of partly accomplishing this goal.

PUBLICATIONS

The considerable developments in ocular toxicology over the past few years are exemplified by the appearance of Fraunfelder's book (Fraunfelder, 1989) on drug-induced ocular side effects, which discusses probable and possible medication-induced side effects and drug interactions. This burgeoning area of oculotoxicity is replete with possible drug-induced effects. It is the previous reports of drug effects or interactions that may alert the ophthalmologist or other physicians to make the connection between drug use and drug-related effects. This book, in addition to including many references of observations, contains compilations of reports from the National Registry of Drug-Induced Ocular Side Effects, which was organized in 1976 to act as a resource for reports of ocular toxicity (Fraunfelder, 1978; Fraunfelder and Meyer, 1982). Data is reported by physicians who suspect adverse reactions secondary to drug therapy. The National Registry located at the Casey Eye Institute in Portland, Oregon, serves as a focal point for all physicians to report possible cause-and-effect relationships between drugs and unwanted side effects. At the national level, accumulation of data can occur at a vastly enhanced rate compared with that which would occur in individual groups of physicians in a common setting, such as in an academic department or group practice. When associations are found, they are reported back to the physicians regarding the use and concentration of drugs, or interaction of drugs with each other, so that appropriate adjustments can be made in drug use by patients. The data bank is also accessible by telephone where enquiries can be made for comparisons of observations with those reported by others.

While an earlier book (Dikstein, 1977), which was the result of a meeting, addressed drug effects on the eye and eye tissues, the focus was more on physiological and pharmacological events, although the responses to excess concentrations (toxicity) was also discussed. Another book assembled information on the newer technologies and approaches available for the study of ocular toxicity (Hockwin et al., 1992). The intent was to provide a presentation of modern methods and models for different ocular tissues.

Over the past 12 years a series of meetings has been held on Drug-Induced Ocular Side Effects and Ocular Toxicology at various locations. The initial meeting of an assembly of those with an interest in ocular toxicity (1977) was in Little Rock, Arkansas, and was organized by F.T. Fraunfelder. This was followed by meetings in Portland, Oregon (1980; Fraunfelder), Milwaukee, Wisconsin (1982; H.F. Edelhauser), Augusta, Georgia (1984; D.S. Hull and K. Green), Bonn, West Germany (1986; O. Hockwin), Toronto, Canada (1988; P.K. Basu), and Deidesheim, West Germany (1990; Hockwin).

Beginning with the Toronto meeting, the International Society of Ocular Toxicology was formally founded. The proceedings of the 1986 meeting, which was the 5th International Symposium on the subject of ocular toxicology, was published (Hockwin, 1987) in book form. The Deidesheim meeting proceedings were published in 1990 as an issue of the journal *Lens and Eye Toxicity Research* (volume 7). The 1992 meeting was held in Sedona, Arizona (S. Lerman and K. Green), with the proceedings also published in an issue of *Lens and Eye Toxicity Research* (volume 9). This meeting included a workshop on alternatives to the Draize test that incorporated evaluations of newer techniques.

The 1994 meeting of the International Society of Ocular Toxicology, held in Annecy, France (I. Weisse and O. Hockwin), had drug pharmacokinetics and experimental electroretinography (ERG) as its themes. The many papers on ERG established standardized laboratory methods for retinal toxicity studies using this sensitive technique. These proceedings were published in book form (Weisse et al., 1995) with over 100 pages devoted to ERG technology. The latest meeting, held in Asheville,

North Carolina (Green), during October 1996, had several themes, including updates on drug metabolism, ocular nitric oxide effects, and the increased use of cell cultures (Green et al., 1997), but the primary focus was a workshop on in vitro versus in vivo methodologies for eye irritancy testing (Edelhauser and Green, 1997). A spectrum of standard as well as newer techniques were discussed against the background of regulatory requirements on different continents. Topics included products, contact lenses, costs of tests, and other devices.

The proceedings of future meetings of the International Society of Ocular Toxicology will appear in the *Journal of Toxicology—Cutaneous and Ocular Toxicology*, which is the official journal of the Society. The *Journal of Ocular Pharmacology and Therapeutics*, which is the official journal of the Association for Ocular Pharmacology and Therapeutics, is also devoted to the publication of papers concerned with toxicology aspects of the eye.

Publications also occur from the National Registry when sufficient data is available on a particular topic or when a specific drug side effect occurs within the reporting system with a greater than usual frequency. These papers have addressed subjects as diverse as the ocular use of topical phenylephrine at high (Fraunfelder and Scafidi, 1978) or low (Fraunfelder and Meyer, 1985) concentrations, to the systemic side effects of beta-adrenergic blockers (Van Buskirk, 1980; Van Buskirk and Fraunfelder, 1984) and carbonic anhydrase inhibitors (Fraunfelder and Meyer, 1987). Other authors have addressed the side effects of beta-adrenergic blockers (Novack and Leopold, 1987) and systemic drug interactions with topical glaucoma medications (Gerber et al., 1990) while yet others, for example, have addressed drug-induced side effects reported in Japan (Sasaki and Yamamura, 1987).

FUTURE AREAS FOR DEVELOPMENT

Although the Draize ocular irritation test has been subject to criticism and modification over the past 40 years, discussions on the use and validity of this test have increased recently. A considerable amount of the discussion has been driven by the concern of investigators, manufacturing or distributing companies, and citizens to reduce the number of animals used in eye irritation testing. This is, of course, but one aspect of ocular toxicity that excludes examination of what are probably the most susceptible tissues to toxic effects of drugs, namely, the lens and retina. The emphasis of the Draize test on external eye tissues, plus the iris, represents only immediate tissue reactions when materials contact the ocular surface. The overall view of ocular toxicity, while incorporating the testing of agents and products to which consumers are exposed, must encompass all drugs, chemicals, agents, and devices as well as all eye tissues because no eye tissue is free from the induction of such effects (Green, 1998).

In vitro techniques cannot completely replace in vivo testing because of their inability to reflect all of the potential parallel and integrated manifestations of irritancy. As has been pointed out, however, perhaps a battery of in vitro tests, each addressing specific response situations may one day replace the Draize test (Holden, 1982;

Swantson, 1983). Acceptance of standards for procedures and scoring systems by all regulatory agencies worldwide would certainly be a major achievement, even though the immediate possibility of such unanimity seems remote. Certainly refinement of the in vivo test procedure is required with acceptance by the appropriate agencies of lower doses and fewer animals per test material. An alteration in the emphasis of the scoring system from the cornea to more susceptible tissues, such as conjunctiva, especially for ophthalmic products, seems desirable (Green, 1998). Similarly, the use of precedent should be allowable on a larger scale; such a maneuver would limit the need to test yet another material for which the ingredients have been sufficiently tested in the past. The use of in vitro techniques to screen materials that have a high irritancy potential would eliminate the need for a number of in vivo tests, and eliminate materials which show eye irritancy potential.

Succeeding chapters in this volume address several aspects of ocular toxicology, providing an overview of where this science stands as applied to different tissues of the eye, the methods used to assess toxicity, and the various sources of toxic effects ranging from drugs administered to alleviate a disease to air pollutants. To date, the history of ocular toxicology is brief and somewhat narrowly focused. Recent years have seen an expansion of interests into many diverse areas despite the lack of funding for such approaches by government agencies. An assessment after the next decade will provide a better perspective on whether or not ocular toxicology has assumed a greater role in the marketing of all products, whether designed for systemic or topical use or reaching the eye accidentally. If progress continues at the recent rate, then assessment of ocular toxicity will use greatly refined methods in vivo for the evaluation of new drugs, agents, or devices, such as contact lenses.

The five years since the original chapter was written on this topic have seen great strides in the use of in vitro methods to restrict eye irritancy testing. This is strongly indicated by the continued decline in the use of rabbits in ocular toxicity tests with the use of in vitro models to evaluate and eliminate potentially hazardous materials before exposure to the eye. The divergence of results concerned with attempts at validating certain in vitro systems does not offer, however, great hope for a rapid resolution to the difficulties associated with these techniques; this despite pressures of governmental and animal welfare constituencies who have exerted influence on the use of animals in the testing procedures. Unfortunately, the very complexity of the responses of ocular tissues to stimuli represents the major stumbling block to the development of even a simple battery of tests that might substitute for the Draize test. A highly modified Draize test using smaller volumes or masses of test product, far fewer animals, and more quantitative and sensitive measurement techniques that allow lower doses to be used is still the mainstay of eye irritation testing.

The transition from an ocular irritation test, which was initially applied to the evaluation of products that are taken either topically or systemically as therapeutic agents or reach the eye from either topical or systemic sources on a more continuous basis, to a sophisticated, quantitatively oriented approach is occurring. Toxicologists have realized the quantum leap between ocular irritancy testing, with its limits on product application to one time, limitation to only three eye tissues, limitation to gross examination techniques, and limitation to observation times, and ocular toxicology when *all* eye tissues can be quantitatively examined (Green, 1998). Increasingly, therefore, techniques such as specular and confocal microscopy, fluorophotometry, electroretinography, Scheimpflug imagery, and other techniques, are being employed to provide the necessary toxicology data. Irritation testing for ophthalmic products is done early in their development to eliminate those compounds or products that would not make it through all the testing protocols. The Draize test is still useful for ocular irritation tests but is restricted as a predictor of ocular toxicology per se.

The use of quantitative and technically sensitive methods for ocular irritancy and/or toxicity evaluation means that the application of chemicals, drugs, or devices to the eye can be achieved in a majority of cases without inducing overt signs of irritancy. This use of very low doses of agents or drugs alleviates the concerns of both researchers and lay public alike in that no reaction occurs or is visible, yet the sophisticated technology allows an evaluation of the physiological and biochemical processes involved in the tissue–drug interaction. This alleviation of the occurrence, or even the suggestion, of pain or discomfort to the test animal also means that any observed tissue responses that require sophisticated technology to detect any changes are not influenced by the presence of any possible occurrence of discomfort or pain. Tissue responses thus reflect true drug–tissue interaction without outside influences. Recommendations, such as those in Europe, that eye irritation testing cease in the very near future will probably have to be amended until appropriate in vitro techniques have been appropriately validated.

The changes that have occurred, with the recognition of the inability of the irritation test to predict real ocular toxicology, have been and will continue to be revolutionary. No longer will we see attempts to modify the Draize test to fulfill the role of a toxicological study. It is incapable of allowing such a process because of its inherent limitations, especially in the tissues examined and the model. Use of animals under more quantitative conditions has allowed ocular toxicology to be determined and has provided impetus for revision of the Draize test to bring greater objectivity to this test.

ACKNOWLEDGMENTS

Some of the work reported herein from the author's laboratory was supported in part by an Unrestricted Departmental Award from Research to Prevent Blindness, Inc. (RPB), and in part by a Senior Scientific Investigator Award from RPB. I thank Brenda Sheppard for her valuable secretarial assistance. This chapter is dedicated to the Kidney Transplant Unit at the Medical College of Georgia, who, for the past 14 years or so, have provided a dedicated level of medical and surgical skills and care that has gone far beyond the norm and allows me to give a historical perspective on anything. In alphabetical order, they are: J.E. Barnett, PA; P.A. Bowen III, MD; A.L. Humphries, MD; J. Hertel, MD; L.L. Mulloy, DO; B.S. Newby, RN; W.H. Wolff, PA; and J.J. Wynn, MD. Without their input into my health care and their responsiveness to acute and chronic difficulties, the outcomes would have been quite different.

REFERENCES

Allgood, G.S. 1989. Use of animal eye test data and human experience for determining the ocular irritation potential of shampoos. *Journal of Toxicology—Cutaneous and Ocular Toxicology* 8:321–326.

Arthur, B.H., Pennisi, S.C., DiPasquale, L.C., Re, T., Dinardo, J., Kennedy, G.L., North-Root, H., Penney, D.A., and Sekerke, H.J. 1986. Effects of anesthetic pretreatment and low volume dosage on ocular irritancy potential of cosmetics: a collaborative study. *Journal of Toxicology—Cutaneous and Ocular Toxicology* 5:215–227.

Avalos, J., Jacobs, A., and Wilkin, J.K. 1997. Toxicity testing for ocular drug products. In *Advances in Ocular Toxicology*, eds. K. Green, H.F. Edelhauser, R.B. Hackett, D.S. Hull, D.E. Potter, and R.C. Tripathi, pp. 261–268. New York: Plenum Press.

Bagley, D.M., Bruner, L.H., de Silva, O., Cottin, M., O'Brien, K.A.F., Uttley, M., and Walker, A.P. 1992. An evaluation of five potential alternatives *in vitro* to the rabbit eye irritation test *in vivo*. *Toxicology In Vitro* 6:275–284.

Baldinger, J., Doft, B.H., Burns, S.A., and Johnson, B. 1986. Retinal toxicity of amphotericin B in vitrectomised versus non-vitrectomised eyes. *British Journal of Ophthalmology* 70:657–661.

Baldwin, H.A., McDonald, T.O., and Beasley, C.H. 1973. Slit-lamp examination of experimental animal eyes. II. Grading scales and photographic evaluation of induced pathological conditions. *Journal of the Society of Cosmetic Chemistry* 24:181–195.

Balls, M., and Fentem, J.H. 1997. Progress towards the validation of alternative tests. *Alternatives to Laboratory Animals* 25:33–43.

Bartlett, J.D., and Jaanus, S.D. 1989. Ocular effects of systemic drugs. In *Clinical Ocular Pharmacology*, eds. J.D. Bartlett and S.D. Jaanus, pp. 801–842. Boston: Butterworth's.

Beckley, J.H. 1965. Comparative eye testing: man vs. animal. *Toxicology and Applied Pharmacology* 7(suppl):93–101.

Bito, L.Z. 1984. Species differences in the responses of the eye to irritation and trauma: a hypothesis of divergence in ocular defense mechanisms, and the choice of experimental animals for eye research. *Experimental Eye Research* 39:807–829.

Blain, L., Lachapelle, P., and Molotchnikoff, S. 1990. The effect of acute triethylene exposure on electroretinogram components. *Neurotoxicology and Teratology* 12:633–636.

Bours, J., Ahrend, M.H.J., and Hockwin, O. 1990. Crystallin profiles of calf and bovine lens in microsections stained for free sulfhydryl groups and proteins. *Lens and Eye Toxicity Research* 7:531–545.

Bracher, M., Faller, C., Spengler, J., and Reinhardt, C.A. 1987/8. Comparison of *in vitro* cell toxicity with *in vivo* eye irritation. *Molecular Toxicology* 1:561–570.

Bradlaw, J.A., and Wilcox, N.L. 1997. Workshop on eye irritation testing: practical applications of non-whole animal alternatives. *Food and Chemical Toxicology* 35:1–11.

Bron, A.J. 1979. Mechanisms of ocular toxicity. In *Drug Toxicity*, ed. J.W. Gorrod, pp. 229–253. London: Taylor & Francis.

Brown, G.C., Eagle, R.C., Shakin, E.P., Gruber, M., and Arbizio, V.V. 1990. Retinal toxicity of intravitreal gentamicin. *Archives of Ophthalmology* 108:1740–1744.

Bruner, L.H., Carr, G.J., Chamberlain, M., and Curren, R.D. 1996. Validation of alternative methods for toxicity testing. *Toxicology In Vitro* 10:479–501.

Bruner, L.H., Kain, D.J., Roberts, D.A., and Parker, R.D. 1991. Evaluation of seven *in vitro* alternatives for ocular safety testing. *Fundamental and Applied Toxicology* 17:136–149.

Burton, A.B.G. 1972. A method for the objective assessment of eye irritation. *Food and Cosmetic Toxicology* 10:209–217.

Burton, A.B.G., York, M., and Lawrence, R.S. 1981. The *in vitro* assessment of severe eye irritants. *Food and Cosmetic Toxicology* 19:471–480.

Carroll, F.D. 1945. Visual symptoms caused by digitalis. *American Journal of Ophthalmology* 28:373–376.

Chamberlain, M., Gad, S.C., Gautheron, P., and Prinsen, M.K. 1997. Organotypic models for the assessment/prediction of ocular irritation. *Food and Chemical Toxicology* 35:23–37.

Chan, P.K., and Hayes, A.W. 1988. Principles and methods for acute toxicity and eye irritancy. In *Principles and Methods of Toxicology*, ed. A.W. Hayes, pp. 169–220. New York: Raven Press.

Christian, M.S., and Diener, R.M. 1996. Soaps and detergents: alternatives to animal irritation tests. *Journal of the American College of Toxicology* 15:1–44.

Code of Federal Regulations. 1979. Title 16, part 1500.42. Washington, DC: U.S. Government Printing Office.

Committee for the Revision of NAS Publication 1138. 1977. Dermal and eye toxicity tests. In *Principles and Procedures for Evaluating the Toxicity of Household Substances*, pp. 41–54. Washington, DC: National Academy of Sciences.

Consumer Product Safety Commission. 1979. *Hazardous Substances Labeling Guide*, Appendix 1, pp. 29, 53. Washington, DC.

D'Amico, D.J., Caspers-Velu, L., Libert, J., Shanks, E., Schrooyen, M., Hanninen, L.A., and Kenyon, K.R. 1985. Comparative toxicity of intravitreal aminoglycoside antibiotics. *American Journal of Ophthalmology* 100:264–275.

Davies, R.E., Kynoch, S.R., and Liggett, M.P. 1976. Eye irritation tests—an assessment of the maximum delay time for remedial irrigation. *Journal of the Society for Cosmetic Chemistry* 27:301–306.

de Silva, O., Cottin, M., Dami, N., Roguet, R., Catroux, P., Toufic, A., Sicard, C., Dossou, K.G., Gerner, I., Schleck, E., Spielmann, H., Gupta, K.C., and Hill, R.N. 1997. Evaluation of eye irritation potential: statistical analysis and tier testing strategies. *Food and Chemical Toxicology* 35:159–164.

Dikstein, S., ed. 1977. *Drugs and Ocular Tissues*. Basel: Karger.

Dragomirescu, V., Hockwin, O., Koch, H.R., and Sasaki, K. 1978. Development of a new equipment for rotating slit image photography according to Scheimpflug's principle. In *Gerontological Aspects of Eye Research*, ed. O. Hockwin, pp. 118–130. Basel: Karger.

Draize, J.H. 1959. Dermal toxicity. In *Appraisal of the Safety of Chemicals in Foods, Drugs and Cosmetics*, pp. 46–59. Austin, TX: Association for Food and Drug Officials of the United States.

Draize, J.H., and Kelley, E.A. 1952. Toxicity to eye mucosa of certain cosmetic preparations containing surface-active agents. In *Proceedings of the Scientific Section of the Toilet Goods Association*, 17:1–4.

Draize, J.H., Woodard, G., and Calvery, H.O. 1944. Methods for the study of irritation and toxicity of substances applied topically to the skin and mucous membranes. *Journal of Pharmacology and Experimental Therapeutics* 82:377–390.

Duke-Elder, S. 1972. Injuries, part 2, non-mechanical injuries. In *System of Ophthalmology*. St. Louis: C.V. Mosby.

Eckerskorn, U., Hockwin, O., Chen, T.T., Knowles, W., and Dobbs, R.E. 1987. Contribution of cataract epidemiological studies to the evaluation of cataractogenic risk factors. In *Drug-Induced Ocular Side Effects and Ocular Toxicology*, ed. O. Hockwin, pp. 71–78. Basel: Karger.

Edelhauser, H.F., and Green, K. 1997. Workshop on *in vitro* versus *in vivo* models for ocular toxicity testing. In *Advances in Ocular Toxicology*, eds. K. Green, H.F. Edelhauser, R.B. Hackett, D.S. Hull, D.E. Potter and R.C. Tripathi, pp. 207–259. New York: Plenum Press.

Edelhauser, H.F., and Ubels, J. 1992. Models and methods for oculotoxicity testing—tear film and cornea. In *Manual of Oculotoxicity Testing of Drugs*, eds. O. Hockwin, K. Green and L. Rubin, pp. 195–218. Stuttgart: G. Fischer-Verlag.

Federal Hazardous Substances Act Regulations. 1982. *Code of Federal Regulations* 16: part 1500.

Federal Register. September 17, 1964;29:1300.

Fiscella, R., Peyman, G.A., Kimura, A., and Small, G. 1988. Intravitreal toxicity of cotrimoxazole. *Ophthalmic Surgery* 19:44–46.

Food and Drug Administration. 1965. *Illustrated Guide for Grading Eye Irritation by Hazardous Substances*. Washington, DC: U.S. Government Printing Office.

Fraunfelder, F.T. 1978. What's new in ocular toxicology? *Sightsaving Reviews* 48:53–58.

Fraunfelder, F.T. 1989. *Drug-Induced Ocular Side Effects and Drug Interactions*, 3rd ed. Philadelphia: Lea & Febiger.

Fraunfelder, F.T., and Meyer, S.M. 1982. The National Registry of drug-induced ocular side effects. *Journal of Toxicology—Cutaneous and Ocular Toxicology* 1:65–70.

Fraunfelder, F.T., and Meyer, S.M. 1985. Possible cardiovascular effects secondary to topical ophthalmic 2.5% phenylephrine. *American Journal of Ophthalmology* 99:362–363.

Fraunfelder, F.T., and Meyer, S.M. 1987. Recent advances in ocular drug toxicity. In *Drug-Induced Ocular Side Effects and Ocular Toxicology*, ed. O. Hockwin, pp. 30–39. Basel: Karger.

Fraunfelder, F.T., and Scafidi, A. 1978. Possible adverse effects from topical ocular 10% phenylephrine. *American Journal of Ophthalmology* 85:447–453.

Freeberg, F.E., Griffith, J.F., Bruce, R.D., and Bay, P.H.S. 1984. Correlation of animal test methods with human experience for household products. *Journal of Toxicology—Cutaneous and Ocular Toxicology* 1:53–64.

Freeberg, F.E., Hooker, D.T., and Griffith, J.F. 1986. Correlation of animal eye test data with human experience for household products: an update. *Journal of Toxicology—Cutaneous and Ocular Toxicology* 5:115–123.

Freeberg, F.E., Nixon, G.A., Reer, P.J., Weaver, J.E., Bruce, R.D., Griffith, J.F., and Sanders, L.W., III. 1986. Human and rabbit eye responses to chemical insult. *Fundamental and Applied Toxicology* 7:626–634.

Friedenwald, J.S., Hughes, W.F., and Hermann, H. 1944. Acid-base tolerance of the cornea. *Archives of Ophthalmology* 31:279–283.

Gerber, S.L., Cantor, L.B., and Brater, D.C. 1990. Systemic drug interactions with topical glaucoma medications. *Survey of Ophthalmology* 35:205–218.

Goldberg, A.M., ed. 1983. *Product Safety Evaluation*. New York: Mary Ann Liebert.

Goldberg, A.M., ed. 1984. *Acute Toxicity Testing: Alternative Approaches*. New York: Mary Ann Liebert.

Goldberg, A.M., ed. 1985. *In Vitro Toxicology: A Progress Report from The Johns Hopkins Center for Alternatives to Animal Testing*. New York: Mary Ann Liebert.

Goldberg, A.M., ed. 1987a. *A Critical Evaluation of Alternatives to Acute Ocular Irritation Testing*. New York: Mary Ann Liebert.

Goldberg, A.M., ed. 1987b. *In Vitro Toxicology: Approaches to Validation*. New York: Mary Ann Liebert.

Goldberg, A.M., ed. 1988. *Progress in In Vitro Toxicology*. New York: Mary Ann Liebert.

Goldberg, A.M., ed. 1989. *In Vitro Toxicology: New Directions*. New York: Mary Ann Liebert.

Gordon, V.C., and Bergman, H.C. 1987. Eyetex: an *in vitro* method for evaluation of ocular irritancy. In *In Vitro Toxicology: Approaches to Validation*, ed. A.M. Goldberg, pp. 293–302. New York: Mary Ann Liebert.

Gordon, V.C., and Bergman, H.C. 1988. External evaluation of the standard Eyetex system in six laboratories to determine intra- and inter-laboratory accuracy and precision. In *Progress in In Vitro Toxicology*, ed. A.M. Goldberg, pp. 317–323. New York: Mary Ann Liebert.

Gordon, V.C., Kelly, C.P., and Bergman, H.C. 1990. Applications of the Eyetex method. *Toxicity In Vitro* 4:314–317.

Grant, W.M. 1974. *Toxicology of the Eye*, 2nd ed. Springfield, IL: Charles C. Thomas.

Grant, W.M., and Schuman, J.S. 1993. Toxicology of the Eye, 4th ed. Springfield, IL: Charles C. Thomas.

Green, K. 1991. Corneal endothelial structure and function under normal and toxic conditions. *Cell Biology Reviews* 25:169–207.

Green, K. 1992a. History of ophthalmic toxicology. In *Ophthalmic Toxicology*, 1st ed., ed. G.C.Y. Chiou, pp. 1–16. New York: Raven Press.

Green, K. 1992b. Models and methods for testing toxicity with aqueous humor, iris and ciliary body. In *Manual of Oculotoxicity Testing of Drugs*, eds. O. Hockwin, K. Green, and L. Rubin, pp. 219–242. Stuttgart: G. Fischer-Verlag.

Green, K. 1992c. Models and methods for testing toxicity on intraocular pressure. In *Manual of Oculotoxicity Testing of Drugs*, eds. O. Hockwin, K. Green, and L. Rubin, pp. 243–253. Stuttgart: G. Fischer-Verlag.

Green, K. 1998. *In vivo* eye irritation test methods. In *Ophthalmic Toxicology*, 2nd ed., ed. G.C.Y. Chiou, pp. 115–163. Washington, DC: Taylor & Francis.

Green, K., Bowman K.A., Elijah, R.D., Mermelstein, R., and Kilpper, R.W. 1985. Dose–effect response of the rabbit eye to cetylpyridinium chloride. *Journal of Toxicology—Cutaneous and Ocular Toxicology* 4:13–26.

Green, K., Cheeks, L., Slagle, T., Paul, H., and Trask, D.K. 1993. Blood–ocular barrier permeability and electroretinograms after intravitreal silicone oils of varying composition. *Journal of Ocular Pharmacology* 9:355–363.

Green, K., Crosby, V.A., and Cheeks, L. 1990. Toxicity of intracameral thymoxamine. *Lens and Eye Toxicity Research* 7:121–132.

Green, K., Edelhauser, H.F., Hackett, R.B., Hull, D.S., Potter, D.E., and Tripathi, R.C., eds. 1997. *Advances in Ocular Toxicology*. New York: Plenum Press.

Green, K., Sobel, R.E., Fineberg, E., Wynn, H.R., and Bowman, K.A. 1981. Subchronic ocular and systemic toxicity of topically applied Δ9-tetrahydrocannabinol. *Annals of Ophthalmology* 13:1219–1222.

Green, W.R., Sullivan, J.B., Hehir, R.M., Scharpf, L.G., and Dickinson, A.W. 1978. *A Systematic Comparison of Chemically Induced Eye Injury in the Albino Rabbit and Rhesus Monkey*. New York: The Soap and Detergent Association.

Griffith, J.F., Nixon, G.A., Bruce, R.D., Reer, P.J., and Bannan, E.A. 1982. Dose-response studies with chemical irritants in the albino rabbit eye as a basis for selecting optimum testing conditions for predicting hazard to the human eye. *Toxicology and Applied Pharmacology* 55:501–513.

Hackett, R.B. 1990. Nonclinical study requirements for ophthalmic drugs and devices in the United States. *Lens and Eye Toxicity Research* 7:181–205.

Havener, W. 1983. *Ocular Pharmacology*, 5th ed. St. Louis: C.V. Mosby.

Hennekes, R., Janssen, K., Muñoz, C., and Winneke, G. 1987. Lead-induced ERG alterations in rats at high and low levels of exposure. In *Drug-Induced Ocular Side Effects and Ocular Toxicology*, ed. O. Hockwin, pp. 193–199. Basel: Karger.

Himber, J., Andermann, G., Erhart, M., Leclerc, G., and Bouzoubaa, M. 1985. *In vitro* potential measurement, anaesthetic and antimicrobial effects as indications of beta-blocker toxicity of the cornea. *Methods and Findings in Experimental Clinical Pharmacology* 7:195–201.

Hockwin O., ed. 1987. *Drug-Induced Ocular Side Effects and Ocular Toxicology*. Basel: Karger.

Hockwin, O., Green, K., and Rubin, L.F., eds. 1992. *Manual of Oculotoxicity Testing of Drugs*, pp. 1–435. Stuttgart: G. Fischer-Verlag.

Holden, C. 1982. New focus on replacing animals in the lab. *Science* 215:35–38.

Jackson, E.M. 1984. Ocular irritancy: the search for acceptable and humane test methods. In *The Cosmetic Industry: Scientific and Regulatory Foundations* ed. N.F. Estrin, pp. 437–464. New York: Marcel Dekker.

Jackson, E.M. 1992. Animal testing in biomedical research. In *Manual of Oculotoxicity Testing of Drugs*, eds. O. Hockwin, K. Green, and L. Rubin, pp. 1–8. Stuttgart: G. Fischer-Verlag.

Jackson, E.M., Hume, R.D., and Wallin, R.F. 1988. The agarose diffusion method for ocular irritancy screening: cosmetic products, part II. *Journal of Toxicology—Cutaneous and Ocular Toxicology* 7:187–194.

Kemp, R.B., Meredith, R.W., and Gamble, S.H. 1985. Toxicity of commercial products on cells in suspension culture: a possible screen for the Draize eye irritation test. *Food and Chemical Toxicology* 23:267–270.

Kemp, R.B., Meredith, R.W., Gamble, S., Frost, M. 1983. A rapid cell culture technique for assessing the toxicity of detergent-based products *in vitro* as a possible screen for eye irritancy *in vivo*. *Cytobios* 36:153–159.

Kennah, H.E., Hignet, S., Laux, P.E., Dorko, J.D., and Barrow, C.S. 1989. An objective procedure for quantitating eye irritation based upon changes of corneal thickness. *Fundamental and Applied Toxicology* 12:258–268.

Kojima, M., Hockwin, O., Rao, G.S., and Garcia, J. 1990. Investigations on the presence of 3-hydroxy-3-methylglutaryl coenzyme—a reductase (HMG- CoA-reductase, E.C. 1.1.1.34) in lenses of various animal species. *Lens and Eye Toxicity Research* 7:605–623.

Kulkarni, P.S., Fleisher, L., and Srinivasan, B.D. 1984. The synthesis of cyclooxygenase products in ocular tissues of various species. *Current Eye Research* 3:447–452.

Leahy, D.E., Duncan, R., Ahr, H.J., Bayliss, M.K., de Boer, A. (Bert) G., Darvas, F., Fentem, J.H., Fry, J.R., Hopkins, R., Houston, J.B., Karlsson, J., Kedderis, G.L., Pratten, M.K., Prieto, P., Smith, D.A., and Straughan, D.W. 1997. Pharmacokinetics in early drug research. The report and recommendations of ECVAM workshop 22. *Alternatives to Laboratory Animals* 25:17–31.

Lehnert, T., Grosdanoff, P., and Hockwin, O. 1987. Assessment of drug-induced oculotoxicity by animal models. In *Drug-Induced Ocular Side Effects and Ocular Toxicology*, ed. O. Hockwin, pp. 232–340. Basel: Karger.

Lehnert, T., and Ulrich, B. 1990. Requirements of preclinical examinations. *Lens and Eye Toxicity Research* 7:207–219.

Leighton, J., Nassaeur, J., and Tchao, R. 1985. The chick embryo in toxicology: an alternative to the rabbit eye. *Food and Chemical Toxicology* 23:293–298.

Lerman, S. 1987. *In vivo* methods to evaluate ocular drug efficacy and side effects. In *Drug-Induced Ocular Side Effects and Ocular Toxicology*, ed. O. Hockwin, pp. 87–104. Basel: Karger.

Lerman, S. 1990. Biophysical methods to monitor lens aging and pre-cataractous changes *in vivo*. *Lens and Eye Toxicity Research* 7:243–249.

Luepke, N.P. 1985. Hen's egg chorioallantoic membrane test for irritation potential. *Food and Chemical Toxicology* 23:287–291.

Marzulli, F.N. 1965. New data on eye and skin tests. *Toxicology and Applied Pharmacology* 7(suppl):79–85.

Maurice, D., and Singh, T. 1986. A permeability test for acute corneal toxicity. *Toxicology Letters* 31:125–130.

McDonald, T.O., Hiddeman, J.W., Howe, W.E., and Robertson, S.M. 1987. Ocular safety evaluation: alternatives and the future. In *Dermatotoxicology*, 3rd ed., eds. F.N. Marzulli and H.I. Maibach, pp. 679–710. Washington, DC: Hemisphere.

McDonald, T.O., Seabaugh, V., Shadduck, J.A., and Edelhauser, H.F. 1987. Eye irritation. In *Dermato-toxicology*, 3rd ed., eds. F.N. Marzulli and H.I. Maibach, pp. 641–696. Washington, DC: Hemisphere.

McDonald, T.O., and Shadduck, J.A. 1977. Eye irritation. In *Dermatotoxicology and Pharmacology, Advances in Modern Toxicology*, vol. 4., eds. F.N. Marzulli and H.I. Maibach, pp. 139–191. Washington, DC: Hemisphere.

Meyer, S.M., and Fraunfelder, F.T. 1987. National registry of drug-induced ocular side effects. In *Drug-Induced Ocular Side Effects and Ocular Toxicology*, ed. O. Hockwin, pp. 40–44. Basel: Karger.

Morgan, R.L., Sorenson, S.S., and Castles, T.R. 1987. Prediction of ocular irritation by corneal pachymetry. *Food and Chemical Toxicology* 25:609–613.

Muir, C.K. 1983. The comparative toxic effects of proprietary antidandruff, adult and baby shampoos on rabbit ileum. *Toxicology Letters* 18:227–230.

Muir, C.K. 1985. Opacity of bovine cornea *in vitro* induced by surfactants and industrial chemicals compared with ocular irritancy *in vivo*. *Toxicology Letters* 24:157–162.

Nardone, R.M., and Bradlaw, J.A. 1983. Toxicity testing with *in vitro* systems. 1. Ocular tissue culture. *Journal of Toxicology—Cutaneous and Ocular Toxicology* 2:81–98.

Newcomb, R.D., and Priest, M.L. 1989. Systemic effects of ocular drugs. In *Clinical Ocular Pharmacology*, eds. J.D. Bartlett and S.D. Jaanus, pp. 843–862. Boston: Butterworth's.

North-Root, H., Yackovich, F., Demetrulias, J., Gacula, M., and Heinze, J.E. 1982. Evaluation of an *in vitro* cell toxicity test using rabbit corneal cells to predict eye irritation potential of surfactants. *Toxicology Letters* 14:207–212.

North-Root, H., Yackovich, F., Demetrulias, J., Gacula, M., and Heinze, J.E. 1985. Prediction of the eye irritation potential of shampoos using the *in vitro* SIRC cell toxicity test. *Food and Chemical Toxicology* 23:271–273.

Novack, G.D., and Leopold, I.H. 1987. The toxicity of topical ophthalmic beta blockers. *Journal of Toxicology—Cutaneous and Ocular Toxicology* 6:283–297.

O'Brien, K.A.F., Dixit, M.B., McCall, J.C., Botham, P.A., and Lewis, R.W. 1992. An interlaboratory assessment of the Eyetex system. *Toxicology In Vitro* 6:549–556.

Parish, W.E. 1985. Ability of *in vitro* (corneal injury—eye organ—and chorioallantoic membrane) tests to represent histopathological features of acute eye inflammation. *Food and Chemical Toxicology* 23:215–227.

Paylor, R., Peyman, G.A., and Badri, S. 1987. Effects of intravitreal injection of fluorosilicone oil after vitrectomy in the rabbit eye. *Canadian Journal of Ophthalmology* 22:251–253.

Physicians' Desk Reference. 1996. Oradell, NJ: Medical Economics Co. Inc.

Physicians' Desk Reference for Ophthalmology. 1996. Oradell, NJ: Medical Economics Co. Inc.

Price, J.B., and Andrews, I.J. 1985. The *in vitro* assessment of eye irritancy using isolated eyes. *Food and Chemical Toxicology* 23:313–315.

Ramselaar, J.A.M., Boot, J.P., van Haeringen, N.J., van Best, J.A., and Oosterhuis, J.A. 1988. Corneal epithelial permeability after instillation of ophthalmic solutions containing local anaesthetics and preservatives. *Current Eye Research* 7:947–950.

Rink, H., and Hockwin, O. 1987. Tissue culture in toxicological research applied to lens epithelial cells. In *Drug-Induced Ocular Side Effects and Ocular Toxicology*, ed. O. Hockwin, pp. 368–375. Basel: Karger.

Roberts, J.E., and Dillon, J. 1990. Screening for potential *in vivo* phototoxicity in the lens/retina. *Lens and Eye Toxicity Research* 7:655–666.

Rubin, L.F. 1990. Albino versus pigmented animals for ocular toxicity testing. *Lens and Eye Toxicity Research* 7:221–230.

Santoul, C., Decrouez, E., Droit, J.Y., and Bonne, C. 1990. Use of a specular microscope with pachymeter in ocular tolerance studies of eye drops in the rabbit. Evaluation of ocular tolerance of benzalkonium chloride (BAK) in aqueous solution, 0.01% and 0.1%. *Lens and Eye Toxicity Research* 7:359–369.

Sasaki, K., and Yamamura, T. 1987. A review of drug-induced ocular side effects in Japan. In *Drug-Induced Ocular Side Effects and Ocular Toxicology*, ed. O. Hockwin, pp. 21–29. Basel: Karger.

Scaife, M.C. 1985. An *in vitro* cytotoxicity test to predict the ocular irritation potential of detergents and detergent products. *Food and Chemical Toxicology* 23:253–258.

Schmitt, C., Schmidt, J., and Hockwin, O. 1990. Ocular drug-safety study with the HMG-CoA reductase inhibitor Pravastatin. *Lens and Eye Toxicity Research* 7:631–641.

Schnieders, B. 1987. Recommendations concerning toxicity tests on medical products. State of affairs within the European Community. In *Drug-Induced Ocular Side Effects and Ocular Toxicology*, ed. O. Hockwin, pp. 1–8. Basel: Karger.

Simmons, S.J., Jumblatt, M.M., and Neufeld, A.H. 1987. Corneal epithelial wound closure in tissue culture: an *in vitro* model of ocular irritancy. *Toxicology and Applied Pharmacology* 8:13–23.

Small, G.H., Peyman, G.A., Srinivasan, A., Smith, R.T., and Fiscella, R. 1987. Retinal toxicity of combination antiviral drugs in an animal model. *Canadian Journal of Ophthalmology* 22:300–303.

Spielmann, H., Gerner, I., Kalweit, S., Moog, R., Wirnsberger, T., Krauser, K., Kreiling, R., Kreuzer, H., Lüpke, N.-P., Miltenberger, H.G., Müller, N., Mürmann, P., Pape, W., Siegemund, B., Spengler, J., Steiling, W., and Wiebel, F.J. 1991. Interlaboratory assessment of alternatives to the Draize eye irritation test in Germany. *Toxicology In Vitro* 5:539–542.

Spielmann, H., Liebsch, M., Moldenhauer, F., Holzhütter, H.-G., Bagley, D.M., Lipman, J.M. Pape, W.J.W., Miltenberger, H., de Silva, O., Hofer, H., and Steiling, W. 1997. CAM-based assays. *Food and Chemical Toxicology* 35:39–66.

Swantson, D.W. 1983. Eye irritancy testing. In *Animals and Alternatives in Toxicity Testing*, eds. M. Balls, R.J. Riddell, and A.N. Worden, pp. 337–366. New York: Academic Press.

Talsma, D.M., Leach, C.L., Hatoum, N.S., Gibbons, R.D., Roger, J.C., and Garvin, P.J. 1988. Reducing the number of rabbits in the Draize eye irritancy test: a statistical analysis of 155 studies conducted over 6 years. *Fundamental and Applied Toxicology* 10:146–153.

Van Buskirk, E.M. 1980. Adverse reactions from timolol administration. *Ophthalmology* 87:447–450.

Van Buskirk, E.M., and Fraunfelder, F.T. 1984. Ocular beta-blockers and systemic effects. *American Journal of Ophthalmology* 98:623–624.

Wallin, R.F., Hume, R.D., and Jackson, E.M. 1987. The agarose diffusion method for ocular irritancy screening: cosmetic products, part I. *Journal of Toxicology—Cutaneous and Ocular Toxicology* 6:239–250.

Ward, S.L., Walker, T.L., and Dimitrijevich, S.D. 1997. Evaluation of chemically induced toxicity using an *in vitro* model of human corneal epithelium. *Toxicology In Vitro* 11:121–139.

Wegener, A., and Hockwin, O. 1987. Animal models as a tool to detect the subliminal cocataractogenic potential of drugs. In *Drug-Induced Ocular Side Effects and Ocular Toxicology*, ed. O. Hockwin, pp. 250–262. Basel: Karger.

Wegener, A., Laser, H., and Hockwin, O. 1987. Measurement of lens transparency changes in animals. Comparison of the Topcon SL-45 combined with linear microdensitometry and the Zeiss SLC system. In *Drug-Induced Ocular Side Effects and Ocular Toxicology*, ed. O. Hockwin, pp. 263–275. Basel: Karger.

Weisse, I., Hockwin, O., Green, K., and Tripathi, R.C., eds. 1995. *Ocular Toxicology*, pp. 1–378. New York: Plenum Press.

Weisse, I., Loosen, H., and Peil, H. 1990. Age-related retinal changes—a comparison between albino and pigmented rabbits. *Lens and Eye Toxicity Research* 7:717–739.

Weltman, A.S., Sparber, S.B., and Jurtshuk, T. 1965. Comparative evaluation and the influence of various factors on eye-irritation scores. *Toxicology and Applied Pharmacology* 7:308–319.

Withering, W. 1785. *An Account of the Foxglove and Some of Its Medical Uses: With Practical Remarks on Dropsy and Other Diseases*. Birmingham: Broomsleigh Press.

Yousufzai, S.Y.K., Chen, A.L., and Abdel-Latif, A.A. 1988. Species differences in the effects of prostaglandins on inositol triphosphate accumulation, phosphatidic acid formation, myosin light chain phosphorylation and contraction in iris sphincter of the mammalian eye: interaction with the cyclic AMP system. *Journal of Pharmacology and Experimental Therapeutics* 247:1064–1072.

Zlioba, A., Peyman, G.A., and Nikoleit, J. 1988. Retinal toxicity study of intravitreal carboplatin and iproplatin. *Annals of Ophthalmology* 20:71–72.

Ophthalmic Toxicology
Edited by George C. Y. Chiou
Copyright © 1999 Taylor & Francis

2

Molecular Basis of Ophthalmic Toxicology

Z. H. Song and Ann Schroeder

*Department of Medical Pharmacology and Toxicology, Texas A&M University Health
Science Center, College Station, Texas, USA*

To deal with the stress of foreign substances (xenobiotics), the body has developed enzyme-mediated transformations. These transformations can be divided into two phases. Phase 1 reactions include hydroxylation, oxidation, and reduction, while phase-2 reactions include conjugation reactions, such as glucuronidation, acetylation, and sulfation. These biotransformation reactions generally increase the polarity of xenobiotics. Through these reactions, the xenobiotics are made less hydrophobic and more easily excretable. However, toxic compounds, such as free radicals, are sometimes generated from these reactions. The eye is especially sensitive to the toxic species produced from the metabolic reactions. This is because the eye is exposed extensively to light each day, and a large amount of oxygen is consumed by the retina.

In this chapter, we will first try to provide an overview of the processes involved in the biotransformation of xenobiotics, particularly biooxidation reactions. We will then try to provide some examples of these reactions that are relevant to ophthalmic toxicology.

XENOBIOTIC METABOLISM

Xenobiotics are foreign substances, such as drugs and pesticides. By metabolizing the xenobiotics through an enzymatic pathway, the body can eliminate these foreign substances and limit the amount of toxic exposure. The enzymes that transform xenobiotics have the daunting challenge of metabolizing a variety of foreign compounds. Therefore, these enzymes usually are present in very large amounts, and many of these enzymes have overlapping-substrate specificities.

Phase-1 Transformations

Cytochrome P-450 System

A distinguishing feature of the cytochrome P-450 enzymes, which accounts for their name, is their spectroscopic property. The reduced carbon monoxide complexes of P-450 enzymes possess an absorption maximum at approximately 450 nm (Omura and Sato, 1962; Omura and Sato, 1964a,b).

The cytochrome P-450 system provides a crucial pathway for xenobiotic metabolism. Cytochrome P-450 enzymes are involved in both detoxifying and bioactivating exogenous and endogenous substances (Schenkman and Griem, 1993; Lewis, 1996). Most of the identified P-450 enzymes are membrane bound and are located in the endoplasmic reticulum of the hepatocyte. In addition, P-450 enzymes involved in xenobiotic metabolisms are found in a variety of organs, including kidney, lung, gut, and eye, whereas P-450 enzymes involved in steroid biosynthesis are located in the adrenals, testes, and ovaries (Schenkman and Griem, 1993; Lewis, 1996).

Cytochrome P-450 enzymes are classified as monooxygenases in which one oxygen atom of molecular oxygen is added to the substrate while the other atom of oxygen is reduced to water (Mueller et al., 1995). There are multiple forms of P-450 enzymes with different catalytic activities (Nelson et al., 1993). To date, the P-450 enzyme family consists of at least 36 families. The cytochrome P-450 enzymes catalyze a wide array of reactions, including hydroxylation, oxidation, and reduction (Gonzales, 1988; Lewis, 1996). Through the reduction of the ferric heme, these enzymes activate oxygen. Since the heme iron in P-450 enzymes accept only one electron at a time, electron transport proteins, such as the NADPH–cytochrome c reductase system, are used to deliver a single electron to the iron while accepting paired electrons (Strobel et al., 1995; Lewis, 1996). These transport proteins use flavin-containing coenzymes. The body has developed an efficient way to respond to foreign substances in that the activity of P-450 enzymes can be induced through exposure to xenobiotics (Whitlock and Denison, 1995).

Phase-2 Transformations

Glucuronidation

One of the most important means of xenobiotic metabolism is glucuronidation (Mulder et al., 1990; Mulders et al., 1993). The reaction proceeds as an SN2 displacement with the xenobiotic acting as the nucleophile. The nucleophile attacks UDP-glucuronate with the catalytic assistance of the enzyme UDP-glucuronyl transferase. The resulting product is a glucuronide. Through glucuronidation, in most cases xenobiotics are transformed into more hydrophilic, less active compounds. The enzymes involved in glucuronidation, UDP-glucuronyltransferases (UGTs) are known to be endoplasmic reticulum integral membrane proteins (Tephly and Burchell, 1990). The enzymes can be classified into two families: UGT1 and UGT2 (Burchell et al., 1991; Clarke and Burchell, 1994).

Endogenous substances, such as heme, also undergo glucuronidation (Ostrow, 1986). Free heme are originated from the catabolism of hemoglobin of red blood cells that are removed from the circulation. Due to its toxicity, the free heme must be degraded. Heme is first broken down to biliverdin through a heme oxygenase-catalyzed reaction. Biliverdin is further reduced to bilirubin, which is toxic at high concentrations. At this point, glucuronidation takes effect. Through the action of bilirubin-UDP-glucuronyltransferase, bilirubin is transferred to bilirubin diglucuronide, a water-soluble compound that can be easily excreted from the body (Hauser and Gollan; 1986; Crawford et al., 1992). Jaundice results from excessive accumulation of bilirubin. The hallmark of jaundice is the yellowing of the whites of the eye. Neonatal jaundice is a result of low bilirubin-UDP-glucuronyltransferase activity in newborns (Lee and Gartner, 1986).

Arylamine N-Acetylation

Another important aspect of xenobiotic metabolism involves arylamine N-acetylation (Evans, 1989; Vatsis and Weber, 1994). Many compounds, including drugs and carcinogens such as isoniazid and benzidine use N-acetylation as their means of metabolism. The enzyme that catalyzes the N-acetylation of arylamine is arylamine N-acetyltransferase. This enzyme is acetyl CoA–dependent. The reaction carries out through a nucleophilic displacement on the carbonyl carbon of the acetyl CoA oxyester, with the thiolate anion of acetyl CoA as the leaving group (Andres et al., 1988). The result is that an acetyl group is transferred from acetyl CoA to an acceptor arylamine.

Molecular cloning has uncovered two genes encoding two forms of N-acetyltransferases, NAT1 and NAT2 (Blum et al., 1990; Ohsako and Deguchi, 1990). It has been found that NAT2 is the locus for human polymorphism of arylamine N-acetyltransferases. Due to mutations on the genes for this enzyme, the capacity for arylamine N-acetylation varies among individuals (Blum et al., 1989; Grant et al.,

1990). Therefore, one is genetically predetermined to be a "slow" or "fast" acetylator. In addition to detoxication, it should be mentioned that in some cases the *N*-acetyltransferase pathway can also activate the arylamine carcinogens (Weber et al., 1990).

Sulfation

The process of sulfation provides an additional pathway for the body to transform and ultimately eliminate xenobiotics (Mulder, 1981; Weinshilboum and Otterness, 1994). In sulfation, the metabolic donor of sulfate is 3-phosphoadenosine-5′-phosphosulfate. It reacts with a variety of substrates in a reaction catalyzed by the enzyme sulfotransferase. Examples of substrates for sulfation are phenols, alcohols, and aromatic amines. Molecular cloning studies have identified multiple forms of sulfotransferases (Weinshilboum, 1990).

Drugs that use the route of sulfation for their metabolism include steroidal oral contraceptives and anabolic steroids used by athletes (Weinshilboum, 1990; Weinshilboum and Otterness, 1994). In addition to xenobiotics, several endogenous compounds, including steroids and bile salts, can also be metabolized by sulfotransferase. The metabolite products of these compounds are excreted in the urine. Although sulfation is used primarily as a detoxication pathway, it can also activate certain toxic compounds (Miller and Surh, 1994).

BIOOXIDATION

Oxidative reactions occur frequently in cells (Malmström, 1982; Southorn and Powis, 1988; Sies, 1991; Rice-Evans et al., 1995). Oxygen radicals are formed through these reactions and contribute to oxygen toxicity. Understanding the molecular basis of these oxidative reactions are important in appreciating their significance.

Superoxide

Due to the short lifespan of superoxide $O_2^{\cdot-}$, it has been difficult to detect its formation. Despite this problem, strong clues for its genesis have been obtained. For example, using the techniques of electron paramagnetic resonance (EPR), the appearance of superoxide has been observed when mitochondrial membrane preparations are exposed to oxygen and electrons are supplied with NAD(P)H (Beauchamp and Fridovich, 1971; Kirby and Fridovich, 1982).

The discovery of enzyme, superoxide dismutase, highlighted the biological significance of its substrate, superoxide (Bannister et al., 1987; McCord and Fridovich, 1988). Superoxide dismutase catalyzes the dismutation of the oxygen radical superoxide anion according to the equation

$$O_2^{\cdot-} + O_2^{\cdot-} + 2H^+ \rightarrow H_2O_2 + O_2$$

Since the superoxide would cause the formation of radicals OH· and singlet oxygen, this reaction prevents the buildup of these damaging radicals. The importance of the enzyme is reflected by the fact that the steady-state concentration of superoxide can be maintained at a much lower value inside the cell by the enzyme as opposed to nonenzyme dismutations (Bannister et al., 1987; McCord and Fridovich, 1988). In kinetic terms, the enzymatic dismutation is a first-order reaction, whereas nonenzymatic dismutation is a second-order reaction with respect to superoxide. Superoxide dismutases are metalloenzymes (Bannister et al., 1987; Stallings et al., 1992). They can be classified into three classes according to their metal content, that is, Cu,Zn-containing, Mn-containing, and Fe-containing superoxide dismutases.

Hydrogen Peroxide

Another significant biooxidation reaction involves hydrogen peroxide H_2O_2 (Diplock, 1994; Liebler and Reed, 1997; Boveris and Cadenas, 1997). Hydrogen peroxide is generated either as the product of oxygen reduction by certain oxidases or as a product of superoxide dismutation. Catalases and peroxidases, referred to collectively as hydroperoxidases, function as the enzymes that break down hydrogen peroxide in the body. Catalase is a specific type of peroxidase in which hydrogen peroxide acts as both oxidant and reductant (Diplock, 1994; Gaetani et al., 1994). Catalase catalyzes the following net reaction:

$$H_2O_2 + H_2O_2 \rightarrow 2H_2O + O_2$$

Other organic or inorganic substrates are oxidized by peroxidases (Saunders et al., 1964; Everse et al., 1991). Peroxidases catalyze the formation of substrate-derived radicals in substances, such as hydrogen peroxide. The net reaction is

$$H_2O_2 + 2RH_2 \rightarrow 2H_2O + 2RH$$

It has been suggested that both catalase and glutathione peroxidase are involved in scavenging hydrogen peroxide (Diplock, 1994; Liebler and Reed, 1997).

Mammalian catalase is a protein composed of four identical subunits, each consisting of one tightly bound molecule of NADPH (Kirkman and Gaetani, 1984). Catalase is compartmentalized in the liver and many other tissues in the peroxisomes. The presence of peroxisomes is indicative of large amounts of localized hydrogen peroxide production. In red blood cells, catalases exist in the cytosol. The human gene encoding catalases has been cloned and sequenced, thereby facilitating further research of their structure and function (Korneluk et al., 1984).

An example of mammalian peroxidases is glutathione peroxidase. Glutathione peroxidase is selenium-dependent, and multiple forms of glutathione peroxidases have been discovered. However, some glutathione transferases can perform peroxidase activities independent of selenium.

Lipid Peroxidation

Lipid peroxidation provides a path through which free radicals operate in a toxic manner (Porter, 1984; Gardner, 1989). It refers to the process of incorporating molecular oxygen into the polyunsaturated fatty acids. If lipid peroxidation is left unchecked due to large amounts of free-radical production, the biological membranes will begin to break down. Normal aerobic metabolism, ischemia–reperfusion conditions, the activation of phagocytes, and certain exogenous compounds, including drugs, are all contributors of the free radicals superoxide and hydrogen peroxide that can initiate the lipid peroxidative processes.

Lipid peroxidation has significant biological ramifications (Nigam et al., 1988). By damaging the lipid bilayer structure in the cell membrane, the membrane becomes "leaky", and important Na^+ and K^+ concentration gradients cannot be maintained.

Glutathione Oxidation

Superoxide, hydrogen peroxide, and lipid peroxidation are all means of oxidative stress in the cell. Glutathione oxidation provides a major pathway to relieve oxidative stress.

The evolution of GSH (reduced glutathione) primarily occurred as a defensive maneuver of the body against toxic oxygen products (Larsson et al., 1983; Sies and Ketterer, 1988; Reed, 1990). GSH is present intracellularly in virtually all aerobic organisms at high concentrations. The sulfhydryl group, -SH, functions as a good nucleophile for reacting with electrophilic chemical compounds, such as those produced by potentially toxic oxidative processes.

GSH is used as a reductant to combat the toxic oxidants (Mannervik et al., 1989; Forman et al., 1997). For example, in the case of free-radicals, GSH reacts with the radical and forms a glutathione radical. Before this new radical can trigger free radical damages, it rapidly reacts with a thiol radical forming glutathione disulfide (GSSG), the oxidized form of GSH:

$$GSH + R^{\cdot} \rightarrow RH + GS^{\cdot}$$

$$GS^{\cdot} + GS^- \rightarrow (GSSG^{\cdot})^-$$

$(GSSG^{\cdot})^-$ rapidly reduces oxygen to superoxide, which is consequently detoxified by superoxide dismutase. GSSG is then reduced back to GSH by an important enzyme, glutathione reductase. Hence, a recycling of GSH is achieved.

Another mechanism of detoxification by GSH involves a set of enzymes known collectively as the glutathione transferases (Tew et al., 1993; Vermeulen et al., 1996). These enzymes catalyze the conjugation of GSH with a wide variety of electrophilic substances that may be cytotoxic. The GSH conjugation product may then be further metabolized or excreted from the cell. Therefore, through the conjugation process, GSH has intercepted the potential toxic effects of the electrophiles. There are four classes of glutathione transferases, which are classified according to their primary structure: Alpha, Mu, Pi, and Theta (Vermeulen et al., 1996). The specificities of the four enzymes are not altogether distinct from one another; this perhaps occurred due to the fact that these enzymes must target a wide range of toxic substances.

Since GSH works to eliminate cellular toxic oxidants, it can also reduce the effectiveness of anticancer drugs (Hayes et al., 1990). Therefore, manipulating the amount of GSH plays an important role in drug therapy. Intracellular GHS levels can be reduced by inhibitors of GSH biosynthesis. By reducing the amount of GSH available, tumors that were previously nonresponsive to certain drugs, will be sensitized to treatment.

To summarize biooxidation reactions, most free-radical generation of the cell is diverted to superoxide, where superoxide dismutase and catalase dispose of the radical products. In this pathway, glutathione acts as a general repair molecule for radical damages. If, however, the supply of glutathione or superoxide dismutase is depleted, the resulting accumulation of superoxide radicals would cause oxidative stress in the cell. This oxidative stress leads to consequences such as lipid peroxidation and toxicity in the cell.

XENOBIOTIC METABOLISM, BIOOXIDATION, AND OPHTHALMIC TOXICOLOGY

Ocular Xenobiotic Metabolism

While the liver is a well-known site for xenobiotic metabolism, similar biotransformations occur in the eye as well (Shichi, 1984). Several biotransformation enzymes have been located in various ocular tissues, including nonpigmented ciliary epithelium, retinal pigmented epithelium, and corneal epithelium (Shichi et al., 1975; Kishida et al., 1986; Schwartzman et al., 1987; Shichi et al., 1991; Zhao and Shichi, 1995). The localization of the enzymes in these sites may serve to protect the eye by detoxifying xenobiotics. Two examples are (1) the enzymes located at the nonpigmented ciliary epithelium may function to prevent toxic compounds from entering the aqueous filtrate and (2) the enzyme located at the retinal pigmented epithelium may act to protect retina from toxic compounds.

Similar to the situation in liver, the activity of biotransformation enzymes in the eye can be induced by certain compounds. For example, it has been shown that in certain strains of mice the activity of aryl hydrocarbon hydroxylase can be induced up to 10-fold higher by the administration of beta-naphthoflavone (Shichi et al., 1975). In addition, a recent immunocytochemical study demonstrated that the level of cytochrome P450 (1A1/1A2) immunoreactivity is markedly increased in the ocular tissues of responsive C57BL/6 mice by treatment with beta-naphthoflavone (Zhao and Shichi, 1995). In mouse cross-breeding experiments, it was demonstrated that the enzyme inducibility is an autosomal dominant trait (Hankinson, 1995). It was hypothesized that this genetic locus (Ah locus) encodes a receptor (AH receptor) that is capable of binding inducers. Using a radiolabeled inducer, the AH receptor can be detected in the livers of responsive mice. In contrast, nonresponsive mice have much lower levels of the AH receptor. To date, the gene for AH receptor has been cloned (Burbach et al., 1992; Ema et al., 1992). It encodes a DNA binding protein that belongs to a family of helix-loop-helix proteins. Interestingly, it has been suggested that, in mice, certain ocular pathological conditions, such as cataract and retinal degeneration, may correlate with genetic differences between different strains in aryl hydrocarbon hydroxylase inducibility (Shichi et al., 1976; Shichi and Nebert, 1982). It was hypothesized that the metabolites produced from the phase-1 transformation may react with cell membrane, protein, and DNA, and eventually destroy visual cells.

Nonpigmented ciliary epithelium has cytochrome P-450 enzyme systems (Shichi et al., 1991; Zhao and Shichi, 1995). Experimental studies using cultured cells as well as in animals have indicated that this biotransformation system may play a role in preventing toxicants from entering aqueous humor.

Nonpigmented ciliary epithelium has cytochrome P-450 enzyme systems (Shichi et al., 1991; Zhao and Shichi, 1995). Experimental studies using cultured cells as well as in animals have indicated that this biotransformation system may play a role in preventing toxicants from entering aqueous humor. Therefore, these enzymes work as a defense mechanism to protect those tissues that are in close contact with aqueous humor.

In the retina, cytochrome P-450 monooxygenase is responsible for aromatic hydroxylation (Shichi et al., 1976; Shichi and Nebert, 1982). Similar to the case of liver, there seem to be genetic variations in the ocular expression of aryl hydrocarbon hydroxylase activity. On one hand, this enzymatic system acts to eliminate toxic compounds that tend to accumulate in the retina. On the other hand, data from animal experiments have suggested that induction of aryl hydrocarbon hydroxylase activity in retinal pigmented epithelium seems to be correlated to retinal degeneration (Shichi et al., 1976; Shichi and Nebert, 1982).

Corneal epithelium also possesses the cytochrome P-450 enzyme systems (Schwartzman et al., 1990). These enzymes play an important role in endogenous arachidonic acid metabolism. In fact, the cytochrome P-450-mediated metabolism is the major pathway of arachidonic acid metabolism in cornea. Because of physical trauma (such as contact lens wear) and/or hypoxic stress, the potent mediators of inflammation, 12-HETEs, are generated from this metabolic pathway (Conners et al., 1995a,b). The 12-HETEs cause vasodilation, chemotaxis, inhibition of Na–K ATPase, and changes in ion pumps (Schwartzman et al., 1990; Conners et al., 1995a,b). These will cause inflammation and damage of the tissue.

Ocular Biooxidation

Light and oxygen are essential for the normal functions of the eye. However, when the excess amount of light and oxygen are present in an uncontrolled fashion, they will have damaging effects on different tissues of the eye. Some of these effects are irreversible and may lead to pathological conditions, such as degeneration of retina and cataract formation in the lens.

Retina

Since the retina is exposed to copious amounts of light daily, and the retina has high levels of long-chain polyunsaturated fatty acids, this tissue is particularly subjective to the formation of free radicals and lipid peroxidation (Fliesler and Anderson, 1983; Green, 1995). Convincing evidences have shown that the products of lipid peroxidation are formed when the retina is exposed to constant light, and the reduction in retinal function is correlated with the light-induced lipid peroxide formation (Wiegand et al., 1986). Furthermore, the presence of molecular photosensitizers that absorb light and generate reactive oxygen species facilitate lipid peroxidation (Andley and Chylack, 1990). These molecular photosensitizers have the ability to react with polyunsaturated lipids to form lipid hydroperoxides, which will damage cell membranes. It has been hypothesized that the damage of retina cells are mediated by endogenous photosensitizers. These potential mediators of light damage include visual pigments, cytochromes, and melanin. The precise molecular mechanisms for biooxidation-induced retinal damage have not been elucidated. It has been suggested that lipid peroxide will form bifunctional compounds that will cross-link lipids and proteins in photoreceptor membranes.

For the purpose of antioxidation, the retina has high levels of glutathione, glutathione-coupled enzymes, and superoxide dismutase (Hall and Hall, 1975; Rapp et al., 1985; De La Paz et al., 1996). Glutathione peroxidase and superoxide dismutase work to detoxify lipid hydroperoxide and superoxide radicals, respectively. The retina also has high levels of vitamin E and vitamin C, which are endogenous scavengers of free radicals (Organisciak et al., 1984; Friedrichson et al., 1995). Studies have shown that they may protect the retina against light stress. For example, it has been shown in rats that increased retinal vitamin C levels resulted in a reduction in light-induced photoreceptor cell damage and in light-induced loss of polyunsaturated fatty acid contents in the retina (Organisciak et al., 1985; Li et al., 1985; Organisciak et al., 1990). In contrast, it has been shown that the diet lacking vitamin E can induce degenerative alterations in rats (el-Hifnawi et al., 1995).

Macular degeneration is characterized by the loss of central vision. Age-related macular degeneration is a major vision problem for people over 65 years old. There are reports of epidemiological and experimental studies that support the theory that light-induced lipid peroxidation leads to age-related macular degeneration (Hyman et al., 1983; Goldberg et al., 1988; Eye Disease Case–Control Group, 1992, 1993; Snodderly, 1995). However, until now the role of antioxidants and mineral supplements in the treatment of age-related macular degeneration has not been firmly established (Bressler and Bressler, 1995).

Lens

Cataract is one of the leading causes of blindness in the elderly. Oxidative stress has been implicated as an important step toward the formation of cataracts (Taylor and Davies, 1987; Davies, 1990; Spector; 1990). During the formation of cataracts, hydrogen peroxide, one of the main sources of ocular oxidative stress, damages the lens proteins by oxidizing sulfhydryl groups in lens proteins. This causes the polymerization of lens proteins and accumulation of insoluble materials in the lens.

The exposure of the eye to phototoxins or photosensitizers, has been implicated in the formation of cataracts (Andley and Chylack, 1990). Photosensitizers include various drugs and dyes. These compounds absorb radiation and undergo photochemical reactions, which result in the formation of free radicals. Due to the slow metabolism of lens proteins, the photodamage is accumulated, and eventually leads to cataract formation. Drugs that act as photosensitizers include allopurinol, which is used to treat gout. Cataract formation has been observed in relatively young patients who have been taking the drug. 8-Methoxypsoralaen and related compounds are used by dermatologists for phototherapy of psoriasis and vitiligo. It has been demonstrated that these compounds can also cause cataract formation.

The lens has very high levels of antioxidants, vitamin C and glutathione (Reddy, 1990; Berman, 1991). It has been reported that young and clear lenses have more of these antioxidants than old and cataractous lenses. The major enzyme that metabolizes hydrogen peroxide in the eye is glutathione peroxidase (Reddy, 1990; Berman 1991). It has been proposed that older lenses have reduced activities of this and other enzymes involved in the oxidative defense, and thus are more susceptible to cataract (Xie et al., 1991; Green, 1995). It has been shown in organ culture experiments that antioxidants can prevent or reverse opacification of the lens (Spector et al., 1993). Several studies in humans also indicate that the intake of antioxidants, such as vitamins C and E and carotenoids, can reduce the risk of cataract (Robertson et al., 1989; Knekt et al., 1992; Varma et al., 1995). In contrast, cigarette smoke and free radicals generated from it contribute to increased incidence of cataracts (Christen et al., 1992).

In summary, considerable evidence suggests that free radicals resulting from the events of ocular biooxidation play an important role in retinal degeneration and cataract formation. During aging or some pathological conditions, the diminished antioxidant enzymes or antioxidants will enhance the risk of retinal degeneration and cataract formation. Diet rich in vitamins, such as fruits and vegetables, may delay the ocular damages caused by oxidative stress.

REFERENCES

Andley, U.P., and Chylack, L.T., Jr. 1990. Recent studies on photodamage to the eye with special reference to clinical phototherapeutic procedures. *Photodermatology, Photoimmunology and Photomedicine* 7(3):98–105.

Andres, H.H., Klem, A.J., Schopfer, L.M., Harrison, J.K., and Weber, W.W. 1988. On the active site of liver acetyl CoA: Arylamine *N*-acetyltransferase from rapid acetylator rabbits. (III/J). *Journal of Biological Chemistry* 263:7521–7527.

Bannister, J.V., Bannister, W.H., and Rotilio, G. 1987. Aspects of the structure, function, and applications of superoxide dismutase. *CRC Critical Reviews in Biochemistry* 22:111–180.

Beauchamp, C., and Fridovich, I. 1971. Superoxide dismutase: improved assays and an assay applicable to acrylamide gels. *Analytical Biochemistry* 44:276–287.

Berman, E.R., ed. 1991. *Biochemistry of the Eye.* New York: Plenum Press.

Blum, M., Grant, D.M., Demierre, A., and Meyer, U.A. 1989. *N*-Acetylation pharmacogenetics: a gene deletion causes absence of arylamine *N*-acetyltransferase in liver of slow acetylator rabbits. *Proceedings of the National Academy of Sciences* 86:9554–9557.

Blum, M., Grant, D.M., McBride, O.W., Heim, M., and Meyer, U.A. 1990. Human arylamine-acetyltransferase genes: isolation, chromosomal localization and functional expression. *DNA and Cell Biology* 9:193–203.

Boveris, A., and Cadenas, E. 1997. Cellular sources and steady-state levels of reactive oxygen species. In *Oxygen, Gene Expression, and Cellular Function,* eds. L.B. Clerch and D.J. Massaro, pp. 1–25. New York: Marcel Dekker.

Bressler, N.M., and Bressler, S.B. 1995. Preventative ophthalmology. Age-related macular degeneration. *Ophthalmology* 102(8):1206–1211.

Burbach, K.M., Poland, A., and Bradfield, C.A. 1992. Cloning of the Ah-receptor cDNA reveals a distinctive ligand-activated transcription factor. *Proceedings of the National Academy of Sciences* 89:8185–8189.

Burchell, B., Nebert, D.W., Nelson, D.R., Bock, K.W., Iyanagi, T., Jansen, P.L.M., Lancet, D., Mulder, G.J., Chowdhury, R.J., Siest, G., Tephly, T.R., and MacKenzie, P.I. 1991. The UDP-glucuronosyltransferase gene superfamily: suggested nomenclature based on evolutionary divergence. *DNA and Cell Biology* 10:487–494.

Christen, W.G., Manson, J.E., Seddon, J.M., Glynn, R.J., Buring, J.E., Rosner, B., and Hennekens, C.H. 1992. A prospective study of cigarette smoking and risk of cataracts in men. *Journal of the American Medical Association* 268:989–993.

Clarke, D.J., and Burchell, B. 1994. The uridine diphosphate glucuronosyltransferase multigene family: function and regulation. In *Conjugation–Deconjugation Reactions in Drug Metabolism and Toxicity,* ed. F.C. Kauffman, pp. 3–43. Berlin: Springer-Verlag.

Conners, M.S., Stoltz, R.A., Webb, S.C., Rosenberg, J., Dunn, M.W., Abraham, N.G., and Laniado-Schwartzman, M. 1995a. A closed eye contact lens model of corneal inflammation. Part 1: Increased synthesis of cytochrome P450 arachidonic acid metabolites. *Investigative Ophthalmology and Visual Science* 36:828–840.

Conners, M.S., Stoltz, R.A., Davis, K.L., Dunn, M.W., Abraham, N.G., Levere, R.D., and Laniado-Schwartzman, M. 1995b. A closed eye contact lens model of corneal inflammation. Part 2: Inhibition of cytochrome P450 arachidonic acid metabolism alleviates inflammatory sequelae. *Investigative Ophthalmology and Visual Science* 36:841–850.

Crawford, J.M., Ransil, B.J., Narciso, J.P., and Gollan, J.L. 1992. Hepatic microsomal bilirubin UDP-glucuronosyltransferase. The kinetics of bilirubin mono- and diglucuronide synthesis. *Journal of Biological Chemistry* 267:16943–16950.

Davies, K.J. 1990. Protein oxidation and proteolytic degradation. General aspects and relationship to cataract formation. *Advances in Experimental Medicine and Biology* 264:503–511.

De La Paz, M.A., Zhang, J., and Fridovich, I. 1996. Antioxidant enzymes of the human retina: effect of age on enzyme activity of macula and periphery. *Current Eye Research* 15:273–278.

Diplock, A.T. 1994. Antioxidants and free radical scavengers. In *Free Radical Damage and Its Control.* Amsterdam: Elsevier.

el-Hifnawi, el-S., Lincoln, D.T., and Dashti, H. 1995. Nutritionally induced retinal degeneration in rats. *Nutrition* 11:705–707.

Ema, M., Sogawa, K., Watanabe, N., Chujoh, Y., Matsushita, N., Gotoh, O., Funae, Y., and Fujii-Kuriyama, Y. 1992. cDNA cloning and structure of mouse putative Ah receptor. *Biochemical and Biophysical Research Communications* 184:246–253.

Evans, D.A. 1989. *N*-Acetyltransferase. *Pharmacology and Therapeutics* 42:157–234.

Everse, J., Everse, K.E., and Grisham, M.B., eds. 1991. *Peroxidases in Chemistry and Biology.* Boca Raton, FL: CRC Press.

Eye Disease Case–Control Study Group. 1992. Risk factors for neovascular age-related macular degeneration. *Archives of Ophthalmology [Chicago]* 110:1701–1708.

Eye Disease Case–Control Study Group. 1993. Antioxidant status and neovascular age-related macular degeneration. *Archives of Ophthalmology* 111:104–109.

Fliesler, S.J., and Anderson, R.E. 1983. Chemistry and metabolism of lipids in the vertebrate retina. *Progress in Lipid Research* 22:79–131.

Forman, H.J., Liu, R.M., and Tian, L. 1997. Glutathione cycling in oxidative stress. In *Oxygen, Gene Expression, and Cellular Function*, eds. L.B. Clerch and D.J. Massaro, pp. 99–121. New York: Marcel Dekker.

Friedrichson, T., Kalbach H.L., Buck, P., and van Kuijk, F.J. 1995. Vitamin E in macular and peripheral tissues of the human eye. *Current Eye Research* 14:693–701.

Gaetani, G.F., Kirkman, H.N., Mangerini, R., and Ferraris, A.M. 1994. Importance of catalase in the disposal of hydrogen peroxide within human erythrocytes. *Blood* 84:325–330.

Gardner, H.W. 1989. Oxygen radical chemistry of polyunsaturated fatty acids. *Free Radical Biology and Medicine* 7:65–86.

Goldberg, J., Flowerdew, G., Smith, E., Brody, J.A., and Tso, M.O. 1988. Factors associated with age-related macular degeneration. An analysis of data from the first National Health and Nutrition Examination Survey. *American Journal of Epidemiology* 128:700–710.

Gonzales, F.J. 1988. The molecular biology of cytochrome P450s. *Pharmacological Reviews* 40:243–288.

Grant, D.M., Morike, K., Eichelbaum, M., and Meyer, U.A. 1990. Acetylation pharmacogenetics: the slow acetylator phenotype is caused by decreased or absent arylamine acetyltransferase in human liver. *Journal of Clinical Investigation* 85:968–972.

Green, K. 1995. Free radicals and aging of anterior segment tissues of the eye: a hypothesis. *Ophthalmic Research* 27 (Suppl)1:143–149.

Hall, M.O., and Hall, D.O. 1975. Superoxide dismutase of bovine and frog rod outer segments. *Biochemical and Biophysical Research Communications* 67:1199–1204.

Hankinson, O. 1993. Research on the aryl hydrocarbon (dioxin) receptor is primed to take off. *Archives of Biochemistry and Biophysics* 300:1–5.

Hankinson, O. 1995. The aryl hydrocarbon receptor complex. *Annual Review of Pharmacology and Toxicology* 35:307–340.

Hauser, S.C., and Gollan, J.L. 1986. Hepatic UDP-glucuronyltransferase and the conjugation of bile pigments. In *Bile Pigments and Jaundice*, ed. J.D. Ostrow, pp. 211–241. New York: Marcel Dekker.

Hayes, J.D., Pickett, C.B., and Mantle T.J., eds. 1990. *Glutathione S-Transferases and Drug Resistance*. London: Taylor & Francis.

Hyman, L.G., Lillienfeld, A.M., Ferris, F.L., and Fine, S.L. 1983. Senile macular degeneration: a case–control study. *American Journal of Epidemiology* 118:213–227.

Kirby, T.W., and Fridovich, I. 1982. A picomolar spectrophotometric assay for superoxide dismutase. *Analytical Biochemistry* 127:435–440.

Kirkman, H.N., and Gaetani, G.F. 1984. Catalase: a tetrameric enzyme with four tightly bound molecules of NADPH. *Proceedings of the National Academy of Sciences* 81:4343–4347.

Kishida, K., Matsumoto, K., Manabe, R., and Sugiyama, T. 1986. Cytochrome P450 and related components of the microsomal electron transport system in the bovine ciliary body. *Current Eye Research* 5:529–533.

Knekt, P., Heliövaara, M., Rissanen, A., Aromaa, A., and Aaran, R.K. 1992. Serum antioxidant vitamins and risk of cataract. *British Medical Journal* 305:1392–1394.

Korneluk, R.G., Quan, F., Lewis, W.H., Gusie, K.S., Willard, H.F., Holmes, M.T., and Gravel, R.A. 1984. Isolation of human fibroblast catalase cDNA clones. *Journal of Biological Chemistry* 259:13819–13823.

Larsson, A., Orrenius, S., Holmgren, A., and Mannervik, B., eds. 1983. *Functions of Glutathione. Biochemical, Physiological, Toxicological and Clinical Aspects*, New York: Raven Press.

Lee, K., and Gartner, L.M. 1986. Fetal bilirubin metabolism and neonatal jaundice. In *Bile Pigments and Jaundice*, ed. J.D. Ostrow, pp. 373–394. New York: Marcel Dekker.

Lewis, D.F.V., ed. 1996. *Cytochromes P450, Structure, Function and Mechanism*. Basingstoke, Hants: Taylor & Francis.

Li, Z.Y., Tso, M.O.M., Wang, H.M., and Organisciak, D.T. 1985. Amelioration of photic injury in rat retina by ascorbic acid: a histopathologic study. *Investigative Ophthalmology and Visual Science* 26:1589–1598.

Liebler, D.C., and Reed, D.J. 1997. *Free-radical defense and repair mechanisms. In Free Radical Toxicology*, ed. K.B. Wallace, pp. 141–171. London: Taylor & Francis.

Malmström, B.G. 1982. Enzymology of oxygen. *Annual Review of Biochemistry* 51:21–59.

Mannervik, B., Carlberg, I., and Larson, K. 1989. Glutathione: general review of mechanism of action. In *Glutathione: Chemical, Biochemical and Medical Aspects*, eds. D. Dolphin, R. Poulson, and O. Avramovic, pp. 475–516. New York: Wiley.

McCord, J.M., and Fridovich, I. 1988. Superoxide dismutase: the first twenty years (1968–1988). *Free Radical Biology and Medicine* 5:363–369.

Miller, J.A., and Surh, Y.-J. 1994. Sulfonation in chemical carcinogenesis. In *Conjugation-Deconjugation Reactions in Drug Metabolism and Toxicity*. pp. 429–457. Springer-Verlag.

Mueller, E.J., Loida, P.J., and Sligar, S.G. 1995. Twenty-five years of P450$_{cam}$ research: mechanistic insights into oxygenase catalysis. In *Cytochrome P450, Structure, Mechanism, and Biochemistry*, 2nd ed., pp. 83–124. New York: Plenum Press.

Mulder, G.J., ed. 1981. *Sulfation of Drugs and Related Compounds*. Boca Raton, FL: CRC Press.

Mulder, G.J., Coughtrie, M.W.H., and Burchell, B. 1990. Glucuronidation. In *Conjugation Reactions in Drug Metabolism: An Integrated Approach*, ed. G.J. Mulder, pp. 51–105. London: Taylor & Francis.

Mulders, T.M.T., Breimer, D.D., and Mulder, G.J. 1993. Glutathione conjugation in man. In *Human Drug Metabolism*, ed. E.H. Jeffery, pp. 133–142. Boca Raton, FL: CRC Press.

Nelson, D.R., Kamataki, T., Waxman, D.J., Guengerich, F.P., Estabrook, R.W., Feyereisen, R., Gonzalez, F.J., Coon, M.J., Gunsalus, I.C., and Gotoh, O. 1993. The P450 superfamily: update on new sequences, gene mapping, accession numbers, early trivial names of enzymes, and nomenclature. *DNA and Cell Biology* 12:1–51.

Nigam, S.K., McBrien, D.C.H., and Slater, T.F., eds. 1988. *Eicosanoids, Lipid Peroxidation, and Cancer*. Berlin: Springer-Verlag.

Ohsako, S., and Deguchi, T. 1990. Cloning and expression of cDNAs for polymorphic and monomorphic arylamine *N*-acetyltransferases from human liver. *Journal of Biological Chemistry* 265:4630–4634.

Omura, T., and Sato, R. 1962. A new cytochrome in liver microsomes. *Journal of Biological Chemistry* 237:1375–1376.

Omura, T., and Sato, R. 1964a. The carbon monoxide–binding pigment of liver microsomes. I. Evidence for its hemoprotein nature. *Journal of Biological Chemistry* 239:2370–2378.

Omura, T., and Sato, R. 1964b. The carbon monoxide–binding pigment of liver microsomes. II. Solubilization, purification, and properties. *Journal of Biological Chemistry* 239:2378–2385.

Organisciak, D.T., Wang, H.M., and Kou, A.L. 1984. Ascorbate and glutathione levels in the developing normal and dystrophic rat retina: effect of intense light exposure. *Current Eye Research* 3(1):257–267.

Organisciak, D.T., Wang, H.M., Li, Z.Y., and Tso, M.O.M. 1985. The protective effect of ascorbate in retinal light damage of rats. *Investigative Ophthalmology and Visual Science* 26:1580–1588.

Organisciak, D.T., Jiang, Y.L, Wang, H.M., and Bicknell, I. 1990. The protective effect of ascorbic acid in retinal light damage of rats exposed to intermittent light. *Investigative Ophthalmology and Visual Science* 31:1195–1202.

Ostrow, J.D., ed. 1986. *Bile Pigments and Jaundice*. New York: Marcel Dekker.

Porter, N.A. 1984. Chemistry of lipid peroxidation. *Methods in Enzymology* 105:273–282.

Rapp, L.M., Naash, R.D., Weigand, R.D., Joel, C.D., Nielsen, J.D., and Anderson, R.E. 1985. Morphological and biochemical comparisons between retinal regions having differing susceptibility to photoreceptor degeneration. In *Retinal Degeneration*, ed. M.M. LaVail, pp. 421–431. New York: Alan R. Liss.

Reddy, V.N. 1990. Glutathione and its function in the lens—an overview. *Experimental Eye Research* 150:771–778.

Reed, D.J. 1990. Glutathione: toxicological implications. *Annual Review of Pharmacology and Toxicology* 30:603–631.

Rice-Evans, C., Halliwell, B., and Lunt, G.G., eds. 1995. *Free Radicals and Oxidative Stress: Environment, Drugs and Food Additives*. London: Portland Press.

Robertson, J.M., Donner, A.P., and Trevithick, J.R. 1989. Vitamin E intake and risk of cataracts in humans. *Annals of the New York Academy of Sciences* 570:372–382.

Saunders, B.C., Holmes-Siedle, A.G., and Stark, B.P., eds. 1964. *Peroxidase: The Properties and Uses of a Versatile Enzyme and of Some Related Catalysts*. London: Butterworths.

Schenkman, J.B., and Griem, H., eds. 1993. *Cytochrome P450*. Heidelberg: Springer-Verlag.

Schwartzman, M.L., Balazy, M., Masferrer, J., Abraham, N.G., McGiff, J.C., and Murphy, R.C. 1987. 12(R)hydroxyeicosatetraenoic acid: a cytochrome-P450-dependent arachidonate metabolite that inhibits Na,K-ATPase in the cornea. *Proceedings of the National Academy of Sciences of the United States of America* 84:8125–8129.

Schwartzman, M.L., Davis, K.L., Nishimura, M., Abraham, N.G., and Murphy, R.C. 1990. The cytochrome P450 metabolic pathway of arachidonic acid in the cornea. *Advances in Prostaglandin, Thromboxane, and Leukotriene Research* 21A:185–192.

Shichi, H. 1984. Biotransformation and drug metabolism. In *Pharmacology of the eye*, ed. M. Sears, pp. 117–148. New York: Springer-Verlag.

Shichi, H., and Nebert, D.W. 1982. Genetic differences in drug metabolism associated with ocular toxicity. *Environmental Health Perspectives* 44:107–117.

Shichi, H., Atlas, S.J., and Nebert, D.W. 1975. Genetically regulated aryl hydrocarbon hydroxylase induction in the eye: possible significance of the drug-metabolizing enzyme system for the retinal pigmented epithelium-choroid. *Experimental Eye Research* 21:557–567.

Shichi, H., Mahalak, S.M., Sakamato, S., and Sugiyama, T. 1991. Immunocytochemical study of phenobarbital- and 3-methylcholanthrene-inducible cytochrome P450 isozymes in primary cultures of porcine ciliary epithelium. *Current Eye Research* 10:779–788.

Shichi, H., Tsunematsu, Y., and Nebert, D.W. 1976. Aryl hydrocarbon hydroxylase induction in retinal pigmented epithelium: possible association of genetic differences in a drug metabolizing enzyme system with retinal degeneration. *Experimental Eye Research* 23:165–176.

Sies, H., ed. 1991. *Oxidative Stress: Oxidants and Antioxidants*. London: Academic Press.

Sies, H., and Ketterer, B., eds. 1988. *Glutathione Conjugation. Mechanisms and Biological Significance*. San Diego: Academic Press.

Snodderly, D.M. 1995. Evidence for protection against age-related macular degeneration by carotenoids and antioxidant vitamins. *American Journal of Clinical Nutrition* 62:1448S–1461S.

Southorn, P.A., and Powis, G. 1988. Free radicals in medicine. I. Chemical nature and biologic reactions. *Mayo Clinic Proceedings* 63:381–389.

Spector, A. 1990. Oxidation and aspects of ocular pathology. *CLAO Journal* 16(1 Suppl):S8–10.

Spector, A., Wang, G.M., Wang, R.R., Garner, W.H., and Moll, H. 1993. The prevention of cataract caused by oxidative stress in cultured rat lenses. H_2O_2 and photochemically induced cataract. *Current Eye Research* 12:163–179.

Stallings, W.C., Bull, C., Fee, J.A., Lah, M.S., and Ludwig, M.L. 1992. Iron and manganese superoxide dismutases: catalytic inferences from the structures. In *Molecular Biology of Free Radical Scavenging Systems*, ed. J.G. Scandalios, pp. 193–211. Cold Spring Harbor, NY: Cold Spring Harbor Laboratory Press.

Strobel, H.W., Hodgson, A.V., and Shen, S. 1995. NADPH cytochrome P450 reductase and its structural and functional domains. In *Cytochrome P450, Structure, Mechanism, and Biochemistry*, 2nd ed., pp. 225–244. New York: Plenum Press.

Taylor, A., and Davies, K.J. 1987. Protein oxidation and loss of protease activity may lead to cataract formation in the aged lens. *Free Radical Biology and Medicine* 3(6):371–377.

Tephly, T.R., and Burchell, B. 1990. UDP-glucuronosyltransferases: a family of detoxifying enzymes. *Trends in Pharmacological Sciences* 11:276–279.

Tew, K.D., Pickett, C.B., Mantle, T.J., Mannervik, B., and Hayes, J.D., eds. 1993. *Structure and Function of Glutathione Transferases*. Boca Raton, FL: CRC Press.

Varma, S.D., Devamanoharan, P.S., and Morris, S.M. 1995. Prevention of cataracts by nutritional and metabolic antioxidants. *Critical Reviews in Food Science & Nutrition* 35(1–2):111–129.

Vatsis, K.P., and Weber, W.W. 1994. Human N-acetyltransferases. In *Conjugation–Deconjugation Reactions in Drug Metabolism and Toxicity*, pp. 109–130. Springer-Verlag.

Vermeulen, N.P.E., Mulder, G.J., Nieuwenhuyse, H., Peters, W.H.M., and Van Bladeren, P.J., eds. 1996. *Glutathione S-Transferases. Structure, Function and Clinical Implications*. London: Taylor & Francis.

Weber, W.W., Levy, G.N., and Hein, D.W. 1990. Acetylation. In *Conjugation Reactions in Drug Metabolism: An Integrated Approach*, pp. 163–191. London: Taylor & Francis.

Weinshilboum, R. 1990. Sulfotransferase pharmacogenetics. *Pharmacology and Therapeutics*. 45:93–107.

Weinshilboum, R., and Otterness, D. 1994. Sulfotransferase enzymes. In *Conjugation-Deconjugation Reactions in Drug Metabolism and Toxicity*, pp. 45–78. Berlin: Springer-Verlag.

Whitlock, J.P., and Denison, M.S. 1995. Induction of cytochrome P450 enzymes that metabolize xenobiotics. In *Cytochrome P450, Structure, Mechanism, and Biochemistry*, 2nd ed., pp. 367–390. New York: Plenum Press.

Wiegand, R.D., Joel, C.D., Rapp, L.M., Nielsen, J.C., Maude, M.B., and Anderson, R.E. 1986. Polyunsaturated fatty acids and vitamin E in rat rod outer segments during light damage. *Investigative Ophthalmology and Visual Science* 27:727–733.

Xie, P.Y., Kanai, A., Nakajima, A., Kitahara, S., Ohtsu, A., and Fujii, K. 1991. Glutathione and glutathione-related enzymes in human cataractous lenses. *Ophthalmic Research* 23:133–140.

Zhao, C., and Shichi, H. 1995. Immunocytochemical study of cytochrome P450 (1A1/1A2) induction in murine ocular tissues. *Experimental Eye Research* 60(2):143–52.

Ophthalmic Toxicology
Edited by George C. Y. Chiou
Copyright © 1999 Taylor & Francis

3

Toxicity in Specific Ocular Tissues

Nicholas J. Millichamp

*Department of Small Animal Medicine and Surgery, College of Veterinary Medicine,
Texas A&M University, College Station, Texas, USA*

Toxins may affect all parts of the eye. Topical substances tend to have more local effects in the eyelids, conjunctiva, and cornea, whereas systemic drugs often have diffuse effects in several parts of the eye. Some drugs have more specific effects on a particular ocular structure. Most of the drugs that cause ocular toxicity cause some degree of visual dysfunction. Many visual disturbances have been reported and are beyond the scope of this review.

This chapter is intended as an introduction to some of the effects of toxins in the eye of humans and animals. This is in no way an attempt at an exhaustive review. For readers who wish to obtain more information either on drugs and effects discussed here or to determine if other less common drug reactions or toxicities occur with a particular agent, other sources of information are available. In particular, the National Registry of Drug-Induced Ocular Side Effects has been incorporated into the comprehensive text by Fraunfelder and Grove (1999). This provides a listing with some indication of significance for every reported ocular side effect in man. This is a valuable source to determine whether a drug has ever caused a particular toxic reaction.

Grant's fourth edition of *Toxicology of the Eye* (Grant and Schuman, 1993) remains the most comprehensive source of detailed information on topical and systemic toxic reactions in the eye. This text is very thorough, presenting worldwide literature in a very complete and readable manner.

Throughout this chapter reference is made to ocular structures and some aspects of ocular physiology. The reader is referred to more detailed texts on these subjects for further information (Prince, 1956; Hogan et al., 1971; Walls, 1942; Duke-Elder, 1958; Prince et al., 1960; Samuelson, 1991; Davson, 1990; Berman, 1991; Ozanics and Jakobiec, 1986; Wilkie and Wyman, 1991).

EYELIDS

The eyelids can be divided into outer skin and orbicularis layers and inner fibrous connective tissue lined by the palpebral conjunctiva. The connective tissue layer in primates forms a semirigid curved tarsal plate in the upper eyelid that conforms to the shape of the globe. The levator palpebrae superioris muscle and sympathetically innervated Müller's muscle insert into the tarsal plate and effect elevation of the upper lid. The eyelids are variably pigmented in different species. Cilia arise at the margins of the eyelids of upper and/or lower lids associated with modified sweat glands. Glands in the tarsal plate (meibomian glands) contribute to the lipid layer of the tear film. In animals, hair covers the eyelids extending onto the face. In humans, cilia are also located at the eyebrow. Closure of the eyelids is largely caused by contraction of the orbicularis oculi muscle, which encircles the eyelid margins.

The eyelids may be affected by toxins in various ways. Neurological effects on levator palpebrae superioris muscle or sympathetically innervated muscle of the upper lid result in ptosis, whereas contraction of these muscles will retract the upper lid. Blepharospasm is a nonspecific response of the eyelids to any painful or irritating stimulus, including conjunctival or corneal irritation or injury, or deeper injury or inflammation in the uvea. Drugs that cause corneal epithelial injury, uveitis, or elevated intraocular pressure and cause a painful sensation in the eye will cause blepharospasm.

Ptosis and Lid Retraction

Drooping of the upper eyelid is seen with several systemic agents. Ptosis or blepharoplegia is a common feature of **venomous snakebite**, being caused by most types of snake venom but especially that of **elapid** and some **viperids. Snake venoms** act like **curariform drugs** to reduce muscle end-plate potentials and prevent action potentials spreading into the muscle. Depolarizing neuromuscular blocking drugs like **succinylcholine** also cause lid drooping (Hardman and Limbird, 1996). The venom of the **black widow spider** also may cause ptosis, along with eyelid edema (Edwards et al., 1980). **Botulinus toxin** causes ptosis by inhibiting acetylcholine release at the muscle ending (Hardman and Limbird, 1996).

Tetraethylammonium, a ganglion blocking agent, causes ptosis. **Guanethidine,** a sympatholytic drug used to reduce lid retraction reduces tone in the sympathetically innervated upper eyelid muscle fibers, causing ptosis. **Mephenesin** is a muscle relaxant that causes ptosis. The metal-chelating agent **penicillamine** has caused toxicity that has often presented with ptosis (Grant and Schuman, 1993).

Sedatives and related drugs including **barbiturates, primidone,** and **alcohol** often cause ptosis (Fraunfelder and Grove, 1996; Grant and Schuman, 1993). **Vincristine** causes ptosis in patients by inducing a neuropathy of peripheral motor nerves (Sandler et al., 1969).

Retraction of the upper eyelid occurs with drugs that stimulate the sympathetic innervation of the upper eyelid, including **phenylephrine, amphetamine,** and **cocaine** (Grant and Schuman, 1993).

Blepharitis

Inflammation of the eyelids has been described with numerous topical drugs, including the antivirals **vidarabine, idoxuridine,** and **trifluridine,** and ophthalmic drug preservatives **(benzalkonium, thimerosal)**. Reactions to most topically applied ophthalmic preparations, as well as numerous systemic drugs, appear to have been reported on occasion as a cause of blepharoconjunctivitis (Fraunfelder and Grove, 1996).

Alopecia and Poliosis

Grant and Schuman (1993) and Fraunfelder and Grove (1996) list various drugs that have caused hair loss or depigmentation of the eyelashes or eyebrows. Most notable in causing alopecia are **actinomycin D, triparanol, thallium,** and **vitamin A** (Grant and Schuman, 1993).

Poliosis has been reported to occur with **corticosteroids, chloroquine, hydroxychloroquine, amodiaquine,** and **triparanol** (Fraunfelder and Grove, 1996; Grant and Schuman, 1993).

LACRIMAL SYSTEM

Many substances cause increased lacrimation and are discussed under corneal and conjunctival irritation. Decreased lacrimation occurs as a side effect of many human drugs (Fraunfelder and Grove, 1996), and may occur due to pharmacological blockage of secretion in the lacrimal gland. A component of this innervation is from the parasympathetic system. Parasympatholytic drugs, including **atropine,** and **scopolamine,** reduce tearing in this manner.

Other compounds have been reported to be toxic to the lacrimal gland in animals and potentially capable of causing clinical keratoconjunctivitis sicca. Drugs toxic to the canine lacrimal gland include **phenazopyridine, sulfadiazine,** and **salicylazosulfapyridine** (Bryan and Slatter, 1973; Slatter, 1973; Kaswan and Salisbury, 1990). **Phenazopyridine** causes necrosis and fibrosis of lacrimal gland acini (Slatter, 1973).

CORNEA AND CONJUNCTIVA

The cornea comprises the anterior 1/4 to 1/16 of the outer fibrous tunic of the eye (depending upon the species), and functions as the major refractive surface of the eye. The cornea is made up of four main layers, excluding the precorneal tear film. The outer epithelium is several cells thick, with columnar germinal cells resting on a basement membrane. The cells become nonkeratinized, stratified squamous as they are displaced superficially and eventually lost into the tear film. The stroma, which lies beneath the epithelial basement membrane, comprises 90% of the total corneal thickness. This layer is made up of layers of corneal lamellae that span the entire corneal surface. The lamellae comprise regularly arranged bundles of collagen fibrils maintained evenly spaced by a proteoglycan ground substance. The water content of the cornea is maintained at 78%. Few keratocytes (specialized fibroblasts) are found in the corneal stroma. Noncollagenous protein, lipids, and glycoproteins comprise the rest of the biochemical makeup of the cornea.

At the inner face of the stroma is a highly elastic layer, Descemet's membrane, which is the basement membrane of the posterior endothelium of the cornea; it apposes the anterior chamber. The endothelial layer is one cell in thickness and has the important function of maintaining corneal hydration and detumescence by pumping water that has leaked into the stroma back into the anterior chamber. This leak pump mechanism is an active process that provides for corneal nutrition from the aqueous humor while maintaining normal stromal hydration. Normal stromal hydration ensures that the collagen fibrils maintain regular spacing, an important feature in maintaining corneal transparency and preventing the development of corneal edema. Focal loss of either the corneal epithelium and to an even greater extent the corneal endothelium results in edema accumulation in the corneal stroma and epithelial layers. Polymorphonuclear leukocytes (PMNs), which may reach the site of epithelial injury, have significant potential to slow epithelial wound healing.

Erosions of the corneal epithelium are healed by rapid sliding of adjacent cells into the defect followed by mitosis of the basal germinal cells to thicken the epithelial layer. Epithelial cells will attach to undamaged basement membrane. If the basement membrane is also damaged (corneal ulcer), epithelial attachment may take several weeks to be complete, pending reformation of an underlying basement membrane.

Stromal lacerations initially fill with fibrin and PMNs attracted to the site of injury to provide phagocytosis of infectious agents that may be present. Keratocytes become activated and produce new collagen into the area of the fibrin clot. Neovascularization of the stroma with granulation tissue production occurs in cases of severe stromal injury. Epithelial cells cover the area of the defect and stromal scarring is eventually remodeled over many months. In some instances PMNs, corneal breakdown products, or toxins may cause rapid dissolution of the stromal collagen and ground substance, which may result in ulceration to Descemet's membrane or perforation of the cornea.

The conjunctiva is a thin mucous membrane that extends from the limbus of the eye to the margin of the eyelids. The conjunctiva that covers the anterior portion of the sclera is the bulbar conjunctiva. It is reflected at the conjunctival fornix to line the inner surface of the eyelids as the palpebral conjunctiva and to cover the third eyelid in species where this structure is found. The space bounded by the conjunctival and corneal surfaces is the conjunctival sac. The conjunctiva is divided histologically into two layers: a superficial layer of stratified columnar epithelium, which is continuous with the stratified squamous epithelium of the cornea, and a deeper substantia propria. The palpebral conjunctival epithelium contains goblet cells, which are particularly numerous at the fornices and over the base of the anterior surface of the third eyelid. The conjunctival epithelium is variably pigmented in different species, particularly near the limbus.

The substantia propria has a superficial glandular layer and a deeper layer of loose fibrous tissue. Two layers of lymphatics are present—one at the depth of the superficial blood vessels and the other in the deep fibrous layer. Lymph follicles are especially numerous in the bulbar conjunctiva of the third eyelid and fornices. The blood supply of the conjunctiva is derived from the anterior ciliary arteries, and the vascular arcades of the eyelids. The conjunctiva and cornea are innervated by the trigeminal nerve.

Corneal and Conjunctival Chemical Burns

Chemical burns to the cornea are due to either acids or alkalis. Acids that may be involved include **sulfuric** and **sulfurous acids, hydrochloric acid, hydrofluoric acid, chromic acid, nitric acid, sulfur dioxide**, and **silver nitrate**. Acids cause coagulation and precipitation of proteins. This occurs in both the epithelium and stroma; however, precipitation of protein in the more superficial layers tends to prevent acid from reaching deeper layers of the cornea and thus the severity of at least weak acid burns is not usually as great as alkali burns, where no such superficial protection occurs. With strong acids, the protective effect may not be particularly significant, and the eye may sustain severe injury. Acids coagulate the epithelial cells and cause contraction (shrinkage) of stromal collagen fibrils. Proteoglycan matrix is precipitated by acids (Friedenwald et al., 1946).

In mild acid burns, the initial changes are turbidity and dulling of the conjunctival surface, possibly with corneal epithelial erosion. The conjunctiva becomes hyperemic and petechial hemorrhages may be seen. With stronger acids, the cornea and conjunctiva immediately become opaque (usually white). Necrotic epithelium is lost within a few days, but will regenerate rapidly in mild cases. In severe cases, the stroma may be clear or becomes thinner and a descemetocele may develop or the cornea may perforate. Healing is by neovascularization with extensive scarring in severe cases (Grant and Schuman, 1993).

Alkalis that may burn the cornea and conjunctiva include **hydroxides of sodium, ammonium, calcium, magnesium**, and **potassium**. Several other hydroxide-containing substances are known to cause ocular damage (Grant and Schuman, 1993). Most severe injury occurs with alkalis at pH over 12 (Grant and Kern, 1955). Variations in the severity of corneal injury appear to correlate with the differences in the epithelial damaging potential of the various alkalis (Grant and Schuman, 1993).

Alkalis cause fatty acid saponification and dissociation in cell membranes. This causes cell destruction allowing penetration of the epithelial layer. In the stroma, the alkali causes swelling of the collagen fibrils, either directly or after hydrolyzation of proteoglycans, and renders the stromal collagen more susceptible to enzymes (particularly collagenase). Collagenases are produced by PMNs (Kao et al., 1986) that enter the cornea in response to high molecular weight substances and collagen breakdown products, which act as PMN chemoattractants (Elgebaly et al., 1987). Collagenase further degrades collagen, causing a melting appearance to the stroma. Plasmin from damaged epithelial cells and fibroblasts (Berman et al., 1980) may additionally retard epithelial healing and potentiate a cascade of events resulting in further collagen and stromal breakdown (Berman, 1991).

Corneal Epithelial Defects and Erosions

Minor defects or erosions in the corneal epithelium, which may heal rapidly, have been described after exposure to several groups of toxins. These are reviewed extensively by Grant and Schuman (1993). Epithelial erosions may occur secondary to impaired sensory innervation of the cornea (neurotropic keratitis). This may occur in acid and alkali burns, or with exposure to carbon or hydrogen disulfide.

Elapid venoms cause excessive lacrimation, conjunctival hyperemia, and corneal edema and may damage the epithelium, causing erosions (Brown, 1980). In severe cases ulceration, perforation, and uveitis occur (Payne and Warrell, 1976; Warrell and Ormerod, 1976).

Solvents cause irritation and pain and loss of epithelium, which in most cases will regenerate again rapidly (Grant and Schuman, 1993).

Surfactants are used as surgical preoperative antiseptic agents and in topically applied ophthalmic drops as preservatives. Benzalkonium chloride is a cationic surfactant commonly used to increase the penetration of certain drugs into the eye. Dodecyl sodium sulfate and soaps are examples of anionic surfactants, and Tween is a nonionic surfactant. Cationic surfactants are in general more injurious to the conjunctiva and cornea than anionic or nonionic types, although the concentration applied to the eye is a more important determinant of the severity of injury. Surfactants cause conjunctival hyperemia, corneal opacification, and epithelial edema, with occasional epithelial erosions.

Chloroacetophenone is a component of a solvent spray tear gas used for self-defense. This agent causes extensive lacrimation, and epithelial erosions or loss with stromal edema. Epithelial lesions usually heal rapidly (MacLeod, 1969). Numerous other related agents that cause excessive lacrimation and epithelial damage have been described by Grant and Schuman (1993). These agents at low concentrations cause marked stimulation of the trigeminal nerve endings in the cornea, and only at higher concentrations cause epithelial damage.

Local anesthetics such as lidocaine, proparacaine, and butacaine cause epithelial damage and retard epithelial healing. These drugs should not be used therapeutically where ocular pain is present (Smelser and Ozanics, 1945).

Epithelial injury occurs with many substances applied topically to the eyes. Hydrogen sulfide gas and sulfur dust cause conjunctival hyperemia and epithelial cell loss, which may be due to the inhibition of cytochrome oxidase in the epithelium. Surfactants such as benzalkonium chloride cause slight damage to epithelial cells and have been used to promote drug penetration into the eye (Havener, 1983). Vinblastine applied topically to the human cornea causes a punctate epithelial keratopathy and erosions (McLendon and Bron, 1978). Low concentrations of mustard gas applied topically to the rabbit eye cause epithelial edema and conjunctival hyperemia several hours after topical application. Longer contact with the irritant can result in stromal ulceration (Kinsey and Grant, 1946). Nitrogen mustard has similar, although more rapid, effects on the conjunctiva and corneal epithelium when applied topically in experimental animals or with exposure in humans. Additionally, acute ocular irritation occurs in the anterior uvea (Mann et al., 1948; Jampol et al., 1976). Allyl alcohol causes conjunctival hyperemia and chemosis and reversible corneal opacification due to epithelial damage and edema (Carpenter and Smyth, 1946). Colchicine causes stromal edema and will reduce the rate of epithelialization of epithelial defects (Grant and Schuman, 1993; Gipson et al., 1982). Other agents that have been found to be toxic to the corneal epithelium include **emetine, dimethyl sulfoxide diisopropylamine in various dyes**, and **formaldehyde** in various concentrations (Grant and Schuman, 1993).

Conjunctivitis and keratitis have been described with many drugs given systemically. These include **phenylbutazone, sulfonamides** (Grant and Schuman, 1993), **cytarabine** (Kaufman et al., 1964), **methotrexate** (Fraunfelder and Grove, 1996), **β-blockers** (Fraunfelder and Grove, 1996), and **phenazopyridine** (Bryan and Slatter, 1973).

Follicular conjunctivitis may occur with topical use of several ophthalmic drugs, including **idoxuridine, vidarabine, pilocarpine,** and **atropine** (Wilson, 1979).

The corneal endothelium may be damaged by air or intraocular irrigating solutions used for cataract surgery (Waltman et al., 1975). Certain preservatives **(benzalkonium chloride)** may be very destructive when applied to the corneal endothelium (Maurice and Perlman, 1977). Damage may occur from certain photosensitizing agents. In cattle, **phenothiazine** causes photosensitization and corneal endothelial damage resulting in severe corneal edema (Whitman and Filmer, 1974). **Dichloroethane,** a solvent, is selectively toxic to the canine corneal endothelium, either after parenteral administration or inhalation. Endothelial cells become swollen and detach from the endothelium and later attempt to cover the defect by sliding from adjacent undamaged areas (Kuwabara et al., 1968).

Deposits in the corneal epithelium, which appear as fine gray granules (cornea verticillata), have been described in humans with several systemic drugs, including **clofazimine, amiodarone, chloroquine,** and **triparanol. Chlorpromazine** causes fine deposits both deep in the stroma and in the epithelium with chronic use, as well as conjunctival pigmentation (Fraunfelder and Grove, 1996; Grant and Schuman, 1993). **Epinephrine** used topically causes fine multifocal pigmented deposits in the conjunctiva and sometimes in the corneal stroma if the epithelial surface is damaged. The deposits are oxidized epinephrine (Reinecke and Kuwabara, 1963).

Corneal Lipidosis

Amphiphilic cationic substances cause lipid deposition in the cornea in several species. In man, **chloroquine** and **amiodarone** cause whorl- or streak-like lipid deposits in the epithelium (Grant and Schuman, 1993). Topical applications of **amiodarone** to rats result in cytoplasmic lipid inclusions in all corneal layers (Bockhardt et al., 1978; Drenckhahn et al., 1983; Lullmann-Rauch, 1991a). Corneal lipidosis has also been caused in rats by **chlorphentermine, iprindole, tamoxifen,** and **chloroquine** (Lullmann-Rauch, 1991a).

Corneal Mucopolysaccharidosis

Glycosaminoglycans (GAGS) may accumulate in keratocytes and the endothelium and basal layers of the epithelium of rats treated with the dicationic amphiphilic drug **tilorone** (Lullmann-Rauch, 1991a).

ANTERIOR UVEA

The anterior uvea comprises the iris and ciliary body. The iris comprises an anterior stroma of collagen fibers, melanocytes, and fibroblasts. The anterior border is made up of fibroblasts and melanocytes. The posterior aspects of the iris is made up of two epithelial layers; the anterior forms the myoepithelial-type dilator muscle and continues as the anterior pigmented epithelium of the ciliary body. The posterior pigmented layer of iris epithelium continues into the ciliary body as the nonpigmented layer of ciliary epithelium. The iris also has a smooth iridal sphincter muscle near the margin of the pupil in the stroma. The ciliary body extends posteriorly from the iris base to the retina. The most anterior aspect of the ciliary body forms the iridocorneal angle, the site of most aqueous humor drainage from the eye. The ciliary body comprises the ciliary muscle, which inserts into the region of the iridocorneal angle, and the ciliary processes, which project inward from the ciliary body toward the lens. The ciliary processes are histologically divided into a highly vascular collagenous stroma, which is separated from the posterior chamber by the two layers of ciliary epithelium. The ciliary epithelium is the cell layer responsible for active secretion of aqueous humor. The zonule fibers that support the lens arise from between adjacent ciliary processes.

Acute Ocular Irritative Response and Uveitis

The most significant ocular pathological responses of the uvea are the acute ocular irritative response and uveitis (inflammation of the uvea). The ocular irritative response consists of miosis, disruption of the blood–aqueous barrier, and changes in the intraocular pressure of the eye in response to various noxious substances, trauma, radiation, cr paracentesis of the anterior chamber. The mechanisms whereby the ocular irritative responses develop and their variation in different species are discussed in the chapter by Millichamp, "Species Specificity."

Numerous toxic substances can potentially cause disruption of the blood–aqueous barrier. In several species irritation of the cornea with compounds such as **nitrogen mustards** will cause breakdown of the blood–aqueous barrier and miosis. Clinically, treatment with miotics may cause dilatation of iris blood vessels, pigment dispersion in the aqueous, and, occasionally, iritis (Grant and Schuman, 1993). Several related substances including organophosphates (irreversible acetylcholinesterase inhibitors) have similar effects. There appears to be little specificity as to which substances that cause ocular surface irritation will also affect the ocular barriers. Variations are more closely tied to the species being tested.

Iris Cysts

Cysts of the pupillary margin occur in patients treated for long periods with **miotics,** including **pilocarpine, demecarium, and echothiophate** (Havener, 1983).

LENS

The lens of the eye is a clear spheroidal structure, composed of an inner, embryolog-ically older nucleus surrounded by a cortex. The whole structure is enclosed by the lens capsule. The anterior lens capsule is lined as far as the lens equator by a single layer of epithelial cells, the continued division of which results in the deposition of successive layers of anucleate lens fibers around the outside of the cortex like the layers of an onion. Consequently, the lens increases in size throughout life. The main biochemical components of the lens are protein and water. The protein fractions are both soluble and insoluble, the latter increasing in proportion to the former with age or in the development of cataract. The lens is suspended behind the iris by zonular fibers that arise from the ciliary body and insert onto the lens capsule circumfer-entially at the lens equator. Lens protein turnover is limited within the lens fibers, most of the metabolic and synthetic activity of the lens taking place in the anterior epithelium (Davson, 1990; Berman, 1991).

Nuclear Sclerosis

Aging changes in animals referred to as nuclear sclerosis involve a change in the refractive properties of the nucleus. These have also been seen as a reversible change in experimental species, including dogs and rabbits but not man, systemically ad-ministered **dimethylsulfoxide** (Rubin, 1975; Wood and Wirth, 1969).

Cataract

Cataract is the most common and significant abnormality of the lens. A cataract is defined as any opacity or loss of transparency, partial or complete, of the lens. The metabolic causes of cataracts have been reviewed elsewhere (Harding and Crabbe, 1984). Changes in lens proteins during cataract formation are similar to those seen in aging. These include tryptophan oxidation, deamination, development of lens pig-mentation, increase in fluorescence, formation of disulfide bonds, cross linking, in-crease in insoluble protein, glycation, and formation of high molecular weight ag-gregates (Berman, 1991). The appearance of cataracts varies considerably among species, and differences in the metabolism of the lens in different species may ac-count for particular sensitivity of one species to toxic cataract development over another.

Numerous topical and systemic drugs have been reported to cause cataracts in man and animals. Complete lists are available in Grant and Schuman (1993) and Fraunfelder and Grove (1996). The various toxic agents that cause cataracts have been thoroughly reviewed in a systematic manner by Harding and Crabbe (1984). This section lists some of the better known toxic causes of cataracts.

Many photosensitizing agents have been described as causes of cataracts (Grant and Schuman, 1993). Light (including sunlight and ultraviolet light [UVL]), although often cited as a cause of cataracts, is probably not able to cause cataracts alone without some photosensitizing agent (Harding and Crabbe, 1984). **8-Methoxypsoralen** (methoxsalen) causes anterior cortical cataracts in mice and guinea pigs with UVL exposure (Cloud et al., 1960, 1961). Other agents that may cause cataracts associated with photosensitization in various species include **nafoxidine, hematoporphyrin, 1,4-bis-(phenylisopropyl)-piperazine,** and **bleomycin (antineoplastic** and **antibiotic)** (Grant and Schuman, 1993).

Various drugs produce cataracts that resemble those caused by ionizing radiation. These cataracts often affect the actively mitotic cells at the lens equator, thus forming equatorial cataracts in the early stages (Grant and Schuman, 1993). **4-(p-Dimethylaminostyryl) quinoline** produces such cataracts in mice (Christenberry et al., 1963). Systemic **iodoacetate** causes posterior polar cataracts in rabbits when given systemically or by intracameral injection (Cibis, 1957). Other agents that have produced cataracts resembling radiation damage include **nitrogen mustard** (Grant and Schuman, 1993). Various antimitotic and antineoplastic drugs cause cataracts in man and animals that resemble radiation cataracts. **Busulfan** affects lens epithelial nucleic acid and reduces mitosis and causes cataracts in rats and humans (Grimes et al., 1965; Hamming et al., 1976). **p-Chlorophenylalanine,** an antimetabolite, may cause cataracts in rats by reducing entry of amino acids into the aqueous or lens (Gralla and Rubin, 1970; Rowe et al., 1973). **Triethylenemelamine** (tretamine) causes cataracts when administered systemically to mice (Christenberry et al., 1963). **Myleran** causes cataracts in rats, presumably by preventing division of lens epithelial cells (Grimes and Von Sallmann, 1966).

Cataracts may result from interference with protein synthesis and metabolism and interference with enzyme systems in the lens. **Naphthalene** and related compounds produce cataracts in rabbits and rats and possibly humans. The drug was used as an antiseptic and anthelminthic. Cataracts are seen with systemic but not intraocular administration (Grant and Schuman, 1993). Both albino and pigmented rabbits are equally affected, whereas pigmented rats are more likely to be affected than albinos due to enzyme differences between the strains. Cataracts can develop to maturity in 2 weeks in rabbits fed naphthalene. Breakdown of the blood–aqueous barrier in rabbits apparently enhances development of cataracts (Hockwin et al., 1969). Naphthalene is probably metabolized to toxic products, in particular **1-2-naphthoquinone,** that reach the eye and cause changes in lens electrolytes (reduced potassium, increased sodium and chloride, and reduced gluthathione and amino acids), all of which have been associated with cataract development (van Heyningen, 1979). **Methionine sulfoxime** interferes with protein synthesis and causes cataracts in rats fed a low-protein diet (Bagchi, 1959). **Mimosine,** a plant extract that affects protein metabolism and enzyme activity, causes various ocular changes when fed to rats, including cataracts, which appear to be a primary effect (Von Sallmann et al., 1959). Lens vacuolation and epithelial hyperplasia also occur in cattle fed a diet of *Leucaena leucocephala,* due to its high mimosine content (Holmes et al., 1981). **2,4-Dinitrophenol** was used orally for weight reduction in humans, and cataracts were seen as a common complication. Cataracts have variously been described in some experimental animals (Grant and Schuman, 1993). The drug uncouples oxidative phosphorylation, which might be expected to increase the lens consumption of oxygen, although this is not the case with incubated lenses in vitro (Kleifeld and Hockwin, 1956). Other mechanisms suggested include a reduction of lens glutathione, although this is not particularly specific and occurs in most cataract formations (Miyata, 1968). Both the anterior capsule and anterior and posterior cortices around the lens sutures were initially involved with progressing to a complete intumescent cataract (Harding and Crabbe, 1984).

Galactose can cause cataracts when given in high doses to experimental animals (Grant and Schuman, 1986). In humans with hereditary galactosemia and in macropods (kangaroos, wallabies, etc.), the enzymes galactose 1-phosphate-uridyltransferase and galactokinase are usually absent. Galactose and galactose-1-phosphate saturate the lens and are converted to galactitol, or dulcitol, which accumulates in lens cells. Cow's milk (high in lactose and galactose) will cause cataracts in these species. Accumulated sugars in the lens (as in diabetes) cause cataracts by exerting an osmotic effect, drawing water into the lens and causing hydropic degeneration. Additionally, protein synthesis and lens enzyme systems may be affected and contribute to cataract development (Harding and Crabbe, 1984). A similar type of sugar cataract is caused by **xylose** toxicity in weanling rats, with accumulation of sorbitol in the lens cells (van Heyningen, 1969). **Arabinose** produces cataracts similar to those caused by galactose and xylose (Grant and Schuman, 1993). **Alloxan** causes cataracts in rabbits and rats, and although it also causes diabetes mellitus, which could contribute to cataract development, it may have a direct antimitotic effect on the lens epithelial cells (Bernat and Bombicki, 1968; Patterson et al., 1965). Cataracts develop in rats within 2 weeks of a single injection of **streptozotocin,** which destroys pancreatic β-cells and causes diabetes (Von Sallmann and Grimes, 1971). Interestingly, cataract development in this case can be reduced by aldose reductase inhibitors, suggesting that the streptozotocin cataracts are secondary to the diabetes induced by the drug (Arison et al., 1967; Poulsom et al., 1982). Oral hypoglycemic drugs such as **carbutamide, tolbutamide,** and **chlorpropamide,** have induced cataracts in rats (Wright, 1963).

Chronic dosing with topical or systemic **corticosteroids** have, on several occasions, resulted in posterior subcapsular cataracts in humans (Black et al., 1960). The same does not always appear to occur in experimental animals (Grant and Schuman, 1993), although cataracts possibly induced by corticosteroids have been reported in adult rabbits and neonatal mice (Render and Carlton, 1991). Various mechanisms have been suggested for corticosteroid cataracts, including elevation of glucose in the plasma and aqueous, increased cation permeability, inhibition of glucose-6-phosphate dehydrogenase, inhibition of RNA synthesis, loss of lens adenosine triphosphate (ATP), and covalent binding of steroid to lens proteins. It is suggested that steroid cataract could have a multifactorial etiology (Harding and Crabbe, 1984). **Clomiphene,** used as a hormonal treatment, has produced cataracts in rats (Newberne et al., 1966).

Triparanol and **diazocholesterol** block the conversion of desmosterol to cholesterol by inhibiting the enzyme desmosterol reductase. Cataracts have been reported in various species, including man, dog, and rat. Affected lenses accumulate abnormally high concentrations of desmosterol, which presumably is associated with the changes of permeability and with sodium and water accumulation in the lens. Opacities are seen initially in the anterior and posterior subcapsular regions, followed by cortical clouding progressing to total opacification (Kirby, 1967; Mizuno et al., 1974).

Various drugs may cause cataracts by producing damaging free radicals in the eye. **Diquat** causes initially posterior subcapsular cataracts that progress to involve the nucleus and, later, the entire lens in the rat (Pirie et al., 1969). Glutathione concentrations are unaffected, but the production of diquat free radical might have a damaging effect on the lens by conversion to superoxide radicals (Stancliffe and Pirie, 1971). However, superoxide can usually be destroyed by several substances present in the lens (including glutathione and ascorbate) and therefore the concept of superoxide damage in diquat toxicity is still unresolved (Harding and Crabbe, 1984). **Hydrogen peroxide** has been found in high concentrations in the aqueous of humans with senile nuclear cataract. Since nuclear proteins become oxidized with aging, it has been suggested that increased concentrations of hydrogen peroxide might be etiologic in causing these aging changes (Spector and Garner, 1981). Hydrogen peroxide, which reduces lens superoxide dismutase, making the lens more prone to damage from free radicals formed in response to sunlight (UVL), might be involved in causing these changes. **Aminotriazole** causes cataracts in the rabbit, possibly by reducing lens catalase concentrations, and increasing local hydrogen peroxide concentrations (Bhuyan et al., 1973; Bhuyan and Bhuyan, 1978).

Miotic anticholinesterase drugs (usually used in man for glaucoma therapy), including **demecarium bromide** and **phospholine iodide,** have caused cataracts in man and monkeys (Axelsson, 1971; Kaufman et al., 1977). Cataracts in man begin as anterior subcapsular vacuoles and progress to involve the nucleus and posterior cortex and, ultimately, the entire lens. In vitro studies of rabbit lenses show a fall in potassium and a rise of sodium and water concentration in the lens (Michon and Kinoshita, 1968a,b). **Epinephrine** given in large doses causes transient lens opacities in rodents (Scullica et al., 1968), although these may be more related to a decrease in blinking, and corneal exposure with subsequent lens dehydration. Cataracts have similarly been produced in rodents with **opiates, phenelzine** combined with **serotonin** (Grant and Schuman, 1993; Fraunfelder and Burns, 1966).

Hygromycin B, an anthelminthic, has caused cataracts in sows when fed in the diet. Lesions are posterior subcapsular cataracts with lens fiber swelling, with cortical vacuolation and degeneration (Sanford and Dukes, 1979; Sanford et al., 1981; Creighton et al., 1982). **Disophenol,** when used in puppies, may cause transient lens opacities (Martin et al., 1972; Martin and Chambreau, 1982). **Rafoxanide** induces equatorial cataracts and papilledema in dogs (Rubin, 1974; Brown et al., 1971). Reversible lens opacities have been seen in dogs administered the systemic antihypertensive agents **diazoxide** (Schiavo et al., 1975) and **dichloroacetate** (Stacpoole et al., 1979).

Thallium, a heavy metal, causes cataracts in experimental animals. The metal is concentrated in lenses in vitro (Grant and Schuman, 1993).

Chlorphentermine is an amphiphilic catatonic drug that causes subcapsular lens opacities in rats by upsetting lipid metabolism (Drenckhahn and Lullmann-Rauch, 1977; Lullmann-Rauch, 1976).

Cyanate has caused posterior subcapsular cataracts in dogs and in humans treated for sickle-cell anemia (Kern et al., 1977; Nicholson et al., 1976). Raised aqueous concentrations of **urea** have been suggested as the cause of cataracts occasionally seen in uremic patients due to **ammonium cyanate** carbamylation of lens proteins (Harding and Crabbe, 1984).

Boron hydride disulfide causes cataracts in mice, possibly by inactivating **Na-adenosine triphosphatase** (ATPase) and reducing water pumping across the anterior lens epithelium, resulting in increased lens hydration (Fukui et al., 1977).

Selenium causes nuclear and later cortical cataracts in rats, possibly by depressing lens glutathione, catalase, and superoxide dismutase, which normally provide protection against free radical damage (Bhuyan et al., 1981a,b; Bunce and Hess, 1981). **Sulfaethoxy-pyridazine,** an antimicrobial drug, has caused cataracts in dogs and rats (Grant and Schuman, 1993).

Trinitrotoluene (TNT) causes equatorial cataracts in humans chronically exposed to its dust or vapor (Grant and Schuman, 1993).

Verapamil, a calcium blocker, has occasionally been reported to cause cataracts in dogs when given at toxic doses (Grant and Schuman, 1993).

The metal chelator **dithizone** causes equatorial cataracts in rats (Grant and Schuman, 1993) and may cause cataracts in dogs along with severe fundus pathology (Budinger, 1961; Delahunt et al., 1962). Cataracts may also occur with the chelators **deferoxamine** and **pyrithione** (Bruckner et al., 1967). Since these agents cause severe inflammatory changes elsewhere in the eye, the cataracts are likely to be secondary occurrences (Grant and Schuman, 1993).

Lens Deposits

Lamellated inclusions and vacuoles formed in the lens epithelium appear as lens opacities in the anterior and posterior cortex in rats fed amphiphilic cationic agents **chloroquine, chlorphentermine,** or **iprindole** (Drenckhahn and Lullmann-Rauch, 1977).

Deposits (presumably of the particular toxin) may occur beneath the anterior lens capsule with systemic toxicity from several **metals** and chronic use of **chlorpromazine** and, possibly, **thiothixene** (Grant and Schuman, 1993).

INTRAOCULAR PRESSURE AND GLAUCOMA

The intraocular pressure (IOP) is maintained within normal limits by an equal rate of secretion and ultrafiltration of aqueous from the ciliary processes and outflow of aqueous via the iridocorneal angle (comprising particularly the trabecular meshwork) and uveoscleral pathway (across the iris and ciliary body into the suprachoroidal space). Drugs may affect the production or drainage of aqueous by systemic peripheral or central effects on the cardiovascular system (for instance by increasing or lowering the intraarterial or intravenous pressure, which is directly reflected in alterations of IOP) or by affecting central control of IOP. Outflow from the anterior chamber via the trabecular meshwork is facilitated by contraction of the ciliary muscle. Drugs may reduce this effect.

Reduction in intraocular pressure is a desired effect of many topical and systemic drugs, including **carbonic anhydrase inhibitors, miotics** (parasympathomimetic drugs), **adrenergics, β-blockers,** and **osmotic agents.** Since these are used clinically in the treatment of glaucoma in man and animals, these drugs rarely lower intraocular pressure to such an extent that it affects ocular function or results in ocular pathology. For this reason, lowering of intraocular pressure is not considered a toxic reaction in the eye. Numerous drugs have the potential to reduce IOP and are listed in Grant and Schuman (1993) and Fraunfelder and Grove (1996).

Elevation of IOP is, however, a significant toxic effect of some drugs that may be used in clinical therapy and is therefore a toxic reaction. Glaucoma may arise as a primary disease or secondary to other ocular pathology such as uveitis, lens luxation, neoplasia, or drug effects in the eye. Obviously there may be interaction between these etiologies—for instance a drug that causes breakdown of the blood–aqueous barrier (BAB), cellular infiltrate into the eye, could result in reduced aqueous outflow due to inflammatory debris clogging the trabecular meshwork and thus cause a secondary rise of IOP. In rabbits, use of drugs that cause disruption of the blood–aqueous barrier **(nitrogen mustard, acids, alkalis)** may cause a rise of IOP associated with disruption of the BAB and changes in the blood flow within the eye. Conversely, in some situations, drugs used to treat uveitis might potentiate a rise in IOP; this occurs in man with atropine. In dogs with acute uveitis, inflammatory debris may obstruct the trabecular meshwork and elevate IOP. Use of a nonsteroidal anti-inflammatory drug, **flurbiprofen,** reduces prostaglandin (PG) production in the eye and further elevates IOP (Millichamp and Dziezyc, 1991). This probably occurs because PGs act as a safety valve in ocular inflammation to increase uveoscleral outflow to compensate for any reduction in iridocorneal outflow.

Parasympatholytic drugs such as **atropine, homatropine, scopolamine, cyclopentolate,** and **tropicamide** paralyze the ciliary muscle and may in some species (certainly man, dog, cat, and horse) increase IOP. Elevated IOP occurs in humans with open-angle glaucoma and can precipitate angle closure in individuals with narrow angles (Mandelkorn and Zimmerman, 1989). Several mechanisms may be involved, including the formation of peripheral anterior synechiae in noninflamed eyes as the base of the iris is dilated into the angle region, and reduced outflow through the ciliary muscle due to paralysis of the ciliary muscle.

Corticosteroids may cause glaucoma in man when used either systemically or topically. A genetic predisposition is seen in man in sensitivity to corticosteroid-induced glaucoma (Armaly, 1967). Corticosteroids have been suggested as affecting intraocular pressure by various mechanisms. The most frequently cited cause of glaucoma is that corticosteroids increase the amounts of glycosaminoglycans (GAG) in the trabecular meshwork possibly by limiting degradation of GAG by lysosomal enzymes. Lysosome membranes are stabilized by corticosteroids. Other possible pathogenetic mechanisms include corticosteroid reduction of phagocytosis by the trabecular meshwork and accumulation of debris (cells) in the meshwork, which blocks flow (Berman, 1991; Bill, 1975). Corticosteroids have been shown in vitro to reduce prostaglandin production by trabecular meshwork cells. If PGs are acting to fine-tune IOP in the eye through the uveoscleral outflow pathway, a reduction of PG in the eye might cause reduced uveoscleral outflow and, thus, a rise in IOP (Weinreb et al., 1983).

In other species, it has been more difficult to demonstrate any effect of corticosteroids on IOP. In rabbits prolonged therapy with doses high enough to cause systemic toxicity do transiently elevate IOP (Grant and Schuman, 1993). In cats, IOP elevation has been reported with topically applied **dexamethasone** (Zhan et al., 1989). The tricyclic antidepressant **amitriptyline** has caused angle-closure glaucoma at high doses (Steele et al., 1967). The H_2-blockers **cimetidine** and **ranitidine** cause elevation of IOP when injected into the cerebral ventricles of rabbits, suggesting an action via the CNS regulatory mechanisms for IOP (Trzeciakowski, 1987).

Acetazolamide reduces intraocular pressure by reducing aqueous secretion, due to its action as a carbonic anhydrase inhibitor (CAI). Cases have been reported in man, however, where the IOP was increased, associated with swelling of the lens and transient myopia (Mandelkorn and Zimmerman, 1989). Despite the normal effect of the CAI-type drug in reducing IOP, swallowing of the anterior chamber induced by lens swelling might be a significant precipitating factor in narrow-angle glaucoma in man.

Several agents including the vasodilator **tolazoline** and sympathomimetics **epinephrine, ephedrine,** and **amphetamine** dilate the pupil and thus might potentiate angle-closure glaucoma in susceptible individuals. Subconjunctival injections of vasodilators are more likely to produce IOP increases than systemic administration (Fraunfelder and Grove, 1996; Grant and Schuman, 1993; Mandelkorn and Zimmerman, 1989).

Parasympathomimetic drugs such as **pilocarpine, carbachol,** and **demecarium,** although indicated for treating open-angle glaucoma, may cause dilatation of iridal vessels and swelling of the iris and ciliary body, and the increased curvature of the lens may displace the iris anteriorly, reducing the depth of the anterior chamber and narrowing the angle. In humans predisposed to narrow-angle glaucoma, this may precipitate angle closure. Additionally, the miotic pupil induced by these drugs may limit aqueous flow from the posterior to the anterior chamber and cause pupil block with iris bombe, thus further narrowing the angle (Grant and Schuman, 1993; Mandelkorn and Zimmerman, 1989).

Viscoelastic substances injected into the eye during intraocular surgery to protect the corneal endothelium and facilitate intraocular lens implantation have been associated with a significant rise in IOP after surgery in humans and dogs. Presumably these agents, which are viscous, interfere with aqueous outflow through the angle (Binkhorst, 1980). Several other examples of fine particulate matter causing elevation of the IOP have been cited (Grant and Schuman, 1993).

RETINA AND CHOROID

The retina is a multilayered structure that lines the posterior segment of the eye. During embryonic development, the optic cup, an evagination of neuroectoderm from the diencephalon, forms inner and outer layers. The cells of the inner layer undergo division and differentiation into the perikarya of the neural retina, whereas the outer layer becomes the retinal pigment epithelium (RPE). The neural retina (hereafter referred to as retina) and RPE become apposed, although a potential intraretinal or subretinal space remains as a site for retinal detachment later in life (Hewitt and Adler, 1989).

Ten layers of RPE and retina are recognized. The RPE is a single layer of cuboidal cells. The folded basal surface of each cell lies on Bruch's membrane, adjacent to the vascular choroid, which provides a blood supply to the outer retina. In some species (such as the guinea pig), most of the retinal nutrition comes from this source. The apical surface of each cell forms elongated processes that extend between the outer segments of the photoreceptors of the retina. The RPE is variably pigmented depending upon the species, the position in the retina, and, in some animals, the age.

The photoreceptors make up the outermost layer of the neural retina. Two main photoreceptor types are recognized—the rods and cones. The proportions of these cell types vary between species and at different geographic locations in the posterior segment. Rod outer segments (ROS) are tubular in shape. The plasma membrane encloses a stack of membrane-bound discs, each held separate from the next and the plasma membrane by a cytoskeletal array of filaments. Cone outer segments are generally shorter than those of rods, and have a more conical shape. The cone plasma membrane forms membranous lamellae by continuous infolding throughout the outer segment. The cytoplasm of the outer and inner segments is continuous through a connecting cilium.

An interphotoreceptor matrix (IPM) fills the potential subretinal space between the RPE cells, photoreceptor outer segments, and glia of the neurosensory retina. The IPM is biochemically composed of carbohydrates (glycosaminoglycans and sialic acid–containing molecules) mostly linked to glycoproteins. The IPM functions may include transfer of retinoids between the photoreceptors and RPE (via the interphotoreceptor retinol-binding protein [IBRP]), maintenance of retinal attachment to the RPE, and support of retinal development and maturation via trophic factors in the IPM (Hewitt and Adler, 1989).

The inner segments of the photoreceptors are highly metabolically active, containing numerous mitochondria. The perikarya of the photoreceptor cells lie in the outer nuclear layer, comprising from 5 to 12 nuclear layers in the peripheral and central retina, which again varies with species. Axons of the photoreceptors terminate in rod spherules and cone pedicles, which synapse with bipolar and horizontal cells in the outer plexiform layer (OPL) (Dowling, 1987).

Nuclei of the bipolar, horizontal, amacrine, and retinal glial (Müller) cells are located in the inner nuclear layer (INL).

The ganglion cell layer comprises mainly ganglion cells, of which as many as 23 different morphological types may occur in the cat retina. The ganglion cell processes project into the nerve fiber layer, the fibers of which radiate toward the optic nerve papilla and leave the eye through the lamina cribrosa of the sclera (Blanks, 1989).

The internal limiting membrane is formed by flat expansions of the Müller cells at the vitreal surface.

The blood supply to the retina comes from two sources. The choroidal circulation provides oxygen and other nutrients to the outer part of the retina, including the photoreceptors. The retinal pigment epithelium controls the flow of nutrients and metabolites into and out of the neurosensory retina. In man, the central artery of the retina forms the ophthalmic artery, which crosses the subarachnoid space and penetrates the optic nerve ventrally and enters the retina with the nerve. In dogs, approximately 20 retinal arteries branch from the short posterior ciliary arteries at the optic disc and supply blood to the inner retinal layers. Choroidal vessels are fenestrated and therefore contribute little to the blood–retinal barrier. Retinal vessels are nonfenestrated and along with tight junctions between RPE cells provide a blood–retinal barrier to limit the size of molecules that can gain access to the neurosensory retina (Samuelson, 1999).

The choroid in several domestic species is modified anteriorly by the presence of a tapetum lucidum. This is cellular in carnivores (cat, dog, ferret) and fibrous in herbivores (cattle, horse). The tapetum as seen ophthalmoscopically varies in color and surface area depending upon the species, the breed or strain, age, and extent of pigmentation elsewhere in the skin and eye. In carnivores, the tapetal cells are packed with elongated rods of modified melanin granules and vary in the concentrations of trace elements or other constituents. The presence of a tapetum and its interspecies variations may affect the response of the retina in tapetal species to various toxins (Samuelson, 1999).

Toxicity may occur at various sites in the retina and choroid. Drugs that affect the cardiovascular system elsewhere in the body may affect the retinal or choroidal circulations. The retinal pigment epithelium may be the primary site of a toxin's actions, possibly determined by the presence or absence of pigment in this layer to which the toxin may bind and become concentrated. Within the retina itself, the photoreceptors, ganglion cells or other neurons, synaptic junctions, or glial cells may be the primary targets of toxins.

Tapetal Color Change and Choroidal Edema

Changes in the appearance or color of the tapetum have been described in dogs due to either the action of systemic vasodilator or drugs with toxic effects in the tapetum itself, the retina, RPE, or underlying choroid. Many of the effects reflect choroidal edema, necrosis, or degeneration of the tapetum and choroid. **Vasodilating agents** produce reversible color changes along a horizontal meridian of the canine tapetum superior to the optic nerve, without histological abnormalities. This site corresponds to the position of the long posterior retinal arteries and may simply be an optical effect due to distortion of retinal and choroidal blood vessels (Rubin, 1974). **Trans-11-amino-10,11-dihydro-5-(3-dimethylaminopropyl)-5,10-epoxy-5-H-dibenzo[a,d]cycloheptene** causes reduced visual acuity and tapetal color reduction, apparently due to tapetal necrosis and resorption in the beagle (Rubin, 1974). Another compound has been described that causes pigmentation of the RPE in dogs over the normally nonpigmented tapetal area (Rubin, 1974). **Ethambutol** and other **ethylenediamenes** also discolor the tapetum of dogs and possibly cats, causing a fluffy-white appearance (Rubin, 1974). The changes, which are reversible after discontinuing drug treatment, may be due to altered refraction by the tapetal cell rodlets, which lose osmophilia and longitudinal orientation in the cell and become swollen. The color changes may reflect a loss in zinc content of the tapetal cells (Grant and Schuman, 1993; Vogul and Kaiser, 1963). Tapetal discoloration also occurs with the zinc chelator **diphenylthiocarbazone (dithizone)** toxicity in dogs due to retinal, choroidal, and tapetal edema associated with necrosis and degeneration of the choroid and tapetum (Budinger, 1961; Delahunt et al., 1962; Weitzel and Strecker, 1954). Another chelating agent, **pyrithione,** also causes tapetal necrosis and choroidal, tapetal, and retinal edema (Delahunt et al., 1962; Moe et al., 1960; Snyder et al., 1965). It would be reasonable to assume that the tapetal damage from these drugs in dogs is due to zinc chelation, since that metal occurs in high concentration in the tapetal cells. However, both **pyrithione** and **zinc pyridinethione** (which does not cause chelation and has a high zinc concentration) also cause severe tapetal edema, degeneration, retinal edema, and detachment in dogs and tapetal atrophy in cats (Cloyd and Wyman, 1978). These changes seem specific for species with a tapetum since no retinal changes are seen in primates, rats, or rabbits, or in beagles with an inherited absence of a tapetum (Grant and Schuman, 1993). Additionally, **ethambutol,** which is also a chelating agent, causes far less severe effects in tapetal species. It has been suggested that some of the severe toxic effects on the tapetum of agents such as zinc pyrithione and dithizone may be partly due to zinc chelation (like ethambutol effects) and partly due to reaction with sulfydryl groups necessary for tapetal metabolic processes (Cloyd and Wyman, 1978).

Retinal Edema

Retinal edema may arise from breakdown of the blood–retinal barrier (BRB) or from edema in the optic nerve. This comprises the tight junctions between adjacent endothelial cells of retinal blood vessels and between retinal pigment epithelial cells (the choroidal vessels are fenestrated and thus are not a barrier to quite large molecules). These two barriers are, respectively, the inner and outer blood retinal barriers. Disruption of either may result in protein and water loss into the retinal extracellular space, seen clinically as retinal edema. In man and other primates with a macula, the latter is often the site of edema (macular edema), especially in the outer plexiform or inner nuclear layers. In some instances, the edema may be seen as clear cystic spaces in the macula (cystoid macular edema) (Jampol, 1989).

Naphthalene causes edema of the retina in rabbits. Small doses cause deposition of calcium oxalate crystals in the retina and vitreous. Larger doses produce the appearance of small circular white lesions, initially in the periphery of the fundus. The edema eventually causes splitting of the retinal layers and detachment above and below the medullary rays (Rubin, 1974; Pirie, 1968; Adams, 1930).

Intracarotid injections of **triaziquone (Treminon)** in rabbits, used to achieve high ocular concentrations, will cause initial retinal edema either in sharply delineated spots or diffuse cloudiness throughout the fundus, and later retinal degeneration and pigment dispersion (Apponi et al., 1964).

Dithizone, a metal chelator, causes retinal edema in rabbits and dogs. Edema in dogs occurs in the retina and tapetum. The changes in the rabbit fundus are less than in the dog, which may in part be due to the lower concentration of zinc in the tapetum of the rabbit (Budinger, 1961; Delahunt et al., 1962; Weitzel and Strecker, 1954; Butturini et al., 1953; Babel and Ziv, 1957).

Fluoride has been reported to cause retinal edema when given intravenously to rabbits (Sorsby and Harding, 1960, 1966). This does not appear to be a significant problem in humans receiving high doses of fluoride for osteoporosis (Grant and Schuman, 1993).

Glutamate causes massive retinal edema in neonatal mice until 10 days after birth associated with damage to ganglion cells and cells in the inner nuclear layer (Cohen, 1967; Olney, 1969).

Sheep and cattle grazing *Helichrysum argyrosphaerum* may develop retinal edema associated with optic nerve edema and hemorrhage, photoreceptor degeneration, and blindness (Basson and Kellerman, 1975).

Iminodipropionitrile causes various ocular lesions in different species. In rats, systemic administration causes retinal edema associated with endothelial proliferation and microaneurysm formation in retinal vessels (Paterson, 1968; Selye, 1957; Wang and Heath, 1968).

Methanol causes nerve fiber layer edema in humans, monkeys, and primates associated with the major toxic action of methanol in the eye—papilledema (Potts et al., 1955; Gilger et al., 1956, 1959).

Iodopyracet, a radiopaque contrast medium, has occasionally caused retinal edema in humans after intracarotid injection (Walsh and Hoyt, 1969). Retinal or macular edema is a reported side effect of several radiographic contrast media.

Retinal edema may occur after intravitreal injection of various substances, including **streptomycin** (Gardiner and Michaelson, 1948).

Macular and retinal edema may occur in cases of severe **quinine** toxicity in humans (Brinton et al., 1980). Cystoid macula edema (CME) may develop in aphakic eyes. It is suggested that surgical inflammation involves production of prostaglandins, which disrupt the perifoveal capillary endothelial cells, and breakdown of the perifoveal BRB. This may be exacerbated by free radicals released in the eye in response to ultraviolet light reaching the macula in the absence of the lens (Jampol, 1989). Epinephrine use for glaucoma has been associated with aphakic CME, possibly by causing prostaglandin production (Thomas et al., 1978). Transient CME occurs in humans treated with nicotinic acid used to reduce serum lipid levels (Gass, 1973). The antiestrogen, **tamoxifen,** used to treat breast cancer has caused CME with prolonged high doses (Kaiser-Kupfer and Lippman, 1978).

Retinal and macular edema has also been described as a side effect of many drugs, including carbonic anhydrase inhibitors, corticosteroids, tranquilizers, diuretics, and amebicides (Fraunfelder and Grove, 1996).

Retinal Detachment

The normal retina adheres to the apical processes of the retinal pigment epithelium due to various adhesive forces, mechanical properties of the photoreceptor outer segments, and the presence of an interphotoreceptor matrix in the subretinal space (Marmor, 1989). The majority of retinal detachments in man arise from peripheral retinal tearing and vitreous flow into the subretinal space (rhegmatogenous detachments). Detachments may also arise from traction of fibrous strands in the vitreous, or serous exudate from the retina or choroid associated with disruption of the blood–retinal barriers, which enters the subretinal space pushing the retina from the underlying pigment epithelium. Most retinal detachments caused by toxins in animals are exudative. Such detachments may be seen with several of the agents described as causing retinal or choroidal edema or tapetal changes.

Retinal detachment associated with retinal folds and subretinal transudate is seen in cats poisoned with **ethylene glycol** (antifreeze) (Barclay and Riis, 1979). **Iodate** causes toxic effects on the RPE and disrupts the BRB, which may present as serous detachment in various experimental animals and man (Grant and Schuman, 1993). Serous retinal detachments have been rarely reported associated with several systemic drugs in man, including **corticosteroids** and **penicillamine** (Fraunfelder and Grove, 1996). **Dithizone** may cause bullous retinal detachments in dogs (Delahunt et al., 1962).

Topical use of various miotics for glaucoma, including **pilocarpine, demecarium bromide,** and **echothiophate,** has been suggested as a cause of retinal detachment, and although circumstantial evidence suggests that this may be the case, examination of available evidence does not confirm the hypothesis that the occurrence of detachments is more than coincidental (Havener, 1983; Beasley and Fraunfelder, 1979).

Premature newborn humans and experimental animals exposed to high **oxygen** concentrations during late stages of retinal development respond with initial cessation of peripheral retinal vascularization, followed by the formation of peripheral retinal neovascularization and fibrotic bands in the vitreous. Retinal detachment occurs associated with traction of fibrotic bands on the peripheral retina and subretinal exudate formation (Garner et al., 1975; Foos, 1985). Oxygen toxicity (pure oxygen) in adult dogs has appeared as choroidal and retinal exudative detachment (Beeler et al., 1964).

Retinal Hemorrhage

Retinal hemorrhage is a commonly reported feature of retinal toxicosis in man, less so in animals. It has been suggested that this is because humans more frequently undergo ocular examination (Grant and Schuman, 1993), although it could also reflect the greater incidence of retinovascular disease in man (and thus some peculiarities of the human retinal vasculature) as compared with domestic or laboratory species in which it is rarely seen. Hemorrhage may result from toxin-induced retinal vasculitis, plasma hyperviscosity, hypertension, neovascularization, or coagulopathies.

Dicumarol, warfarin, and other anticoagulant drugs may occasionally cause retinal hemorrhage by reducing blood clotting mechanisms (Grant and Schuman, 1993). **Viper** and **rattlesnake** bites have caused retinal hemorrhages (Guttman-Friedmann, 1956; McLane, 1943). These venoms contain anticoagulant factors (Mebs, 1978). Retinal hemorrhage has occasionally been reported in animals administered **alloxan** to induce diabetes mellitus. Changes at most are comparable to the background retinopathy described in man without vascular proliferative changes (Grant and Schuman, 1993). **Carbon disulfide** is a volatile liquid that may cause formation of retinal microaneurysms and hemorrhage without retinal neovascularization (Hotta and Goto, 1970). **Chloramphenicol** administration in children has resulted in hemorrhage of the optic papilla associated with optic neuritis (Kittell and Cornelius, 1969). Plasma hyperviscosity induced by intravenous **dextrans** in monkeys has caused retinal hemorrhages (Maurolf and Mesher, 1973).

Dithizone, pyrithione, and **zinc pyrithione** cause retinal hemorrhage in dogs associated with severe exudative changes in the posterior segment and choroidal degeneration (Budinger, 1961; Delahunt et al., 1962; Cloyd and Wyman, 1978).

Retinal hemorrhages in the retinal nerve fiber layer are seen in some aphakic patients with **epinephrine**-induced cystoid macular edema (Kolker and Becker, 1968). **Systemic lead** or **phosphorus** toxicity may result in retinal hemorrhages, either associated with optic neuritis or due to vasculitis, sclerosis, or degeneration of retinal vessels (Grant and Schuman, 1993; Lobeck, 1936). Occasional case reports of retinal hemorrhage have been described in humans or animals administered **aspirin, benzene, dapsone, diquat, ethambutol, hexachlorophene, methyl bromide,** or **radiopaque x-ray media** (Grant and Schuman, 1993).

Retinal Vessel Abnormalities

Toxins may cause various changes in retinal blood vessels, most notably narrowing, which may occur acutely due to undefined mechanisms, or occur secondary to retinal or optic atrophy due to reduced demand in the degenerate tissue for nutrients. This appears to be the reason for retinal vessels narrowing with a considerable number of toxins (see retinal degeneration). **Quinine** and some of its derivatives cause acute narrowing of retinal arterioles. These changes occur later than the acute and reversible blindness that occurs with quinine toxicity and thus probably do not contrast to the loss of visual acuity (Brinton et al., 1980). **Ergotamine** has also been associated with visual deficits and retinal arteriole narrowing in humans that persisted after other funduscopic and visual signs improved (Mindel et al., 1981). **Oxygen** causes retinal vasoconstriction in adult humans (Anderson, 1968). Various anesthetic agents, including **barbiturates,** also cause retinal vasoconstriction (Fraunfelder and Grove, 1996).

Occlusion of central retinal arteries or veins has been described in many reports of women taking **oral contraceptives,** although as pointed out by Grant and Schuman (1993) there is no evidence that vascular occlusions occurred more frequently in these patients than the general population (Grant and Schuman, 1993; Swartz, 1989). Thrombosis may occur in retinal vessels in humans treated with **phenylpropanolamine hydrochloride** (Gilmer et al., 1986).

Carbon dioxide, amyl nitrate, and **hypoxia** cause vasodilation of retinal blood vessels.

Engorgement of retinal vessels may be seen in **methanol toxicosis** (Grant and Schuman, 1993).

Retinal Pigment Epithelium

The retinal pigment epithelium (RPE) serves an important function both in providing a means for nutrition and waste removal (phagocytosis of the photoreceptor outer segments) in the outer layers of the retina. It also forms an integral part of the outer blood–retinal barrier. Toxins that damage the RPE often have functional and morphological effects on the neural retina. Several groups of compounds have been found to have toxic effects that may involve the RPE, most notably the **quinolines** and **phenothiazines** (Zinn and Marmor, 1979). Changes in the RPE are clinically manifest as pigmentary retinopathy with either a decrease or increase of pigmentation.

Primary toxic effects on the RPE appearing as RPE degeneration with secondary effects on the neural retinal have been reported with several agents. **Sodium iodate** given intravenously causes selective damage to the RPE with swelling of the cells, with later degeneration of the photoreceptors and pigment migration and proliferation (Noell, 1951, 1953; Nilsson et al., 1977). Electrophysiological data in sheep demonstrate that the earliest functional changes are in the RPE (Nilsson et al., 1977). **Sodium azide** does not specifically damage the RPE cells, although it does change the standing potential across the retina (attributable to RPE) (Noell, 1952). This effect can be abolished by sodium iodate (Graymore, 1970). **Aminophenoxyalkanes** cause retinal degeneration in several species (**aminophenoxyalkanes** in cats and rabbits [Ashton, 1957; Sorsby and Nakajima, 1958], **diaminodiphenoxy(heptane)** in monkeys, cats, and dogs [Ashton, 1957; Edge et al., 1956; Orzalesi et al., 1967], and **diaminodiphenoxyheptane** in humans [Zinn and Marmor, 1979]). These appear clinically as pigmentary retinopathies. The RPE cells become swollen and proliferate, causing retinal distortion and then photoreceptor outer segment loss. RPE over the tapetal fundus undergoes reactionary pigmentation. **Urethane** damages the RPE in rats possibly by effects on RPE mitochondria (Bellhorn et al., 1973; Amemiya, 1968). **Oxalate** metabolized from **methoxyflurane** results in deposition of oxalate crystals in the RPE (Bullock et al., 1974). The RPE atrophies or undergoes peripheral proliferation and hyperpigmentation in response to intravitreal iron damage to retinal photoreceptors (Barber et al., 1971). **Systemic lead** toxicity in rabbits results in RPE cell swelling due to accumulation of phagosomes and lipofuscin (Brown, 1975). *N*-**Methyl-*N*-nitrosourea** causes swelling of RPE cells with pigment dispersion and later degeneration of photoreceptors, seen clinically as a pigmentary retinopathy in hamsters (Herrold, 1967).

   Chloroquine in high doses causes retinopathy in man. The main lesion appears to be in the photoreceptors and ganglion cells (Abraham and Hendy, 1970; Ramsey and Fine, 1972; Rosenthal et al., 1978). The drug is concentrated in melanin-containing RPE cells, which may provide a reservoir for release of the drug into and toxic effects on the retinal neurons (Bernstein et al., 1963). RPE changes consist of variable depigmentation and hyperpigmentation (macular "bull's-eye" lesion) (Zinn and Marmor, 1979), hyperplasia, and migration of pigment into the retina (Berstein and Ginsberg, 1964). In other species, similar pigmentary changes occur in RPE cells (Rubin, 1974). **Amopyroquin** causes pigment proliferation from the RPE in beagles (Kurtz et al., 1967). **Hydroxychloroquine** and **diiodohydroxyquin** have similar effects on the RPE (Zinn and Marmor, 1979). **Quinine** causes blindness and changes in the electroretinogram (ERG) c-wave and electrooculogram (EOG) during the acute phases of toxicity, which suggests that the RPE may be primarily affected (Hommer, 1968; Cibis et al., 1973).

   Phenothiazines are also concentrated in RPE melanin and persist in RPE cells for long periods of time (Ullberg et al., 1970). Overdosage with **thioridazine** causes a pigmentary retinopathy with visual loss in man. Irreversible black pigmentary stippling is seen throughout the posterior fundus, which may progress to RPE atrophy and patchy depigmentation (Zinn and Marmor, 1979; Davidorf, 1973). **Piperidylchlorophenothiazine** selectively damages rods, resulting in excessive accumulation of outer segment lamellar debris and inclusions in the RPE, which appears as a pigmentary retinopathy in humans and cats (Goar and Fletcher, 1956; Burian and Fletcher, 1958; Cerletti and Meier-Ruge, 1968). **Dithizone** toxicity in dogs may result in RPE hypertrophy, which gives the tapetum a granular appearance (Rubin, 1974). **Sparsomycin** causes primary clumping of RPE pigment with degeneration of adjacent photoreceptors (McFarlane et al., 1966). **Intravitreal cephaloridine** causes photoreceptor degeneration and degeneration of the RPE (Vlchek and Peyman, 1975). **Amphiphilic cationic compounds** cause the formation of membrane-bound crystalloid or lamellar inclusions in the RPE and ganglion cells in rats (Drenckhahn and Lullmann-Rauch, 1978). **Fenthione** causes retinal degeneration in rats associated with swelling and disorganization of RPE cells (Imai et al., 1983).

Photoreceptor Degeneration

Degeneration of the retinal rods and cones may occur from primary action of a toxin on the cells, damage to the RPE or choroid and outer blood–retinal barrier with secondary photoreceptor degeneration, or following extensive damage and degeneration in the inner retinal layers.

Piperidylchlorophenothiazine (NP-207) causes retinal toxicity in man and cats although not in several other species (Grant and Schuman, 1993). The drug accumulates in the melanin of the choroid. In man, NP-207 affects dim light vision and later visual acuity (Verrey, 1956). Its effects may be partially reversible. Electrophysiological studies identify the site of toxicity as the photoreceptor layer (Bornschein et al., 1974). The ophthalmoscopic appearance in the cat is of a pigmentary retinopathy that develops after 4 to 6 weeks of treatment, spreading as a horizontal band from the area centralis (Rubin, 1974). Pigmentary changes deep in the retina also occur in man. In both species, the drug causes disruption of the rod outer segments and may activate photoreceptor shedding. The excess membranous lipid material engulfed by the RPE produces the clinical appearance of pigmentation. NP-207 acts on the ellipsoids of the rods and probably inhibits oxidative phosphorylation by inhibiting flavine nucleotides (Cerletti and Meier-Ruge, 1968; Meier-Ruge and Cerletti, 1966; Meier-Ruge et al., 1966).

Ammeline, a herbicide, causes degeneration of photoreceptors secondary to histological degeneration of the RPE. **Aramite,** a plant pesticide, causes electroretinographic signs of photoreceptor damage in mice. **Benzoic acid** causes exudative retinal detachment and degeneration of rods and cones (Grant and Schuman, 1993).

"Bright blindness" is seen in sheep fed bracken fern (*Pteridium aquilinum*). Tapetal hyperreflectivity is seen due to thinning of the overlying retina. Degeneration initially affects the rods and cones, the outer segments of which become fragmented and vesicular, and later the nuclear layers (Barnett and Watson, 1970; Barnett et al., 1972). The plant *Stypandra imbricata* or blindgrass, causes degeneration of photoreceptors and optic neuritis in sheep that graze it. Similar lesions are seen in rats fed blindgrass (Huxtable et al., 1980; Main et al., 1981).

Several cardiac glycosides, including **digitalis** and **digoxin,** have been shown to have toxic effects in the eye. The most commonly reported are central and paracentral scotomas, reduced visual acuity, and color vision deficits. These are reversible when the drug is discontinued and may be associated with a reduction of the ERG amplitude. This suggests that the toxic effects are probably at the level of the outer retina. No histological degeneration of the photoreceptors has been reported (Grant and Schuman, 1993).

Colchicine, an antimitotic agent, causes photoreceptor degeneration and blocks axonal transport in rats when administered intravitreally.

Ethylenimine, an alkylating agent and a related compound, **4,4′-diamino-diphenylmethane,** causes specific atrophy of rods and cones in cats, but not in man or other species tested (von Canstatt et al., 1966).

Sodium fluorescein and **hematoporphyrin** have been reported to act as photosensitizing agents in albino mice and pigmented rabbits, causing photoreceptor damage (Grant and Schuman, 1993).

Vitamin A causes retinal damage in rats, with signs of mitochondrial damage evident both in the photoreceptors and RPE (Amemiya, 1967).

Sodium fluoride causes outer segment disorganization and loss following changes in the RPE in rabbits given high doses of the drug intravenously (Sorsby and Harding, 1960; Vanysek et al., 1969).

Hexachlorophene causes photoreceptor outer segment disorganization and degeneration, and optic atrophy and retinal hemorrhage. Photoreceptor degeneration appears to be distinct from changes in the optic nerve and ganglion cells (Rose et al., 1981).

Sodium iodate causes photoreceptor degeneration secondary to damage to the RPE and blood–retinal barrier (Nilsson et al., 1977).

Iodoacetate causes rapid and selective toxicity on the photoreceptors when administered by intravenous or intraarterial injection. Rods are more sensitive to iodoacetate than cones. Within a few hours of injection, swelling of mitochondria in the rod inner segments is seen, with rapid progression of photoreceptor and RPE disorganization and degeneration (Grignolo, 1969; Reading and Sorsby, 1966). **Bromoacetate** causes a similar retinal degeneration in rabbits (Lucas et al., 1957).

N-Methyl-N-nitrosourea, a carcinogenic agent, causes retinal degeneration (RPE and photoreceptors) in the hamster when given intravenously (Herrold, 1967).

Quinine appears to have several effects in the retina at the level of the photoreceptors, RPE, ganglion cells, and optic nerve fibers. In reviewing the literature, Grant and Schuman (1993) concluded that electrophysiological data points to early toxicity in the RPE and photoreceptors with later changes in the optic nerve, ganglion cells, and inner retinal vasculature.

Quinoline and its derivatives have caused retinal degeneration and optic nerve atrophy in several species (Fraunfelder and Grove, 1996; Grant and Schuman, 1993).

Sodium azide causes changes in the ERG that point to the RPE as the primary site of damage. Photoreceptors can be shown to undergo degeneration, which is probably secondary to RPE degeneration (Hansson, 1966).

Sucrose causes specific degeneration of the rods and cones that does not affect the RPE or inner retinal neurons. Retinal vascular changes are reminiscent of background retinopathy in man (Cohen et al., 1972).

Urethane administered parenterally to pigmented rats causes photoreceptor degeneration and growth of new vessels into the retinal pigment epithelium (Bellhorn et al., 1973).

Guanosine 3′,5′-cyclic monophosphate (cyclic GMP) has been shown to be toxic to photoreceptors, causing disorganization and breakup of outer segments in retinas in vitro (Ulshafer et al., 1980). This is believed to be involved in the pathogenesis of certain inherited photoreceptor degenerations in rodents, dogs, and cats (Aguirre et al., 1982).

Tunicamycin causes photoreceptor-specific degeneration by suppressing the renewal mechanisms of the photoreceptor outer segments (Fliesler et al., 1984).

Vincristine, an antineoplastic agent, causes photoreceptor inner segment degeneration when injected into the vitreous in rats (Hansson, 1972), whereas in a human who became night blind after vincristine therapy, the normal a-wave and abnormally small b-wave suggested that the drug might cause a neurotransmission defect in the outer plexiform layer (Ripps et al., 1984).

Vitamin A inhibits the alcohol dehydrogenase systems of the photoreceptors and RPE with disruption of mitochondrial membranes in the photoreceptor inner segments (Amemiya, 1967).

Ganglion Cells and Inner Retina

Ganglion cells can be damaged by toxins that exert their effects directly on these proximal retinal neurons, through damage to the optic nerve into which they project and by toxic effects on the other retinal neurons and glia or retinal pigment epithelium. In many cases, it is difficult to separate these actions and determine that the ganglion cell is the primary target of a toxin. Other cells in the inner retina (bipolar, horizontal, or amacrine cells) may be affected, particularly by neurotransmitter-like substances.

Doxorubicin causes neurofilament accumulation in the cell body and central axon of ganglion cells and then loss of ganglion cells in the rat retina possibly by inhibiting slow axoplasmic flow, causing axon swelling and death (Parhad et al., 1984).

Arsanilic acid causes degeneration of the ganglion cells in humans (Grant and Schuman, 1993). In pigs, this compound causes blindness due to optic nerve atrophy without any evident retinal lesions (Witzel et al., 1976). Ducks fed *Ammi majus* seeds develop vacuolation and degeneration of the ganglion cells (Barishak et al., 1976). *Dryopteris felix mas* toxicity causes blindness in cattle that feed upon the plant. Histology reveals the main lesion to be ganglion cell and optic nerve fiber degeneration (Rosen et al., 1970). Similar findings occur in **chloramphenicol** toxicity causing optic atrophy and ganglion cell loss (Kittell and Cornelius, 1969; Cogan et al., 1973). **Carbon dioxide** toxicity in man may cause degeneration of ganglion cells and associated blindness. Dogs are very sensitive to the effects of quinine and cinchona derivatives. The drug selectively causes degeneration of retinal ganglion cells and subsequent optic atrophy. Ophthalmoscopically, cinchona toxicity causes retinal arteriolar vasoconstriction and pallor of the optic disc (Rubin, 1974).

Carbon disulfide appears to cause primary damage to the ganglion cells with associated retrobulbar optic neuritis (Grant and Schuman, 1993). In rats, it causes acute ganglion cell degeneration (Ide, 1958).

L-**Cysteine** is selectively toxic to ganglion cells and amacrine cells in the rat retina (Pederson and Karlsen, 1980; Karlsen and Pederson, 1982).

Glutamate is a neurotransmitter in the retina. At toxic doses, it causes very specific degeneration of ganglion cells in rat neonates with destruction of the inner retinal layers by 17 days of age. The glial cells and inner nuclear layer later degenerate (Lucas et al., 1957; Sisk and Kuwabara, 1985).

Trimethyltin causes most degeneration in the inner retinal layers with pyknosis seen in the inner and outer nuclear layers and swelling of the photoreceptor inner segments (Bouldin et al., 1984).

Locoweed (*Astragalus mollissimus*) causes vacuolation of ganglion and bipolar cells in cattle and sheep (Van Kampen and James, 1972) by suppressing the enzyme α-mannosidase. Oligosaccharides accumulate in and affect the function of ganglion cells and neurons in the central nervous system (CNS) (Dorling et al., 1978).

Methanol poisoning in man presents typically with blindness due to optic atrophy. In acute cases, optic nerve edema is seen. Histologically, in advanced cases, optic and ganglion cell atrophy is detected, although these are not seen in acute cases. In monkeys, the earliest signs of methanol toxicity are optic nerve edema. Ganglion cell degeneration occurs secondary to restricted axoplasmic flow because of swollen optic nerve oligodendroglia (Grant and Schuman, 1993).

Quinine toxicity results in vacuolation of ganglion cells and associated optic atrophy (as well as outer retinal degeneration and later vascular attenuation) (Grant and Schuman, 1993).

Orthochromic granules are seen in the ganglion cells of rats treated with **chloroquine** apart from its toxic effects of the RPE and photoreceptors (Thompson, 1975).

As in other sites in the retina and cornea, **amphiphilic cationic compounds** may cause accumulation of lipids in ganglion cells (Drenckhahn and Lullmann-Rauch, 1978).

Kainic acid causes pyknosis of amacrine cells and edema in the inner plexiform layer possibly by causing persistent depolarization of the neurons (Lessell et al., 1980).

Retinal Lipidosis

Lipid deposits in the retina occur with **cationic amphiphilic drugs** such as **chlorphentermine, triparanol,** and **1-chloroamitriptyline** administered to rats. These cause no significant pathology and are only diagnosed by ultrastructural examination of the RPE, ganglion cells, Müller cells, and neurons of the inner nuclear layer (Lullmann et al., 1978; Lullmann-Rauch, 1991b). Retinal lipidosis occurs in several other species treated long-term with **chloroquine** (Lullmann-Rauch, 1991b).

OPTIC NERVE

The ganglion cell's central axons pass into the nerve fiber layer of the retina and converge to a point just below and medial to the posterior pole of the eye to form the optic nerve at the optic disc or papilla.

The optic nerve may be considered to consist of three portions: (a) ocular, the part seen within the eye and composed of retina, choroidal, and scleral portions; (b) orbital, which extends from the lamina cribrosa of the sclera to the optic foramen; and (c) intracranial, which passes from the optic foramen to the optic chiasm.

The optic nerve is formed by ganglion cell axons, glia (astrocytes and microglia), collagenous setae arising from the ensheathing pia mater, blood vessels, and in the retrobulbar part of the nerve myelin.

The site in the sclera where the nerve fibers leave the eye is the lamina cribrosa, a sieve-like arrangement of scleral collagen through which fascicles of nerve fibers and ensheathing glia pass.

In dogs, the entire optic nerve, extending up into the peripapillary area of the retina, may be myelinated. In man, cats, and horses, the nerve becomes myelinated after it exits through the lamina cribrosa.

The orbital and intracranial portions of the optic nerve are invested by the outer dura mater, subarachnoid, and pia mater.

The blood supply to the optic nerve is from the internal ophthalmic artery in domestic species, whereas the blood supply to the choroid and retina is derived from the external maxillary artery via the external ophthalmic artery and long and short posterior ciliary arteries. In primates, by contrast, both the anterior and posterior segment are supplied by the internal carotid artery via the internal ophthalmic artery. The central retinal artery in primates penetrates the dura mater and crosses the subarachnoid space to form the central retinal artery. In animals, the long posterior ciliary arteries, giving rise to cilioretinal arteries, pierce the globe around the periphery of the optic nerve.

Toxic influences on the nerve may be a reflection of processes occurring in the retina and particularly the ganglion cells or CNS disease. Specific toxic disorders may be caused by demyelinating drugs. The most common lesions caused by drug toxicity are optic neuritis (often loosely referred to as optic neuropathy) and (often as a consequence) optic atrophy. The optic nerve may become inflamed in association with chorioretinitis or meningoencephalitis and undergo atrophy secondary to retinal (or chorioretinal) degeneration.

Optic Neuritis, Neuropathy, and Atrophy

Optic neuritis may be seen within the eye or occur in any part of the nerve as far back as the chiasm. Lesions behind the eye are referred to as retrobulbar optic neuritis. In man, this involves, in particular, ganglion cell fibers from the papillomacular bundle. Optic neuritis may result in various disturbances of vision, although a central scotoma, complete loss of vision, and color deficiencies are commonly reported.

Hexachlorophene causes signs of intraocular or retrobulbar optic neuritis in man (Grant and Schuman, 1993). In rats, there is demyelination and degeneration of axons of the optic nerve and pathways, associated with severe lesions in the white matter of the brain. Optic nerve destruction precedes ganglion cell loss.

Arsanilic acid and its derivatives, including **acetarsone**, cause optic neuritis and atrophy in humans and pigs. The damage to the nerve causes sudden blindness (Witzel et al., 1976).

Poisoning with *Dryopteris felix mas*, the active ingredient of which is **felicin**, causes retrobulbar neuropathy in man, cattle, and dogs. In man, ophthalmoscopic signs of optic neuritis have been described progressing to optic atrophy. In dogs and rabbits, histologic evidence of ganglion cell death and axon degeneration is seen without signs of neuronal inflammation, although endovasculitis and perivasculitis are described (Grant and Schuman, 1993). In cattle, hemorrhages and edema are seen at the optic disc, and optic atrophy ensues. Histologically, axons persist in areas devoid of myelin, suggesting that medullary sheaths and oligodendrocytes may be more susceptible to the toxin due to their high lipid content (Rosen et al., 1970). In sheep and goats grazed on *Stypandra glauca* (blindgrass), similar optic neuropathy affects the intracranial and intracanalicular portions of the nerve (Main et al., 1981). *Stypandra imbricata* consumed by sheep, goats, or rats causes blindness due to vacuolation of optic nerve myelin, degeneration of the axons, and gliosis. The orbital and intracranial nerves in the rats were considerably swollen (Huxtable, 1980). *Helichrysum argyrosphaerum* causes almost identical lesions in cattle (Basson and Kellerman, 1975).

Carbon disulfide may cause retrobulbar neuritis and atrophy in man and, experimentally, in rabbits and mice ganglion cell, and optic nerve fiber degeneration is seen (Grant and Schuman, 1993).

Chronic **thallium** toxicosis causes optic neuritis and atrophy with relative sparing of the outer retina (Manschot, 1969).

Chloramphenicol has caused optic neuritis and atrophy in children treated for cystic fibrosis (Kittell and Cornelius, 1969). Atrophy of ganglion cells in the macular region and optic nerve fibers is seen histologically (Cogan et al., 1973).

Clioquinol, an antiamebic drug, exerts a very specific toxic effect on the long tracts of the spinal cord and the optic nerves. The disease has been seen in humans and reproduced in dogs and cats. Degeneration of the nerve may extend from the ganglion cells to the lateral geniculate synapse (Committee on Drugs, 1974; Tateishi et al., 1973; Worden et al., 1978; Krinke et al., 1979).

Cyanides in near-lethal doses will cause retrobulbar optic atrophy in rats, possibly associated with a paucity of capillaries at this site, which would render the tissue more susceptible to the acidotic effects of cyanide (Lessell, 1971; Lessell and Kuwabara, 1974).

Dinitrobenzene and related compounds are believed (based on the signs of central scotomas and color deficiencies) to cause retrobulbar neuropathy in man (Fraunfelder and Grove, 1996; Grant and Schuman, 1993).

Disulfiram has caused several cases of bilateral optic neuritis in humans (Grant and Schuman, 1993). **Penicillamine** has caused several cases of optic neuritis in man (Grant and Schuman, 1993). Several **monoamine oxidase inhibitors (isoniazid, octamoxin, pheniprazine)** have caused cases of optic neuritis and atrophy in man (Grant and Schuman, 1993; Levy and Michel-Ber, 1968). **Plasmocid,** an 8-

aminoquinoline, has caused optic neuritis and atrophy in humans, cats, dogs, and rabbits (Grant and Schuman, 1993).

Lead toxicity in man has caused optic neuropathy. Optic atrophy may result from increased intracranial pressure (affecting the pressure around the optic nerve via the subarachnoid) or as a direct toxic effect of lead on the optic nerve. Papilledema is a consistent feature due to raised intracranial pressure (Grant and Schuman, 1993).

The antitubercular drug **ethambutol,** specifically causes chiasmal retrobulbar neuritis in monkeys and rats (Schmidt and Schmidt, 1966; Lessell, 1976) and, based upon clinical findings, also in humans. In rabbits, the drug causes demyelination of the optic nerve (Matsuoka et al., 1972).

Ethylene glycol, when ingested, causes acidosis, and clinical signs suggestive of retrobulbar neuropathy have been described in man (Beasley and Buck, 1980; Berger and Ayyar, 1981).

Glutamate administered to rats or mice during the first 10 postnatal days causes specific ganglion cell degeneration that progresses to optic atrophy (Olney, 1969; Freedman and Potts, 1963; Hansson, 1970).

In **methanol** toxicity in humans, an early change appears to be demyelinization of the retrolaminar portion of the optic nerve (Sharpe et al., 1982). Later findings are of optic nerve atrophy and ganglion cell death. Clinically, patients initially have evidence of retinal and optic nerve edema, from which they may recover or progress to optic atrophy and blindness (Benton and Calhoun, 1953).

Optic Nerve Edema

In dogs, oral **rafoxanide** causes edema and vacuolation of the optic nerve and chiasm. Edema of the optic disc may be due to edema in the ocular and retrobulbar portion of the nerve as well as raised intracranial pressure due to edema of the white matter of the brain (Brown et al., 1971). **Hexachlorophene** which has been used to treat liver fluke causes transient edema of the optic nerve in sheep between 24 and 72 hr of administration, followed by irreversible loss of the pupillary light reflexes. Affected animals have hydrocephalus and optic nerve edema and vacuolation progressing to gliosis (Rubin, 1974).

Optic neuritis and atrophy have been described along with peripapillary edema, and retinal hemorrhages associated with impaired central vision in children treated for several weeks with high doses of **chloramphenicol.** Many cases proceed to optic atrophy. Degenerative changes are confined to ganglion cells and optic nerve.

EXTRAOCULAR MUSCLES

Paralysis of extraocular muscles (EOM) may arise in some toxicities. Signs include strabismus, restricted eye movement, diplopia, and, occasionally, complete external ophthalmoplegia. Toxicity may be due to local action of toxins at the muscle end plate or associated with central nervous system toxicity.

EOM weakness has been described with various animal venoms and plant toxins, including **elapid snake venoms,** *Amanita* **mushrooms, scorpion venom, botulinus toxin,** *d***-tubocurarine,** and *Gelsemium sempervirens.*

Partial paralysis of EOM may occur in humans some days after receiving **spinal anesthetics** (Walsh and Hoyt, 1969).

Primidone, an anticonvulsant, causes occasional cases of ophthalmoplegia, mainly in association with phenytoin (Grant and Schuman, 1993).

EOM paralysis usually assumed to be due to the CNS effects of the toxin have been reported with **carbamazepine, arsphenamine, barbiturates, lead** (which is unusual in that it may also cause local signs of pathology in the EOM), and **nalidixic acid** (Bockhardt et al., 1978).

Neurotoxicity with effects on EOM have been described with various antibiotics, including furmethanol and streptomycin.

Toxins that have caused total EOM paralysis include **amitriptyline.**

Pamaquine, an 8-aminoquinoline antimalarial, has caused damage to the EOM nuclei in dogs and possible sympathetic effects that appear as divergent strabismus, mild enophthalmos, and miosis (Schmidt and Schmidt, 1948). **Plasmocid,** another 8-aminoquinoline antimalarial, causes selective injury to the third, fourth, and sixth nerve nuclei, thus affecting extraocular muscle function (Grant and Schuman, 1993).

Thallium poisoning causes a polyneuropathy that presents with strabismus, ptosis, and paralysis of the extraocular muscles. Degeneration of nerve fibers of the extraocular muscles has been reported (Cavanagh et al., 1974).

Trichloroethylene causes neuritis affecting cranial nerves resulting in EOM palsy (Buxton and Hayward, 1967; Feldman et al., 1970). Grant and Schuman (1993) points out that this toxicity is probably associated with decomposition products of trichloroethylene (especially dichloracetylene), which might be the toxic principle.

Vincristine can cause a neuropathy that may involve nerves innervating EOM, causing EOM paralysis (Albert et al., 1967).

Nystagmus has occurred with several toxins. The site of action is usually not the eye but the CNS (Fraunfelder and Grove, 1996; Grant and Schuman, 1993).

ORBIT

The most commonly reported toxic orbital abnormality is exophthalmos (Fraunfelder and Grove, 1996; Grant and Schuman, 1993). This has been reported commonly as a side effect of various **corticosteroids** in man (Slansky et al., 1967; Hiroz et al., 1981).

Lithium, used as an anti-manic depressive therapy in man, causes thyroid dysfunction and an associated exophthalmos (Segal et al., 1973). **Methyl cyanide** injected into rabbits causes thyroid hyperplasia and exophthalmos (Marine et al., 1933).

Vitamin A toxicity has caused exophthalmos in dogs and guinea pigs when administered in high doses. In the guinea pig, malformation of the orbit has been shown to be the cause of exophthalmos (Maddock et al., 1949; Robens, 1970).

Aminocaproic acid injected intravenously in cats causes contraction of sympathetically innervated muscle in the orbital cone, resulting in mild exophthalmos (Cummings and Welter, 1966).

OCULAR TERATOGENESIS

The normal development of the eye may be affected in the uterus by a variety of toxins. The most common ocular malformations reported are varying degrees of microphthalmia to anophthalmia, colobomatous defects, and vitreoretinal dysplasia.

Selenium toxicity in sheep during early embryonic development causes microphthalmia with cysts and normal-sized eyes with microcornea or in which the cornea and iris are missing, with ectopia lentis or aphakia. Other structures may have colobomas. The failure of sclera to form enables the forming vitreous to flow into adjacent mesectodermal tissue to form cysts (Miller and Gelatt, 1991).

Maternal ingestion of the plant *Veratrum californicum* by sheep on the 14th day of gestation produces cyclopia in the offspring. Various alkaloids, **cyclopamine, veratrosine, jervine, cycloposine, pseudojervine,** and **isorubijervine,** have been found to be the toxic agents. In severe cases, bones of the upper jaw and cranium were distorted with fusion of the cerebral hemispheres, hydrocephalus, cyclopia, and anophthalmia (Babbott et al., 1962; Mulvihill, 1972; Binns et al., 1963; Keeler and Binns, 1966; Binns et al., 1965).

Vitamin A causes various ocular malformations that have included lens and retinal defects, microphthalmia, and colobomas in rabbits, rats, and chickens (Grant and Schuman, 1993). In hamsters and guinea pigs, abnormal growth of the orbital bones may result in abnormally shallow orbits and exophthalmos.

Apholate, an alkylating agent used as an insect chemosterilant, may cause anophthalmia and defective development of cranial and facial bones with absence of the orbital cavities in sheep (Younger, 1965).

Griseofulvin administered to cats in the first half of gestation causes anophthalmia, cyclopia, and optic nerve aplasia in the kittens (Scott, 1975).

Anticoagulants, such as **warfarin,** taken by humans during pregnancy have caused microphthalmia or abnormally large eyes, optic atrophy, and lens opacities (Shaul and Hall, 1977).

Chlorambucil, an antineoplastic drug, causes retinal dysplasia in mice, rats, and monkeys, and lens and optic nerve malformations in mice (Calvert and Gabriel, 1974; Rugh and Skaredoff, 1965). **Vinblastine** has produced anophthalmia, microphthalmia, and other developmental defects in hamsters (Ferm, 1963). **Cyclophosphamide** used in several species has caused congenital malformation of the nasolacrimal ducts (Calvert and Gabriel, 1974; Singh et al., 1976; Stuhltrager, 1982). **Alloxan,** has caused teratogenic defects of the lens and iris in mice. **Busulfan** has caused congenital malformations in humans (Grant and Schuman, 1993).

Felicin, the toxic principle of *Dryopteris felix mas*, has caused microphthalmia, anophthalmia, and dysplastic development of the retina and optic nerves when administered to mice (Grant and Schuman, 1993).

Salicylate produces anophthalmia, microphthalmia, and apparent exophthalmia in rats (Goldman and Yakovac, 1964).

Azathioprine causes ocular malformations, including defects in the lens in rabbits (Tuchmann-Duplessis and Mercier-Parot, 1965).

The antioxidant food additive, **butylated hydroxytoluene,** causes anophthalmia in rats (Johnson, 1965).

2,4-Dichlorophenyl-*p*-nitrophenyl ether causes hypoplasia of the harderian gland. The eyes may be normal in size or larger than usual. The enophthalmos, due to absence of the harderian gland, may resemble microphthalmia (Gray et al., 1982).

Idoxuridine causes retinal dysplasia and defects in the iris and ciliary body when administered to rabbits (Itoi et al., 1975).

The alkaloid, **caffeine,** has caused lens abnormalities in developing rat lenses (Pitel and Lerman, 1964).

Corticosteriods applied topically to the eyes of pregnant mice have caused congenital abnormalities in the offspring (Ballard et al., 1977).

Isotretinoin causes ocular teratogenesis in man—defects ranging from microphthalmia to abnormal development of central projections of the visual pathway (Benke, 1984; Hill, 1984).

Trypan blue, an anionic dye, causes anophthalmia and microphthalmia in rats (Beck and Lloyd, 1963).

Lysergic acid diethylamide (LSD) has produced lens epithelial abnormalities similar to those caused by radiation in mice (Hanaway, 1969) and multiple ocular anomalies in man (Apple and Bennett, 1974; Chan et al., 1978).

1-Methyl-3-nitro-1-nitrosoguanidine causes dysgenesis of the anterior segment, hypoplasia of the iris stroma, and ectopia of the ciliary body in rabbits (Alfieri and Alfieri-Rolla, 1973).

Abnormal facial development with shortening of the palpebral fissure has been described in humans with fetal alcohol syndrome (Miller et al., 1981). Attempts to reproduce a model of the human syndrome in mice has demonstrated that **ethanol** causes microphthalmia (Cook et al., 1987).

Nickel carbonyl has caused anophthalmia and microphthalmia in rats exposed to it in early gestation.

Acute **quinine** toxicity associated with high doses taken during pregnancy has caused optic nerve hypoplasia in humans (McKinna, 1966).

Tetracycline has resulted in corneal and lens discoloration in fetuses of mice and rabbits when fed to the dams during gestation, although this cannot be considered a malformation (Grant and Schuman, 1993).

Thalidomide causes various ocular malformations in humans, and some defects have been duplicated in rabbits. Abnormal development of extraocular muscles is commonly reported (Laszczyk et al., 1976). Other abnormalities include microphthalmia and colobomas of the iris, choroid, retina, and lenticular and retinal dysplasia (Cullen, 1966a,b).

Ocular teratogenic effects in various animal species have also been described with **cyclizine**, an antihistamine, and **colchicine** (Grant and Schuman, 1986).

REFERENCES

Abraham, R., and Hendy, R.J. 1970. Irreversible lysosomal damage induced by chloroquine in the retinae of pigmented and albino rats. *Experimental Molecular Pathology* 12:185–200.

Adams, D.R. 1930. The nature of the ocular lesions produced experimentally by naphthalene. *British Journal of Ophthalmology* 14:49–60.

Aguirre, G.D., Farber, D.B., Lolley, R.N., et al. 1982. Retinal degenerations in the dog. III. Abnormal cyclic nucleotide metabolism in rod–cone dysplasia. *Experimental Eye Research* 35:625–642.

Albert, D.M., Wong, V., and Henderson, E.S. 1967. Ocular complications of vincristine therapy. *Archives of Ophthalmology* 78:709–713.

Alfieri, G., and Alfieri-Rolla, G. 1973. Ocular alterations in the newborn rabbit after treatment of the mother during gestation with *N*-methyl-*N*-nitro-*N*-nitrosoguanidine. *Archivio e Rassegna Italiana di Ottalmologia* 3:247–256.

Amemiya, T. 1967. Cytochemical and electron microscopic examination of the retina of rats with hypervitaminosis A. *Acta Societatis Ophthalmologicae Japonicae—Japan* 71:2236–2251.

Amemiya, T. 1968. Electron microscopic study of the retina of rats repeatedly treated with urethane. *Ophthalmology Japan* 72:293–298.

Anderson, B., Jr. 1968. Ocular effects of changes in oxygen and carbon dioxide tension. *Transactions of the American Ophthalmology Society* 66:423–474.

Apple, D.J., and Bennett, T.O. 1974. Multiple systemic and ocular malformations associated with maternal LSD usage. *Archives of Ophthalmology* 92:301–303.

Apponi, G., Tieri, O., and Rinaldi, E. 1964. The retinotoxic action of Trenimon. *Acta Ophthalmology* 42:64–67.

Arison, R.N., Ciaccio, E.L., Glitzer, M.S., Cassaro, J.A., and Pruss, M.P. 1967. Light and electron microscopy of lesions in rats rendered diabetic with streptozotocin. *Diabetes* 16:51–56.

Armaly, M.F. 1967. Inheritance of dexamethasone hypertension and glaucoma. *Archives of Ophthalmology* 77:747.

Ashton, N. 1957. Degeneration of the retina due to 1,5-bis(*p*-aminophenoxy) pentane dihydrochloride. *Journal of Pathology and Bacteriology* 74:103–112.

Axelsson, U. 1971. Cataracts following the use of long-acting cholinesterase inhibitors in glaucoma. *Proceedings of the European Society for the Study of Drug Toxicity* 12:199–203.

Babbott, F.L., Binns, W., and Ingalls, T.H. 1962. Field studies of cyclopian malformations in sheep. *Archives of Environmental Health* 5:109–113.

Babel, J., and Ziv, B. 1957. The action of dithizone on the retina of the rabbit. *Experientia* 13:122–123.

Bagchi, K. 1959. The effects of methionine sulphoximine induced by methionine deficiency on the crystalline lens of albino rats. *Indian Journal of Medicine Research* 47:437–447.

Ballard, P.D., Hearney, E.F., et al. 1977. Comparative teratogenicity of selected glucocorticoids applied ocularly in mice. *Teratology* 16:175–180.

Barber, A.N., Catsulis, C., and Cangelosi, R.J. 1971. Studies on experimental retinitis light and electron microscopy. *British Journal of Ophthalmology* 55:91–105.

Barclay, S.M., and Riis, R.C. 1979. Retinal detachment and reattachment associated with ethylene glycol intoxication in a cat. *Journal of the American Animal Hospital Association* 15:719–724.

Barishak, Y.R., Beemer, A.M., et al. 1976. Histology of the retina and choroid in ducklings photosensitized by feeding *Ammi majus* seeds. *Ophthalmic Research* 8:169–178.

Barnett, K.C., Blakemore, W.F., and Mason, J. 1972. Bracken retinopathy in sheep. *Transactions of the Ophthalmology Society UK* 92:741–744.

Barnett, K.C., and Watson, W.A. 1970. Bright blindness in sheep. *Research Veterinary Science* 11:289.

Basson, P.A., and Kellerman, T.S. 1975. Blindness and encephalopathy caused by *Helichrysum argyrosphaerum* DC (Compositae) in sheep and cattle. *Onderstepoort Journal of Veterinary Research* 42:135–147.

Beasley, H., and Fraunfelder, F.T. 1979. Retinal detachments and topical ocular miotics. *American Academy of Ophthalmology* 86:95–98.

Beasley, V.R., and Buck, W.B. 1980. Acute ethylene glycol toxicosis: a review. *Veterinary and Human Toxicology* 22:255-263.

Beck, F., and Lloyd, J.B. 1963. The preparation and teratogenic properties of pure trypan blue and its common contaminants. *Journal of Embryology and Experimental Morphology* 11:175–184.

Beeler, C.C., Newton, N.L., et al. 1964. Retinal detachment in adult dogs resulting from oxygen toxicity. *Archives of Ophthalmology* 71:665–670.

Bellhorn, R.W., Bellhorn, M.S., Friedman, A.J., and Henkind, P. 1973. Urethane-induced retinopathy in pigmented rats. *Investigative Ophthalmology and Visual Science* 12:65–76.

Benke, P.J. 1984. The isotretinoin teratogen syndrome. *Journal of the American Medical Association* 251:3267–3269.

Benton, C.D., Jr., and Calhoun, F.P., Jr. 1953. The ocular effects of methyl alcohol poisoning: report of a catastrophe involving 320 persons. *American Journal of Ophthalmology* 36:1677–1685.

Berger, J.R., and Ayyar, D.R. 1981. Neurological complications of ethylene glycol intoxication. *Archives of Neurology* 38:724–726.

Berman, E.R. 1991. *Biochemistry of the Eye.* New York: Plenum Press.

Berman, M., Leary, R., and Gage, J. 1980. Evidence for a role of the plasminogen activator–plasmin system in corneal ulceration. *Investigative Ophthalmology and Visual Science* 19:1204–1221.

Bernat, R., and Bombicki, K. 1968. Changes in the concentration of glutathione, ascorbic acid, and sulfhydryl amino acids in experimental cataracts. *Acta Physiologica Polonica* 19:205–215.

Bernstein, H., Zvaifler, N., et al. 1963. The ocular deposition of chloroquine. *Investigative Ophthalmology* 2:384–391.

Berstein, H.N., and Ginsberg, J. 1964. The pathology of chloroquine retinopathy. *Archives of Ophthalmology* 71:238–245.

Bhuyan, K.C., and Bhuyan, D.K. 1978. Regulation of hydrogen peroxide in aqueous humors. *Biochemistry Biophysics Acta* 542:28–38.

Bhuyan, K.C., Bhuyan, D.K., and Katzin, H.M. 1973. Amizol-induced cataract and inhibition of lens catalase in rabbit. *Ophthalmic Research* 5:236–247.

Bhuyan, K.C., Bhuyan, D.K., and Podos, S.M. 1981a. Cataract induced by selenium in the rat I. Effect on the lenticular protein and thiols. *IRCS Medical Science* 9:194–195.

Bhuyan, K.C., Bhuyan, D.K., and Podos, D.M. 1981b. Selenium-induced cataract; biochemical mechanisms. In *Proceedings of the 2nd International Symposium on Selenium in Biological Medicine*, eds. J.E. Spallholz, J.L. Martin, and H.E. Ganther, pp. 403–412. Westport.

Bill, A. 1975. The drainage of aqueous humor. *Investigative Ophthalmology and Visual Science* 14: 1.

Binkhorst, C.G. 1980. Inflammation and intraocular pressure after the use of Healon in intraocular lens surgery. *American Intra-Ocular Implant Society Journal* 6:340.

Binns, W., et al. 1963. A congenital cyclopian-type malformation in lambs induced by material ingestation of a range plant, *Veratrum californicum. American Journal of Veterinary Research* 24:1164.

Binns, W., et al. 1965. Chronologic evaluation of teratogenicity in sheep fed *Veratrum californicum. Journal of the American Veterinary Medical Association* 147:839.

Black, R.L., Oglesby, R.B., Von Sallmann, L., and Bunim, J.J. 1960. Posterior subcapsular cataracts induced by corticosteroids in patients with rheumatoid arthritis. *Journal of the American Medical Association* 174:166–171.

Blanks, J.C. 1989. Morphology of the retina. In *Retina*, vol. 1., eds. S.J. Ryan and T.E. Ogden, pp. 37–52. St. Louis: C.V. Mosby.

Bockhardt, H., Drenckhahn, D., and Lullmann-Rauch, R. 1978. Amiodarone-induced lipidosis-like alterations in ocular tissues of rats. *Graefes Archives of Clinical Experiments in Ophthalmology* 207:91–96.

Bornschein, H., Hoyer, J., et al. 1974. Animal experimental study with a substance harmful to the visual system (NP 207). *Graefes Archives of Clinical Experiments in Ophthalmology* 190:13–25.

Bouldin, T.W., Goines, N.D., and Krigman, N.R. 1984. Trimethyltin retinopathy. Relationship of subcellular response to neuronal subspecialization. *Journal of Neuropathology and Experimental Neurology* 43:162–174.

Brinton, G.S., Norton, E.W.D., et al. 1980. Ocular quinine toxicity. *American Journal of Ophthalmology* 90:403–410.

Brown, C.J. 1980. Ocular envenomization by the West African spitting cobra. *Annals of Ophthalmology* 12:868–870.

Brown, D.V.L. 1975. Reaction of the rabbit retinal pigment epithelium to systemic lead poisoning. *Transactions of the American Ophthalmology Society* 72:404–447.

Brown, W.R., Rubin, L., Hite, M., and Zwickey, R.E. 1971. Experimental papilledema in the dog induced by a salicylanilide. *Toxicology in Applied Pharmacology* 21:532–541.

Bruckner, R., Hess, R., Keberle, H., Pericin, C., and Tripod, J. 1967. Tierexperimentelle pathologische Linsenveränderungen nach langdauernder Verabreichung höher Dosen von desferal hely. *Acta Physiology and Pharmacology* 25:62–77.

Bryan, G.M., and Slatter, D.H. 1973. Keratoconjunctivitis sicca induced by phenazopyridine in dogs. *Archives of Ophthalmology* 90:310–311.

Budinger, J.M. 1961. Diphenylthiocarbazone blindness in dogs. *Archives of Ophthalmology* 71:304–310.

Bullock, J.D., Albert, D.M., Skinner, C.W., Miller, W.H., and Galla, J.H. 1974. Calcium oxalate retinopathy associated with generalized oxalosis: x-ray diffraction and electron microscopic studies of crystal deposits. *Investigative Ophthalmology* 13:256–265.

Bunce, G.E., and Hess, J.L. 1981. Biochemical changes associated with selenite-induced cataract in the rat. *Experimental Eye Research* 33:504–514.

Burian, H.M., and Fletcher, M.C. 1958. Visual functions in patients with retinal pigmentary degeneration following the use of NP 207. *Archives of Ophthalmology* 60:612–629.

Butturini, U., Grignolo, A., and Baronchelli, A. 1953. "Diabetes" from dithizone: metabolic, ocular and histologic aspects. *General Clinical Medicine* 34:1253–1347.

Buxton, P.H., and Hayward, M. 1967. Polyneuritis cranialis associated with industrial trichloroethylene poisoning. *Journal of Neurology and Neurosurgery Psychiatry* 30:511–518.

Calvert, A., and Gabriel, R.O. 1974. Eye defects induced by chlorambucil in the mouse. *Compes Rendus des Seances de la Societe de Biologie et de Ses Filiates* 168:1115–1118.

Carpenter, C.P., and Smyth, H.F. 1946. Chemical burns of the rabbit cornea. *American Journal of Ophthalmology* 29:1363-1374.

Cavanagh, J.B., Fuller, N.H., et al. 1974. The effects of the thallium salts, with particular reference to the nervous system changes. *Quarterly Journal of Medicine* 43:293–319.

Cerletti, A., and Meier-Ruge, W. 1968. Toxicological studies on phenothiazine induced retinopathy. *Proceedings of the European Society for the Study of Drug Toxicity* 9:170–188.

Chan, C.C., Fishman, M., and Egbert, P.R. 1978. Multiple ocular anomalies associated with maternal LSD ingestion. *Archives of Ophthalmology* 96:282–284.

Christenberry, K.W., Conklin, J.W., et al. 1963. Induction of cataracts in mice by 4-(*p*-dimethylaminostyryl) quinoline. *Archives of Ophthalmology* 70:250–252.

Cibis, P.A. 1957. Ocular lesions produced by iodoacetate. *Archives of Ophthalmology* 57:509–519.

Cibis, G.W., Burian, H.M., and Blodi, F.C. 1973. Electroretinogram changes in acute quinine poisoning. *Archives of Ophthalmology* 90:307–309.

Cloud, T.M., Hakim, R., and Griffin, A.C. 1960. Photosensitization of the eye with methoxsalen. I. Acute effects. *Archives of Ophthalmology* 64:346–351.

Cloud, T.M., Hakim, R., and Griffin, A.C. 1961. Photosensitization of the eye with methoxsalen. II. Chronic effects. *Archives of Ophthalmology* 66:689–693.

Cloyd, G.G., and Wyman, M. 1978. Ocular toxicity studies with zinc pyridinethione. *Toxicology and Applied Pharmacology* 45:771–782.

Cogan, D.G., Truman, J.T., and Smith, T.R. 1973. Optic neuropathy, chloramphenicol and infantile genetic agranulocytosis. *Investigative Ophthalmology* 12:534–537.

Cohen, A.I. 1967. An electron microscopic study of the modification by monosodium glutamate of the retinas of normal and "rodless" mice. *American Journal of Anatomy* 120:319.

Cohen, A.M., Michaelson, I.C., and Yanko, L. 1972. Retinopathy in rats with disturbed carbohydrate metabolism following a high sucrose diet. *American Journal of Ophthalmology* 73:863–875.

Committee on Drugs. 1974. Blindness and neuropathy from diiodohydroxyquin-like drugs. *Pediatrics* 54:378–379.

Cook, C.S., Nowotny, A.Z., and Sulik, K.K. 1987. Fetal alcohol syndrome: eye malformation in a mouse model. *Archives of Ophthalmology* 105:1576–1581.

Creighton, M.O., Trevithick, J.R., Sanford, S.E., and Dukes, T.W. 1982. Modeling cortical cataractogenesis IV. Induction by hygromycin B in vivo (swine) and in vitro (rat lens). *Experimental Eye Research* 34:467–476.

Cullen, J.F. 1966a. Teratogenic agents and thalidomide. *Transactions of the Ophthalmology Society UK* 86:101–113.

Cullen, J.F. 1966b. Clinical anophthalmos in a thalidomide child. *Journal of Pediatric Ophthalmology* 3:10–14.

Cummings, J.R., and Welter, A.N. 1966. Cardiovascular studies on aminocaproic acid. *Toxicology and Applied Pharmacology* 9:57–69.

Davidorf, F.H. 1973. Thioridazine pigmentary retinopathy. *Archives of Ophthalmology* 90:251–255.

Davson, H. 1990. *Physiology of the Eye*, 5th ed. New York: Pergamon Press.

Delahunt, C.S., Stebbins, R.B., Anderson, J., and Bailey, J. 1962. The cause of blindness in dogs given hydroxypyridinethione. *Toxicology Applications in Pharmacology* 4:286–291.

Dorling, P.R., Huxtable, C.R., and Vogel, P. 1978. Lysosomal storage in *Swainsona* spp. toxicosis, an induced mannosidosis. *Neuropathology and Applied Neurobiology* 4:285–295.

Dowling, J.E. 1987. *The Retina: An Approachable Part of the Brain.* Cambridge, MA: Belknap Press of Harvard University Press.

Drenckhahn, D., Jacobi, B., and Lullmann-Rauch, R. 1983. Corneal lipidosis in rats treated with amphiphilic cationic drugs. *Arzneimittelforschung* 33:827–831.

Drenckhahn, D., and Lullmann-Rauch, R. 1977. Lens opacities associated with lipidosis-like ultrastructural alterations in rats treated with chloroquine, chlorphentermine, or iprindole. *Experimental Eye Research* 24:621–632.

Drenckhahn, D., and Lullmann-Rauch, R. 1978. Drug-induced retinal lipidosis: differential susceptibilities of pigment epithelium and neuroretina toward several amphiphilic cation drugs. *Experimental Molecular Pathology* 28:360–371.

Duke-Elder, S. 1958. The eye in evolution. In *System of Ophthalmology*, vol. 1. St. Louis: C.V. Mosby.

Edge, N.D., Mason, D.F.J., Wien, R., and Ashton, N. 1956. The pharmacological effects of certain diaminodiphenoxy alkanes. *Nature* 178:806–807.

Edwards, J.J., Anderson, R.L., and Wood, J.R. 1980. Loxoscelism of the eyelids. *Archives of Ophthalmology* 98:1997–2000.

Elgebaly, S.A., Downes, R.T., Bohr, M., Forouhar, F., O'Rourke, J., and Kreutzer, D.L. 1987. Inflammatory mediators in alkali-burned corneas: preliminary characterization. *Current Eye Research* 6:1263–1274.

Feldman, R.G., Mayer, R.M., and Taub, A. 1970. Evidence for peripheral neurotoxic effect of trichloroethylene. *Neurology* 20:599–606.

Ferm, V.H. 1963. Congenital malformations in hamster embryos after treatment with vinblastine and vincristine. *Science* 141:126.

Fliesler, S.J., Rapp, L.M., and Hollyfield, J.G. 1984. Photoreceptor-specific degeneration caused by tunicamycin. *Nature* 311:575–577.

Foos, R.Y. 1985. Chronic retinopathy of prematurity. *Ophthalmology* 92:563–574.

Fraunfelder, F.T., and Burns, R.P. 1966. Effect of lid closure in drug-induced experimental cataracts. *Archives of Ophthalmology* 76:599–601.

Fraunfelder, F.T., and Meyer, S.M. 1983. Ocular toxicity of antineoplastic agents. *Ophthalmology* 90:1–3.

Fraunfelder, F.T., and Grove, I.A. 1996. *Drug-Induced Ocular Side Effects and Drug Interactions*, 4th ed. Baltimore, Williams and Wilkins.

Freedman, J.K., and Potts, A.M. 1963. Repression of glutaminase 1 in the rat retina by administration of sodium-*L*-glutamate. *Investigative Ophthalmology* 2:252–258.

Friedenwald, J.S., Hughes, W.F., and Herrmann, H. 1946. Acid burns of the eye. *Archives of Ophthalmology* 35:98–108.

Fukui, H.N., Iwata, S., Epstein, D.L., and Merola, L.O. 1977. Cataractogenic effects of a boron hydride disulfide compound. *Investigative Ophthalmology* 16:654–657.

Gardiner, P.A., and Michaelson, I.C. 1948. Intravitreous streptomycin: its toxicity and diffusion. *British Journal of Ophthalmology* 32:449–456.

Garner, A., Ashton, N., Tripathi, R., Kohner, E.M., Bulpitt, C.J., and Dollery, C.T. 1975. Pathogenesis of hypertensive retinopathy: an experimental study in the monkey. *British Journal of Ophthalmology* 59:3–44.

Gass, J.D.M. 1973. Nicotinic acid maculopathy. *American Journal of Ophthalmology* 76:500–510.

Gilger, A.P., Farkas, I.S., and Potts, A.M. 1959. Studies on visual toxicity of methanol. *American Journal of Ophthalmology* 48:153–160.

Gilger, A.P., Potts, A.M., and Farkas, I.S. 1956. Studies on the visual toxicity of methanol. *American Journal of Ophthalmology* 42:244–251.

Gilmer, G., Swartz, M., Teske, M., and Crandall, A.S. 1986. Over-the-counter phenylpropanolamine: a possible cause of central retinal vein occlusion. *Archives of Ophthalmology* 104:642.

Gipson, I.K., Westcott, M.J., and Brooksby, N.G. 1982. Effects of cytochalasins B and D and colchicine on migration of the corneal epithelium. *Investigative Ophthalmology and Visual Science* 22:633–642.

Goar, E.F., and Fletcher, M.C. 1956. Toxic chorioretinopathy following the use of NP 207. *American Journal of Ophthalmology* 44:603–608.

Goldman, A.S., and Yakovac, W.C. 1964. Salicylate intoxication and congenital anomalies. *Archives of Environmental Health* 8:648–656.

Gralla, E.J., and Rubin, L. 1970. Ocular studies with parachlorophenylalanine in rats and monkeys. *Archives of Ophthalmology* 83:734–740.

Grant, W.M. and Schuman, I.S. 1993. *Toxicology of the Eye*, 4th ed. Springfield: Charles C. Thomas.

Grant, W.M., and Kern, H.L. 1955. Action of alkalies on the corneal stroma. *Archives of Ophthalmology* 54:931–939.

Gray, L.E.J., Kavlock, R.J., et al. 1982. Prenatal exposure to the herbicide 2,4-dichlorophenyl-*p*-nitrophenyl ether destroys the rodent Harderian gland. *Science* 215:293–294.

Graymore, C.N. 1970. *Biochemistry of the Eye*. New York: Academic Press.

Grignolo, A. 1969. Rhodopsin cycle and fine structure of rabbit retina in experimental degeneration induced by retinotoxic agents. *Experimental Eye Research* 8:254.

Grimes, P., and Von Sallmann, L. 1966. Interference with cell proliferation and induction of polyploidy in rat lens epithelium during prolonged myleran treatment. *Experimental Cell Research* 42:265–273.

Grimes, P., Von Sallmann, L., and Frichette, A. 1965. Influence of Myleran on cell proliferation in the lens epithelium. *Investigative Ophthalmology* 3:566–576.

Guttman-Friedmann, A. 1956. Blindness after snakebite. *British Journal of Ophthalmology* 40:57–59.

Hamming, N.A., Apple, D.J., and Goldberg, M.F. 1976. Histopathology and ultrastructure of busulfan-induced cataract. *Graefes Archives of Ophthalmology* 200:139–147.

Hanaway, J.K. 1969. Lysergic acid diethylamide: effects on the developing mouse lens. *Science* 164:574–575.

Hansson, H.A. 1966. Selective effects of metabolic inhibitors on retinal cultures. *Experimental Eye Research* 5:335–354.

Hansson, H.A. 1970. Ultrastructural studies on the long term effects of sodium glutamate on the rat retina. *Virchows Archives (B)* 6:1–11.

Hansson, H.A. 1972. Retinal changes induced by treatment with vincristine and vinblastine. *Documenta Ophthalmologica* 31:65–88.

Harding, J.J., and Crabbe, M.J.C. 1984. The lens: development, proteins, metabolism and cataract. In *The Eye*, vol. 1B, 3rd ed., ed. H. Davson, pp. 207–492. Orlando, FL: Academic Press.

Hardman, J.G., and Limbird, L.E. 1996. *The Pharmacological Basis of Therapeutics*, 9th ed. New York: Pergamon Press.

Havener, W.H. 1983. *Ocular Pharmacology*, 5th ed. St. Louis: C.V. Mosby.

Herrold, K.M. 1967. Pigmentary degeneration of the retina induced by *N*-methyl-*N*-nitrosourea. *Archives of Ophthalmology* 78:650–653.

Hewitt, A.T., and Adler, R. 1989. Retinal pigment epithelium and interphotoreceptor matrix: structure and specialized functions. In *Retina*, vol. 1, eds. S.J. Ryan and T.E. Ogden, pp. 57–64. St. Louis: C.V. Mosby.

Hill, R.M. 1984. Isotretinoin teratogenicity. *The Lancet* 112:1465.

Hiroz, C.A., Assimacopoulos, T., et al. 1981. Ophthalmologic side effects of lithium. *Encephale* 7:123–128.

Hockwin, O., Okamoto, T., et al. 1969. Genesis of cataracts: cumulative effects of subliminal noxious influences. *Annals of Ophthalmology* 1:321–325.

Hogan, M.J., Alvarado, J.A., and Weddell, J.E. 1971. *Histology of the Human Eye*. Philadelphia: W.B. Saunders.

Holmes, J.H.C., Humphrey, J.D., Walton, E.A., and O'Shea, J.D. 1981. Cataracts, goiter and infertility in cattle grazed on an exclusive diet of *Leucaena leucocephala*. *Australian Veterinary Journal* 57:257–261.

Hommer, K. 1968. The effects of quinine, chloroquine, iodoacetate, and chlorodiazepoxide on the ERG of the isolated rabbit retina. *Graefes Archives of Ophthalmology* 175:111–120.

Hotta, R., and Goto, S. 1970. A fluorescein angiographic study on microangiopathia sulfocarbonica. *Acta Society of Ophthalmology—Japan* 74:1463–1467.

Huxtable, C.R., Dorling, P.R., and Slatter, D.H. 1980. Myelin oedema, optic neuropathy and retinopathy in experimental *Stypandra imbricata* toxicosis. *Neuropathology and Applied Neurobiology* 6:221–232.

Ide, T. 1958. Histopathological studies on retina, optic nerve and arachnoidal membrane of mouse exposed to carbon disulfide poisoning. *Acta Society Letter of Ophthalmology—Japan* 62A:85–108.

Imai, H., Miyamata, M., Uga, S., and Ishikawa, S. 1983. Retinal degeneration in rats exposed to an organophosphate pesticide (Fenthion). *Environmental Research* 30:453.

Itoi, M., Gefter, J.W., et al. 1975. Teratogenicities of ophthalmic drugs. *Archives of Ophthalmology* 93:46–51.

Jampol, L.M. 1989. Macular edema. In *Retina*, vol. 2, eds. S.J. Ryan, A.P. Schachat, R.P. Murphy, et al., pp. 81–88. St. Louis: C.V. Mosby.

Jampol, L.M., Axelrod, A., and Tessler, H. 1976. Pathways of the eye's response to topical nitrogen mustard. *Investigative Ophthalmology and Visual Science* 15:486–489.

Johnson, A.R. 1965. A re-examination of the possible teratogenic effects of butylated hydroxytoluene (BHT). *Food and Cosmetic Toxicology* 3:371–375.

Kaiser-Kupfer, M.I., and Lippman, M.E. 1978. Tamoxifen retinopathy. *Cancer Treatment Review* 62:315–320.

Kao, W.W-Y., Ebert, J., Kao, C.W-C., Covington, H., and Cintron, C. 1986. Development of monoclonal antibodies recognizing collagenase from rabbit PMN: the presence of this enzyme in ulcerating corneas. *Current Eye Research* 5:801–815.

Karlsen, R.L., and Pederson, O.O. 1982. A morphological study of the acute toxicity of *L*-cysteine on the retina of young rats. *Experimental Eye Research* 34:65–69.

Kaswan, R.L., and Salisbury, M.A. 1990. A new perspective on canine keratoconjunctivitis sicca: treatment with ophthalmic cyclosporine. *Veterinary Clinic of North America [Small Animal Practice]* 20:583–613.

Kaufman, H.E., Capella, J.A., et al. 1964. Corneal toxicity of cytosine arabinoside. *Archives of Ophthalmology* 72:535–540.

Kaufman, P.L., Axelsson, U., and Barany, E.H. 1977. Induction of subcapsular cataracts in cynomolgus monkeys by echothiophate. *Archives of Ophthalmology* 95:499–504.

Keeler, R.F., and Binns, W. 1966. Teratogenic compounds of *V. californicum. Canadian Veterinary Journal* 44:819.

Kern, H.L., Bellhorn, R.W., and Peterson, C.M. 1977. Sodium cyanate induced ocular lesions in the beagle. *Journal of Pharmacology and Experimental Therapeutics* 200:10–16.

Kinsey, V.E., and Grant, W.M. 1946. Determination of the rate of disappearance of mustard gas and mustard intermediates in the corneal tissue. *Journal of Clinical Investigation* 25:776–779.

Kirby, T.J. 1967. Cataracts produced by triparanol. *Transactions of the American Ophthalmology Society* 65:493–543.

Kittell, V., and Cornelius, C. 1969. Optic nerve injury by chloramphenicol. *Klinische Monatsblaetter fuer Augenheilkunde* 155:83–87.

Kleifeld, O., and Hockwin, O. 1956. The effect of dinitrophenol (DNP), ethylenediamine tetra-acetic acid, diamox and butazolidin on the metabolism of the lens. *Graefes Archives of Ophthalmology* 158:54–63.

Kolker, A.E., and Becker, B. 1968. Epinephrine maculopathy. *Archives of Ophthalmology* 79:552–562.

Krinke, G., Schaumburg, H.H., et al. 1979. Clioquinol and 2,5-hexanedione induce different types of distal axonopathy in the dog. *Acta Neuropathology* 47:213–221.

Kurtz, S.M., Kaump, D.H., Schardein, J.L., Roll, D.E., Reutner, T.F., and Fisken, R.A. 1967. The effect of long-term administration of amopyroquin, a 4-aminoquinoline compound, on the retina of pigmented and nonpigmented laboratory animals. *Investigative Ophthalmology* 6:420.

Kuwabara, T., Quevedo, A.T., and Cogan, D.G. 1968. An experimental study of dichloroethane poisoning. *Archives of Ophthalmology* 79:321–330.

Laszczyk, W.A., et al. 1976. Changes in the visual system of rabbit fetuses after thalidomide administration. *Ophthalmic Research* 8:146–151.

Lessell, S. 1971. Experimental cyanide optic neuropathy. *Archives of Ophthalmology* 86:194–204.

Lessell, S. 1976. Histopathology of experimental ethambutol intoxication. *Investigative Ophthalmology and Visual Science* 15:765–769.

Lessell, S., Craft, J.L., and Albert, D.M. 1980. Kainic acid induces mitoses in mature retinal neurones in rats. *Experimental Eye Research* 30:731–738.

Lessell, S., and Kuwabara, T. 1974. Fine structure of experimental cyanide optic neuropathy. *Investigative Ophthalmology and Visual Science* 13:748–756.

Levy, J., and Michel-Ber, E. 1968. Difficulties and complications caused in man by monoamine oxidase (MAO) inhibitors, with special reference to their specific and secondary pharmacological effects. *Proceedings of the European Society for the Study of Drug Toxicity* 9:189–245.

Lobeck, E. 1936. On knowledge of retinal changes in chronic lead poisoning. *Graefes Archives of Ophthalmology* 135:165–168.

Lucas, D.R., Newhouse, J.P., and Davery, J.B. 1957. Experimental degeneration of the retina. *British Journal of Ophthalmology* 41:313–316.

Lullmann, H., Lullmann-Rauch, R., and Wassermann, O. 1978. Lipidosis induced by amphiphilic cationic drugs. *Biochemistry Pharmacology* 27:1103–1108.

Lullmann-Rauch, R. 1976. Retinal lipidosis in albino rats treated with chlorpentermine and with tricyclic antidepressants. *Acta Neuropathology* 35:55–67.

Lullmann-Rauch, R. 1991a. Lipidosis and mucopolysaccharidosis of the cornea due to cationic amphiphilic drugs, rat. In *Eye and Ear*, eds. T.C. Jones, U. Mohr, and R.D. Hunt, pp. 25–29. Berlin: Springer-Verlag.

Lullmann-Rauch, R. 1991b. Lipidosis of the retina due to cationic amphiphilic drugs, rat. In *Eye and Ear*, eds. T.C. Jones, U. Mohr, and R.D. Hunt, pp. 87–92. Berlin: Springer-Verlag.

MacLeod, I.F. 1969. Chemical mace: ocular effects in rabbits and monkeys. *Journal of Forensic Science* 14:34–47.

Maddock, C.L., Wolbach, S.B., and Maddock, S. 1949. Hypervitaminosis A in the dog. *Journal of Nutrition* 39:117.

Main, D.C., Slatter, D.H., and Huxtable, C.R. 1981. *Stypandra imbricata* ("blind grass") toxicoses in goats and sheep—clinical and pathologic findings in 4 field cases. *Australian Veterinary Journal* 57(3):132–135.

Mandelkorn, R.M., and Zimmerman, T.J. 1989. Effects of nonsteroidal drugs on glaucoma. In *The Glaucomas*, eds. R. Ritch, B.M. Shields, and T. Krupin, pp. 1169–1184. St. Louis: C.V. Mosby.

Mann, I., Pirie, A., and Pullinger, B.D. 1948. An experimental and clinical study of the reaction of the anterior segment of the eye to chemical injury, with special reference to chemical warfare agents. *British Journal of Ophthalmology* 13(suppl):1–171.

Manschot, W.A. 1969. Ophthalmic pathological findings in a case of thallium poisoning. *Ophthalmologica* 158:348–349.

Marine, D., Rosen, S.H., and Cipra, A. 1933. Further studies on the exophthalmos in rabbits, produced by methyl cyanide. *Proceedings of the Society of Experimental Biology and Medicine* 30:649–651.

Marmor, M.F. 1989. Mechanisms of normal retinal adhesion. In *Retina*, vol. 3, ed. S.J. Ryan, pp. 71–87. St. Louis: C.V. Mosby.

Martin, C.L., and Chambreau, T. 1982. Cataract production in experimentally orphaned puppies fed a commercial replacement for bitch's milk. *Journal of the American Animal Hospital Association* 18:115–119.

Martin, C.L., Christmas, R., and Leipold, H.W. 1972. Formation of temporary cataracts in dogs given a disophenol preparation. *Journal of the American Veterinary Medical Association* 161:294–300.

Matsuoka, Y., Mukoyama, M., and Sobue, I. 1972. Histopathological study of experimental ethambutol neuropathy. *Clinical Neurology* 12:453–459.

Maurice, D., and Perlman, M. 1977. Permanent destruction of the corneal endothelium in rabbits. *Investigative Ophthalmology* 16:646.

Maurolf, F.A., and Mesher, J.H. 1973. Experimental hyperviscosity retinopathy. *Annals of Ophthalmology* 5:205–209.

McFarlane, J.R., Yanoff, M., and Sheie, H.G. 1966. Toxic retinopathy following sparsomycin therapy. *Archives of Ophthalmology* 76:532–540.

McKinna, A.J. 1966. Quinine induced hypoplasia of the optic nerve. *Canadian Journal of Ophthalmology* 1:261–266.

McLane, J. 1943. Retinal hemorrhage in case of rattlesnake bite. *Journal of the Florida Medical Association* 30:22–25.

McLendon, B.F., and Bron, A.J. 1978. Corneal toxicity from vinblastine solution. *British Journal of Ophthalmology* 62:97–99.

Mebs, D. 1978. Pharmacology of reptilian venoms. In *Biology of the Reptilia, vol. 8. Physiology B*, ed. C. Gans, pp. 437–530. New York: Academic Press.

Meier-Ruge, W., and Cerletti, A. 1966. On the experimental pathology of phenothiazine retinopathy. *Ophthalmology* 151:512–533.

Meier-Ruge, W., Kalberer, F., and Cerletti, A. 1966. Microhistoautoradiographic investigations of the distribution of tritium-labeled phenothiazine derivatives in the eye. *Experientia* 22:153–155.

Michon, J., Jr., and Khloshita, J.H. 1968a. Experimental miotic cataract I. *Archives of Ophthalmology* 79:79–86.

Michon, J., Jr., and Khloshita, J.H. 1968b. Experimental miotic cataract II. *Archives of Ophthalmology* 79:611–616.

Miller, M., Israel, J., and Cuttone, J. 1981. Fetal alcohol syndrome. *Journal of Pediatric Ophthalmology Strabismus* 18:6–15.

Miller, T.R., and Gelatt, K.N. 1991. Food animal ophthalmology. In *Veterinary Ophthalmology*, 2nd ed., ed. K.N. Gelatt, pp. 611–655. Philadelphia: Lea & Febiger.

Millichamp, N.J., and Dziezyc, J.D. 1991. Control of the ocular irritative response in the dog: a comparison of flunixin meglumine and flurbiprofen. *American Journal of Veterinary Research* 52:1452–1455.

Mindel, J.S., Rubenstein, A.E., and Franklin, B. 1981. Ocular ergotamine tartrate toxicity during treatment of Vacor-induced orthostatic hypotension. *American Journal of Ophthalmology* 92:492–496.

Miyata, A. 1968. Studies on the experimental dinitrophenol cataract. *Acta Society of Ophthalmology—Japan* 72:2307–2324.

Mizuno, G., Ellison, E., et al. 1974. Lipids of the triparanol cataract in the rat. *Ophthalmic Research* 6:206–215.

Moe, R.A., Kirpan, J., and Linegar, C.R. 1960. Toxicology of hydroxypyridinethione. *Toxicology and Applied Pharmacology* 2:156–170.

Mulvihill, J.J. 1972. Congenital and genetic disease in domestic animals. *Science* 176:132–137.

Newberne, J.W., Kuhn, W.L., and Elsea, J.R. 1966. Toxicologic studies on clomiphene. *Toxicology Applications in Ophthalmology* 9:44–56.

Nicholson, D.H., Harkness, D.R., Benson, W.E., and Peterson, C.M. 1976. Cyanate induced cataracts in patients with sickle cell hemoglobinopathies. *Archives of Ophthalmology* 94:927–930.

Nilsson, S.E.G., Knave, B., and Persson, H.E. 1977. Changes in ultrastructure and function of the sheep pigment epithelium and retina induced by sodium iodate II. Early effects. *Acta Ophthalmologica* 55:1007–1026.

Noell, W.K. 1951. The effect of iodoacetate on the vertebrate retina. *Journal of Cellular Comparative Physiology* 37:283–307.

Noell, W.K. 1952. Azide sensitive potential difference across the eye bulb. *American Journal of Physiology* 170:217.

Noell, W.K. 1953. Experimentally induced toxic effects on structure and function of visual cells and pigment epithelium. *American Journal of Ophthalmology* 36:103–116.

Olney, J.W. 1969. Glutamate-induced retinal degeneration in neonatal mice. *Journal of Neuropathology and Experimental Neurology* 28:455–474.

Orzalesi, N., Grignolo, A., Calabria, G.A., and Castellazzo, R.A. 1967. A study on fine structure and the rhodopsin cycle of the rabbit retina in experimental degeneration induced by diaminodiphenoxypentane. *Experimental Eye Research* 6(4):376–382.

Ozanics, V., and Jakobiec, F.A. 1986. Prenatal development of the eye and its adnexa. In *Biomedical Foundations of Ophthalmology*, vol. I, eds. T.D. Duane and E.A. Jaeger, pp. 9–86. Philadelphia: Harper & Row.

Parhad, I.M., Giffin, J.W., Clark, A.W., and Koves, J.F. 1984. Doxorubicin intoxication: neuro-filamentous axonal changes with subacute neuronal death. *Journal of Neuropathology and Experimental Neurology* 43:188–200.

Paterson, R.A. 1968. The effect of hydroxyethyl-substituted rutosides on the B,B-iminodipropionitrile-induced retinopathy in the rat. *British Journal of Experimental Pathology* 49:283–287.

Patterson, J.W., Patterson, M.E., Kinsey, V.E., and Reddy, D.V.N. 1965. Lens assays on diabetic and galactosemic rats receiving diets that modify cataract development. *Investigative Ophthalmology* 4:98–103.

Payne, Y., and Warrell, D.A. 1976. Effects of venom in eye from spitting cobra. *Archives of Ophthalmology* 94:1803.

Pederson, O.O., and Karlsen, R.L. 1980. The toxic effect of *L*-cysteine on the rat retina. *Investigative Ophthalmology and Visual Science* 19:886–892.

Pirie, A. 1968. Pathology in the eye of the naphthalene-fed rabbit. *Experimental Eye Research* 7:354–357.

Pirie, A., Rees, J.R., and Holmberg, N.J. 1969. Diquat cataract in the rat. *Biochemistry Journal* 89:114.

Pitel, M., and Lerman, L. 1964. Further studies on the effects of intrauterine vasoconstrictors on the fetal rat lens. *American Journal of Ophthalmology* 58:464–470.

Potts, A.M., Praglin, J., and Farkas, I. 1955. Studies on the visual toxicity of methanol. *American Journal of Ophthalmology* 40:76–83.

Poulsom, R., Boot Hanford, R.P., and Heath, H. 1982. Some effects of aldose reductase inhibition upon the eyes of long-term streptozotocin-diabetic rats. *Current Eye Research* 2:351–355.

Prince, J.H. 1956. *Comparative Anatomy of the Eye*. Springfield: Charles C. Thomas.

Prince, J.H., Diesem, C.D., Eglitis, I., and Ruskell, G.L. 1960. *Anatomy and Histology of the Eye and Orbit in Domestic Animals*. Springfield: Charles C. Thomas.

Ramsey, M.S., and Fine, B.S. 1972. Chloroquine toxicity in the human eye. *American Journal of Ophthalmology* 73:229–235.

Reading, H.W., and Sorsby, A. 1966. Retinal toxicity and tissue-SH levels. *Biochemistry and Pharmacology* 15:1389–1393.

Reinecke, R.D., and Kuwabara, T. 1963. Corneal deposits secondary to topical epinephrine. *Archives of Ophthalmology* 70: 170–172.

Render, J.A., and Carlton, W.W. 1991. Induced cataracts, lens, rat. In *Eye and Ear*, eds. T.C. Jones, U. Mohr and R.D. Hunt, pp. 63–70. Berlin: Springer-Verlag.

Ripps, H., Carr, R.E., et al. 1984. Functional abnormalities in vincristine-induced night blindness. *Investigative Ophthalmology and Visual Science* 25:787–794.

Robens, J.F. 1970. Teratogenic effects of hypervitaminosis A in the hamster and in the guinea pig. *Toxicology and Applied Pharmacology* 16:88–99.

Rose, A.L., Wen, G.Y., and Cammer, W. 1981. Hexachlorophene retinopathy in suckling rats. *Journal of Neurological Science* 52:163–178.

Rosen, E.S., Edgar, J.T., and Smith, J.L.S. 1970. Male fern retro-bulbar neuropathy in cattle. *Journal of Small Animal Practice* 10:619–625.

Rosenthal, A.R., Kolb, H., Bergsma, D., Huxsoll, D., and Hopkins, J.L. 1978. Chloroquine retinopathy in the rhesus monkey. *Investigative Ophthalmology and Visual Science* 17:1158–1175.

Rowe, V.D., Zigler, S., Andersen, A.E., Sidbury, J.B., and Guroff, G. 1973. Some characteristics of the p-chlorophenylalanine-induced cataract. *Experimental Eye Research* 17:245–250.

Rubin, L.F. 1974. *Atlas of Veterinary Ophthalmoscopy*. Philadelphia: Lea & Febiger.

Rubin, L.F. 1975. Toxicity of dimethyl sulfoxide, alone and in combination. *Annals of the New York Academy of Science* 243:98–103.

Rugh, R., and Skaredoff, L. 1965. Radiation and radiomimetic chlorambucil and the fetal retina. *Archives of Ophthalmology* 74:382–393.

Samuelson, D.A. 1999. Ophthalmic anatomy. In *Veterinary Ophthalmology*, 3rd ed., ed. K.N. Gelatt, pp. 31–150. Philadelphia: Lippincott, Williams, and Wilkins.

Sandler, S.G., Tobin, W., and Henderson, E.S. 1969 Vincristine-induced neuropathy. *Neurology* 19:367–374.

Sanford, S.E., and Dukes, T.W. 1979. Acquired bilateral cortical cataracts in mature sows. *Journal of the American Veterinary Medical Association* 173:852–853.

Sanford, S.E., Dukes, T.W., Creighton, M.O., and Trevithick, J.R. 1981. Conical cataracts induced by hygromycin B in swine. *American Journal of Veterinary Research* 42:1534–1537.

Schiavo, D.M., Field, W.E., and Vymetol, F.J. 1975. Cataracts in beagle dogs given diazoxide. *Diabetes* 24:1041.

Schmidt, I.G., and Schmidt, L.H. 1948. Neurotoxicity of the 8-aminoquinolines. *Journal of Neuropathology and Experimental Neurology* 7:368–398.

Schmidt, I.G., and Schmidt, L.H. 1966. Studies of the neurotoxicity of ethambutol and its racemate for the rhesus monkey. *Journal of Neuropathology and Experimental Neurology* 25:40–67.

Scott, F.W. 1975. Teratogenesis in cats associated with griseofulvin therapy. *Teratology* 11:79.

Scullica, L., Bisantis, C., and Pezzi, P.P. 1968. Effects of epinephrine on the mitotic activity of the lens epithelium. *Bolletino di Oculistica* 47:561–567.

Segal, R.L., Rosenblatt, S., and Eliasoph, I. 1973. Endocrine exophthalmos during lithium therapy of manic-depressive disease. *New England Journal of Medicine* 289:136–138.

Selye, H. 1957. Prevention by thyroxine of the ocular changes normally produced by B,B-iminodipropionitrile (IDNP). *American Journal of Ophthalmology* 44:763–765.

Sharpe, J.A., Hostovsky, M., et al. 1982. Methanol optic neuropathy: a histopathological study. *Neurology* 32:1093–1100.

Shaul, W.L., and Hall, J.G. 1977. Multiple congenital anomalies associated with oral anticoagulants. *American Journal of Obstetrics and Gynecology* 127:191–198.

Singh, S., et al. 1976. Eye anomalies induced by cyclophosphamide in rat fetuses. *Acta Anatomy* 94:490–496.

Sisk, D.R., and Kuwabara, T. 1985. Histological changes in the inner retina of albino rats following intravitreal injection of monosodium *L*-glutamate. *Graefes Archives of Clinical Experiments in Ophthalmology* 223:250–258.

Slansky, H.H., Kolbert, G., and Gartner, S. 1967. Exophthalmos induced by corticosteroids. *Archives of Ophthalmology* 77:579–581.

Slatter, D.H. 1973. Keratoconjunctivitis sicca in the dog produced by oral phenazopyridine hydrochloride. *Journal of Small Animal Practice* 14:749–771.

Smelser, G., and Ozanics, V. 1945. Effect of local anesthetics on cell division and migration following thermal burns of the cornea. *Archives of Ophthalmology* 34:271–277.

Snyder, F.H., Buehler, E.F., and Winek, C.L. 1965. Safety evaluation of zinc 2-pyridinethiol 1-oxide in a shampoo formulation. *Toxicology and Applied Pharmacology* 7:425–437.

Sorsby, A., and Harding, R. 1960. Experimental degeneration of the retina. *British Journal of Ophthalmology* 44:213–224.

Sorsby, A., and Harding, R. 1966. Oxidizing agents as potentiators of the retinotoxic action of sodium fluoride, sodium iodate, and sodium iodoacetate. *Nature* 210:997–998.

Sorsby, A., and Nakajima, A. 1958. Experimental degeneration of the retina IV. Diaminodiphenoxy alkanes as inducing agents. *British Journal of Ophthalmology* 42:563–570.

Spector, A., and Garner, W.H. 1981. Hydrogen peroxide and human cataract. *Ceskoslovenska Oftalmologie* 33:673–681.

Stacpoole, P.W., Moore, G.W., and Kornhauser, D.M. 1979. Toxicity of chronic dichloracetate. *New England Journal of Medicine* 300:372.

Stancliffe, T.C., and Pirie, A. 1971. Production of superoxide radicals in reactions of the herbicide diquat. *Federation of the European Biochemistry Society Letter* 17:297–299.

Steele, C.M., O'Duffy, J., and Brown, S.S. 1967. Clinical effects and treatment of imipramine and amitriptyline poisoning in children. *British Medical Journal* 3:663.

Stuhltrager, U. 1982. Cyclophosphamide-induced developmental disturbances of the nasolacrimal ducts in the mouse. *Folio Ophthalmology* 7:207–211.

Swartz, M. 1989. Other diseases: drug toxicity and metabolic and nutritional conditions. In *Retina*, vol. 2, eds. S.J. Ryan, A.P. Schachat, R.P. Murphy, et al., pp. 737–748. St. Louis: C.V. Mosby.

Tateishi, J., Kuroda, S., et al. 1973. Experimental myelo-optic neuropathy induced by clioquinol. *Acta Neuropathology* 24:304–320.

Thomas, J.V., Gragoudas, E.S., Blair, N.P., and Lapus, J.V. 1978. Correlation of epinephrine use and macular edema in aphakic glaucomatous eyes. *Archives of Ophthalmology* 96:625–628.

Thompson, S.W. 1975. Chloroquine toxicity in the rat. *Veterinary Pathology* 12:71.

Trzeciakowski, J.P. 1987. Review: central control of intraocular pressure. *Journal of Ocular Pharmacology* 3:367–377.

Tuchmann-Duplessis, H., and Mercier-Parot, L. 1965. Dissociation of antitumor and teratogenic properties of a purine antimetabolite, azathioprine. *Comple Rendus des Seances de la Societe de Biologie et de Ses Filiates* 159:2290–2294.

Ullberg, S., Linquist, N.G., and Sjostrand, S.E. 1970. Accumulation of chorioretinotoxic drugs in the foetal eye. *Nature* 227:1257–1258.

Ulshafer, R.J., Garcia, C.A., and Hollyfield, J.G. 1980. Elevated levels of cGMP destroy rod photoreceptors in the human retina. *Investigative Ophthalmology and Visual Science* 38.

van Heyningen, R. 1969. Xylose cataract: a comparison between the weanling and the older rat. *Experimental Eye Research* 8:379–385.

van Heyningen, R. 1979. Naphthalene cataract in rats and rabbits: a resume. *Experimental Eye Research* 28:435–439.

Van Kampen, K.R., and James, L.F. 1972. Sequential development of the lesions in locoweed poisoning. *Clinical Toxicology* 5:575–580.

Vanysek, J., Anton, M., et al. 1969. Some metabolic disturbances of the retina due to the effect of natrium fluoride. *Ophthalmologica* 158:684–690.

Verrey, F. 1956. Pigmentary degeneration of the retina of drug origin. *Ophthalmology* 131:296–303.

Vlchek, J.K., and Peyman, G.A. 1975. Cephaloridine-induced retinopathy by intravitreal infection: an ultrastructural study. *Annals of Ophthalmology* 7:903–914.

Vogul, A., and Kaiser, J. 1963. Ethambutol induced transient change and reconstitution (*in vivo*) of the tapetum lucidum color in the dog. *Experimental Molecular Pathology* 2(suppl):136–149.

von Canstatt, B.S., Hofmann, H.T., et al. 1966. Disturbances of the cat retina by poisoning with perorally or percutaneously administered chemicals. *Verhandlungen der Deutschen Gesellschaft für Pathologie* 50:429–435.

Von Sallmann, L., and Grimes, P. 1971. Eye changes in streptozotocin diabetes in rats. *American Journal of Ophthalmology* 71(1–part 2):312–319.

Von Sallmann, L., Grimes, P., and Collins, E. 1959. Mimosine cataract. *American Journal of Ophthalmology* 47:107–117.

Walls, G.L. 1942. *The Vertebrate Eye and Its Adaptive Radiation*. Bloomfield Hills, MI: Cranbrook Institute of Science.

Walsh, F.B., and Hoyt, W.F. 1969. *Clinical Neuro-ophthalmology*, 3rd ed. Baltimore: Williams & Wilkins.

Waltman, S.R., Carroll, D., Schimmelpfennig, W., and Okun, E. 1975. Intraocular irrigation solutions for clinical vitrectomy. *Ophthalmic Surgery* 6:90.

Wang, M.K., and Heath, H. 1968. Effect of B,B-iminodipropionitrile and related compounds on the electroretinogram and the retinal vascular system of the rat. *Experimental Eye Research* 7:56–61.

Warrell, D.A., and Ormerod, L.D. 1976. Snake venom ophthalmia and blindness caused by the spitting cobra (*Naja nigricollis*) in Nigeria. *American Journal of Tropical Medical Hygiene* 25:525–529.

Weinreb, R.N., Mitchell, M.D., and Polansky, J.R. 1983. Prostaglandin production by human trabecular cells: in vitro inhibition by dexamethasone. *Investigative Ophthalmology and Visual Science* 24:1541–1545.

Weitzel, G., and Strecker, F.J. 1954. Zinc in the tapetum lucidum. *Zeitschrift für Physiologische Chemie* 296:1930.

Whitman, L.K., and Filmer, D.B. 1974. A photosensitized keratitis in young cattle following the use of phenothiazine as an anthelmintic. *Australian Veterinary Journal* 23:336–340.

Wilkie, D.A., and Wyman, M. 1991. Comparative anatomy and physiology of the mammalian eye. In *Dermal and Ocular Toxicology: Fundamentals and Methods*, ed. D.W. Hobson, pp. 433–491. Boca Raton, CRC Press.

Wilson, F.M., II. 1979. Adverse external ocular effects of topical ophthalmic medications. *Survey of Ophthalmology* 24:57.

Witzel, D.A., Smith, E.L., et al. 1976. Arsanilic acid-induced blindness in swine. *American Journal of Veterinary Research* 37:521–524.

Wood, D.C., and Wirth, N.V. 1969. Changes in rabbit lenses following DMSO therapy. *Ophthalmology* 158:488–493.

Worden, A.N., Heywood, R., et al. 1978. Clioquinol toxicity in the dog. *Toxicology* 9:227–238.

Wright, H.N. 1963. Corneal and lenticular opacities in eyes of rats following long-term administration of sulfonylurea derivatives. *Diabetes* 12:550–554.

Younger, R.L. 1965. Probable induction of congenital anomalies in a lamb by apholate. *American Journal of Veterinary Research* 26:991.

Zhan, G.L., Miranda, O.C., and Bito, L.Z. 1989 Steroid-induced ocular hypertension in cats. *Investigative Ophthalmology and Visual Science* 30:445.

Zinn, K.M., and Marmor, M.F. 1979. Toxicology of the human retinal pigment epithelium. In *The Retinal Pigment Epithelium*, eds. K.M. Zinn, and M.F. Marmor, pp. 395–412. Cambridge, MA: Harvard University Press.

Ophthalmic Toxicology
Edited by George C. Y. Chiou
Copyright © 1999 Taylor & Francis

4

Species Specificity

Factors Affecting the Interpretation of Species Differences in Toxic Responses of Ocular Tissues

Nicholas J. Millichamp

Department of Small Animal Medicine and Surgery, College of Veterinary Medicine, Texas A&M University, College Station, Texas, USA

- **Eyelids**
- **Lacrimal System**
- **Conjunctiva and Cornea**
- **Anterior Uveal Vascular Changes and the Blood–Aqueous Barrier**
- **Cellular Infiltration Into the Anterior Chamber**
- **Miosis**
- **Changes in Intraocular Pressure**
- **Aqueous Humor**
- **Lens**
- **Retina and Choroid**
- **Ocular Albinism**
- **References**

The manner in which the eye responds to chemicals, radiation, and other toxic insults is influenced by many factors, some of which are described elsewhere in this book. Variations in morphology, physiology, biochemistry, and pharmacology of the eye in different species of animal may have a significant effect on the reaction of the eye to injury or toxins. Even within a particular species, difference in age and degree of ocular pigmentation may affect the eye's response to, and recovery or repair from, noxious substances. The area of the eye in which most differences are seen and about which most is known is the anterior uvea and the response of the iris sphincter muscle and blood–aqueous barrier to toxic substances. For this reason, the anterior uvea will receive most attention.

Both humans and animals are affected by a number of inherited ocular diseases. Since many of these may mimic the response of the eye to toxic substances, it is important that the toxicologist be aware of which inherited eye diseases occur in the species being used in any study. It is important that both human and veterinary ophthalmologists are able to differentiate between toxic reactions in the eye and inherited diseases, since this will profoundly influence the course any planned therapy will take.

Additionally, most of the species used in ocular toxicity testing are prone to various infectious ocular diseases. Although these are beyond the scope of this chapter, details may be found in veterinary ophthalmologic texts (Slatter, 1990; Gelatt, 1999). Certain species have been used to develop models of infectious and metabolic ocular diseases (Tabbara and Cello, 1984).

This chapter examines some of the considerations that affect species specificity in ocular toxic reactions. Most of the reported toxic reactions of the eyes in animals have been the result of experimental studies; whereas, in man, the preponderance of toxic reactions are noted as accidental occurrences or the side effects of drugs in use for other purposes. It is usually difficult to make meaningful direct comparisons between species in the reaction to a particular toxin due to differences in experimental protocols, routes of administration, dose of drug, and duration of the study. Rarely is information available about the pharmacokinetics of absorption, distribution, biotransformation, and excretion of drugs in the eye of even one test species, let alone controlled comparative studies in several species. Thus, in many instances we are unable to say that a particular species significantly differs in the type of ocular response to a toxin when compared with another species. There are few examples of well-controlled studies between particular species or strains to demonstrate differences in toxic effects. The varying susceptibilities of different strains of mice to light-induced retinal damage is one example (Naash et al., 1989).

The species of animal that are most commonly used in toxicological and pharmacological studies and thus are most frequently compared to man are the rabbit, rat, cat, dog, and monkey. Little is known of toxic reactions in the eye of other domestic species.

A detailed review of comparative ocular anatomy, histology, physiology, biochemistry, and pharmacology is beyond the scope of this chapter. The reader is referred to appropriate publications in the reference list that cover these aspects in some depth (Gelatt, 1999; Walls, 1942; Duke-Elder, 1958; Prince et al., 1960; Berman, 1991; Davson, 1990; Havener, 1984). Aspects of comparative anatomy and physiology relevant to toxicological studies has recently been reviewed (Wilkie and Wyman, 1991). Other aspects of spontaneous or experimental ocular disease in laboratory animals have been reviewed elsewhere (Bellhorn, 1991; Peiffer et al., 1981).

EYELIDS

The eyelids can be divided into two layers—an outer layer of skin and muscle and an inner layer of fibrous connective tissue lined by the palpebral conjunctiva. The skin is variably pigmented and has hair follicles and associated sebaceous and sweat glands. The fibrous layer of the upper eyelid is especially well developed into a tarsal plate in primates; however, this is poorly developed in other laboratory and domestic species. The perimarginal tarsal plate in all species contains modified sebaceous tarsal or meibomian glands that contribute lipid to the tear film. Several muscles are present in the lids. The orbicularis muscle encircles the margin and closes the lids. The upper lid is elevated primarily by the levator palpebrae superioris muscle with a contribution from the deeper, sympathetically innervated Müller's muscle.

Cilia arising at the lid margins are present in most species but are absent in the cat and only found on the upper eyelid of the dog and horse.

The shape of the palpebral fissure varies among species, being almond shaped in carnivores and man, and more circular in rodents, rabbits, and some subhuman primates. The lids are pigmented in most species, although not in albinos, which may affect the response of the eyelids to toxins.

There are relatively few specific conditions affecting the eyelid that may mimic toxic effects in different species. Drooping of the upper eyelid (ptosis) is reported in man in response to several systemic drugs and toxins (Grant and Schuman, 1993; Fraunfelder and Grove, 1996), and may develop with advancing age in man and occasionally in dogs. In dogs, the ptotic upper eyelid cilia may contact and irritate the cornea (trichiasis). Ptosis of the upper eyelid may be seen in man, cat, and dog as part of Homer's syndrome due to denervation of the sympathetic innervation to the upper eyelid. Sagging of the lower eyelid (ectropion), which may become more marked with age, may be seen in certain canine breeds.

The presence of the third eyelid in laboratory species has been considered a factor that would affect the ocular response to drugs compared with primates by trapping test substances in the conjunctival fornix. Studies in monkeys and rabbits in which the nictitans was removed from the latter do not suggest this to be a significant factor in the differential response to irritants (Buehler and Newmann, 1964), although entrapment may be more of a factor when using viscous formulations of drugs (Durand-Cavagna et al., 1989).

LACRIMAL SYSTEM

The precorneal tear film is secreted by a variety of glands in the eyelids and orbital region in all laboratory and domestic species and man. The lipid portion of tears is secreted by meibomian glands in the fibrous tarsal region of the upper and lower lid, the mucous portion by goblet cells in the conjunctiva. These components of the tear film appear to differ little between species. The major portion of the tear film is made up of an aqueous component that maintains wetting and lubrication of the lids, cornea, and conjunctiva, provides nutrition to and removes waste products from the corneal epithelium and anterior corneal stroma, and provides specific and nonspecific defense mechanisms against infectious disease. This serous portion of the tear film is secreted by the lacrimal gland in most species and by various auxiliary glands in several species. In man and other primates, only a lacrimal gland is present; in dogs and cats, a lacrimal and nictitating membrane occurs. In mice, a harderian gland is found in addition to the lacrimal gland; in rats, there are three lacrimal glands, the intra- and extraorbital glands and a harderian gland, and in rabbits, lacrimal, nictitans, and harderian glands occur. Tear volumes produced vary between the species. In man, 15 μl of tears are produced in 5 min with the stimulus of a Schirmer tear test strip. In dogs, the same volume is produced in 1 min (Wilkie and Wyman, 1991). The tear film turnover rate in rabbits is approximately half that in man despite the presence of three lacrimal glands (Prince, 1964; Hackett and Stern, 1991).

Tears are lost from the ocular surface by evaporation and drainage through the nasolacrimal system. The contact time of tears at the ocular surface may be affected by the rate of production, extent of evaporation, which may be greater in species like rabbits that have protruding eyes and blink infrequently, and the rate of drainage. Drainage may be influenced by the rate of blinking, by the lacrimal pump action of the eyelids, and by the presence of one or two lacrimal puncta (rabbits and pigs have only one punctum; rodents, carnivores, and primates have two). Tear film pH is similar in laboratory species and man, averaging 7.5; however, the pH of the rabbit tear film at 8.2 falls well outside the 6.6 to 7.8 considered the nonirritating range in man (Wilkie and Wyman, 1991; Hackett and Stern, 1991).

Dog and man are species in which a deficiency of the aqueous portion of the tears (keratoconjunctivitis sicca [KCS]) occurs with some frequency. In dogs, the disease may be an autoimmune disorder, and there are particular breeds and families that are more predisposed than others. This may interfere with drug toxicity studies since several drugs, including phenazopyridine and sulfonamides, can result in KCS due to toxic effects on the lacrimal gland (Kaswan and Salisbury, 1990).

In rats, viral sialodacryoadenitis is a common disease. Clinical signs may vary and include exophthalmos, epiphora, and blood staining of the tears and nares, keratoconjunctivitis, iritis, chorioretinitis, and retinal degeneration. These may be confusing in toxicological studies where similar ocular toxic responses are seen. The disease appears at 6 to 12 months of age (Lai et al., 1976; Hunt, 1963; Weissbroth and Peress, 1977).

CONJUNCTIVA AND CORNEA

Despite reported differences in the response of various species to surface irritants, there is no evidence to suggest that these are due to differences in the anatomy or morphology of the conjunctiva or cornea. The relevance of differences in the size, thickness, and curvature of the cornea in different species in responses to surface irritants has not been demonstrated (Wilkie and Wyman, 1991). Similarly, although presumably any differences must reflect interspecies variation in conjunctival and corneal innervation, no comparative studies of the nerve supply or the neuropharmacology exist. It is likely that factors that affect the uveal response of the eye to irritation in various species (see below) may also play some as yet undefined part in variable response of the ocular surface. Comparative studies are needed in particular to determine the ability of the corneal epithelium to resist surface-acting toxins and to examine healing rates of the corneal surface in different species. The corneal endothelium by contrast does vary in its reparative capacity. Endothelial healing capacity is greatest in young animals and in rabbits and to a lesser extent in dogs (Samuelson, 1991).

The cornea varies in thickness in different species as does the number of cell layers in the epithelium. One might speculate that this could affect the resistance of the eye of some species to certain epithelial-damaging toxins or caustic substances, although this is unproven. It has been suggested that the rabbit, which has a thin layer of epithelial cells, would be more sensitive to topically applied irritants since these would penetrate the epithelium more readily than in species such as the cat or dog with thicker layers of epithelial cells (Daston and Freeberg, 1991). However, any differences in sensitivity might lie in pharmacological differences in the cornea or conjunctiva or differences in the density of nerve endings in the epithelium in different species.

Several studies have attempted to compare the sensitivity of the cornea and conjunctiva to ocular irritants (gases, surfactants, or detergents). In one early study, it was concluded that corneal sensitivity declines in the following order: bovine, man, rabbit, dog, and cat (Hellauer, 1950). Various studies have found in comparisons of rabbits, monkeys, and man that the rabbit is the most sensitive species, with monkeys and man showing similar responses to topical detergents and surfactants (Beckley,1965; Beckley et al., 1969). Similar observations of increased ocular sensitivity in rabbits compared with monkeys have been described using surfactants or sodium hydroxide topically (Buehler and Newmann, 1964). One study utilizing surfactants in a number of laboratory species found that the rabbit, hamster, and mouse showed the most sensitivity, followed by the guinea pig and rat, with the dog, cat, rhesus monkey, and chicken showing the least sensitivity (Gersbein and McDonald, 1992). Interestingly, one of these studies found that if the irritant was confined to the rabbit cornea and did not contact the conjunctiva, the degree of ocular irritation was less than when the conjunctiva was also irritated and the degree of response more closely resembled that seen in the monkey. This would suggest that irritation of the conjunctiva plays a significant role in determining the frequently observed sensitivity of the rabbit to ocular toxins (Buehler and Newmann, 1964).

There is also evidence that the rabbit cornea may be more easily traumatized by irritants than other species. Benzalkonium chloride (BAK) 0.01%, when applied to the cornea of the rabbit in a hydroxyethylcellulose vehicle, causes corneal epithelial damage that is not seen in dogs. In part, this may relate to the contact time achieved using a viscous vehicle, since neither BAK nor the vehicle alone causes corneal injury in either species (Durand-Cavagna et al., 1989).

Despite the studies mentioned above, other studies have found that rabbits have a low sensitivity to certain soaps (Gaunt and Harper, 1964), and that the human eye is considerably more sensitive to the riot-control substances dibenzoxazepine (CR) and o-chlorobenzylidine malononitrile (CS) than rabbits, guinea pigs, or rats (Ballantyne and Swanston, 1973; Ballantyne et al., 1974; Ballantyne and Swanston, 1974). It therefore appears that although species differences exist in responses of the cornea and conjunctiva to topically applied toxins, this may be influenced by the type and formulation of toxin used. In general, however, the response of the monkey eye to surface-applied toxins is most similar to that in man.

Little is known of the neural reflexes and inflammatory mediators involved in producing the signs of ocular inflammation observed in the conjunctiva or cornea when toxins are applied to the ocular surface. Even less is known about species differences. As Bito (1984) has pointed out, there are differences in the appearance of perilimbal hyperemia in response to corneal irritation in different species. Some differences may be less real than easy to observe, as in monkeys where the perilimbal conjunctiva may be more difficult to see than in rabbits or rodents because of the narrow primate palpebral fissure and ocular pigmentation in the primate eyelids and uvea. The time course of development of perilimbal hyperemia (involving the conjunctival or episcleral vasculature) in humans after corneal irritation may parallel the time course of development of uveal hyperemia in rabbits associated with blood–aqueous barrier breakdown. Similar axon reflexes with release of neuropeptides and other inflammatory mediators might be involved in causing conjunctival and episcleral hyperemia as are involved in the anterior uvea (see below) (Unger, 1989).

Inflammatory mediators involved in conjunctival vasodilatation that might therefore act as inflammatory mediators released in response to ocular irritation include histamine in man, rabbit, and guinea pig (Eakins and Bhattacherjee, 1977; Abelson, Allansmith, et al., 1980; Abelson, Sofer, et al., 1977; Stock et al., 1990), some arachidonic acid metabolites including certain prostaglandins in the guinea pig (Woodward and Ledgard, 1985b; Woodward et al., 1990), and sulfido-leukotrienes in the guinea pig and hamster (Woodward et al., 1990; Woodward and Ledgard, 1985a; Garceau and Ford-Hutchinson, 1987; Gary et al., 1988). Most studies of conjunctival inflammatory mediators have centered on allergic responses and there is no certainty that the same mediators are involved or are involved to the same extent in toxic reactions of the conjunctiva.

In the cornea, there is evidence that cyclooxygenase and lipoxygenase, products of arachidonic acid metabolism (prostaglandins, hydroperoxy acids, and leukotrienes), are produced in the cornea after cryogenic injury or herpes infections. Although there are suggestions that some of these products may be involved in stimulating polymorphonuclear (PMN) chemotaxis and angiogenesis in the cornea, the exact role of these mediators is largely unresolved (Bazan, 1987; Bazan, Birkle, et al., 1985; Birkle et al., 1986; Srinivasa and Kulkarni, 1980; Benezra, 1978). Platelet activating factor (PAF) is produced in the alkali-burned rabbit cornea (Bazan and Reddy, 1989), and a PAF antagonist will reduce corneal edema, chemotaxis, and activation on PMNs in the alkali-burned cornea (Bazan, Braquet, et al., 1987; Bazan, Sridevi, et al., 1987).

Infiltrates or metabolic by-products have been reported as opacities in the cornea in response to many drugs in various species (Grant, 1986; Fraunfelder and Meyer, 1982). Interpretation of these findings may be complicated in various species by the occurrence of inherited dystrophies and age-related degenerations (Bellhorn, 1991; Kenyon et al., 1986; Cooley and Dice, 1990; Whitley, 1991; Nasisse, 1991; Crispin, 1982). In rodents, spontaneously occurring mineralization and degeneration has been reported. These changes may be inherited or related to environmental factors other than toxins (Bellhorn et al., 1988; Losco and Troup, 1988; Van Winkle and Balk, 1986).

In dogs and cats, various types of corneal dystrophies are known to occur. In most, inheritance is the suspected etiology, and this has been proven in several instances. Epithelial dystrophies may present with epithelial erosions or nonhealing ulcers. These may be initiated by slight trauma to the epithelial surface, which subsequently fails to heal normally. Stromal deposits of lipids are commonly seen as an inherited disease in several canine breeds, including the beagle. The deposits often are arranged in a particular geographic pattern and may develop at particular ages in specific breeds, which may help in differentiating them from toxic reactions in the cornea. Progressively worsening corneal edema and bullous keratopathy occur in several canine breeds due to endothelial dystrophy. Both stromal and endothelial dystrophies causing corneal edema have been described in cats (Cooley and Dice, 1990; Nasisse, 1991). Other deposits occasionally seen include mucopolysaccharides and minerals.

Degenerations of the cornea occur in rodents, cats, and dogs. These present as corneal opacification due to mineral or lipid deposits with or without loss of thickness in the corneal stroma (Bellhorn, 1991; Whitley, 1991).

ANTERIOR UVEAL VASCULAR CHANGES AND THE BLOOD–AQUEOUS BARRIER

The area of the eye that has received the most study in relation to species differences is the anterior uvea, comprising the iris and ciliary body. The eye responds to many physical and noxious chemical stimuli with an acute irritative response that may persist as anterior uveitis if the stimulus persists. It has become apparent that considerable variation exists between different species in these responses determined by anatomical and pharmacological differences of the anterior segment of the eye (Bito, 1984; Unger, 1989).

The ocular irritative response of the eye consists of anterior uveal hyperemia, constriction of the iris sphincter muscle causing a reduction in pupil size (miosis), breakdown of the blood–aqueous barrier (BAB), and a change (usually a rise) in intraocular pressure (Unger, 1989). Later components of ocular inflammation may represent a continuation of these effects as well as cellular infiltration into the anterior segment of the eye.

The irritative response can be induced by many physical (traumatic), thermal, and chemical stimuli. These include trauma to the eye and paracentesis, chemical irritants such as nitrogen mustard (Jampol et al., 1976) and formaldehyde (Butler et al., 1979) applied to the cornea, alkali and acid burns of the cornea, and topically applied potential chemical inflammatory mediators such as prostaglandins and arachidonic acid. The same responses can be achieved by laser and x-ray irradiation of the iris or lens (Unger et al., 1974; Stjernschantz, von Dickhoff, et al., 1986; Bito and Klein,

1981). Clinically important is the effect of bacterial endotoxins (Eakins, 1977). Considerable variation exists between different species in the pharmacology of the components of the ocular irritative response. Aspects of these differences have been reviewed elsewhere (Unger, 1989; Bhattacherjee and Paterson, 1990b; Millichamp and Dziezyc, 1991a).

The rabbit is the species most sensitive to ocular irritation among laboratory and domestic species. The initial irritative response is mediated by a neural reflex arc in the rabbit. Stimulation of the fifth (trigeminal) cranial nerve results in an acute ocular irritative response (Stjernschantz et al., 1979), which is largely due to the release of substance P (SP), calcitonin gene-related peptide (CGRP), and possibly other neuropeptides from trigeminal nerve endings in the anterior uvea (Bill et al., 1979; Stjernschantz et al., 1982). The effects are reduced, but not abolished, by an SP-inhibitor, suggesting that other chemical mediators may be involved (Stjernschantz, von Dickhoff, et al., 1986). Since the cornea and conjunctiva are densely innervated by the fifth cranial nerve, any irritation of these tissues by chemicals is likely to result in an irritative response in this species. The anatomical components of the neural reflex arc are presumed to be similar in most laboratory and domestic animal species, whereas the magnitude of the response varies widely both experimentally and clinically and is probably determined by differences in the morphology of the blood–aqueous barrier, receptor types in the anterior uvea, and mediators released into the anterior uvea in response to trigeminal stimulation.

The blood–aqueous barrier comprises tight junctions between ciliary and iridal epithelial cells and an endothelial barrier in the iridal capillaries. Together, these structures prevent macromolecules from access to the anterior or posterior chambers. Although the basic pattern is similar in most mammals, some anatomical differences exist that might affect the relative sensitivity of the BAB to breakdown. The rabbit, which has the most sensitive BAB, has well-developed iridial portions of the ciliary processes, which appear to be the site of BAB breakdown in this species. By contrast, this region of the ciliary processes is poorly developed in primates with a more stable BAB (Raviola, 1977; Kozart, 1968; Smelser and Pei, 1965; Ohnishi and Tanaka, 1981; Bartels et al., 1979). Additionally the types of intercellular junctions in the iris vary between species. In the rat, cat, and pig most are of the gap–junction type, whereas in man, monkey, and mouse they are tight junctions (Szalay et al., 1991). Protein accumulation in the aqueous, which is a feature of BAB breakdown, occurs because of disruption of the BAB structures in the rabbit (Unger et al., 1975), whereas in primates it rarely occurs in response to acute ocular irritation. Protein entry into the anterior chamber can be achieved in primates after paracentesis of the anterior chamber, but in this situation, which does not closely mimic irritation of the eye by toxins, the flare primarily results from reflux from the iridocorneal angle and Schlemm's canal (Bito, 1984; Bartels et al., 1979; Raviola, 1974). The extent of protein production in the anterior chamber resulting in flare differs considerably between species. Marked flare develops rapidly in rabbits and guinea pigs, more slowly and of lesser magnitude in cats, and not to any measurable extent in owl monkeys and ducks after the topical application of nitrogen mustard to the eye (Klein and Bito, 1983).

The difference in the stability of the BAB in rabbits compared with other species, and especially primates, has been demonstrated with both noxious chemical and physical stimuli applied to the eye and with aqueous loss from the eye (paracentesis). This is, therefore, not a response that is specific for particular toxic stimuli but does vary considerably between species. The sensitivity of the blood–aqueous barrier to breakdown has been hypothesized to correlate with the extent of lateral positioning and exposure of the eyes in the head and thus exposure of the eye to trauma. This varies in the following manner: rabbit > sheep > pig > dog > cat > primates (Bito, 1989b). The rabbit, which has a protruding eye, would be quite likely to sustain damage to the cornea. This species needs an ocular defense mechanism that results in rapid breakdown of the BAB, allowing protein (including fibrin) to enter the anterior chamber to help seal any breach in the cornea until healing can occur. Primates at the other end of the spectrum of BAB reaction have eyes that receive some protection from the bony orbit and are thus less likely to sustain severe injury. Should injury occur in primates, production of large amounts of protein in the anterior chamber would severely limit visual acuity in species that rely heavily upon vision for survival (Bito, 1984).

Calcitonin gene-related peptide is a potent vasodilator in the rabbit and cat, and will break down the BAB when injected into the anterior chamber of the rabbit, but not of the cat (Unger et al., 1985; Oksala and Stjernschantz, 1988a; Oksala, 1988).

Prostaglandins may contribute to anterior uveal vasodilation and BAB disruption in some species. In the rabbit, disruption of the BAB has been detected with intracameral injection of PGE_2 (Bito et al., 1982; Bhattacherjee and Paterson, 1990a). The production of prostaglandins (PGs) in the aqueous humor may parallel BAB disruption in endotoxin-induced inflammation in the rabbit (Bhattacherjee, 1975; Fleisher and McGahan, 1986), although in at least some studies disruption of the barrier in rabbits and rats precedes production of detectable PG concentrations in aqueous (Csukas et al., 1990; Herbort et al., 1988). PGs probably play a significant, although not exclusive, role in disruption of the BAB in dogs as shown by studies using cyclooxygenase-inhibiting drugs to control BAB breakdown (Millichamp and Dziezyc, 1991a; Regnier et al., 1986; Krohne and Vestre, 1987; Millichamp et al., 1991; Dziezyc et al., 1991). PGs are probably less important in disruption of the primate BAB (Unger, 1989; Bito et al., 1989).

Other mediators including platelet activating factor, interleukin-1_α, and tumor necrosis factor (TNF) cause ocular changes that vary with the chemical and include anterior uveal vasodilatation, disruption of the BAB, or protein extravasation into the aqueous in rabbits. Whether these substances are involved in toxic disruption of the BAB in this species or others and how these substances interact with other inflammatory mediators is largely unknown (Verbey et al., 1989; Bussolino et al., 1990; Rubin and Rosenbaum, 1990; Rubin and Rosenbaum, 1988; Rosenbaum et al., 1988; Fleisher et al., 1990).

CELLULAR INFILTRATION INTO THE ANTERIOR CHAMBER

Cellular infiltration into the anterior uvea and subsequently the aqueous is a common feature of spontaneous and experimental inflammatory disease. Cellular infiltration into the anterior uvea and aqueous may differ in magnitude in different species in much the same manner as BAB breakdown. The pharmacology of chemotaxis of polymorphonuclear leukocytes into the aqueous appears similar in several species studied. In at least rabbits, guinea pigs, and cats, leukotriene B4 (LTB4) injected into the anterior chamber causes marked PMN chemotaxis (Bhattacherjee and Paterson, 1990a; Bhattacherjee et al., 1980; Bhattacherjee, Hammond, et al., 1981; Stjernschantz, Sherk, et al., 1984). In rabbits and rats, the appearance of PMNs in endotoxin uveitis appears to parallel the rise of LTB4 concentrations in the aqueous (Csukas et al., 1990; Herbort et al., 1988). In rabbits, interleukin-1, interleukin-1$_\alpha$, and TNF may cause cellular infiltration (Rubin and Rosenbaum, 1988; Rosenbaum et al., 1988; Fleisher et al., 1990; Bhattacherjee and Henderson, 1987; Kulkarni and Srinivasan, 1988). The role of these mediators in other species is as yet undetermined.

MIOSIS

Constriction of the pupil (miosis) is a characteristic feature of acute ocular irritation and prolonged uveitis in many species. Miosis may be considered an undesirable toxic side effect of various ocular medications in man. For instance, cholinergic drugs (pilocarpine, demecarium bromide) used in glaucoma therapy result in miosis and painful ciliary spasm (Havener, 1966). In evaluating new prostaglandin analogues for glaucoma therapy, an important consideration has been to develop drugs that reduce intraocular pressure without causing toxic side effects including miosis, disruption of the blood–aqueous barrier, and reduced uveoscleral outflow due to ciliary muscle contraction (Bito, 1989a).

Miosis results from contraction of the iris sphincter muscle located around the free margin of the iris. The two major iris muscles are the circular sphincter muscle and the radial dilator muscle. In mammals, the sphincter muscle is a smooth-muscle type with muscarinic cholinergic receptors (unlike lower vertebrates, such as birds and reptiles, where the sphincter has nicotinic cholinergic receptors). There are very considerable differences between vertebrate species in the pharmacology of miosis in response to ocular irritation.

Nitrogen mustard applied to the eyes causes miosis in the rabbit, cat, and owl monkey, but not the guinea pig or duck (Klein and Bito, 1983; Camras and Bito, 1980a,b). Additionally miosis in the cat and to a lesser extent the rabbit is reduced by pretreatment with indomethacin, although this has no effect on miosis in the owl monkey. These observations underlie the very complex differences between various species in the response of the iris sphincter muscle to particular toxic substances that irritate the eye. It seems clear, however, that as with disruption of the BAB, miosis is a nonspecific response of the eye caused by neurotransmitters, neuromodulators, or inflammatory agents released or synthesized in ocular tissues in response to trauma or chemical or physical irritation. Although we are far from a complete understanding of the various interactions between inflammatory mediators that result in irritation-induced miosis, evidence from both in vitro and in vivo experiments is accumulating that suggests interspecies differences in the sensitivity of the iris sphincter to various mediators, in part reflecting species differences in either the presence or density of chemical receptors (Tachado et al., 1991).

The early literature of miosis studied the effects of noxious substances applied to or injected into the eye. Extracts of rabbit, cat, or dog iris with prostaglandin-like activity contracted smooth muscle (Ambache, 1957; Ambache et al., 1965, 1990). PG-like activity was occasionally measured in the aqueous humor at the time miosis was observed, and prostaglandins injected into the eyes of rabbits and cats apparently caused miosis (Eakins et al., 1972; Waitzman and King, 1967; Beitch and Eakins, 1969). Prostaglandins thus became early candidates as mediators of the miotic response. It is now known that miosis is a result of complex interactions that probably involve at least acetylcholine, neuropeptides (particularly the neurotransmitter substance P), norepinephrine, and products of arachidonic acid metabolism (prostaglandins and leukotrienes).

Prostaglandin $F_{2\alpha}$ contracts the iris sphincter muscle in the cow, dog, and cat but not man, pig, or rabbit, whereas PGA_2 causes iris sphincter contraction in the cow and pig, but not man, cat, dog, or rabbit. Among these species, leukotriene D_4 contracts the iris sphincter only in the cow and cat (Yousufzai et al., 1988, 1990). Similarly, in vivo it appears that $PGF_{2\alpha}$ causes miosis when applied topically or injected intracamerally into the canine or feline eye. The bovine iris sphincter muscle is also contracted by PGA_2, PGE_2, and PGE_1. The feline eye is less sensitive to miotic effects of PGE_2 (Bito, Draga, et al., 1983; Bito et al., 1987; Miranda and Bito, 1989). The rabbit pupil is not significantly constricted by prostaglandins (Bito et al., 1982; Kulkarni and Srinivasan, 1982) and, in early studies that suggested otherwise, miosis may have resulted from ocular cannulation or PG-induced release of other mediators, notably neuropeptides from nerve endings of the trigeminal nerve in the uvea (Miranda and Bito, 1989; Unger and Butler, 1988). In vitro studies in the rat also suggest that, although there is no direct miotic effect of PGs, they may cause the release of other sphincter-contracting mediators (Hayashi et al., 1986). In nonhuman primates, $PGF_{2\alpha}$ has either no miotic effect or one that is very slight (Camras et al., 1987; Crawford et al., 1987; Lee et al., 1984). Although miosis has been reported in human eyes in response to topical PGs, there is also evidence that suggests that PGs have little miotic effect in man (Miranda and Bito, 1989; Camras and Miranda, 1989).

Substance P (SP) is present in the uveal tract of several mammalian species. It contracts the iris sphincter muscle in the rabbit, cow, and pig (Soloway et al., 1981; Unger and Tighe, 1984) but not in the cat, dog, or baboon (Unger and Tighe, 1984; Abdel-Latif et al., 1990). In man SP has variable effects, and although alone it does not appear to contract the iris sphincter (Unger and Tighe, 1984), contraction may occur in the presence of an enkephalinase inhibitor, suggesting that the peptide enkephalinase may regulate SP-induced iris sphincter contraction in man (Anderson et al., 1989).

The differences in response of the iris sphincter muscle may reflect the action of these various mediators via specific receptors on second messenger systems in the smooth muscle, which appears to be species dependent. Two second messenger systems are present in the iris sphincter—one involving production of inositol triphosphate (IP3) in the muscle cell, the other production of adenosine 3′,5′-cyclic monophosphate (cAMP). IP3 production mobilizes calcium and causes muscle contraction by myosin light chain (MLC) phosphorylation; cAMP inhibits MLC phosphorylation and thus tends to relax the muscle. Acetylcholine stimulates muscarinic receptors and causes IP3 production in all mammalian iridal sphincter muscles so far tested, thus causing contraction. The differential effects of other agonist or inflammatory mediators on either receptor or second messenger system will determine whether the muscle contracts or relaxes (Yousufzai et al., 1988). Thus, in considering effects of drugs on the pupil only muscarinic cholinergic drugs, inhibitors of their production, or specific receptor antagonists can be expected to universally affect most mammalian species in a similar fashion. The other mediators listed above that cause iris sphincter contraction are also associated with production of IP3 in the muscle cell (Tachado et al., 1991; Yousufzai et al., 1988, 1990; Abdel-Latif et al., 1990), and the variability in receptor and second messenger types among different species will affect the pupil response to particular toxins.

CHANGES IN INTRAOCULAR PRESSURE

Nitrogen mustard applied to the eyes of rabbits, guinea pigs, and cats causes an acute rise of intraocular pressure (IOP), which is biphasic during the first 24 hr in the first two species. A small increase in IOP is also seen in ducks, but not in owl monkeys. These changes in IOP are variably affected by indomethacin, suggesting that prostanoids play at least some role in regulating the changes in IOP in these species, although the exact nature of their involvement differs between species (Klein and Bito, 1983; Camras and Bito, 1980a,b). The rise of IOP is probably not specific for topically applied ocular toxins since similar changes occur in rabbits and dogs following laser damage of the iris or lens (Stjernschantz, von Dickhoff, et al., 1986; Millichamp et al., 1991).

The variation in IOP change in different species probably reflects differences in the mechanisms of aqueous production, anatomy of the anterior uveal vasculature, and aqueous outflow anatomy and pharmacology. The increase in IOP after Nd:YAG lasing of the eye is probably due to increased ocular blood flow causing an increase in the fluid volume of the ciliary processes, increased ultrafiltration of aqueous, and an influx of extravasate into the eye associated with disruption of the blood–aqueous barrier (BAB) (Unger, 1989). Additionally, later in ocular inflammation, the trabecular meshwork of the iridocorneal angle becomes swollen, and protein entering the eye due to disruption of the BAB and inflammatory cells entering the aqueous from the uvea may block outflow through the trabecular meshwork. Subsequent changes in the IOP may reflect the morphological and pharmacological differences in aqueous outflow. In toxicology studies, the effects of drugs on the outflow of aqueous may vary between species.

The outflow of aqueous from the eye is via one of two routes: (a) the conventional or iridocorneal outflow, namely the trabecular meshwork, and some form of scleral venous plexus and aqueous veins into the general venous circulation (Samuelson, 1991); and (b) the uveoscleral route across the iris root and anterior face of the ciliary muscle, between the ciliary muscle bundles, into the suprachoroidal space and out through the sclera (Bill, 1975; Barrie et al., 1985). Differences in the anatomy of the iridocorneal angle exist between the various mammalian species used in experimental studies (Tripathi, 1974).

The relative contribution of these two outflow pathways vary between species, with the uveoscleral accounting for 30% to 65% in nonhuman primates, 13% in rabbits, 3% in cats, 15% in dogs, and 4% to 14% in man (Samuelson, 1991).

It has been speculated that increases in IOP associated with obstruction of iridocorneal outflow in ocular inflammation may be minimized by increasing uveoscleral outflow (Kaufman et al., 1989). The effects of drugs on the IOP must thus be weighed both against the relative contributions of the outflow pathways in different species and the normal pharmacological control of IOP via the two main outflow routes. For instance, $PGF_{2\alpha}$ and its analogues are known to lower IOP in several mammalian species, including the dog, cat, subhuman primates, man, and rabbit, acting primarily by increasing uveoscleral outflow. This effect can be markedly reduced in the dog by cyclooxygenase inhibitors, which reduce PG production in the irritated eye (Millichamp et al., 1991; Millichamp and Dziezyc, 1991b). PGE_2 injected intracamerally will markedly elevate IOP in the rabbit (presumably by increasing uveal vasodilation and disrupting the BAB), but only slightly in monkeys and cats, and in the latter species only with much higher doses than used in the rabbit (Eakins, 1970; Kelly and Starr, 1971). It is possible that in other species drugs that affect PG production may have quantitatively different effects on IOP depending on the uveoscleral contribution to outflow.

Other species differences in IOP regulation in the irritated eye will be determined by other inflammatory mediators released. CGRP is released from trigeminal nerve endings in rabbits in response to ocular irritation (Wahlestedt et al., 1985). CGRP injected into the rabbit eye causes vasodilatation, breakdown of the BAB, and a rise in IOP. Conversely, CGRP injected into the feline eye causes a fall in IOP possibly by increasing outflow facility from the eye (Oksala and Stjernschantz, 1988b). Platelet activating factor applied topically to rabbit eyes also increases IOP, an effect that can be abolished with a PAF receptor antagonist, although no studies have been reported using PAF in other species.

Changes in IOP in response to drugs applied to the eye or given systemically might be affected by the existence or predisposition of existing glaucoma or an anatomical predisposition to develop elevated IOP. Species in which spontaneous, inherited glaucoma occurs include man, dogs, and rabbits. Glaucoma as a primary disease is by contrast very rare in rodents, subhuman primates, and cats, although it may occur secondary to intraocular inflammation (Bellhorn, 1991). In man, the most common form of glaucoma is the chronic, open-angle type. Although this type occurs in some breeds of dog, including beagle, narrow-angle glaucoma is also commonly encountered in this species (Gelatt, 1991a). In New Zealand white rabbits, a recessively inherited glaucoma has been described similar to congenital glaucoma in man due to an abnormally developed anterior chamber angle (Hanna et al., 1963). Dogs and rabbits should be screened for normal IOP and undergo gonioscopic examination of the iridocorneal angle in any studies where drugs might affect IOP.

AQUEOUS HUMOR

The aqueous humor is secreted and drained at equal rates. These are similar for most animals studied, but are highest in cats. Intraocular pressures show slight variations in the different species (Gum, 1991). The biochemical composition of the aqueous humor is generally similar to plasma but with low concentrations of protein. The aqueous is made up of electrolytes, glucose, oxygen, amino acids protein, immunoglobulin, ascorbate, urea, and lactate. Concentrations are similar in most mammals and have been reviewed by Wilkie and Wyman (1991). Amino acid transport systems present in rabbits may be missing in primates, cats, and dogs. Little is known of changes in aqueous humor composition except increased protein concentration in response to toxins.

LENS

The most frequent toxic reaction of the lens is the development of cataracts. Cataracts have been seen in most of the laboratory species, although often the etiology is undetermined. Numerous examples of toxic cataracts are known in many species of animal; however, there is little evidence that any particular species is more prone to develop toxic cataracts than any other (Grant and Schuman, 1993). Some species may be less likely overall to develop cataracts than others, however, and presumably differences in lens biochemistry may account for this. For instance, cataracts of any form are seen less frequently in cats than in dogs, and cats are very rarely affected with diabetic cataracts. The time period required for the lens to develop cataractous change may vary between species with any particular toxin, making direct comparisons difficult (Barnett and Noel, 1968). Differences between species in the development of cataracts may reflect postnatal lens growth. For instance, the lens in dogs and humans continues to grow throughout adult life, whereas the bovine, rabbit, and rat lens changes little in size. Variations in specific sensitivity to cataract development may also reflect differences in lens metabolism and differences in the chemical composition of the lens in different species (Wilkie and Wyman, 1991; van Heyningen, 1976).

Normal variations in the appearance of the lens may be confused with toxic changes, at least in rodents and dogs. The suture lines in dogs, cats, and man have a Y-shaped appearance. In dogs, during the first few months of life, the suture lines may be very prominent and, although this may be less so at a year of age, the posterior sutures may again appear during the second year of life (Bellhorn, 1991). This may be confused with either inherited or toxic cataracts involving the lens sutures.

Inherited cataracts are seen most commonly in dogs and rodents. In rats, cataracts at various locations have been associated with aging (Taradach et al., 1981; Balazs et al., 1970). The incidence of unilateral posterior lens opacities in normal laboratory rats is surprisingly high (5% to 10%) and may increase with age (Bellhorn, 1991). Many opacities in the rat lens appear in the posterior cortex, which may also be the site of development of toxic cataract. Animals must be screened before the study to rule out the presence of any preexisting lesions. Rodents under anesthesia may develop lens opacities of the anterior lens cortex. This may be due to aqueous dehydration or cooling and is reversible when blinking is resumed (Fraunfelder and Burns, 1966). Various inherited cataracts have been described in certain strains of mice, which may become apparent in early postnatal life or in adult animals, depending upon the strain of mouse (Kador et al., 1980; Kuck et al., 1981; Russell et al., 1977).

In dogs, the most common cause of cataracts is inheritance, and a considerable number of different types of cataracts have been reported in particular breeds (Gelatt, 1991b). In some the appearance of the cataract and age of onset are characteristic enough to imply an inherited etiology: for instance, the posterior polar subcapsular cataracts seen in the Labrador or golden retriever at 6 to 8 months of age (Curtis and Barnett, 1989). In other breeds, the appearance and age of onset are not characteristic for inherited cataract, although the frequency with which cataracts occur in the breed would be sufficient to suggest an inherited etiology: for instance, cortical cataracts in the American cocker spaniel (Yakely, 1978). An average incidence of 3.7% of beagles in a research colony were found to have some unilateral or bilateral lens opacities (Rubin, 1989).

RETINA AND CHOROID

Various differences in the anatomy of the retina and choroid in domestic and laboratory species are likely to affect the response of the retina and choroid to toxic injury.

The choroid in several species is modified anteriorly to form a tapetum lucidum. In the dog, cat, and ferret, this is formed by a layer of cells containing electron-dense rods. In horses and other ungulates, the layer is fibrous, comprising layers of collagen. Biochemically, the tapetum varies between species, also. In the cat, the tapetal rods have a high concentration of riboflavin, whereas in the dog and ferret, tapetum has a high concentration of zinc and cysteine (Samuelson, 1991). The tapetum may vary in color, as seen ophthalmoscopically between and within any species and with the age of the animal (Rubin, 1974). This may be significant in toxicity studies since there are drugs, such as ethambutol, that can also cause color changes in the tapetum (Rubin, 1974). An inherited tapetal degeneration has been reported in the beagle (Bellhorn et al., 1975).

The vasculature of the choroid and retina differ between species. In primates the arterial supply to the retina is via a central retinal artery. In other species with retinal vasculature, the retinal arterial supply is via the short posterior ciliary arteries forming cilioretinal arteries. Various retinal patterns are present in mammals: holangiotic vasculature in primates, cats, dogs, rodents, and cattle arises from the central retinal arteries or cilioretinal vessels and extends into the inner retinal layers throughout the retina; merangiotic vasculature arises from cilioretinal vessels and radiates into the horizontal quadrants of the retina; paurangiotic vessels are small and numerous and radiate only a small distance from the optic nerve into the retina; the anangiotic pattern is a retina that lacks blood vessels. The relative contribution of the underlying choroid to retinal nutrition depends upon the extent of retinal vascularization. Animals with minimal retinal vascularization have thinner retinas to facilitate diffusion of nutrients and waste products from the choroid (Wilkie and Wyman, 1991).

Primates possess an area of especially high cone density in the retina—the fovea centralis, which lacks rod photoreceptors and blood vessels. Carnivores have a comparable area of increased cone density temporal to the optic disc.

Retinal degeneration occurs commonly in several laboratory species and man, although very rarely in any other primates. Retinal degeneration may be inherited, age or environment related, or due to nutritional deficiencies. These various etiologies should be recognized as potential causes of retinal atrophy in animals that will be used for any long-term toxicological studies. Inherited retinal degenerations occur in many breeds of dog, cats, rats, and mice. Inherited degenerations can primarily involve the retinal pigment epithelium (RPE) or the neural retina and may develop as disease in early postnatal life and progress rapidly or later in adult animals with slower progression. Most inherited retinal degenerations affect the rod photoreceptors initially and then progress to involve the cones, and ultimately the remaining retinal neurons.

In man, several different types of retinal dystrophy or degeneration have been reported. Some of these have an inherited basis; others are associated with other systemic and metabolic diseases (Weleber, 1989; Bateman et al., 1989).

In the dog and mouse, various primary retinal degenerations involve the photoreceptors. Early-onset retinal degenerations (photoreceptor dysplasia) may vary between breeds or strains in the inheritance locus and biochemical defects involved. Where biochemical abnormalities are known in dogs and rodents, they have been shown to involve the guanosine $3', 5'$-cyclic monophosphate (cGMP) phosphodiesterase involved in visual transduction (Millichamp, 1990; Lee et al., 1985; Woodford et al., 1982). Late-onset retinal degenerations in dogs, which are similar to some forms of inherited retinitis pigmentosa in man, involve the same gene locus in several different breeds (Aguirre and Acland, 1988). Abnormalities of photoreceptor membrane lipids have been detected in some poodles with late-onset retinal degeneration (Wetzel et al., 1989). Similar inherited retinal degenerations are also seen in the cat (Barnett and Curtis, 1985; Narfstrom, 1985).

Retinal degeneration associated with a retinal pigment epithelial dystrophy is also seen in the dog. The diseased RPE accumulates lipopigment, and the neural retina subsequently undergoes slow degeneration (Aguirre and Laties, 1976).

Photoreceptor dysplasia also occurs in mice. As in the dog, these are diseases seen in young animals with rapid progression. The best characterized are the rd and rds strains (Sanyal et al., 1980; Sidman and Green, 1965).

Retinal degenerations have also been reported in the rat. The best documented degeneration is seen in the RCS rat. The disease is a primary retinal pigment epitheliopathy. Failure of the RPE to phagocytose shed photoreceptor outer segments results in accumulation of membranous debris between retina and RPE and subsequent retinal atrophy in the early postnatal period (Dowling and Sidman, 1962). Retinal degenerations have occasionally been reported in other strains of rat that may not be inherited. Defining the etiology of retinal degeneration in this species can be problematic since degenerations associated with old age and exposure to high light levels have also been reported (Bellhorn, 1991).

Phototoxic retinal degeneration may influence the interpretation of toxicologic studies in rodents. Rats and mice are particularly sensitive to light-induced retinal degeneration. In part, this may be due to the prevalence of studies performed in albino strains of these species. Various other factors influencing the rate and severity of light-induced degeneration include the use of mydriatics, age (older animals are more susceptible), sex (females are more susceptible), environmental temperature (retinal degeneration proceeds more rapidly at higher temperatures), and maintenance of the animals on a continuous rather than cyclic lighting regime (Naash et al., 1989; Bellhorn, 1991; Noell et al., 1966; O'Steen et al., 1974).

Other retinal degenerations that may be confused with toxic reactions in the retina of laboratory species include nutritional retinal degeneration due to taurine deficiency in cats (Hayes and Carey, 1975) and vitamin E deficiency in dogs (Riis et al., 1981).

OCULAR ALBINISM

The presence or lack of pigment in the eye may have various effects on the response of the eye to toxins. This becomes significant in that albinism is an inherited trait in several mammalian species, and particularly in some that are routinely used in laboratory studies.

Albinism is inherited in man and among species used for toxicity experiments— rats, mice, and rabbits. Although true, complete albinism does not occur in the dog, cat, or other domestic species, reduced ocular pigmentation does occur in certain breeds and lines. Since albino rabbits and rats are commonly used for testing potentially toxic drugs, it is important to ask whether the lack of pigment will affect the type of reaction that might be expected in man, a species that usually has a well-pigmented eye.

Rubin (1990) has recently thoroughly reviewed the significance of ocular pigmentation in ocular toxicity testing. A lack of melanin pigment has been associated with reduced visual performance in man (Creel et al., 1978), and physiological differences have been observed in experimental animals (Rubin, 1990). For instance, in albino rabbits, mice, and rats, dark adaptation thresholds are higher than in their pigmented counterparts (Balkema, 1988), and albino rats and rabbits lack an electroretinographic c-wave (Weidner, 1976; Graves et al., 1985; Dodt and Echte, 1961; Reuter, 1974).

Toxicological studies on the retina and orbital glands in albino rodents can be affected by the increased sensitivity of the retina in albinos to light-induced degeneration (Williams et al., 1985; Reiter, 1973). Additionally, the effects of aging-related retinal degeneration is more pronounced in albino rats than in pigmented strains (Weisse et al., 1990).

It is known that certain chemicals can be absorbed by pigment and therefore accumulate in pigmented ocular tissues (Potts, 1964; Havener, 1983). This accumulation of chemical in the eye may predispose the pigmented ocular tissue to more injurious effects from the chemical than in nonpigmented albino strains. Various possible effects of the presence or lack of pigment on ocular reactions to chemicals as outlined below are suggested by Rubin (1990).

The albino animal may be more susceptible to chemical toxicity than pigmented animals. For instance, retinal degeneration occurs in albino but not pigmented rats given vinyl δ-aminobutyric acid (GABA) (Butler et al., 1987). Conversely, pigmented animals may be more susceptible to toxic injury than albinos. Pigmented rats are more susceptible to naphthalene cataracts since they possess enzymes required for cataract development that are lacking in albino rats. Uveal degeneration and ocular phthisis has been seen in pigmented rats but not in albinos administered a herbicide (Rubin, 1990).

Although some chemicals may be accumulated in pigmented ocular tissues, toxicity may occur regardless of whether pigment is present or not and also may affect nonpigmented parts of the eye. This is the case with amopyroquin, which causes retinal degeneration in pigmented dogs and albino rats (Kurtz et al., 1967) and in chloroquine-and chlorpromazine-induced keratopathies (Francois and Maudgal, 1965; Rubin et al., 1970).

Finally, there are examples where, despite accumulation of chemicals in pigmented tissue, no ocular toxic reactions are detected in either pigmented or albino animals. This is true for certain antimalarials (Kuhn et al., 1981), beta blockers (Poynter et al., 1976), and certain other drugs in clinical use (Howard et al., 1969).

To avoid the effects of pigmentation or its absence on toxicological studies, it is essential to use both pigmented and albino strains of the test species wherever possible.

There are many unresolved issues in comparative toxicology of the eye. It is obvious that, ideally, studies of ocular drug reactions should be performed in the species to which the information will be most relevantly applied in the clinical setting. Since the primate appears to react like man in most respects, it would seem to be a logical choice as an experimental model for toxicological and drug side effects studies. However, there are considerable ethical and cost considerations in using primates in toxicological research, at least in part due to the often precarious status of many primate species in the wild.

The use of rodents and rabbits should continue to be the mainstay of toxicological research whenever possible. Use of dogs and cats, however, may be considered when the results are applicable to the clinical veterinary situation.

REFERENCES

Abdel-Latif, A.A., Yousufzai, S.Y.K., and Tachado, S.D. 1990. Differential effects of $PGF_2\alpha$, PGA_2, LTD_4, and substance P on formation of cAMP and IP_3 and on contraction in iris sphincters of different mammalian species. *Investigative Ophthalmology and Visual Science* 31(suppl):247.

Abelson, M.B., Allansmith, M.R., and Friedlander, M.H. 1980. Effects of topically applied decongestant and antihistamine. *American Journal of Ophthalmology* 90:254–257.

Abelson, M.B., Soter, N.A., Simon, M.A., Dohlman, J., and Allansmith, M.R. 1977. Histamine in human tears. *American Journal of Ophthalmology* 83:417–418.

Aguirre, G.D., and Acland, G.M. 1988. Variation in retinal degeneration phenotype inherited at the prcd locus. *Experimental Eye Research* 46:663–687.

Aguirre, G.D., and Laties, A. 1976. Pigment epithelial dystrophy in the dog. *Experimental Eye Research* 23:247–256.

Ambache, N. 1957. Properties of irin, a physiological constituent of the rabbit's eye. *Journal of Physiology* 135:114–132.

Ambache, N., Kavanagh, L., and Whiting, J. 1965. Effect of mechanical stimulation on rabbits' eyes: release of active substance in anterior chamber perfusates. *Journal of Physiology* 176:378–408.

Ambache, N., Kavanagh, L., and Whiting, J. 1990. Some differences in uveal reactions between cats and rabbits. *Journal of Physiology* 182:110–130.

Anderson, J.A., Malfroy, B., Richard, N.R., Hernandez, E.V., Lucas, C., and Binder, P.S. 1989. Substance P contracts the human iris sphincter, a response regulated by endogenous enkephalinase. *Investigative Ophthalmology and Visual Science* 30(suppl):269.

Balazs, T., Ohtake, S., and Noble, J.F. 1970. Spontaneous lenticular changes in the rat. *Laboratory Animal Science* 20:215.

Balkema, G.W. 1988. Elevated dark-adapted thresholds in albino rodents. *Investigative Ophthalmology and Visual Science* 29:544–549.

Ballantyne, B., Gazzard, M.F., et al. 1974. Ophthalmic toxicology of *o*-chlorobenzylidene malononitrile (CS). *Archives of Toxicology* 32:149–168.

Ballantyne, B., and Swanston, D.W. 1973. The irritant potential of dilute solutions of ortho-chlorobenzylidene malononitrile (CS) on the eye and tongue. *Acta Pharmacology and Toxicology* 32:266–277.

Ballantyne, B., and Swanston, D.W. 1974. The irritant effects of dilute solutions dibenzoxazepine (CR) on the eye and tongue. *Acta Pharmacology and Toxicology* 35:412–423.

Barnett, K.C., and Curtis, R. 1985. Autosomal dominant progressive retinal atrophy in Abyssinian cats. *Journal of Heredity* 76:168–170.

Barnett, K.C., and Noel, P.R.B. 1968. The eye in general toxicity studies. In *Evaluation of Drug Effects on the Eye*, ed. P.V. Piggot, pp. 23–31. London: F.J. Parsons.

Barrie, K.P., Gum, G.G., and Gelatt, K.N. 1985. Morphological studies of uveoscleral outflow in normotensive and glaucomatous beagles with fluorescein labeled dextran. *American Journal of Veterinary Research* 46:89–97.

Bartels, S.P., Pederson, J.E., Gaasterland, D.E., and Armaly, M.F. 1979. Sites of breakdown of the blood aqueous barrier after paracentesis of the rhesus monkey eye. *Investigative Ophthalmology and Visual Science* 18:1050–1060.

Bateman, J.B., Lang, G.E., and Maumenee, I.H. 1989. Genetic metabolic disorders associated with retinal degenerations/dystrophies. In *Retina*, vol. 1, eds. S.J. Ryan and T.E. Ogden, pp. 421–445. St. Louis: C.V. Mosby.

Bazan, H.E.P. 1987. Corneal injury alters eicosanoid formation in the rabbit anterior segment in vivo. *Investigative Ophthalmology and Visual Science* 28:314–319.

Bazan, H.E.P., Birkle, D.L., Beuerman, R.W., and Bazan, N.G. 1985. Inflammation-induced stimulation of the synthesis of prostaglandins and lipoxygenase-reaction products in rabbit cornea. *Current Eye Research* 4:175–179.

Bazan, H.E.P., Braquet, P., Reddy, S.T.K., and Bazan, N.G. 1987. Inhibition of the alkali burn-induced lipoxygenation of arachidonic acid in the rabbit cornea in vivo by a platelet activating factor antagonist. *Journal of Ocular Pharmacology* 3:357–365.

Bazan, H.E.P., and Reddy, S.T.K. 1989. Production of platelet-activating factor (PAF) in the cornea after stimulation. *Investigative Ophthalmology and Visual Science* 30(suppl):404.

Bazan, H.E.P., Sridevi, T.K., Woodland, J.M., and Bazan, N.G. 1987. The accumulation of platelet activating factor in the injured cornea may be interrelated with the synthesis of lipoxygenase products. *Biochemistry/Biophysics Research Communication* 149:915–920.

Beckley, J.H. 1965. Comparative eye testing: man vs. animal. *Toxicology and Applied Pharmacology* 7:93–101.

Beckley, J.H., Russell, T.J., and Rubin, L.F. 1969. Use of the rhesus monkey for predicting human response to eye irritants. *Toxicology and Applied Pharmacology* 15:1–9.

Beitch, B.R., and Eakins, K.E. 1969. The effects of prostaglandins on the intraocular pressure of the rabbit. *British Journal of Pharmacology* 37:158–167.

Bellhorn, R.W. 1991. Laboratory animal ophthalmology. In *Veterinary Ophthalmology*, 2nd ed., ed. K.N. Gelatt, pp. 656–679. Philadelphia: Lea & Febiger.

Bellhorn, R.W., Bellhorn, M.B., Swarm, R.L., and Impellizzeri, C.W. 1975. Hereditary tapetal abnormality in the beagle. *Ophthalmic Research* 7:250–260.

Bellhorn, R.W., Korte, G.E., and Abrutyn, D. 1988. Spontaneous corneal degeneration in the rat. *Laboratory Animal Sciences* 38:46–50.

Benezra, D. 1978. Neovasculogenic ability of prostaglandins, growth factors and synthetic chemoattractants. *American Journal of Ophthalmology* 86:455–461.

Berman, E.R. 1991. *Biochemistry of the Eye*. New York: Plenum Press.

Bhattacherjee, P. 1975. Release of prostaglandin-like substances by *Shigella* endotoxin and its inhibition by nonsteroidal anti-inflammatory compounds. *British Journal of Pharmacology* 54:489–494.

Bhattacherjee, P., and Henderson, B. 1987. Ocular responses to interleukin-1 injected into the anterior chamber of the rabbit. *Investigative Ophthalmology and Visual Science* 28(suppl):200.

Bhattacherjee, P., and Paterson, C.A. 1990a. Further investigation into the ocular effects of prostaglandin E_2, leukotriene B_4 and formyl-methionyl-leucyl phenylalanine. *Experimental Eye Research* 51:93–96.

Bhattacherjee, P., and Paterson, C.A. 1990b. Inflammatory mediators in models of immunogenic and non-immunogenic inflammation of the anterior segment of the eye. In *Lipid Mediators in Eye Inflammation*, ed. N.G. Bazan, pp. 65–82. Basel: Karger.

Bhattacherjee, P., Eakins, K.E., and Hammond, B. 1980. Chemotactic activity of arachidonic acid lipoxygenase products in the rabbit eye. *British Journal of Pharmacology* 73:254P–255P.

Bhattacherjee, P., Hammond, B., Salmon, J.A., Stepney, R., and Eakins, K.E. 1981. Chemotactic response to some arachidonic acid lipoxygenase products in the rabbit eye. *European Journal of Pharmacology* 73:21–28.

Bill, A. 1975. Blood circulation and fluid dynamics in the eye. *Pharmacology Review* 55:383–417.

Bill, A., Stjernschantz, J., Mandahl, A., Brodin, E., and Nilsson, G. 1979. Substance P: release on trigeminal nerve stimulation effects in the eye. *Acta Physiology Scandinavia* 106:371–373.

Birkle, D.L., Sanitiato, J.J., Kaufman, H.E., and Bazan, N.G. 1986. Arachidonic acid metabolism to eicosanoids in herpes virus–infected rabbit cornea. *Investigative Ophthalmology and Visual Science* 27:1443–1446.

Bito, L.Z. 1984. Species differences in the responses of the eye to irritation and trauma: a hypothesis of divergence in ocular defense mechanisms, and the choice of experimental animals for eye research. *Experimental Eye Research* 39:807–829.

Bito, L.Z. 1989a. A physiologic approach to the development of new drugs for glaucoma. *Ophthalmology Clinics of North America* 2:65–76.

Bito, L.Z. 1989b. A physiological approach to glaucoma management: the use of local hormones and the pharmacokinetics of prostaglandin esters. *Progressive Clinical Biological Research* 312:329–347.

Bito, L.Z., and Klein, E.M. 1981. The unique sensitivity of the rabbit eye to x-ray-induced ocular inflammation. *Experimental Eye Research* 33:403–412.

Bito, L.Z., Baroody, R.A., and Miranda, O.C. 1987. Eicosanoids as a new class of ocular hypotensive agents 1. The apparent therapeutic advantages of derived prostaglandins of the A and B type as compared with primary prostaglandins on the E, F, and D type. *Experimental Eye Research* 44:825–837.

Bito, L.Z., Camras, C.B., Gum, G.G., and Resul, B. 1989. The ocular hypotensive effects and side effects of prostaglandins on the eyes of experimental animals. *Progressive Clinical Biological Research* 312:349–365.

Bito, L.Z., Draga, A., Blanco, J., and Camras, C.B. 1983. Long-term maintenance of reduced intraocular pressure by daily or twice daily topical application of prostaglandins to cat or rhesus monkey eyes. *Investigative Ophthalmology and Visual Science* 24:312–319.

Bito, L.Z., Nichols, P.R., and Baroody, R.A. 1982. A comparison of the miotic and inflammatory effects of biologically active polypeptides and prostaglandin E_2 on the rabbit eye. *Experimental Eye Research* 34:325–337.

Buehler, E.V., and Newmann, E.A. 1964. A comparison of eye irritation in monkeys and rabbits. *Toxicology and Applied Pharmacology* 6:701–710.

Bussolino, F., Carenini, A.B., Carenini, B.B., and Arese, P. 1990. Platelet-activating factor and cytokines mediate and amplify the inflammatory response at site of microvascular injury. In *Lipid Mediators in Eye Inflammation*, ed. N.G. Bazan, pp. 130–148. Basel: Karger.

Butler, J.M., Unger, W.G., and Hammond, B.R. 1979. Sensory mediation of the ocular response to neutral formaldehyde. *Experimental Eye Research* 28:577–589.

Butler, W.H., Ford, G.P., and Newberne, J.W. 1987. A study of the effects of vigabrabin on the central nervous system and retina of Sprague Dawley and Lister-hooded rats. *Toxicology and Pathology* 15:143–148.

Camras, C.B., and Bito, L.Z, 1980a. The pathophysiological effects of nitrogen mustard on the rabbit eye II. The inhibition of the initial hypertensive phase by capsaicin and the apparent role of substance P. *Investigative Ophthalmology and Visual Science* 19:423–428.

Camras, C.B., and Bito, L.Z. 1980b. The pathophysiological effects of nitrogen mustard on the rabbit eye I. The biphasic intraocular pressure response and the role of prostaglandins. *Experimental Eye Research* 30:41–52.

Camras, C.B., and Miranda, O.C. 1989. The putative role of prostaglandins in surgical miosis. *Progressive Clinical Biology Research* 312:197–210.

Camras, C.B., Podos, S.M., Rosenthal, J.S., Lee, P-Y., and Severin, C.H. 1987. Multiple dosing of prostaglandin $F_{2\alpha}$ or epinephrine on cynomolgus monkey eyes 1. Aqueous humor dynamics. *Investigative Ophthalmology and Visual Science* 28:463–469.

Cooley, P.L., and Dice, P.F. 1990. Corneal dystrophy in the dog and cat. *Veterinary Clinic of North America [Small Animal Practice]* 20:681–692.

Crawford, K., Kaufman, P.L., and Gabelt, B.T. 1987. Effects of topical PGF2a on aqueous humor dynamics in cynomolgus monkeys. *Current Eye Research* 6:1035–1044.

Creel, D., O'Donnell, F.E., Jr., and Witkop, C.J., Jr. 1978. Visual system anomalies in human ocular albinos. *Science* 201:931–933.

Crispin, S.M. 1982. Corneal dystrophies in small animals. *Veterinary Annals* 22:298–310.

Csukas, S., Paterson, C.A., Brown, K., and Bhattacherjee, P. 1990. Time course of rabbit ocular inflammatory response and mediator release after intravitreal endotoxin. *Investigative Ophthalmology and Visual Science* 31:382–387.

Curtis, R., and Barnett, K.C. 1989. A survey of cataracts in golden and Labrador retrievers. *Journal of Small Animal Practice* 30:277–286.

Daston, G.P., and Freeberg, F.E. 1991. Ocular irritation testing. In *Dermal and Ocular Toxicology: Fundamentals and Methods*, ed. D.W. Hobson, pp. 509–539. Boca Raton, CRC Press.

Davson, H. 1990. *Physiology of the Eye*, 5th ed. New York: Pergamon Press.

Dodt, E., and Echte, K. 1961. Dark and light adaptation in pigmented and white rat as measured by erg threshold. *Journal of Neurophysiology* 24:427–445.

Dowling, J.E., and Sidman, R.L. 1962. Inherited retinal dystrophy in the rat. *Journal of Cell Biology* 14:73–109.

Duke-Elder, S. 1958. The eye in evolution. In *System of Ophthalmology*, vol. 1. St. Louis: C.V. Mosby.

Durand-Cavagna, G., Delort, P., Duprat, P., Bailly, Y., Plazonnet, B., and Gordon, L.R. 1989. Corneal toxicity studies in rabbits and dogs with hydroxyethylcellulose and benzalkonium chloride. *Fundamental and Applied Toxicology* 13:500–508.

Dziezyc, J., Millichamp, N.J., Keller, C.K., and Smith, W.B. 1992. The effect of $PGF_{2\alpha}$ and LTD4 on pupil size, intraocular pressure and blood–aqueous barrier in the dog. *American Journal of Veterinary Research* 53:1302–1304.

Eakins, K.E. 1970. Increased intraocular pressure produced by prostaglandins PGE_1 and E_2 in the cat eye. *Experimental Eye Research* 10:87–92.

Eakins, K.E. 1977. Prostaglandin and non-prostaglandin mediated breakdown of the blood aqueous barrier. *Experimental Eye Research* 25(suppl):483–498.

Eakins, K.E., and Bhattacherjee, P. 1977. Histamine, prostaglandins and ocular inflammation. *Experimental Eye Research* 24:299–305.

Eakins, K.E., Whitelocke, R.A.F., and Perkins, E.S. 1972. Release of prostaglandins in ocular inflammation in the rabbit. *Nature* 239:248–249.

Fleisher, L.N., and McGahan, M.C. 1986. Time course for prostaglandin synthesis by rabbit lens during endotoxin-induced ocular inflammation. *Current Eye Research* 5:629–634.

Fleisher, L.N., Fenrell, J.B., and McGahan, M.C. 1990. Ocular inflammatory effects of intravitreally injected tumor necrosis factor-alpha and endotoxin. *Inflammation* 14:325–335.

Francois, J., and Maudgal, M.C. 1965. Experimental chloroquine keratopathy. *American Journal of Ophthalmology* 60:459–464.

Fraunfelder, F.T., and Burns, R.P. 1966. Effect of lid closure in drug-induced experimental cataracts. *Archives of Ophthalmology* 76:599–601.

Fraunfelder, F.T., and Grove, I.A. 1996. *Drug-Induced Ocular Side Effects and Drug Interactions*, 4th ed. Baltimore, Williams and Wilkins.

Garceau, D., and Ford-Hutchinson, A.W. 1987. The role of leukotriene D_4 as a mediator of allergic conjunctivitis in the guinea-pig. *European Journal of Pharmacology* 134:285–292.

Gary, R.K., Woodward, D.F., Nieves, A.L., Williams, L.S., Gleason, J.G., and Wasserman, M.A. 1988. Characterization of the conjunctival vasopermeability response to leukotrienes and their involvement in immediate hypersensitivity. *Investigative Ophthalmology and Visual Science* 29:119–126.

Gaunt, F., and Harper, K.H. 1964. The potential irritancy to the rabbit eye of certain commercially available shampoos. *Journal of the Society of Cosmetic Chemistry* 15:209–230.

Gelatt, K.N. 1991a. The canine glaucomas. In *Veterinary Ophthalmology*, 2nd ed., ed. K.N. Gelatt, pp. 396–428. Philadelphia: Lea & Febiger.

Gelatt, K.N. 1991b. The canine lens. In *Veterinary Ophthalmology*, 2nd ed., ed. K.N. Gelatt, pp. 429–460. Philadelphia: Lea & Febiger.

Gelatt, K.N. 1999. *Veterinary Ophthalmology*, 3rd ed. Philadelphia: Lippincott, Williams, and Wilkins.

Gersbein, L.L., and McDonald, J.E. 1992. Evaluation of the corneal irritancy of test shampoos and detergents in various animal species. *Food and Cosmetic Toxicology* 15:131–134.

Grant, W.M. and Schuman I.S. 1993. *Toxicology of the Eye*, 4th ed. Springfield, IL: Charles C. Thomas.

Graves, A., Green, D.G., and Fisher, L.J. 1985. Light exposure can reduce selectively or abolish the c-wave of the albino rat electroretinogram. *Investigative Ophthalmology and Visual Science* 26:388–393.

Gum, G.G. 1991. Physiology of the eye. In *Veterinary Ophthalmology*, 2nd ed., ed. K.N. Gelatt, pp. 124–161. Philadelphia: Lea & Febiger.

Hackett, R.B., and Stern, M.E. 1991. Preclinical toxicology/safety considerations in the development of ophthalmic drugs and devices. In *Dermal and Ocular Toxicology: Fundamentals and Methods*, ed. D.W. Hobson, pp. 607–626. Boca Raton. CRC Press.

Hanna, B.L., Swain, P.B., and Sheppard, B. 1963. Recessive buphthalmos in the rabbit. *Genetics* 47:519–529.

Havener, H.A. 1966. *Ocular Pharmacology*. St. Louis: C.V. Mosby.

Havener, W.H. 1983. *Ocular Pharmacology*, 5th ed. St. Louis: C.V. Mosby.

Havener, W.H. 1984. *Pharmacology of the Eye*. Berlin: Springer-Verlag.

Hayashi, M.T., Miranda, O.C., Bito, L.Z., and Baroody, R.A. 1986. Specific, non-specific, direct, and indirect miotic effects of prostaglandins (PGs). *Investigative Ophthalmology and Visual Science* 27(suppl):248 (abstract).

Hayes, K.C., and Carey, R.E. 1975. Retinal degeneration associated with taurine deficiency in the cat. *Science* 188:949–950.

Hellauer, H.F. 1950. Sensibilität und Acetylcholingehalt der Hornhaut Verschiedener Tiere und des Menschen. *Zeitschrift fuer Vergleichende Physiologie* 32:303–310.

Herbort, C.P., Okumura, A., and Mochizuki, M. 1988. Endotoxin-induced uveitis in the rat. *Graefes Archives of Clinical Experimental Ophthalmology* 226:553–558.

Howard, R.D., McDonald, C.J., Dunn, B., and Creasey, W.A. 1969. Experimental chlorpromazine cataracts. *Investigative Ophthalmology* 8:413–421.

Hunt, R.D. 1963. Dacryoadenitis in the Sprague–Dawley rat. *American Journal of Veterinary Research* 24:638–641.

Jampol, L.M., Axelrod, A., and Tessler, H. 1976. Pathways of the eye's response to topical nitrogen mustard. *Investigative Ophthalmology and Visual Science* 15:486–489.

Kador, P.F., Fukui, H.N., Fukushi, S., Jernigan, H.M., and Kinoshita, J.H. 1980. Philly mouse: a new model of hereditary cataract. *Experimental Eye Research* 30:59–68.

Kaswan, R.L., and Salisbury, M.A. 1990. A new perspective on canine keratoconjunctivitis sicca: treatment with ophthalmic cyclosporine. *Veterinary Clinic of North America [Small Animal Practice]* 20:583–613.

Kaufman, P.L., Crawford, K., and Gabelt, B.T. 1989. The effects of prostaglandins on aqueous humor dynamics. *Ophthalmology Clinics of North America* 2:141–150.

Kelly, R.G.M., and Starr, M.S. 1971. Effects of prostaglandins and a prostaglandin antagonist on intraocular pressure and protein in the monkey eye. *Canadian Journal of Ophthalmology* 6:205–211.

Kenyon, K.R., Fogle, J.A., and Grayson, M. 1986. Dysgeneses, dystrophies and degenerations of the cornea. In *Clinical Ophthalmology*, ed. T.D. Duane, pp. 1–56. Philadelphia: Harper & Row.

Klein, E.M., and Bito, L.Z. 1983. Species variations in the pathophysiologic responses of vertebrate eyes to a chemical irritant, nitrogen mustard. *Investigative Ophthalmology and Visual Science* 24:184–191.

Kozart, D.M. 1968. Light and electron microscopic study of regional morphologic differences in the processes of the ciliary body in the rabbit. *Investigative Ophthalmology and Visual Science* 7:15–33.

Krohne, S.D.G., and Vestre, W.A. 1987. Effects of flunixin meglumine and dexamethasone on aqueous protein values after intraocular surgery in the dog. *American Journal of Veterinary Research* 48:420–422.

Kuck, J.F.R., Kuwabara, T., and Kuck, K.D. 1981. The Emory mouse cataract: an animal model for human senile cataract. *Current Eye Research* 1:643–649.

Kuhn, H., Keller, P., Kovacs, E., and Steiger, A. 1981. Lack of correlation between melanin affinity and retinopathy in mice and cats treated with chloroquine or flunitrazepam. *Graefes Archives of Clinical Experimental Ophthalmology* 216:177–190.

Kulkarni, P.S., and Srinivasan, B.D. 1982. The effect of intravitreal and topical prostaglandins on intraocular inflammation. *Investigative Ophthalmology and Visual Science* 23:383–392.

Kulkarni, P.S., and Srinivasan, B.D. 1988. Cachectin: a novel polypeptide induces uveitis in the rabbit eye. *Experimental Eye Research* 46:631–633.

Kurtz, S.M., Kaump, D.H., Schardein, J.L., Roll, D.E., Reutner, T.F., and Fisken, R.A. 1967. The effect of long-term administration of amopyroquin, a 4-aminoquinoline compound, on the retina of pigmented and nonpigmented laboratory animals. *Investigative Ophthalmology* 6:420.

Lai, Y.L., Jacoby, R., Bhatt, P., and Jonas, A. 1976. Keratoconjunctivitis associated with sialodacryoadenitis in rats. *Investigative Ophthalmology and Visual Science* 15:538–541.

Lee, P., Podos, S.M., and Severin, C. 1984. Effect of prostaglandin $F_{2\alpha}$ on aqueous humor dynamics of rabbit, cat, and monkey. *Investigative Ophthalmology and Visual Science* 25:1087–1093.

Lee, R.H., Lieberman, B.S., Hurwitz, R.L., and Lolley, R.N. 1985. Phosphodiesterase-probes show distinct defects in rd mice and Irish Setter dog disorders. *Investigative Ophthalmology and Visual Science* 26:1569–1579.

Losco, P.E., and Troup, C.M. 1988. Corneal dystrophy in Fischer 344 rats. *Laboratory Animal Sciences* 38:702–710.

Millichamp, N.J. 1990. Retinal degeneration in the dog and cat. *Veterinary Clinics of North America [Small Animal Practice]* 20:799–835.

Millichamp, N.J., and Dziezyc, J. 1991a. Mediators of ocular inflammation. *Progressive Veterinary Comparative Ophthalmology* 1:41–58.

Millichamp, N.J., and Dziezyc, J.D. 1991b. Control of the ocular irritative response in the dog: a comparison of flunixin meglumine and flurbiprofen. *American Journal of Veterinary Research* 52:1452–1455.

Millichamp, N.J., Dziezyc, J.D., Rohde, B.H., Chiou, G.C.Y., and Smith, W.B. 1991. Acute effects of anti-inflammatory drugs in Nd:YAG laser induced uveitis in the dog. *American Journal of Veterinary Research* 52:1279–1284.

Miranda, O.C., and Bito, L.Z. 1989. The putative and demonstrated miotic effects of prostaglandins in mammals. *Progressive Clinical Biological Research* 312:171–195.

Naash, M.I., LaVail, M.M., and Anderson, R.E. 1989. Factors affecting the susceptibility of the retina to light damage. *Progressive Clinical Biology Research* 314:513–522.

Narfstrom, K. 1985. Progressive retinal atrophy in the Abyssinian cat: clinical characteristics. *Investigative Ophthalmology and Visual Science* 26:193–200.

Nasisse, M.P. 1991. Feline ophthalmology. In *Veterinary Ophthalmology*, 2nd ed., ed. K.N. Gelatt, pp. 529–575. Philadelphia: Lea & Febiger.

Noell, W.K., Walker, V.S., Kang, B.S., and Berman, S. 1966. Retinal damage by light in rats. *Investigative Ophthalmology and Visual Science* 5:450–473.

Ohnishi, Y., and Tanaka, M. 1981. Effects of pilocarpine and paracentesis on occluding junctions between the nonpigmented ciliary epithelial cells. *Experimental Eye Research* 32:635–647.

Oksala, O. 1988. Effects of calcitonin gene-related peptide and substance P on regional blood flow in the cat eye. *Experimental Eye Research* 47:283–289.

Oksala, O., and Stjernschantz, J. 1988a. Effects of calcitonin gene-related peptide in the eye. *Investigative Ophthalmology and Visual Science* 29:1006–1011.

Oksala, O., and Stjernschantz, J. 1988b. Increase in outflow facility of aqueous humor in cats induced by calcitonin gene-related peptide. *Experimental Eye Research* 47:787–790.

O'Steen, W.K., Anderson, K.V., and Shear, C.R. 1974. Photoreceptor degeneration in albino rats: dependency on age. *Investigative Ophthalmology and Visual Science* 13:334–339.

Peiffer, R.L., Armstrong, J.R., and Johnson, P.T. 1981. Animals in ophthalmic research: concepts and methodologies. In *Methods of Animal Experimentation*, ed. W.I. Gay, pp. 140–235. New York: Academic Press.

Potts, A.M. 1964. The reaction of uveal pigment in vitro with polycyclic compounds. *Investigative Ophthalmology* 3:405–416.

Poynter, D., Martin, L.E., Harrison, C., and Cook, J. 1976. Affinity of labetalol for ocular melanin. *British Journal of Clinical Pharmacology* 3:711–720.

Prince, J.H. 1964. *The Rabbit in Eye Research*. Springfield, IL: Charles C. Thomas.

Prince, J.H., Diesem, C.D., Eglitis, I., and Ruskell, G.L. 1960. *Anatomy and Histology of the Eye and Orbit in Domestic Animals*. Springfield, IL: Charles C. Thomas.

Raviola, G. 1974. Effects of paracentesis on the blood–aqueous barrier: an electron microscope study on *Macaca mulatta* using horseradish peroxidase as a tracer. *Investigative Ophthalmology and Visual Science* 13:828–858.

Raviola, G. 1977. The structural basis of the blood–ocular barriers. *Experimental Eye Research* 25(suppl):27–63.

Regnier, A., Whitley, R.D., Benard, P., and Bonnefoi, M. 1986. Effect of flunixin meglumine on the breakdown of the blood–aqueous barrier following paracentesis in the canine eye. *Journal of Ocular Pharmacology* 2:165–170.

Reiter, R.J. 1973. Comparative effects of continual lighting and pinealectomy on the eyes, the harderian glands and reproduction in pigmented and albino rats. *Comparative Biochemistry and Physiology* 44A:503.

Reuter, J.H. 1974. The electroretinogram of albino and pigmented rabbits. *Documenta Ophthalmologica* 11:483.

Riis, R.C., Sheffy, B.E., Loew, E., Kern, T.J., and Smith, J.S. 1981. Vitamin E deficiency retinopathy in dogs. *American Journal of Veterinary Research* 42:74–86.

Rosenbaum, J.T., Howes, E., Jr., Rubin, R.M., and Samples, J.R. 1988. Ocular inflammatory effects of intravitreally injected tumor necrosis factor. *American Journal of Pathology* 133:47–53.

Rubin, L.F. 1974. *Atlas of Veterinary Ophthalmoscopy*. Philadelphia: Lea & Febiger.

Rubin, L.F. 1989. *Inherited Eye Diseases in Purebred Dogs*. Baltimore: Williams & Wilkins.

Rubin, L.F. 1990. Albino versus pigmented animals for ocular toxicity testing. *Lens and Eye Toxicity Research* 7:221–230.

Rubin, L.F., Murchison, T.E., and Barron, C.N. 1970. Chlorpromazine and the eye of the dog. A chronic study. *Experimental Molecular Pathology* 13:111–117.

Rubin, R.M., and Rosenbaum, J.T. 1990. The role of platelet activating factor in ocular inflammation. In *Platelet-Activating Factor in Endotoxin and Immune Diseases*, eds. D.A. Handley, R.N. Saunders, W.J. Houlihan, et al., pp. 189–205. New York: Marcel Dekker.

Rubin, R.M., and Rosenbaum, T. 1988. Platelet-activating factor antagonist inhibits interleukin 1-induced inflammation. *Biochemistry Biophysics Research Community* 154:429–436.

Russell, P., Tsunematsu, Y., Huang, F.L., and Kinoshita, J.H. 1977. Tissue culture of lens epithelial cells from normal and Nakano mice. *Investigative Ophthalmology and Visual Science* 16:243–246.

Samuelson, D.A. 1991. Ophthalmic anatomy and embryology. In *Veterinary Ophthalmology*, 2nd ed., K.N. Gelatt, pp. 3–123. Philadelphia: Lea & Febiger.

Sanyal, S., De Ruiter, A., and Hawkins, R.K. 1980. Development and degeneration of retina in rds mutant mice: light microscopy. *Journal of Comparative Neurology* 194:193–207.

Sidman, R., and Green, M. 1965. Retinal degeneration in the mouse. Localization of the rd locus in linkage group XVII. *Journal of Heredity* 56:23.

Slatter, D.H. 1990. *Fundamentals of Veterinary Ophthalmology*, 2nd ed. Philadelphia: W.B. Saunders.

Smelser, G.K., and Pei, Y.K. 1965. Cytological basis of protein leakage into the eye following paracentesis. An electron microscopic study. *Investigative Ophthalmology and Visual Science* 4:249–263.

Soloway, M.R., Stjernschantz, J., and Sears, M. 1981. The miotic effect of substance P on the isolated rabbit iris. *Investigative Ophthalmology and Visual Science* 20:47–52.

Srinivasa, B.D., and Kulkarni, P.S. 1980. The role of arachidonic acid metabolites in the mediation of the polymorphonuclear leukocyte response following corneal injury. *Investigative Ophthalmology and Visual Science* 19:1087–1093.

Stjernschantz, J., Geijer, C., and Bill, A. 1979. Electrical stimulation of the fifth cranial nerve in rabbits: effects on ocular blood flow, extravascular albumin content and intraocular pressure. *Experimental Eye Research* 28:229–238.

Stjernschantz, J., Sears, M., and Mishima, H. 1982. Role of substance P in the antidromic vasodilation, neurogenic plasma extravasation and disruption of the blood–aqueous barrier in the rabbit eye. *Archives of Pharmacology* 321:329–335.

Stjernschantz, J., Sherk, T., Borgeat, P., and Sears, M. 1984. Intraocular effects of lipoxygenase pathway products in arachidonic acid metabolism. *Acta Ophthalmologica* 62:104–111.

Stjernschantz, J., von Dickhoff, K., Oksala, O., and Seppa, H. 1986. A study of the mechanism of ocular irritation following YAG laser capsulotomy in rabbits. *Experimental Eye Research* 43:641–651.

Stock, E.L., Roth, S.I., Kim, E.D., Walsh, M.K., and Thamman, R. 1990. The effect of platelet-activating factor (PAF), histamine, and ethanol on vascular permeability of the guinea pig conjunctiva. *Investigative Ophthalmology and Visual Science* 31:987–992.

Szalay, J., Nunziata, B., and Henkind, P. 1991. Permeability of the iridal blood vessels. *Experimental Eye Research* 1:531–543.

Tabbara, K.F., and Cello, R.M. 1984. *Animal Models of Ocular Diseases.* Springfield, IL: Charles C. Thomas.

Tachado, S.D., Akhtar, R.A., Yousufzai, S.Y.K., and Abdel-Latif, A.A. 1991. Species differences in the effects of substance P on inositol triphosphate accumulation and cyclic AMP formation, and on contraction in isolated iris sphincter of the mammalian eye: differences in receptor density. *Experimental Eye Research* 53:729–739.

Taradach, C., Regnier, B., and Perraud, J. 1981. Eye lesions in Sprague–Dawley rats: types and incidence in relation to age. *Laboratory Animals* 15:285–287.

Tripathi, R.C. 1974. Comparative physiology and anatomy of the aqueous outflow pathway. In *The Eye*, vol. 5, eds. H. Favson and L.T. Graham, p. 163. New York: Academic Press.

Unger, W.G. 1989. Mediation of the ocular response to injury and irritation: peptides versus prostaglandins. *Progressive Clinical Biological Research* 312:293–328.

Unger, W.G., and Butler, J.M. 1988. Neuropeptides in the uveal tract. *Eye* 2:S202–S212.

Unger, W.G., and Tighe, J. 1984. The response of the isolated iris sphincter pupillary muscle to substance P. *Experimental Eye Research* 39:677–684.

Unger, W.G., Cole, D.F., and Hammond, B. 1975. Disruption of the blood–aqueous barrier following paracentesis in the rabbit. *Experimental Eye Research* 20:255–270.

Unger, W.G., Perkins, E.S., and Bass, M.S. 1974. The response of the rabbit eye to laser irradiation of the iris. *Experimental Eye Research* 19:367–377.

Unger, W.G., Terenghi, G., Ghatei, M.A., Butler, J.M., Polak, J.M., and Bloom, S.R. 1985. Calcitonin gene-related polypeptide as a mediator of the neurogenic ocular injury response. *Journal of Ocular Pharmacology* 1:185–195.

van Heyningen, R. 1976. Experimental studies on cataract. *Investigative Ophthalmology and Visual Science* 15:685–697.

Van Winkle, T.J., and Balk, M.W. 1986. Spontaneous corneal opacities in laboratory mice. *Laboratory Animal Sciences* 36:248–255.

Verbey, N.L., Van Delft, J.L., Van Haeringen, N.J., and Braquet, P. 1989. Platelet-activating factor and laser trauma to the iris. *Investigative Ophthalmology and Visual Science* 30:1101–1103.

Wahlestedt, C., Hakanson, R., Beding, B., Brodin, E., Ekman, R., and Sundler, F. 1985. Intraocular effects of CGRP, a neuropeptide in sensory nerves. In *Tachykinin Antagonists*, eds. R. Hakanson and F. Sundler, pp. 137–146. New York: Elsevier Science.

Waitzman, M.B., and King, C.D. 1967. Prostaglandin influences on intraocular pressure and pupil size. *American Journal of Physiology* 212:329–334.

Walls, G.L. 1942. *The Vertebrate Eye and Its Adaptive Radiation.* Bloomfield Hills, MI: Cranbrook Institute of Science.

Weidner, C. 1976. The c-wave in the erg of albino rat. *Vision Research* 16:753–763.

Weissbroth, S.H., and Peress, N. 1977. Ophthalmic lesions and dacryoadenitis: a naturally occurring aspect of sialodacryoadenitis virus infection of the laboratory rat. *Laboratory Animal Sciences* 27:466–473.

Weisse, I., Loosen, H., and Peil, H. 1990. Age-related retinal changes—a comparison between albino and pigmented rats. *Lens and Eye Toxicity Research* 7:717–739.

Weleber, R.G. 1989. Retinitis pigmentosa and allied disorders. In *Retina*, vol. 1, eds. S.J. Ryan and T.E. Ogden, pp. 299–420. St. Louis: C.V. Mosby.

Wetzel, M.G., Fahlman, C., Maude, M.B., et al. 1989. Fatty acid metabolism in normal miniature poodles and those affected with progressive rod–cone degeneration (PRCD). *Progressive Clinical Biological Research* 314:427–440.

Whitley, R.D. 1991. Canine cornea. In *Veterinary Ophthalmology*, 2nd ed., ed. K.N. Gelatt, pp. 307–356. Philadelphia: Lea & Febiger.

Wilkie, D.A., and Wyman, M. 1991. Comparative anatomy and physiology of the mammalian eye. In *Dermal and Ocular Toxicology: Fundamentals and Methods*, ed. D.W. Hobson, pp. 433–491. Boca Raton. CRC Press.

Williams, R.H., Howard, A.G., and Williams, T.P. 1985. Retinal damage in pigmented and albino rats exposed to low levels of cyclic light following a single mydriatic treatment. *Current Eye Research* 4:97–102.

Woodford, B.J., Liu, Y., Fletcher, R.T., et al. 1982. Cyclic nucleotide metabolism in inherited retinopathy in collies: a biochemical and histochemical study. *Experimental Eye Research* 34:703–714.

Woodward, D.F., and Ledgard, S.E. 1985a. Comparison of leukotrienes as conjunctival microvascular permeability factors. *Ophthalmic Research* 17:318–320.

Woodward, D.F., and Ledgard, S.E. 1985b. Effect of LTD_4 on conjunctival vasopermeability and blood–aqueous barrier integrity. *Investigative Ophthalmology and Visual Science* 26:481–485.

Woodward, D.F., Hawley, S.B., Williams, L.S., et al. 1990. Studies on the ocular pharmacology of prostaglandin D2. *Investigative Ophthalmology and Visual Science* 31:138–146.

Yakely, W.L. 1978. A study of hereditary cataracts in the American cocker spaniel. *Journal of the American Veterinary Medical Association* 172:814.

Yousufzai, S.Y.K., Chen, A-L., and Abdel-Latif, A.A. 1988. Species differences in the effects of prostaglandins on inositol triphosphate accumulation, phosphatidic acid formation, myosin light chain phosphorylation and contraction of iris sphincter of the mammalian eye: interaction with the cyclic AMP system. *Journal of Pharmacology and Experimental Therapy* 247:1064–1072.

Yousufzai, S.Y.K., Tachado, S.D., and Abdel-Latif, A.A. 1990. Species differences in the effects of leukotriene D4 on inositol triphosphate accumulation, cyclic AMP formation and contraction in iris sphincter of the mammalian eye. *Prostaglandins* 39:227–240.

Ophthalmic Toxicology
Edited by George C. Y. Chiou
Copyright © 1999 Taylor & Francis

5

In Vivo Eye Irritation Test Methods

Keith Green

*Department of Ophthalmology and Department of Physiology and Endocrinology,
Medical College of Georgia, Augusta, Georgia, USA*

INTRODUCTION

Eye irritation testing of ophthalmic and non-ophthalmic products forms the basis of guidelines and recommendations of worldwide regulatory agencies in the evaluation of product safety to protect and safeguard the health of humans. This public health service covers a complete range of manufactured or raw materials to which humans can be exposed in the home or workplace. These agencies make an analysis of a product or compound proposed for marketing by establishing a safety profile after toxicological evaluations have been conducted. Such evaluations are usually performed by the supplier or manufacturer of the product (or a subcontractor with expertise in this area) under specifically delineated guidelines (GLP, or good laboratory practices, is a widely accepted standard) and submitted to the respective agencies for review. There is frequently an iterative process involved beyond the initial data submission where the agency will ask for further data before re-review and approval or disapproval for human exposure (Green, Sobel, et al., 1981).

Toxicity versus Irritation

It is important to recognize that testing of products was initially designed to assess the ocular effects of substances that would accidentally reach the eye on a one-time basis. Such products included household or office products, agricultural materials, environmental factors, volatile organic compounds such as may exist in newly painted or carpeted buildings, and an entire range of manufactured or raw materials; anything, in fact, that had the potential of gaining access to the human eye. With the advent of eye care products and drugs designed specifically for topical ophthalmic use, sometimes for extended time periods, a choice was apparently made to continue to use the basic test paradigm to assess the ocular irritation potential of these latter materials. It is not clear upon what basis this choice was made, except that a test system already existed that could be used to eliminate compounds from further development. Unfortunately, the in vivo test system is designed to evaluate only short-term ocular irritation responses to agents. Furthermore, ophthalmic products are specifically developed to have zero or minimal induction of ocular irritation since this would be counter to the therapeutic use of any topical drug.

Ocular toxicity, however, goes far beyond immediate irritation responses and may involve longer term tissue reactions. While evaluation of short-term irritation potential is an important component in initially assessing the use, and value, of ophthalmic drug products, the technique falls short of providing a complete evaluation. It is becoming increasingly evident that assessment of ocular tissue toxicity requires a far greater degree of subtlety and longevity than the original test system can provide. There is a considerable difference, therefore, between the acute ocular irritation potential of a product or chemical and the ocular toxicity of the same materials. Ocular toxicity also includes the effects of systemic drugs designed to effect a change in a peripheral system. Examples are cholesterol-reducing agents that might have secondary effects on the lens (Schmitt et al., 1990), calcium-channel blockers for systemic hypertension that may reduce intraocular pressure, and steroids used as anti-inflammatory drugs or as a component of immunosuppressive therapy that can cause cataracts. This distinction between acute irritation and longer-term toxicity induction is vitally important to keep in mind during any discussion of the two situations.

Primary Test System

To ensure that safe and effective drugs and other products are available for any conceivable type or degree of human exposure or use, the evaluations are primarily made with in vivo studies. These determinations lead to acceptance or rejection of a particular product or offer data that can be used for labeling of chemicals or products at various levels of irritancy or corrosiveness. This is particularly important for harsh cleansers or other irritants, for example, which are often labeled for eye care in the case of accidental exposure; liberal washing of the eyes and lids is usually indicated to provide rapid dilution of the product.

Such a testing process minimizes the obvious avoidable health risks, while not entirely evaluating or eliminating potential toxic side effects because of the experimental design and duration of the test system. Some products or compounds are known to induce adverse side effects only after continued use over several years. As one component of the safety profile, ocular and dermal drugs or products, and those materials that may have access to the eye, are evaluated for their potential to cause ocular irritation (Schnieders, 1987; Lehnert and Ulrich, 1990; Wilcox, 1992; Beck et al., 1995). The method most widely employed to determine ocular irritation potential for externally applied materials is the Draize test (Code of Federal Regulations, 1979).

In Vivo versus In Vitro

While there has been a proliferation of in vitro techniques that have been developed as potential alternatives, or supplementary adjuncts, to in vivo test methods (Leighton et al., 1985; Parish, 1985; Frazier, 1989; Wilcox and Bruner, 1990; Bruner et al., 1991; Hagino et al., 1991; Atkinson et al., 1992; Bagley et al., 1992, 1994; Ellingson et al., 1992; Gautheron et al., 1992; Goldberg and Silber, 1992; Hubert, 1992; O'Brien et al., 1992; Rougier et al., 1992; Sina et al., 1992; Goldberg et al., 1993; Green, Chambers, et al., 1993; Rasmussen, 1993; Spielmann et al., 1993; Balls and Straughan, 1996; Christian and Diener, 1996; Ward et al., 1997), the latter still forms the ultimate mainstay of ocular irritation testing. There are several reasons for the continued use of and dependence on in vivo methodologies, but the main one is that none of the in vitro alternatives offers the spectrum of responses that occur in the whole in situ eye, some of which may be interactive.

It is for this reason, too, that complete elimination of in vivo eye irritation testing will not be possible. It will be of widespread interest to monitor the European experience when in vivo experimentation, particularly that associated with product testing, becomes markedly reduced, if not eliminated, by law within the next few years. Those tests concerned with cosmetic evaluation have already been eliminated by the adoption of appropriate laws. The in vitro tests will certainly reduce the numbers of animals involved and confine animal exposure only to materials with limited potential to induce irritancy; nevertheless, reliance will continue upon in vivo test methods. In vitro methods, no matter how good as a test, will never be able to replace the in vivo situation. When the first compound that passes the in vitro tests but fails when placed in the human eye occurs, then perhaps the legislatively driven process will be replaced by one based upon science. No one will surely condone the exposure of humans to materials that have not first been tested in animals, albeit with significant pre-in vivo predictive evaluations of irritancy or toxicity potential by in vitro tests.

Ocular Responses

The complexity of the ocular response to an irritative stimulus involves physiological, pharmacological, biochemical, immunological, and inflammatory reactions and any metabolites produced from the test agent. Alterations in membrane permeability, enzyme reactions, neurogenic and nonneurogenic factors, vascular effects, chemical transmitters, the type and proportion of arachidonic acid metabolites and many other contributing factors are probably all involved in what appears to the observer as a simple tissue reaction, such as conjunctival hyperemia. The tissue reactions may well vary, not only in intensity but also in the degree to which different tissues are affected by any individual stimulus, and in the quantitative contribution of each factor to the final response. Reactions may involve sensitization of tissues to particular types of materials, such as volatile organic solvents. The introduction of a new volatile organic compound after a prior exposure period may then trigger a physiological response even though the exposure limit is below regulatory or recommended levels.

It is important that any testing, from initial evaluative processes to final product evaluations, whether it be structure–activity relationship studies, in vitro tests, or in vivo testing, all make sure that not only is the parent test agent evaluated, but that any metabolites are also tested. In this regard, it is important to verify that the metabolism of the test material in the in vivo model be the same as that in man. If this is not verified then the toxicologist may spend considerable time in vain. This consideration assumes greater importance with increasing use of pro-drugs and "soft" drugs, such as beta-adrenergic blockers, in therapeutic regimens.

It is the very complexity of this integrated system that belies the development of a single in vitro predictive test that can be used to replace what is known as the Draize test. Any individual test may simply reflect a portion of a single different aspect of the complex of responses; thus a battery of in vitro tests will be required to eventually form a pre-Draize screening protocol before eventual limited product testing in an animal model. The in vitro screening will eliminate compounds with substantial irritancy or toxic potential and allow only products or compounds with little predicted potential for the induction of eye irritancy to be tested in vivo. Coupled with the utilization of prior information on the same or similar ingredients in the products, this would be a major step in causing a marked reduction in animal numbers and in subjecting animals only to potentially nonirritant or noncorrosive materials.

The in vitro methodologies will provide a firm basis, once validation of these tests is complete, for reducing animal exposure and use, especially when coupled with the decrease in legislated requirements on the numbers of animals required per test material. In vivo testing would still constitute the final step in irritancy evaluation since it represents the only ultimate test situation that offers predictive value for effects on the human eye. No in vitro test can ever replace the many interactive and integrated components of the in vivo test paradigm. It is the very complexity and interactive nature of each individual component response to a particular stimulus that provides the in vivo reaction. Isolation of even ideal in vivo simulation of individual components fails to include the interactive component.

DRAIZE TEST

Observations were made at the turn of the 20th century concerning cataract formation and other ocular disorders that appeared to be related to the use of systemic medications. This was particularly true for steroids as they became introduced into medicine when the secondary side effects of cataract formation and elevated intraocular pressure were noted and causal relationships established. More recent examples of toxic side effects include the cataract-inducing effects of topical echothiophate, and the occurrence of superficial punctate keratitis caused by preservatives, which are surfactants, in topical medications. Even these very limited examples illustrate why irritation and toxicity testing of drugs and potentially marketed products is essential for establishing the safety of these materials before human exposure. Many other examples exist of systemic effects of topical drugs, ocular effects of systemic drugs, and ocular side effects from topical drugs (Fraunfelder, 1989; Grant and Shuman, 1993).

Society demands that the population not be exposed to agents that are capable of interfering with human health and welfare. On the other hand, considerable concern has been expressed at various levels concerning the use of rabbits and other animals in the test paradigm used in the evaluation of products to which humans are or may be exposed. This apparently irreconcilable difference has had somewhat of a resolution with the initial use of structure–activity relationships to assess the potential of a product, or an ingredient, to cause health problems based upon historical data. Further, the use of progressive and sequential in vitro methodologies offers a means by which all products do not have to be tested in living animals. Elimination of material through the employment of new approaches, while not precisely simulating the in vivo condition, at least offers a means of assessing irritation potential. Without these evaluative and iterative processes human health could be compromised and materials introduced into the marketplace that could jeopardize human well-being. Such a result would not be tolerated; thus some testing paradigms must remain in place.

The need to test various products for eye irritation was also strongly influenced by several incidences of ocular damage after human exposure to improperly tested materials. One such example is an eyelash dye that contained *p*-phenylene-diamine which entered the United States market in the early 1930s. It was quickly established that external structures of the eye developed supersensitivity to this product that led, in some circumstances, to corneal ulceration and loss of vision (McCally et al., 1933). Reaction to these chemicals, and similar incidences, led to the creation of the Food, Drug, and Cosmetic Act in 1938 for the regulation of the safety and labeling of products that would have potential access to humans.

Concurrent with this was the development of ocular irritation or toxicity test methods to predict eye irritation in humans. Numerous adverse side effects have been described more recently after either topical or systemic drug delivery (Fraunfelder and Scafidi, 1978; Van Buskirk, 1980; Van Buskirk and Fraunfelder, 1984; Fraunfelder and Meyer, 1985, 1987; Fraunfelder, 1989; Grant and Shuman, 1993), and the principle behind eye irritation and toxicity testing is to minimize or eliminate such potential responses through testing before human exposure. In this way materials, chemicals, drugs, or devices are either approved or denied for human exposure. In some instances, however, toxicity (as distinct from acute ocular irritancy) is revealed only after months or years of exposure of the eye to a particular agent. It is under these conditions that the testing process is sometimes reversed, with subsequent long-term animal testing after human exposure has occurred in order to identify mechanisms of drug action and the underlying cause for the long-term toxicity.

Method

Friedenwald and co-workers published a method for assessing the acid and base tolerance of the cornea in albino rabbits (Friedenwald et al., 1944). In 1944, Draize, who was at the time a member of the Food and Drug Administration (FDA) staff, and his co-workers published the first standardized method that formed the basis of the most widely used system for studying in vivo eye irritation (Draize et al., 1944). The original method has undergone subtle changes in order to incorporate the ability to test the eye irritation of different types of chemicals (Draize and Kelley, 1952; Draize, 1959; Green, Sullivan, et al., 1978). All of these techniques were designed for the testing of the ocular irritation potential of nonophthalmic products, that is, compounds that may accidentally contact the eye during a manufacturing process or in the home or work environment. Because of the widespread acceptance of this test method, however, it has also been adopted for the testing of ophthalmic products prior to marketing; this, despite the shortcoming of the test system to identify anything but short-term acute ocular irritation. With this limitation, it is surprising how predictive the test is for longer-term human use.

Several major problems exist with the performance of the Draize test:

1. Different people read the same response differently (Weltman et al., 1965; Weil and Scala, 1971; Baldwin et al., 1973). Although standards have been described, and slides made available of different grades of responses (Food and Drug Administration, 1965; Consumer Product Safety Commission, 1976) to provide guidance in evaluating the various grades of reactivity, standardization of the observations has been difficult. Internal consistency of observation within a specific setting may occur, but the subjective nature of the test allows considerable freedom of interpretation.
2. Different methods are used to instill test materials onto the test eyes. Some investigators place the materials into the lower cul-de-sac (as described in the test paradigm [Code of Federal Regulations, 1979]) then allow the animal to blink and spread material across the corneal and conjunctival surfaces, while others may instill the test material directly onto the corneal surface. The latter, obviously, will create a different distribution pattern of the test material that may well result in a different set of responses by different eye tissues as a result of the kinetic changes.
3. Different investigators use different experimental designs, that is, variations in observation times or scoring systems, and so on.

The net result of these three variations is that it is often difficult to compare results from different laboratories or test facilities, and any comparisons frequently can be quite misleading. These differences occur despite the description and publication of the standardized methodology by regulatory agencies, such as the FDA (Code of Federal Regulations, 1979) and the Consumer Product Safety Commission (1976) in the United States, and complete details of the test protocol in other countries.

Test Protocol

The assessment of eye irritation potential of a compound or product usually begins with measurement of pH, if the material is a solution, and other physicochemical parameters including structure–activity relationships based upon the chemical composition (Barratt, 1995a,b; Barratt et al., 1995; Chamberlain and Barratt, 1995; Règnier and Imbert, 1992; Sugai et al., 1990). Values below pH 2.5 and above 11.5 are immediately indicative of ocular damage potential, and further testing is not forthcoming. With a pH within the range indicated, dermal irritation testing would follow. This is performed on the shaved area of a rodent (rat, guinea pig, or rabbit) with observations on inflammatory-type reactions. Severe responses in this dermal test again preclude further testing since experience has shown that compounds inducing marked skin reactions translate that activity to the eye (Hurley et al., 1993).

If a compound or product successfully cleared these hurdles then usually the next stage would be in vivo rabbit eye irritation testing. The advent of in vitro alternatives with their contribution to the test system, however, allows a limited evaluation of irritancy potential at this point. Any of a variety of techniques are available, each with its own limitations. Nevertheless, the use of these approaches, collectively, aids in the elimination of certain products before the need for in vivo irritation testing. Successful passage through this in vitro phase leads to advancement into the eye irritation assessment phase. The amount of test substance applied to the eye is normally 100 μl (or 100 mg for a solid) placed into the lower cul-de-sac, with observations of the various criteria then made at the designated and required intervals of 1 h, 24 h, 48 h, 72 h, and 1 week after administration. The grading system for the responses of various eye tissues (Table 1) is that described by Draize (Draize et al., 1944; Draize and Kelley, 1952; Draize, 1959).

There have been numerous variations on this basic protocol. These include the following: (1) a reduction in volume (or mass) of the test compound to 10 μl (or 10 mg), as recommended by the National Academy of Sciences (1978); (2) the performance of a rinse with saline after instillation of the test product (this is applicable only to nonophthalmic products and even then is limited to a small percentage of the test eyes); (3) use of a slit-lamp or loupes to allow finer assessment of the ocular changes (Baldwin et al., 1973; Green, Sobel, et al., 1981); (4) use of topical fluorescein solution to evaluate corneal epithelial debridement, areas of corneal staining or to measure corneal epithelial permeability; (5) use of an optical or ultrasonic pachymeter to measure corneal thickness; and (6) extension of the test period to 21 days to allow reversal of the irritancy response (NAS Committee for Revisions of NAS Publication 1138, 1978). These, and other, aspects of the Draize test have been discussed widely in a variety of sources (Ballantyne and Swanston, 1977; Chan and Hayes, 1985; McDonald, Hiddeman, et al., 1987; McDonald, Seabaugh, et al., 1987; Gad and Changelis, 1988; Hackett, 1990; Rohde, 1992; Schiavo, 1992; Green, 1992a; Green, Edelhauser, et al., 1997).

TABLE 1. *Scale of weighted scores for grading the severity of ocular lesions*

I.	Cornea		
	A.	Opacity—degree of density (area that is most dense is taken for reading)	
		Scattered or diffuse area—details of iris clearly visible	1
		Easily discernible translucent areas, details of iris slightly obscured	2
		Opalescent areas, no details of iris visible, size of pupil barely discernible	3
		Opaque, iris invisible	4
	B.	Area of cornea involved	
		One-quarter (or less) but not zero	1
		Greater than one-quarter, less than one-half	2
		Greater than one-half, less than three-quarters	3
		Greater than three-quarters up to whole area	4
		Score equals A × B × 5 Total maximum = 80	
II.	Iris		
	A.	Values	
		Folds above normal, congestion, swelling, circumcorneal injection (any one or all of these or combination of any thereof), iris still reacting to light (sluggish reaction is positive)	1
		No reaction to light, hemorrhage; gross destruction (any one or all of these)	2
		Score equals A × 5 Total maximum = 10	
III.	Conjunctiva		
	A.	Redness (refers to palpebral conjunctiva only)	
		Vessels definitely injected above normal	1
		More diffuse, deeper crimson red, individual vessels not easily discernible	2
		Diffuse beefy red	3
	B.	Chemosis	
		Any swelling above normal (includes nictitating membrane)	1
		Obvious swelling with partial eversion of the lids	2
		Swelling with lids about half closed	3
		Swelling with lids about half closed to completely closed	4
	C.	Discharge	
		Any amount different from normal (does not include small amount observed in inner canthus of normal animals)	1
		Discharge with moistening of the lids and hairs just adjacent to the lids	2
		Discharge with moistening of the lids and considerable area around the eye	3
		Score (A + B + C) × 2 Total maximum = 20	

The maximum total score (110) is the sum of all scores obtained for the cornea (80, or 73%), iris (10, or 9%), and conjunctiva (20, or 18%).

Draize Test Difficulties

Problems with the Draize test as described for its use in eye irritancy evaluation include the following: (1) the interspecies transfer of information from the rabbit test model to the human experience (Zbinden, 1991); (2) the difference in blink rate between human and rabbit; (3) the degree of tearing induced by the test agent; (4) the relative area of the conjunctiva relative to the cornea in man versus rabbit; (5) the emphasis of the Draize scoring system on the corneal response relative to that of the conjunctiva; (6) the absence of the use of a slit-lamp, or even loupes, to provide a more detailed examination; and (7) the large amount of test material employed.

Blink Rate

The blink rate in rabbits is about once per minute at best (usually less) compared with 15 times a minute in man. The distribution of material following a blink, therefore, may be quite different between the two species since redistribution would be much more rapid and complete in man, resulting in quite different kinetics of the applied material in the tear film. In contradistinction to this, most applied solid or liquid materials initiate a blink once instillation into the cul-de-sac is complete. This initial blink will influence the first phase of test substance distribution, but subsequent distribution may well be influenced by the species differences in blink rate.

Lacrimation

Adding to this factor is the degree of tearing induced by the test material. If irritation occurs, usually even when quite minor, then the tear flow increases and dilution of the test material occurs. Thus, the availability of the test substance will influence the scores for irritation of the ocular tissues. Some paradoxical responses may occur with large test volumes or amounts initiating a large increase in tear flow which would elute the test material quite quickly from the ocular surface, thereby significantly diminishing any ocular response; smaller volumes or quantities of the same test material might initiate only minor increases in tear flow, thereby allowing a much greater ocular response to occur.

Surface Area and Nictitans

In humans, the distribution of test agent and its longevity on the ocular surface may be an important consideration since conjunctival area is double that of the rabbit, providing a greater expanse for tissue and test substance interaction, thereby adding yet another complicating factor into the interspecies transfer of information. Furthermore, the rabbit has a large nictitating membrane, or nictitans (third eyelid), which can act as a physical barrier to loss of added material by offering a tissue under which test compound, particularly a solid, may be trapped and reside. In addition, it may act as a reservoir for chemicals that are initially absorbed into, or adsorbed onto, the tissue and subsequently returned into the tear film as part of the pharmacokinetic phenomena. The latter process will prolong the time of drug exposure and could influence the interpretation of drug effects. Some investigators have advocated the removal of the nictitans prior to use of the rabbit in toxicity testing but, more frequently, it is left intact.

Drug Absorption

Certain chemicals, such as the preservatives benzalkonium chloride (BAK) and chlorhexidine digluconate, alter corneal epithelial permeability to drugs and other chemicals (Green and Tønjum, 1971; Green, Livingston, et al., 1980; Green, 1993). In addition, BAK is retained by the corneal epithelium for long time periods with slow elution into the tear film (Clayton et al., 1985; Champeau and Edelhauser, 1986; Green and Chapman, 1986; Green, Chapman, et al., 1987). Such behavior not only prolongs the presence of the surfactant in the tears but also allows a large extension of the time available for exertion of physiological effects on membrane permeability. Inclusion of preservatives that are surfactants in products frequently alters the kinetic relationships of drugs with the ocular tissues. The larger conjunctival area of humans also offers a larger reservoir for compounds, such as BAK or other preservatives.

Scoring

The original Draize test was designed for testing nonophthalmic materials, such as soaps, shampoos (Bell et al., 1979), and other household materials; thus a major potential site of irritancy or toxicity was the cornea. Emphasis was therefore placed on this tissue. A glance at the scoring system (Table 1) reveals that 80 of the total of 110 total score is directed toward the cornea (Green, 1992a).

While this may be acceptable for nonophthalmic materials, such as copying machine toners, cosmetics, soaps, shampoos, household products, and so on, it is not truly applicable to ophthalmic products. For an ophthalmic material to reach the stage of in vivo animal testing, initial physicochemical data review and in vitro toxicity testing, as the first two components of the three-tier test system, will, by necessity, have ruled out most of those products or materials likely to involve a corneal response. Thus, the major effects initiated by ophthalmic products are those of conjunctival redness and/or chemosis that may be accompanied by discharge (Green, 1992a; Edelhauser and Green, 1997). The total score for this aspect of the test is only 30 out of the 110 total (27%); thus some revision of the Draize test is required for ophthalmic products where a greater range of scores for hyperemia of the conjunctiva, chemosis, and/or discharge would be welcome. Such revision has not yet occurred yet seems overdue in order that more realistic evaluative criteria, with an emphasis redirected from that of the original Draize test, may be established for assessing the irritation potential of ophthalmic substances.

Observation Times and Animal Numbers

Additional times of observation should be strongly considered, to add significantly to the need for evaluation of potentially irritative effects to be observed during the first few hours after application of the ophthalmic product or other material. It is recommended that, in addition to the 1-hr time currently required, observations and scoring be made at 3, 5, and 7-hr after ophthalmic product administration. These times would cover those hours where an initial response is most likely to be induced by the chemical and would represent no additional hardship or difficulty for the observer when using fewer animals (Edelhauser and Green, 1997). The proposed, and recommended, decrease from six animals to one animal allows the observer an appropriate amount of time to perform in-depth evaluation of tissue responses. Even with an additional two rabbits per observation period (if a positive response is seen in the first rabbit) this is a large reduction in numbers.

Revised Scoring System

A revision and reemphasis of the Draize scoring system is also needed. Such a proposal is made in Table 2. The revised system adds fluorescein staining to the corneal scoring, but removes the emphasis from this tissue from 80 of a total of 110 points (72%) in the original system (see Table 1) to a more realistic 24 of a total of 84 points (or 28%). The iris scores stay the same, while those for the conjunctiva are increased to 60% of the total score.

The conjunctival scores are based on bulbar, not palpebral, scoring since this more realistically represents not only that portion of the conjunctiva likely to respond to a stimulus but also that which is more readily observed. In this investigator's experience, even eversion of the lids to examine the palpebral conjunctiva can induce disturbance of the normal condition. The majority of the descriptive parts of the original Draize test are retained for the sake of historical continuity, but the change in emphasis and observation times represents a recognition of the changes that have occurred in the test system as applied to ophthalmic products.

Despite this reemphasis in the scoring system of the Draize test, there is still no recognition of the potential effects on the lens or retina of applied drugs, chemicals, or devices. These longer-term changes reflect toxicity rather than ocular irritancy and are the sites where, frequently, changes occur in response to drug use. The latter effects happen, however, most often only after longer term use of a drug or chemical than a one-time application and represent another level of assessment of tissue responses.

Reduced Test Volume or Mass Size

The incorporation of the use of smaller volumes or masses of test material relates to the findings that eye irritation, as judged from reports in man, was about 10-fold more intensive in the rabbit relative to man in response to the same stimulus (Beckley, 1965; Griffith et al., 1982; Freeberg, Griffith, et al., 1984; Freeberg, Hooker, et al., 1986; Freeberg, Nixon, et al., 1986; Allgood, 1989; Lambert et al., 1993). Comparisons were made between the limited number of reports of accidental contact of the human eye with substances that also had been fully tested in rabbits. These results, from the files of company adverse-effect reports, formed the basis of the recommendation for lower quantities of test materials to be employed in eye irritation testing by the National Academy of Sciences (NAS Committee for Revisions of NAS Publication 1138, 1978). The use of small volume (10 μl) or mass (10 mg) of material allows a more direct interspecies comparison of the rabbit response with that observed or predicted in man with the same stimulus.

TABLE 2. *Proposed scoring for ophthalmic products; modified from Draize*

I.	Cornea		
	A.	Opacity—degree of density (area that is most dense is taken for reading)	
		Scattered or diffuse area—details of iris clearly visible	1
		Easily discernible translucent areas, details of iris slightly obscured	2
		Opalescent areas, no details of iris visible, size of pupil barely discernible	3
		Opaque, iris invisible	4
	B.	Area of cornea involved	
		One-quarter (or less) but not zero	1
		Greater than one-quarter, less than one-half	2
		Greater than one-half, less than three-quarters	3
		Greater than three-quarters, up to whole area	4
	C.	Fluorescein staining	
		Punctate fluorescein staining	1
		Patches of fluorescein staining	2
		Diffuse staining over entire area	3
		Deep stromal staining	4
		Score equals (A + B + C) × 2 Total maximum = 24	
II.	Iris		
	A.	Values	
		Folds above normal, congestion, swelling, circumcorneal injection (any one or all of these or combination of any thereof), iris still reacting to light (sluggish reaction is positive)	1
		No reaction to light, hemorrhage; gross destruction (any one or all of these)	2
		Score equals A × 5 Total maximum = 10	
III.	Conjunctiva		
	A.	Redness (refers to bulbar conjunctiva only)	
		Vessels definitely injected above normal	1
		More diffuse, deeper crimson red, individual vessels not easily discernible	2
		Diffuse beefy red	3
	B.	Chemosis	
		Any swelling above normal (includes nictitating membrane)	1
		Obvious swelling with partial eversion of the lids	2
		Swelling with lids about half closed	3
		Swelling with lids about half closed to completely closed	4
	C.	Discharge	
		Any amount different from normal (does not include small amount observed in inner canthus of normal animals)	1
		Discharge with moistening of the lids and hairs just adjacent to the lids	2
		Discharge with moistening of the lids and considerable area around the eye	3
		Score (A + B + C) × 5 Total maximum = 50	

The maximum total score (84) is the sum of all scores obtained for the cornea (24, or 28%), iris (10, or 12%), and conjunctiva (50, or 60%).

Local Anesthetic

Another variation in the Draize test has been the use of topical anesthetic prior to the instillation of test material (Arthur et al., 1986; Durham et al., 1992; Seabaugh et al., 1993). The use of in vitro tests prior to entry of chemicals or products into an in vivo test paradigm has alleviated much of the need for this process, since the vast majority of potential severe irritants have been eliminated from in vivo testing. Only in cases where medical treatment modalities are sought for accidental exposure to irritants or corrosives might the use of full-strength test compounds be justified and employed concurrently with simultaneously applied local anesthetics.

Fluorescein

The use of topical fluorescein solution has been recommended as an adjunct to the Draize test to allow visualization of areas of corneal epithelium (see Table 2) that reveal an increased permeability as evidenced by stromal staining (Hickey et al., 1973; Jacobs and Martens, 1989; Edelhauser and Green, 1997). This examination may be extended by applying sufficient fluorescein to allow a quantitative measurement of corneal epithelial permeability (Green, Bowman, et al., 1985; Ramselaar et al., 1988; Edelhauser and Green, 1997; McCarey and Reaves, 1997) using a fluorophotometer. This provides the opportunity to compare either a treated eye with a paired untreated eye or perform sequential measurements pre- and post-test-product application.

Pachymetry

Pachymetry has also been used to measure corneal thickness, thereby providing yet another quantitative evaluation of the effects of a test product or treatment modality on the cornea (Burton, 1972; Meyer et al., 1978; Green, Bowman, et al., 1985; Morgan et al., 1987; Kennah et al., 1989; Green, Crosby, et al., 1990). This measurement is achieved using optical or ultrasonic methods and gives an accurate determination of corneal thickness changes. The method assumes greater importance with the use of the Draize test to evaluate products or chemicals that are less likely, due to prior in vitro testing, to induce overt signs of toxicity or irritancy. Small quantitative increases in corneal thickness may be detected using these sensitive techniques in the absence of frank edema (Green, Bowman, et al., 1985; Green, 1991a).

Specular Microscopy and Endothelial Permeability

The use of specular microscopy to quantitate changes in the corneal endothelium, through morphometric analysis of specular micrographs, has also been added to the arsenal of experimental approaches in the evaluation of eye irritation (Santoul et al., 1990; Edelhauser and Ubels, 1992). Even in the absence of overt signs of ocular irritation, test materials can induce changes in different tissues that may reflect alterations in physiological or biochemical processes, such as membrane permeability or alterations in enzyme activity.

Corneal endothelial permeability in vivo is determined after the topical or iontophoretic application of fluorescein. The dye penetrates the cornea and aqueous humor eventually assuming a steady rate of loss from both tissues; corneal loss occurs across the endothelium into the anterior chamber while aqueous humor fluorescein is replaced by freshly formed, non-dye-containing, aqueous. Calculations can be made of endothelial permeability (and aqueous humor turnover rate) from these values

(Green, 1992b). Over a long-term exposure to a chemical, such tissue changes may result in toxic responses (Green, 1991a).

The corneal endothelium may also serve as a paradigm for ocular toxicity testing in the evaluation of materials that are used elsewhere in the eye. One example consists of silicone oils where a test system of in vivo anterior chamber silicone oil is allowed to remain in place for one week before in vitro measurements of endothelial permeability. This model provides an accurate evaluation of various oil contaminants that might normally be present in contaminated oils used to replace vitreous humor as a retinal tamponade. It has been shown that the shorter time course of the corneal endothelial response reflects the longer-term changes induced by the same deliberately added contaminants, both quantitatively and qualitatively, when the latter were placed in the vitreous where effects were not realized for several months (Norman et al., 1990; Green, Cheeks, et al., 1993b; Green, Cheeks, et al., 1993a). Nevertheless, toxic effects on the corneal endothelium are replicated on the blood–retinal barrier and the retinal photoreceptors. This model, thus, forms an accurate predictive method for the evaluation of various catalysts and low molecular weight compounds that remain in certain oils after polymerization. Using data obtained in these studies enables the definition of compounds that should be removed from oils prior to clinical use.

Confocal Microscopy

Confocal microscopy (Minsky, 1988) allows the examination of structures at different planes within even an opaque tissue, such as a swollen, edematous cornea. From its beginnings in in vitro studies of thick tissues, the technique has become applicable to the in vivo situation with use in both basic and clinical studies (Cavanagh et al., 1993, 1995; Jester et al., 1992a,b). Images can be acquired in real time for the study of physiological or pathophysiological events applied to ocular irritation or toxicity testing. It has potentially a great advantage in viewing ongoing processes of tissue–drug interactions and subsequent recovery. In this instance, in common with many other new techniques, only low levels of test agent need be used, which avoids induction of overt signs of irritation, thereby allowing only the drug–tissue interaction to be quantitated. This apparatus should, therefore, offer another appropriate method of assessing drug or chemical effects on the eye in a noninvasive manner.

Use of Other Methods

The incorporation of both more sensitive and quantitative methods and techniques into test systems offers a means by which evaluation can be made of the potential of a test agent or process to induce subliminal tissue changes that could lead to considerable adverse effects in the long term (Farkas et al., 1983). These evaluations assume greater importance for ocular tissues when consideration is given to the interplay between two unrelated events. The corneal endothelium may first respond to a chemical by becoming more sensitive or showing a decreased cell count per unit area and therefore, secondarily, becoming less able to cope with a further insult (Green, 1991a). Such a change would thereby lead to a more rapid and eventful endothelial decompensation than would normally occur following the "second" insult if it were to be given alone.

Albino versus Pigmented Animals

Not only have albino rabbits been compared with pigmented rabbits with few apparent differences noted in the external ocular responses (Rubin 1990; Weisse et al., 1990), but the time delay from instillation of product to rinsing has also been assessed (Davies et al., 1976; Patton and Robinson, 1976). Binding to, and the kinetics of exchange of chemicals with, intraocular and intratissue melanin can theoretically have a significant impact on the intraocular effects of a particular chemical or its metabolites, but this has not been investigated in great depth for any materials except ophthalmic products. The latter has been studied as part of investigations on drug pharmacokinetics where the binding and release kinetics of adrenergic drugs can play a significant role in determining the final drug effect in the eye (Green, 1991b).

Rinsing

Delays of longer than 30 sec between administration of a stimulant and rinsing of the eye with saline appear to allow the full development of the response as initiated in a nonrinse condition, presumably due to the fact that the arachidonic acid cascade is initiated within this time with activation of the resultant biochemical pathways (Kulkarni et al., 1984; Yousufzai et al., 1988). The degree of response is highly species-specific, with rabbits giving a large response and monkeys a low response to the same stimulus as judged by the overt signs or by biochemical changes (Bito, 1984; Bito and Klein, 1981; Klein and Bito, 1983; Kulkarni et al., 1984; Yousufzai et al., 1988). Animals, such as rats, hamsters, cats, and so on, fall between rabbit and subhuman primate in the response categories. Once initiated, these biochemical events are irreversible and progress to their natural conclusion with production of the end-stage metabolites, such as thromboxanes, leukotrienes, prostaglandins, and HETES.

The local inflammatory and irritancy induced by a test agent may actually enhance the influence of the compound either by increasing local absorption, as a result of altering permeability or generating more dilated blood vessels than normal. In such a case, the initiation of events will actually influence the progression of the response either by exacerbating or attenuating the reaction, depending upon which events prevail. The time course of the entire reaction, therefore, as well as the sequential events, will be affected by the various tissue reactions per se. The effects of such changes are difficult to predict on an a priori basis.

Animal Numbers

The number of animals used in irritancy testing has decreased from nine, as defined in the original test, to six (Code of Federal Regulations, 1979; De Sousa et al., 1984; Talsma et al., 1988; Meyer, 1993; Springer et al., 1993) with even greater reductions planned. Either a single rabbit or three rabbits might be employed (Gupta et al., 1993; Avalos et al., 1997). In the case of a single rabbit, if a positive response is seen in any grade category (Table 1) then another two rabbits would be tested. Two of three animals would need to have a positive response for irritant status to be assigned to the product. Positive effects always lead to further testing in up to six rabbits. When three rabbits are employed, a response in two rabbits indicates a positive response, and the test material would be classified as an irritant (Springer et al., 1993; Avalos et al., 1997).

Interpretation

Usually any ophthalmic product that induces a response of above 1 in the corneal criteria, above 1 for iris, and above a grade of 2 for the conjunctival lesions for anything but a minimal time is considered nonviable for further pursuit in humans. Some degree of irritancy may be acceptable if the prospective use of the product is only for a very brief period of time (local anesthetic, anti-inflammatory) rather than for extended periods (glaucoma medications [although latanoprost, the prostaglandin analog, causes temporary conjunctival hyperemia], dry-eye or contact lens solutions). Nonophthalmic products are simply labeled as possessing one degree of irritancy or another, or being labeled as a corrosive substance when marketed.

Slit-lamp

Use of a slit-lamp in the evaluation of ocular irritancy is almost mandatory (Baldwin et al., 1973; Green, Sobel, et al., 1981). This procedure allows precise observation of blood vessels, conjunctival swelling and corneal lesions (Baldwin et al., 1973; McDonald, Seabaugh, et al., 1987), with a more accurate and, at least, a semiquantitative assessment of any damage to the eye tissues. A slit-lamp offers a blue light for accurate observation of fluorescein staining of the cornea. The magnification offered by a slit-lamp allows a more detailed examination of both extraocular and intraocular tissues. Direct or indirect ophthalmoscopy is also essential for examination of the retina through a dilated pupil (Rubin, 1992; Schiavo, 1992). Permanent records of the appearance of the fundus can be obtained through photography.

Test Agent Loss

Use of the high volume (100 μl) or high mass (100 mg) of test product leads to significant difficulties in accurately determining the actual amount delivered to the eye.

When 100 μl is added to the ocular surface, where the tear film of 7–10 μl normally resides, this most frequently leads to a loss of an unknown volume of fluid onto the cheek. The first blink often causes both this displacement of fluid together with forcing fluid down the lacrimal duct into the canaliculi and hence the nose. This blink causes a further immediate loss of fluid that is dependent upon the added volume (Chrai et al., 1973, 1974). The palpebral fissure of the rabbit eye can comfortably hold a maximum of about 30 μl of fluid. Any volume greater than this is excessive and does not participate in the test.

For example, addition of 100 μl increases the volume on the ocular surface to 110 μl, which, if all of this is retained on the eye (an unlikely event), is reduced to 10 μl after the first couple of blinks. Exposure of ocular tissues to the test agent, therefore, is only to the degree of about 10% of the applied quantity for any time longer than two blinks. If the applied volume is 30 μl, then the first blink reduces the total volume from 40 μl to 10 μl, an exposure to 25% of the applied volume. Obviously, lower applied volumes provide greater exposure to the test agent until one reaches the National Academy of Sciences guidelines of 10 μl. In this instance, assuming complete and immediate mixing of tears and test material, the exposure is as much as 50% of the test agent concentration for longer time periods, since temporal dilution would occur only at the rate governed by new tear secretion.

The situation is equally applicable to solid materials. If 100 mg of any solid material is applied to the eye, the first blink will deposit a large quantity of the test agent onto the cheek. In experiments designed to test for the amounts remaining on the eye after the use of xerographic toners, 100 mg of the black material was placed onto rabbit eyes. Immediately after the first blink the eye surface, bounded by the lid margins, was thoroughly rinsed with saline, with all black particulate matter being easily identified. The toner was dried and weighed; an average of 5 or 6 mg of material was retrieved from the eye. Thus, even with solid test agents there is an enormous loss of test compound, over 90%, after the first blink (Green, Bowman, et al., 1985).

Draize Test Modifications

As indicated above, the Draize test has been modified regarding the scoring system used. Different investigators have expanded the different categories (Table 1) and added new categories, such as fluorescein staining. These changes have been made in an attempt to describe and define the ocular irritation response more precisely, especially as the Draize test has been increasingly used to test ophthalmic, rather than nonophthalmic, products (Edelhauser and Green, 1997).

Fluorescein

The use of fluorescein staining, whether examined with or without the slit-lamp, offers considerable advantages over simple observation of the cornea without dye. Fluorescein allows the identification of areas of corneal epithelial debridement or increased dye permeability as well as permitting a much more accurate measure of the area involved. In this test, however, one must establish a firm baseline in the animals prior to exposure to the product. This is necessary because the rabbit shows some staining even in the absence of application of test material due to surface cell desquamation that occurs as part of the cyclic replacement of the epithelium with a 5- or 6-day periodicity (Edelhauser and Green, 1997). By including the use of a fluorophotometer one can expand the fluorescein portion of the test to include a quantitative measurement of corneal epithelial permeability.

Test Use

In the testing of ophthalmic products, rinsing is not performed. Such action would be counter to the test itself since ophthalmic products are delivered to the eye with the goal of achieving extraocular or intraocular therapeutic drug doses. To this end, ophthalmic solutions or suspensions are manufactured to specifications designed to reduce irritation to a level compatible with the stability and chemical nature of the active ingredient(s). Testing of ophthalmic solutions or compounds usually follows the application regimen for the proposed use of the agent, that is, once to many times per day, depending upon the proposed therapeutic use. This stands in contradistinction to nonophthalmic products where a single application is used to simulate accidental exposure.

Other potential ophthalmic products can be tested and assessed using the Draize test. For example, a series of tests were performed to examine the ocular irritation of a series of chemicals derived from the glue that mussels use to attach to rocks in the tidal zone (Green, 1996). The extremely strong adhesive properties of these compounds and their ability to act as a substrate for ophthalmic cells in tissue culture (Picciano and Benedict, 1986a,b) provided impetus for an examination of their in vivo irritation potential. Compounds were injected in a 13- to 15-μl volume either intracamerally or immediately subepithelially in the cornea in order to reflect their possible intraocular and intratissue use as a tissue glue.

Many compounds were without irritative effects when given subepithelially in the cornea but even several of these compounds caused some minor and quickly reversible effects when given intracamerally (Green, 1996). The difference in response, depending upon the site of administration, is probably related to the fact that subepithelial injections allow polymerization of the injected liquid material before any constituent has the opportunity to reach the anterior chamber. Direct anterior chamber injections, on the other hand, allow access of intraocular tissues to constituents despite rapid polymerization.

These studies indicate that manipulation of the chemical backbone of these materials, by alteration of the L-dopa or amino acid content, could lead to the synthesis of compounds with very low, or even no, ocular irritation capability. Intrastromal use would have much less potential for ocular irritancy. These materials offer a means of sealing eye wounds, offering a substrate upon which cells may grow within the eye or on the ocular surface, or aiding in reepithelialization in corneal ulcers or in diabetics. These experiments also illustrated the value of slit-lamp utilization since several of the compounds formed thin, veil-like areas underlying the epithelium that were invisible to the unaided eye (Green, 1996).

Protocols and test model systems are somewhat negotiable with the FDA within the framework of the designated tests, being dependent on the material and the various constituent chemicals with scientific justification being of uppermost concern (Avalos et al., 1997). Any ingredient that is used in a product that already has a history of inducing eye irritation should be a trigger for the product to undergo a full range of in vitro and, if necessary, in vivo testing prior to admission to the market place. The use of different levels of warning labeling would be dependent upon the reactions induced by such a product.

Contact lenses and their solutions can also be evaluated using standard ocular irritation testing. These tests occur over a 21-day period with readings made at weekly intervals. The test conditions are described with an equal male–female distribution among the test animals, and lens-wearing period of 8 to 16 hours per day. The lenses are cleaned, washed, and stored for the remainder of the 24 h in their usual solutions. The ocular irritation criteria are the same as those employed for any other ophthalmic product (Edelhauser and Green, 1997).

Species Comparisons

Based on the notion that the eyes of animals more closely related to humans could more accurately predict human ocular responses to the identical irritant, the ocular responses of rhesus monkeys have been studied (Beckley et al., 1969; Green, Sullivan, et al., 1978; Swanston, 1983). The results were compared with observations made in rabbits and humans. The compounds instilled into the eyes of rabbits, rhesus monkeys, and human volunteers were a 5% soap suspension and an experimental all-purpose liquid household cleaner (Green, Sullivan, et al., 1978; Swanston, 1983).

A polyethylene cap was fitted over the head and eyes of the test rabbits to prevent pawing at the eyes and thus eliminate any physical trauma. The monkeys were placed in restraining boxes so that only the head protruded. They were fed and watered by hand and were not removed during the observation period. Male adult volunteers (ages 23 to 40) were used to gather human data.

In all three species, 0.1 ml of each test material was instilled directly onto the cornea of one eye without rinsing in rabbits and monkeys (human volunteers were allowed to wash their eyes 1 to 2 min after instillation; as noted above, this time probably exceeds that within which irritation responses are initiated and possibly served no scientific purpose). The paired contralateral eye of each subject served as a control. A slit-lamp biomicroscope was used for pretest examination of all subjects.

The animals and human subjects were graded according to the Draize system (Draize et al., 1944). Examinations were also performed at 1 h and 6 h postinstillation and daily thereafter. For humans, examination was made at 15 min, 1 h, 4 or 6 h, and 24 h postinstillation. Eyes were stained with fluorescein for the examinations. Scores were given according to a system that provided more categories and more divisions than the Draize test (Swanston, 1983). Similarities between the reactions in monkeys and humans, which were much closer to each other than either human or monkey reactions were to rabbit reactions, suggest the usefulness of utilizing nonhuman primates in irritation studies.

Similar experiments were also run by Swanston (1983). Rabbit, monkey, and human ocular reaction to the instillation of a 5% soap solution and a liquid household cleaner were graded and compared according to a scoring system based on the use of slit-lamp biomicroscopy and fluorescein, and also according to the commonly used Draize visual observation method (Draize et al., 1944).

Reactions in monkeys were more comparable to human reactions than were those seen in rabbits, based on biomicroscopic observations. Instillation of a 5% soap solution into rabbit eyes produced a minimal corneal epithelial effect. The same material caused corneal epithelial damage to both monkeys and humans. These lesions were not, however, visible without the use of slit-lamp biomicroscopy and/or fluorescein. The detergent composition used for these studies produced irritation in all three species. However, in this study, the degree of human response predicted by the rabbit was much greater than that predicted by the monkey, which again was more accurate in predicting the nature of the human hazard (Green, Sullivan, et al., 1978; Green, Edelhauser, et al., 1997).

Tear Flow

Test materials ranging from tear gas (Ballantyne et al., 1974) or other chemical constituents of products to solutions of low or high pH can cause increased lacrimation. Determination of tear flow can be achieved by measuring the dilution of tracers, such as fluorescein (Mishima et al., 1966) or technetium, Tc^{99} (Chrai et al., 1973; Patton and Robinson, 1975; Greaves et al., 1991). The tracer is added to the tear film and a baseline dilution established that can then be evaluated after addition of the test material. The volume of tracer solution added to the tear film needs to be as small as possible, preferably no greater than 2 μl, and must itself be at physiologic pH so that it does not induce changes in tear flow per se. Since tear pH is normally between pH 7.3 and 7.7 (Stjernschantz and Astin, 1993), a solution in this range would be considered acceptable. The use of such a solution should not induce increased blinking that can also occur with the addition of even a very slightly irritating solution.

Pain

Newer approaches and test procedures prior to the use of in vivo techniques have led to a marked diminution in the eye irritation testing of compounds that might induce pain. Nevertheless, if pain is considered a likely event, then adequate topical anesthetic must be applied prior to the test material. It is difficult to assess pain in the rabbit model except by observation of complete or partial closure of the eyelids, excessive lacrimation that appears as marked dampness of the area around the eyes, and pawing at the eye. Vocalization may sometimes occur temporarily upon instillation of test agent. The only means to objectively measure pain responses is by electrophysiological techniques (Beuerman et al., 1992) in an anesthetized animal.

Corneal Epithelial Permeability

With the advent of considerable in vitro testing before entering an in vivo test phase, and the widespread use of the Draize test to identify the irritancy potential of ophthalmic products, many test agents do not induce overt ocular effects. Nevertheless, changes may be induced that can be responsible for toxic effects to be realized at a later date. To evaluate this potential, newer techniques have been introduced that allow evaluation of physiological changes in tissue behavior.

Corneal epithelial fluorescein permeability offers a quantitative measure of more subtle changes in this membrane in response to the addition of test products to the eye (Edelhauser and Green, 1997). The permeability can be measured, after one or many applications of the test material, in a noninvasive manner and without the use of local or systemic anesthesia. Stromal fluorescein concentration is measured at intervals after the topical application of dye. Normal physiology is thus sustained as far as the test system is involved, with the product being the only variable. Use of topical fluorescein allows either the semiquantitative or quantitative measure of permeability (Adler et al., 1971; Green, Bowman, et al., 1985; Boets et al., 1988; Ramselaar et al., 1988; Stolwijk et al., 1990; McCarey and Reaves, 1997).

Even when no overt signs of eye irritancy exist, the test product may induce alterations in corneal epithelial permeability, and the technology of fluorophotometry allows the measurement of such changes that indicate effects, usually of ophthalmic products, on the eye. Such responses would normally be undetectable by any other available means. The degree of variability from a single-drop topical dye instillation for the assessment of corneal epithelial permeability has been recently addressed. The single-drop procedure is unreliable for evaluating individual patient changes but has a role in population-based research (McNamara et al., 1997). Determinations can be made, with the appropriate application of sufficient fluorescein or other dye, of corneal endothelial permeability and aqueous humor turnover rate which may also be affected by the intraocular penetration of the test chemical(s) (Green, 1992b).

Corneal Epithelial Reepithelialization

Another in vivo test paradigm for the evaluation of eye irritation is corneal epithelial wound healing. Lesions of a precise area can be created in the epithelium either by mechanical scraping or by chemical methods (Bowman and Green, 1982; Edelhauser and Ubels, 1992). Lesions are created in anesthetized rabbits. In the case of a mechanical lesion, an area, usually about 6 mm in diameter, is delineated using a trephine, and the cells within that region are scraped off with a blade or Gill corneal knife. Remaining cells are removed with a Q-tip or small cotton ball on the end of a toothpick (Ho et al., 1974). For chemical cell removal, a circular piece of filter paper is soaked in *n*-heptanol, and the 6-mm-diameter paper is then placed on the corneal epithelium for 60 sec (Cintron et al., 1979).

In both cases of epithelial debridement, there is usually a period of about 6 h during which little happens except some small cellular rearrangement. After this time, corneal reepithelialization occurs, through the centripetal movement of cells toward the center of the lesion, and this can be quantitated using fluorescein solution topically applied to the eye and photography. Fluorescein stains the area where epithelium is missing, and appropriate color photography using filters allows the lesion to be accurately photographed (Bowman and Green, 1982; Green, Johnson, et al., 1989; Edelhauser and Green, 1997).

Evaluation of the area of the lesion can be made at successive time intervals either by computer analysis of images obtained from a digitizer pad or weighing of paper upon which the corneal image is projected and the lesion area cut out. The rate of closure of epithelial wounds is 60 μm per hour regardless of the initial wound diameter (Crosson et al., 1986). In some instances, for example with sodium lauryl sulfate (Green, Johnson, et al., 1989), lesions may expand before eventually contracting and giving full reepithelialization. In the latter case, complete epithelial wound healing occurred over an 8- or 9-day period relative to the 48 h normally required for covering a 6-mm-diameter lesion (Green, Johnson, et al., 1989). A similar independent finding of initial increased lesion size occurred following the application of sodium dodecyl sulfate, with a very slow rate of reepithelialization (Edelhauser and Ubels, 1992). In these cases of the study of anionic surfactants, at 10% of the concentration predicted to reach the eye, it is to be noted that the effects on reepithelialization occurred in the absence of any overt signs of irritancy.

Systemic Administration or Intake

While the Draize test, in an appropriately modified form, can be employed for externally applied products or materials, it is of little value in the evaluation of the ocular toxicity of systemic medications or the accidental intake of other materials. This is a totally different area of investigation that requires the use of sophisticated techniques (Scheimpflug imagery for the lens, electroretinography for the retina, specular microscopy and pachymetry for the cornea, etc.). The nature of the product and that it is used, or obtains access, systemically means that its systemic toxicity profile is very low, otherwise it could not have reached such a point in its development. Any potential ocular toxicity could usually be investigated following clinical observations of an adverse side effect. Animal studies would then be undertaken using one or more of the refined techniques as needed to specify the site and mode of drug action responsible for the adverse side effect.

Substances, whether medications or other materials, that are ingested orally or absorbed through the skin follow different pathways. Oral intake leads to a first-pass hepatic effect that may provide not only the original compound but also one or more metabolites (Green, 1982) that may contribute to any ocular toxicological response.

Direct absorption through the skin, however, more resembles an intravenous injection since the chemical enters the blood stream directly, before subsequent metabolism.

Evaluations of any ocular effects must take into account that such metabolites may well occur; thus, knowledge of the metabolic breakdown of the test compound is imperative to ascribe any effect to a specific chemical species. Knowledge of the metabolic pathway in the in vivo animal model should obviously parallel that which occurs in man. This is exemplified by chloramphenicol, which is metabolized by the rabbit but not by man, as determined by thin-layer chromatography (Beasley et al., 1975; Green and MacKeen, 1976). Indeed, it has been estimated that the rabbit should receive about 20 times more chloramphenicol to make the rabbit study analogous to the human study (Havener, 1974).

EYE MOVEMENTS

Saccadic Eye Movement

Ocular toxic effects can be realized not only as pain, irritation, and loss of vision, but as dysfunction of the muscles of eye movement or of accommodation, which also leads to impairment of vision (Rohde, 1992). Eye movements can be used to determine the toxic effects of certain chemicals on the eye, particularly those that paralyze muscle movements. Because fine muscle movement is more sensitive to muscle paralyzing agents than is coarse muscle movement (such as that of the limbs), this is a good in vivo model for studying toxic effects of chemicals on the eye.

Studies have been made on human subjects (Levett and Jaeger, 1980). After a 3- to 5-h fast, the subjects were fitted with eyeglass frames on which were mounted two phototransistors and one infrared source, with which eye movements were monitored. The frame permitted the phototransistors to be closely positioned near the limbus on either side of the eye. The phototransistor outputs gave a voltage output proportional to reflected infrared light, which gave an accurate indication of eye position. A dot displayed on an oscilloscope served as the target, which only took one of two positions on the screen during the course of the experiments. The target position and the eye position were continuously recorded. Histograms of saccadic eye movement latency were computed, typically for between 25 and 100 responses.

For a given subject, two to five histograms were collected under control conditions. A prescribed quantity of alcohol was then given, and latency histograms were repeatedly computed at 15-min intervals for periods of 3–5 h. In normal subjects, data showed the most common range for saccadic eye movement latency to be approximately 200–250 msec. The fastest times observed were about 50 msec. In all subjects tested, saccadic eye movement latency increased following administration of alcohol.

This procedure could be used to study the toxicity of other substances that affect eye movement and muscle coordination. Many kinds of medications and drugs have the side effect of drowsiness. This procedure could be a quick, noninvasive means of quantitating those side effects (Rohde, 1992) not only of systemically administered drugs but also of topically applied medications or products.

Smooth Pursuit Eye Movements

This procedure tests the effects of toxic agents on a voluntary neurological function. A monocular eye movement monitor was used in this representative study (Jaeger and Yoo, 1975). A computer presented a target stimulus on a horizontal axis. Each trial consisted of the subject tracking the target for approximately 1 min. Rest periods of 3–5 min were given between trials. The results suggest a general pattern of response. This response indicates that between normal smooth pursuit movements and the saccadic pursuit movements of the severely intoxicated state, there exists a continuum of degraded smooth pursuit movements (Rohde, 1992). Here, also, various test products or drugs could be evaluated for their effects on this parameter.

OCULAR MICROCIRCULATION

Eye irritants frequently cause conjunctival vasodilation and an increase in ocular circulation, which are not quantitatively measured in the Draize test. Indeed, only conjunctival hyperemia receives a qualitative evaluation as does the iris. Several techniques can be used to quantitate the measurement of ocular blood flow, including (a) the microsphere technique (Bill, 1974; Morgan et al., 1981; Chiou and Yan, 1986), (b) laser Doppler velocimetry (Robinson et al., 1986; Yan and Chiou, 1987), and (c) pulsatile blood flow measurement (Raitta and Tolonen, 1980; Chiou et al., 1990).

Microsphere Technique

The microsphere technique can be used to measure blood flow in all parts of the eye tissue (Bill, 1974; Morgan et al., 1981; Chiou and Yan, 1986). Furthermore, any other tissues either immediately extraocular or distant from the eye can be harvested and blood flow calculated on any tissue. However, this technique can be used only in terminal animal experiments. Rabbits are anesthetized with a ketamine/xylazine mixture (Morgan et al., 1981). The left femoral artery is cannulated, while PE 90 tubing is inserted into the left ventricle through the right carotid artery. Heparin is administered intravenously. A bolus of strontium-85 (^{85}Sr)-labeled microspheres or colored microspheres (15.6 ± 0.8 μm diameter) is injected, in a volume of saline containing 1% Tween 80, into the left ventricle. The surfactant, Tween 80, acts as a dispersing agent to prevent microsphere clumping or aggregation. Approximately 1 million microspheres are administered. Blood is collected from the femoral artery for 60 sec immediately after injection of the microspheres to provide a measure of the precapillary, or source, blood flow and microsphere contents. Both blood volume flow for 1 min and number of microspheres passing through the pre-capillary circulation are obtained from these femoral artery values.

The rabbit is then killed with an excess of saturated KCl into the ventricle. The eyes (and any other body tissues, as needed) are removed and dissected into iris, ciliary body, retina, and choroid. Extraocular muscles, conjunctiva, and so on, can also be harvested. The tissues are weighed and, when using ^{85}Sr microspheres, their radioactivities are determined. Other labels are used for microspheres, such as chromium-51 (^{51}Cr) or cerium-141 (^{141}Ce), and through the use of different isotopic labels can be used for pre- and post-drug measurements in the same animal. When using colored microspheres, the number of microspheres in the digested tissues is counted under a microscope using a hemocytometer. The blood flow in the tissues is calculated knowing the rate of untrapped blood flow in the femoral artery and its radioactivity, or the number of colored microspheres, and the relative radioactivity or number of microspheres of the ocular tissues where the microspheres are trapped in the capillaries due to their size; tissue blood flow is calculated by simple proportionality and expressed as microliters per minute per milligram of tissue (Bill, 1974; Green, Wynn, et al., 1978; Morgan et al., 1981, 1983; Jay et al., 1984; Green, Paterson, et al., 1985, 1990; Green and Schermerhorn, 1985; Rohde, 1992).

This technique is the only one of the three listed here that provides values for blood flow through all ocular tissues, including iris and conjunctiva, that are the most likely to be affected by an externally applied agent. Studies can be made after acute (Green, Wynn, et al., 1978; Morgan et al., 1981, 1983; Green, Paterson, et al., 1985, 1990) or subchronic (Green and Schermerhorn, 1985; Green and Hatchett, 1987) drug administration.

Laser-Doppler Velocimetry

Laser-Doppler velocimetry allows the measurement of retinal blood flow in conscious animals and patients. It is widely used in animal experiments (Yan and Chiou, 1987) and in some clinics (Robinson et al., 1986). As indicated, this technique only allows blood flow measurements in the retina.

Although the procedure can be used on conscious animals, rabbits are usually anesthetized to eliminate eye movements. The femoral artery and vein are cannulated to monitor blood pressure and for injection of anesthetic and drugs, respectively. The reflected beam of laser light from the laser-Doppler depends on the average cell velocity and cell density in the measured volume of the blood vessels under investigation.

Pulsatile Blood Flow Method

The pulsatile blood flow measured with oculosphygmography is noninvasive and easily workable (Raitta and Tolonen, 1980; Chiou et al., 1990). Rabbits are placed in restraining boxes and a drop of tetracaine applied to the eye (Chiou et al., 1990). An air applanation tonometer (Walker and Litovich, 1972; Green, 1992c) is applied to the eye. The pulsations in intraocular pressure produced by the flow of blood in the ocular vessels are measured when pressure is applied to the eye. The probe is connected to a pressure transducer, and total ocular blood flow is deduced from the intraocular pressure fluctuations (Yan and Chiou, 1987; Rohde, 1992). The limitation of this approach is that only total ocular blood flow can be determined with no discrimination between the various tissues (retina, choroid, iris, etc.).

AQUEOUS HUMOR AND INTRAOCULAR PRESSURE

Both aqueous humor characteristics and intraocular pressure may be altered by topically applied products or chemicals (Green and Padgett, 1979; Green and Elijah, 1981; Green, Elijah, et al., 1981; Green, Elijah, et al., 1982; Green, Elijah, et al., 1986), and a variety of techniques are available to measure such induced changes (Green, 1992b,c). Aqueous humor composition may be determined, although this is a terminal experiment in rabbits, meaning that different (paired) eyes or different groups of animals (treated versus control) must be compared. The animal must receive topical anesthetic prior to removal of a 100- to 150-μl sample of aqueous humor. Harvesting of greater volumes of aqueous humor leads to breakdown of the blood–aqueous barrier and a marked change in aqueous composition, particularly of protein content, although ions are also altered. Because of the great sensitivity of the rabbit blood–aqueous barrier to any ocular manipulation, suppository aspirin or intraperitoneal indomethacin should be seriously considered as a prophylactic measure when aqueous humor samples are taken in this species. Such pretreatment will, at least, reduce the effects of prostanoid release in the eye.

Aqueous Cell and Protein

In vivo testing can be made of aqueous flare using an instrument designed to use the reflectivity of light from particulate matter as a measure of proteins in the anterior chamber. A commercial laser flare meter (Green, 1992b), as well as laboratory-constructed equipment (Anjou and Krakau, 1961), is available.

Hyphema can be estimated with accuracy using a nomogram that uses the depth of the anterior chamber and the height of the hyphema when both are determined using a slit-lamp (Green, 1992b).

Aqueous Humor Inflow

A measure of the permeability of the blood–aqueous barrier can be obtained through the use of intravenous fluorescein and a fluorophotometer. The rate of fluorescein entry into the eye can be quantitated either in the same animal pre- and post-treatment or in control and experimental groups of animals (Ward et al., 1991; Ward, Ferguson, et al., 1992a; Ward, Ferguson, et al., 1992b; Green, 1992b).

Aqueous humor turnover rate can be determined after either the topical or iontophoretic application of fluorescein to the cornea. Either method will allow the entry of dye into the cornea and anterior chamber where, ultimately, a peak concentration is reached followed by a parallel and linear decline in tissue and fluid concentrations. The rate of dilution of the dye allows the calculation of not only aqueous humor formation rate, which may be altered by an applied toxin, but also of corneal endothelial permeability coefficient (Ward et al., 1991; Ward, Ferguson, et al., 1992a; Ward, Ferguson, et al., 1992b; Green, 1992b). These methods allow the measurement of very subtle alterations in physiological and biochemical processes that govern membrane permeability, even where no overt changes are seen. Changes can also be followed over time of natural changes in these parameters as a function of, for example, the menstrual cycle or pregnancy (Green, Cullen, et al., 1984; Green, Phillips, et al., 1988).

Intraocular Pressure

A variety of instrumentation exists for intraocular pressure determination (Green, 1992c), including the more accurate applanation devices. Regardless of the type of tonometer, however, the chosen apparatus must be calibrated on a regular basis for each test species (Hammond and Bhattacherjee, 1984; Frenkel et al., 1988). Such calibration is especially important in long-term studies (Green, Kim, et al., 1977; Green, Phillips, et al., 1985).

Local anesthetic prior to intraocular pressure measurements in conscious animals should consist of one drop of anesthetic that is washed off after 5–10 sec with 1 ml of saline or a diluted drop of anesthetic that is used without ocular rinsing (Maurice and Singh, 1985). Care should be taken not to manipulate the eye or to add any pressure on the eye during the anesthetic administration, rinsing, or measurement process. Each of these steps could alter the intraocular pressure, which requires time to readjust.

In either case, the absence of epithelial disturbances caused by the choice of the mode of anesthetic application should be established in pretest studies (Green, 1992c).

IRIS

Color

Changes in iris color may occur, as exemplified by the effects of the prostaglandin derivative latanoprost. This compound reduces intraocular pressure through its actions on uveoscleral or uveovortex outflow pathways (unconventional outflow) and, thus, offers a unique intraocular pressure-reducing mechanism (Nilsson et al., 1989; Alm and Villumsen, 1991; Camras et al., 1992; Racz et al., 1993; Toris et al., 1993; Alm et al., 1995; Watson et al., 1996). As indicated, one of the side effects of this new drug is that it induces, over a 6- to 9-month period, an increase in iris color by darkening mixed-color irides. This occurs through an increase in iris pigmentation in about 5–15% of the patients. Such iris color changes can be quantitated using computer technology that provides a much more reliable measurement capacity than does color assessment by the human eye or capture of the color on photographic film (Bee et al., 1997). The computer images are analyzed by an image analysis software package that displays the colors as numerical values when determined in red, green, and blue color strength. The latter procedure obviates changes in development solution, temperature, changes with time and condition of film storage, and so on when dealing with photographic film. In addition, the technology is able to distinguish color changes at a more subtle level than by eye or film.

Pupil Size

Pupil diameter can also be measured. This can be achieved either by direct measurement using a transparent ruler under constant light conditions, after the application of a substance to the ocular surface, or by infrared camera measurements. The latter provides greater accuracy in quantitating changes in pupil diameter without manipulation of the eye or the use of changes in ambient light intensity which would itself change pupil diameter.

Fluorescein Angiography

The intravenous injection of fluorescein can be used to provide information concerning the vascular status of the iris. Comparative measures can be made of the permeability of iridial vessels in both clinical and animal studies (Bergstrom et al., 1976; Van Nerom et al., 1981; Hull et al., 1985; Csukas et al., 1987; Csukas and Green, 1988; Green, Paterson, et al., 1990).

Aging has been shown to increase fluorescein leakage at the pupillary margin in man as well as to increase the time of fluorescein to reach the pupillary margin from the limbus (Van Nerom et al., 1981). Inflammatory effects of a relatively marked nature have also been noted under various stimulating experimental conditions (i.e., an increase in hydrogen peroxide or oxygen free radical products concentration of the anterior chamber [Hull et al., 1985; Csukas et al., 1987; Csukas and Green, 1988]) or after prostaglandin- or endotoxin-induced inflammation (Green, Paterson, et al., 1985, 1990). Analysis of these photographs, taken at short intervals after dye injection, can provide a quantitative measure of the leakiness of iris vessels.

LENS

Accommodation

Accommodation is a combined response of the lens, ciliary muscle, and iris that may be affected by reactions to foreign materials that gain access to the eye. Measurement of accommodation is a sensitive method for detecting the effects of chemical stimuli on the eye (Levett and Jaeger, 1980; Rohde, 1992).

Cataract Formation

Cataracts can be induced by ultraviolet (UV) light (Tuffs et al., 1987), by chemicals (Koch et al., 1976; Lubek et al., 1990; Hockwin, Wegener, et al., 1992), by diseases such as diabetes (Piatigorsky, 1980; Schmidt et al., 1987), and by combinations of stimuli including radiation (Eckerskorn et al., 1987; Hockwin and Wegener, 1987). The latter includes syncataractogenesis, which represents the combined influence of two separate subliminal factors that lead to lens opacities only when in combination. In cocataractogenesis, the direct effect of a toxic agent is potentiated by a subliminal factor that alone has no effect (Hockwin, Green, et al., 1992; Hockwin, Wegener, et al., 1992).

Measurement of Cataract Formation

Several methods exist for the classification and measurement of cataract formation. These range from slit-lamp observations (Hockwin, Green, et al., 1992), to Scheimpflug imagery with subsequent quantitative densitometric analysis of the photographic film or computer images (Dragomirescu et al., 1978; Hockwin, Wegener, et al., 1984–85, 1987; Eckerskorn et al., 1987; Lehnert et al., 1987; Lerman, 1987; Wegener et al., 1987), to the LOC III system proposed and used by Chylack (Chylack et al., 1993), to use of a system that provides an impression of the lens opaque areas from retroillumination (Sparrow et al., 1986). Dilation of the pupil is important to allow the lens normally covered by the iris to be examined; for Scheimpflug imagery, a fully dilated pupil is a necessity for obtaining comprehensive and reproducible images (Cheeks et al., 1992).

Cataractogenesis by UV Irradiation

A study (Tuffs et al., 1987) was undertaken to establish a new cataract model for animal studies in which the cataractogenic agent was short-wave UV radiation (280–315 nm; UV-B). This model has few side effects and does not interfere with the absorption of drugs in the lens (Tuffs et al., 1987; Hockwin, Green, et al., 1992).

Cataractogenesis by Chemicals

Many drugs and environmental chemicals are bioactivated by enzyme systems, such as cytochrome P-450 and prostaglandin synthetase, to potentially toxic reactive intermediates. Naphthalene is one of many polycyclic aromatic hydrocarbons that may be bioactivated by the cytochrome P-450 monooxygenase enzymes to a potentially toxic, reactive arene oxide intermediate. If not immediately detoxified, the arene oxide intermediate, or possibly a quinone derivative, may bind covalently to lenticular macromolecules resulting in cellular toxicity, which may be expressed as a cataract (Tuffs et al., 1987; Hockwin, Wegener, et al., 1992). Oral naphthalene, given every other day to rats, creates a zonular cataract in the lens cortex over a 6-week period (Hockwin, Green, et al., 1992).

Cataractogenesis Due to Diabetes

Diabetes induces substantial lens opacity changes over time, and this has been investigated in several model systems (Hockwin, Green, et al., 1992). In one series of experiments, three groups of Brown–Norway rats were used: group C, control; group D, diabetes; and group DS, diabetes and sorbinil treatment (Bours et al., 1987). Streptozotocin (70 mg/kg) in a single injection was used to induce diabetes in groups D and DS. Sorbinil (25 mg/kg) was given orally every 2 days to group DS. During the entire 6-week experiment, measurements of blood glucose level showed values of at least 280 mg/100 ml in the DS group.

Slit-lamp examinations and Scheimpflug photos were made before, during, and at the end of the experiments. After the experiments were completed, the lenses were dissected from eyes, and lens weights were measured. The lenses were sectioned by a frozen-sectioning technique (Hockwin et al., 1986). Lenses were quick-frozen with dry ice on a microtome sample holder, with the posterior side of the lens facing downward. The lenses were cut into sections in a cryostat at $-20°C$. Thirty to forty sections were united to one fraction. The fractions were homogenized and centrifuged at $11,000 \times g$. Supernatants and sediments of each fraction were lyophilized, and the amounts of water-soluble and water-insoluble crystallins and their ratios determined. The fraction dry weight was calculated by addition of water-soluble and water-insoluble crystallins.

The water-soluble crystallins of each fraction or layer of the three groups were separated by polyacrylamide thin-layer isoelectric focusing. The samples were stained for proteins with Coomassie Brilliant Blue W and for glycoproteins with periodic acid-Schiff reagent. The proteins of each crystallin class were determined by densitometry and calculated in percent from the fraction dry weight.

The lens wet weights of the diabetes (D) group and of the diabetes–sorbinil (DS) group were significantly diminished by 5 mg, partly due to hydration in group D and dehydration in group DS.

The dry weight was lower in groups D and DS than in group C. The percentage dry weight in group D was lower than in groups C and DS. The water content in groups D and DS was lower than in group C, but the percentage lens water was higher in group D but lower in group DS than in the control. The ratio of wet weight over dry weight was higher for group D and for group DS, compared with group C (Bours et al., 1987; Rohde, 1992). These whole-lens results indicate and reflect some of the significant biochemical changes that occur in the rat lens as a result of the induction of diabetes. These include changes in water content, dry weight, and protein composition with aggregation of molecules occurring to create an opacity due to increased light scattering. It is evident that diabetes induces considerable changes in lens protein composition, some of which can be reflected in noninvasive Scheimpflug biomicroscopy.

This is also illustrated by recent studies comparing lens proteins with Scheimpflug imagery and subsequent microdensitometric analysis (Swamy-Mruthinti et al., 1996a,b). Induction of diabetes in albino rats with streptozotocin was associated with only small increases in both lens density and protein glycation for the first 60 days after diabetic onset (blood glucose > 400 mg/dl). Between 60 and 90 days, however, dramatic changes occurred in both measured parameters until lenses became quite opaque with typical diabetic changes. In separate experiments, it proved possible to reduce the degree of cataract density and glycation through the systemic adminis-tration of aminoguanidine (Swamy-Mruthinti et al., 1996b). This response was only possible in moderately (< 350 mg/dl), but not highly (> 350 mg/dl), diabetic animals. The results suggest that some further control can be exerted over cataract formation through the use of antiglycation compounds when the underlying diabetes is not severe.

Animal Models

Various models exist for the determination of the cataractogenic potential of differ-ent drugs and/or products (Wegener and Hockwin, 1987; Bours et al., 1990; Kojima et al., 1990; Lerman 1990, 1992; Roberts and Dillon, 1990; Schmitt et al., 1990; Hockwin, Wegener, et al., 1992; Edelhauser and Green, 1997). Recent studies by Wegener (see Edelhauser and Green, 1997) have examined animal models based on hereditary defects and those due to acquired or induced effects. Mice with a genetic expression of an anterior suture cataract showed enhancement of the defect when irradiated with UV-B. This result indicates the possibility of modulating genetic de-fects, although this area requires considerable exploration.

Induced models, such as those for diabetes, should reflect the clinical condi-tion and subsequent clinical sequelae. Exposure to UV-A, for example, produces only subliminal effects, but responses are realized if the diet of the animal is made vitamin-E deficient. UV-B, on the other hand, produces an anterior polar cataract directly (Edelhauser and Green, 1997). With the diabetic and naphthalene cataracts, there are chemicals that reduce the rate of onset and severity of the cataract, but there are other chemicals that accelerate cataract formation induced by these conditions. A multiplicity of animal models for cataract exist that can be induced or altered by antibiotics, anti-inflammatory agents (including nonsteroidal compounds) and many other drugs used systemically (Edelhauser and Green, 1997).

The lens offers one of the sites within the eye that is extremely sensitive to many chemicals or external influences. For this reason, examination of the lens using quan-titative measures should be undertaken whenever possible during toxicological ex-aminations. Care should be exercised to keep a close watch on any simultaneous factors that may be influencing the lens in order that syn- or co-cataractogenic fac-tors can be minimized.

RETINA

The retina is extremely sensitive to physicochemical stimuli as it contains ample neurons and photoreceptor cells. Drug-induced oculotoxicity is thus detectable by measuring the retinal changes with electroretinography (ERG) (Gramoni, 1980; Rubin, 1992; Zrenner, 1992; Weisse et al., 1995) and visual evoked responses (Cooper et al., 1980). Although this is not a component of the ocular irritancy (Draize) test, full consideration should be given to the use of ERG as a component of toxicological testing on the eye. As with the lens, the retina is very sensitive to extraocular stimuli and provides an excellent means of determining whether a chemical or product has the potential to induce ocular toxicity. If an effect is seen in the retina (or lens), then careful examination should be made of other ocular tissues. If responses occur in either of these two tissues, there is a high probability that toxic effects would be found in other ocular tissues upon careful examination.

Electroretinography

The most important ion in ERG studies is potassium (K^+), and the potassium channel governs much of the neurological behavior of the retina (Miller and Dowling, 1970; Dick and Miller, 1985; Dick et al., 1985; Nilius and Reichenbach, 1988). The b-wave component of the electroretinogram and the subsequent oscillatory b-wave component are both mediated by potassium shifts in the retina. It has been found that the b-wave is a Müller glial cell response (Miller and Dowling, 1970) and that there are a variety of changes in extracellular potassium in the retina in response to various stimuli.

Various mammalian models exist for determining the potential retinal neurotoxicity of different chemicals or products. The ERG, electrooculogram (EOG) (Gouras and Gunkel, 1963), and visual evoked potential (VEP) aid considerably in characterizing the effects of compounds on the visual system since each test targets a different portion of the visual pathway (Geller et al., 1995). Each test can be administered noninvasively in animals and humans. Use of the pigmented rat allows at least a comparison between the ERG and VEP even though latencies and amplitudes differ. Albino rats have an associated problem of susceptibility to phototoxic degeneration of the outer nuclear layer (Geller et al., 1995) that makes this model less than satisfactory.

Other models include the dog, cat, and monkey (Bee et al., 1995; Clerc and Sayn, 1995; Weisse et al., 1995; Edelhauser and Green, 1997), all of which use methods adapted from clinical electroretinography (Marmor et al., 1989; Zrenner, 1992; Jacobi et al., 1993). Both photopic and scotopic procedures may be employed (Bee et al., 1995), although some authors have suggested that sufficiently complete toxicity information can be obtained without the prerequisite of dark adaptation (Clerc and Sayn, 1995). Corneal contact lens electrodes are used in rabbit, cat, dog, and monkey with wick electrodes used in mice, and a reference electrode attached to a shaved area of skin in all species. A Ganzfeld stimulus is best since this allows both eyes to be tested simultaneously. Several arrangements of detection systems exist, but a good commercial one is made by Nicolet (Bee et al., 1995; Edelhauser and Green, 1997). A Ganzfeld stimulus is difficult in animals with eyes on the side of their heads (i.e., mice, rabbits, etc.), but is easy with subhuman primates. In the former animals, an arrangement of the light stimulus should be sought where the eye-to-light distance is equal for each eye to ensure that the delivered stimulus from photoflood lights is the same for each eye.

The primary difference between the clinical measurement setup and that for an animal is that the latter are usually anesthetized. Usually, this is accomplished with intramuscular ketamine (Clerc and Sayn, 1995; Edelhauser and Green, 1997), although other sedatives may be used, especially a combination of ketamine and benzodiazepam. Other anesthetics, such as barbiturates or halothane, induce changes in the ERG per se that can override the delineation of toxic drug effects. Anesthesia may not be necessary, or desirable, in beagle dogs or micropigs (Loget and Saint-Macary, 1995).

The retinal toxicity of intravitreal, topical or systemic chemicals has been widely determined using the measurement of ERG (D'Amico et al., 1985; Baldinger et al., 1986; Hennekes et al., 1987; Paylor et al., 1987; Small et al., 1987; Fiscella et al., 1988; Zlioba et al., 1988; Blain et al., 1990; Brown et al., 1990; Green, Slagle, et al., 1992a; Green, Slagle, et al., 1992b; Green, Cheeks, et al., 1993a; Green, Slagle et al., 1993; Shirao and Kawasaki, 1995). These studies include organic and inorganic chemicals ranging from antibiotics to silicone oil. The techniques for ERG are, therefore, well described in the literature and have assumed a standard type of protocol which allows results from different laboratories to be directly compared. Decreases in the b-wave after light stimulation under dark-adapted conditions are indicative of photoreceptor toxicity as long as appropriate care is taken to ensure that the light stimulation is well standardized and calibrated.

The adoption of uniform procedures and standards for ERG determination has provided this technique with a powerful influence in determining retinal toxicity (Zrenner, 1992). The standards were derived from clinical ERG, where uniformity is a prerequisite for comparisons of ERG performed temporally, that allow ERGs taken at different times to be evaluated in order to detect disease progression.

Blood–Retinal Barrier Permeability

Measurement of blood–retinal barrier permeability can be made using a fluorophotometer such as the Ocumetrics Fluorotron Master, in its vitreous mode through the dilated pupil of a test eye. Fluorescein is given intravenously after an initial ocular scan to determine background fluorescence. Scans are then made at predetermined intervals (5 min and 60 min) after fluorescein injection as designated by the built-in software, and calculations are made of the rate of entry of dye into the vitreous. In this way, the dye concentration can be measured in different ocular compartments as a function of time and treatment (Jones et al., 1982; Cunha-Vaz, 1985; Gray et al., 1985; Green, Slagle, et al., 1992a; Green, Slagle, et al., 1992b; Green, Slagle, et al.,

1993; Green, Cheeks, et al., 1993a). This sensitive and accurate technique can be used to evaluate and compare paired eyes or eyes in different animals that receive different treatments.

Fluorescein Angiography

This procedure is used to illustrate vascular flow, leakage, and the general appearance of vascular trees in the fundus. Photographic records are obtained for later evaluation. Fluorescein is injected intravenously and appears in the eye within 5–20 sec, and cameras with rapid recycling capacity are vital to provide records of the early phases of vessel filling.

Indocyanine green dye is often used to evaluate choroidal vascular bed filling and circulation since it can be detected through the retinal pigmented epithelium in the early phases of ocular circulation.

SKIN TESTS

Good correlation of dermal irritation and ocular irritation would allow a reasonable prediction of eye irritation from skin irritation tests (Gilman et al., 1983). As a result, eye irritation tests could be avoided for chemicals that would potentially cause severe eye damage. Draize testing would be carried out only if the eye irritation of a chemical is predicted to be mild or nonirritating. It should be used mainly for safety assurance rather than for toxicity determination (Williams, 1984; Avalos et al., 1997; Edelhauser and Green, 1997). Unfortunately, people are likely to come in contact with irritants (such as pesticides, household cleaners) and even corrosives (such as oven cleaners) in their daily life and work, so a knowledge of the kind of ocular damage these chemicals produce is needed to predict the best form of emergency treatment. An example is the use of citrate/acetate solutions for eye wash after an alkali burn of the eye, which is more efficacious in curtailing damage than water alone (Pfister et al., 1981, 1991).

Acute Toxicity

Typically, animals are prepared by clipping the skin of the trunk free of hair and may be further prepared by making epidermal abrasions longitudinally 2 cm apart over the area of exposure. Twenty-four hours later, doses of liquids or solutions, or solids, are introduced for a 24-h exposure. At the end of the 24-h period of exposure, any sleeves or screens over the test material are removed, and the skin reactions noted immediately. The animals are checked for gross symptoms and are then transferred to individual metabolism cages where they are observed for a minimal period of two weeks. Body weight, food consumption, and gross symptoms of systemic effects are checked daily. Observations for changes in blood morphology are made (Rohde, 1992).

Subacute Toxicity (20- or 90-Day Experiments)

In these experiments, relatively large doses are applied daily to an uncovered area of the clipped skin. The area exposed is approximately 10% of the total surface of the animal. The material is gently rubbed into the skin with a glass rod. The animals are observed for two weeks following the final exposure. The same observations for gross symptoms, urine, tissues, and so on are made as in the acute experiments. These test protocols are frequently used to establish the potential ocular toxicity of compounds prior to any eye irritancy testing (Hackett, 1990) and form part of the preocular testing system. Corrosive and highly irritant chemicals may, thus, be eliminated from eye testing. It must be kept in mind, however, that even these products must be tested in the rabbit model at least once in order to determine the best conditions for neutralization or limitation of their damaging effects. This is well-illustrated in the case of alkali burns to the eye, where experimental procedures indicated that immediate rinsing of the eye with citrate-containing solution offered a superior treatment modality (Pfister et al., 1981, 1991; Haddox et al., 1989) relative to water rinsing alone.

SUMMARY

As evidenced by the above, a variety of techniques are available in the evaluation of the ocular toxicity of potential drugs, products, or devices. The originally designated paradigm, the Draize test, serves the purpose for non-ophthalmic and even, in initial test phases, for ophthalmic products, of assessing the ocular irritation potential of materials. For ophthalmic products, however, sufficient pre-Draize in vitro testing should have occurred to indicate whether a compound had any irritation potential; if so, it should have been eliminated at an early stage.

Use of the Draize test for ophthalmic toxicity testing is almost redundant, both for the reasons given above and that only one drop of a solution, or a single amount of dry substance, is applied to the ocular surface. The latter does not reflect the majority of typical ophthalmic product use. Furthermore, the Draize test only assesses the irritation potential of the cornea, conjunctiva, and iris, with limited scope within these guidelines. The Draize test provides a valuable evaluative method for nonophthalmic substances that allows labeling of materials that may accidentally come into contact with the eye.

For the evaluation of ocular toxicity of ophthalmic products (or even long-term use of non-ophthalmic products, such as systemic drugs or other compounds), more subtle methodology is required. This methodology has been developed to allow biochemical and physiological processes to be further understood in many eye tissues (cornea, lens, retina, iris, ciliary body, trabecular meshwork, etc.) and provides a quantitative assessment of tissue responses. The increased value of these methodologies is immediately obvious with the provision of better evaluations.

The application of these sophisticated techniques, such as corneal endothelial morphological studies using either specular or confocal microscopy, quantitative densitometric examination of lens photographs (Scheimpflug biomicroscopy), electroretinography, fluorophotometry, and so on, to ocular toxicological studies has provided impetus to this burgeoning area (Hockwin, Green, et al., 1992). The inclusion of all eye tissues in the evaluation process of ocular toxicology of products, drugs, and devices has brought an understanding of effects in these tissues that was previously absent. It is apparent, therefore, that the evaluation of ocular toxicity has undergone a major alteration in terms of assessment criteria, quantitation of responses, and the tissues that are examined. The realization has occurred that ocular toxicity is not limited to specific ocular tissues but may affect both intra- and extra-ocular structures. As described herein, a large variety of in vivo techniques are available for the quantitation of ocular tissue responses.

The legislatively driven European guidelines that originally called for the cessation of animal testing of cosmetics and their ingredients, as well as other aspects of animal research, appear to have undergone considerable restructuring. The original amendment seems to have been rejected and apparently will be replaced by new legislation that addresses areas of restraint-of-trade and the relative slowness of adoption of in vitro alternative technologies. Those laws concerning cosmetics testing will apparently be unaltered. These changes reflect the realization that public safety is at risk with the immediate elimination of adequate in vivo testing protocols. The in vitro test procedures simply are not at a stage where reliance can be placed upon their predictive capacity. Validation of the in vitro tests will take several more years and even then only fragments of the attempted simulation of the complex, integrated in vivo ocular response will be possible. Pursuit of the ideal goal is to be actively encouraged and supported, as it is vigorously in Europe, but the process has to be recognized as being slow.

It remains our responsibility, as ocular toxicologists, to protect human health by providing appropriate testing of agents, products, devices, and so on, to eliminate compounds that may adversely affect the eye. This step should occur early in the evaluative process in order to preserve human and other resources. We should ensure that adequate initial physicochemical data is evaluated (such as structure–activity relationships), that in vitro testing is performed to eliminate undesirable materials and, finally, that in vivo testing be performed using reduced numbers of animals, better technology to evaluate any toxic responses in all eye tissues, low doses of agents to reflect the human experience, and humane care and treatment of animals. By following these progressive steps, we use a scientific basis for decision-making concerning any restriction of a product for human exposure. As investigators who have the responsibility for the conduct of these tests, the onus is on our shoulders to perform those evaluations using the best approach that we deem acceptable for a complete analysis of the toxicity of the product under test.

We must also be at the forefront of efforts to bring attention to the difference between the ocular irritation response (with its inherent limitations to specific tissues, times of examination, examination criteria, etc.) and ocular toxicology. The latter includes *all* eye tissues, intra- and extra-ocular, and thus encompasses much more than irritation per se. It is imperative that this distinction be sustained and made clear to the appropriate authorities that one test cannot suffice for ophthalmic and non-ophthalmic compounds or products. The two evaluative processes are designed for two entirely different reasons and must not be considered equal. No concept of ocular toxicity can be obtained from a crude examination of cornea, conjunctiva, and iris (irritation test). The methodology required for toxicity studies is sophisticated and frequently requires modern computer technology for data analysis compared with a qualitative judgment using a scale of 0 to 4 that is observer-dependent.

ACKNOWLEDGMENTS

Some of the work reported here from my laboratory was supported by an unrestricted departmental award from Research to Prevent Blindness, Inc., New York, New York. The author is the recipient of a Senior Scientific Investigators Award from Research to Prevent Blindness, Inc. Brenda Sheppard provided valuable secretarial assistance.

REFERENCES

Adler, C.A., Maurice, D.M., and Paterson, M.E. 1971. The effect of viscosity of the vehicle on the penetration of fluorescein into the human eye. *Experimental Eye Research* 11:34–42.

Allgood, G.S. 1989. Use of animal eye test data and human experience for determining the ocular irritation potential of shampoos. *Journal of Toxicology—Cutaneous and Ocular Toxicology* 8:321–326.

Alm, A., Stjernschantz, J., and The Scandinavian Latanoprost Study Group. 1995. Effects on intraocular pressure and side effects of 0.005% latanoprost applied once daily, evening or morning: a comparison with timolol. *Ophthalmology* 102:1743–1752.

Alm, A., and Villumsen, J. 1991. PhXA34, a new potent ocular hypotensive drug. A study on dose–response relationship and on aqueous humor dynamics in healthy volunteers. *Archives of Ophthalmology* 109:1564–1568.

Anjou, C.I.N., and Krakau, C.E.T. 1961. Aqueous flare and protein content in the anterior chamber of normal rabbits' eyes. *Acta Ophthalmologica* 39:95–101.

Arthur, B.H., Pennisi, S.C., DiPasquale, L.C., Re, T., Dinardo, J., Kennedy, G.L., North-Root, H., Penney, D.A., and Sekerke, H.J. 1986. Effects of anesthetic pretreatment and low volume dosage on ocular irritancy potential of cosmetics: a collaborative study. *Journal of Toxicology—Cutaneous and Ocular Toxicology* 5:215–227.

Atkinson, K.A., Fentem, J.H., Clothier, R.H., and Balls, M. 1992. Alternatives to ocular irritation testing in animals. *Lens and Eye Toxicity Research* 9:247–258.

Avalos, J., Jacobs, A., and Wilkin, J.K. 1997. Toxicity testing for ocular drug products. In *Advances in Ocular Toxicology*, eds. K. Green, H.F. Edelhauser, R.B. Hackett, D.S. Hull, D.E. Potter, and R.C. Tripathi, pp. 261–268. New York: Plenum Press.

Bagley, D., Booman, K.A., Bruner, L.H., et al. 1994. The SDA Alternatives Program Phase III: comparison of in vitro data with animal eye irritation data on solvents, surfactants, oxidizing agents, and prototype cleaning products. *Journal of Toxicology—Cutaneous and Ocular Toxicology* 13:127–155.

Bagley, D.M., Bruner, L.H., de Silva, O., Cottin, M., O'Brien, K.A.F., Uttley, M., and Walker, A.P. 1992. An evaluation of five potential alternatives in vitro to the rabbit eye irritation test in vivo. *Toxicology In Vitro* 4:275–284.

Baldinger, J., Doft, B.H., Burns, S.A., and Johnson, B. 1986. Retinal toxicity of amphotericin B in vitrectomized versus non-vitrectomized eyes. *British Journal of Ophthalmology* 70:657–661.

Baldwin, H.A., McDonald, T.O., and Beasley, C.H. 1973. Slit-lamp examination of experimental animal eyes. II. Grading scales and photographic evaluation of induced pathological conditions. *Journal of the Society of Cosmetic Chemistry* 24:181–195.

Ballantyne, B., Gazzard, M.F., Swanston, D.W., and Williams, P. 1974. The ophthalmic toxicology of *o*-chlorobenzylidine malononitrile (CS). *Archives of Toxicology* 32:149–168.

Ballantyne, B., and Swanston, D.W. 1977. The scope and limitations of acute eye irritation tests. In *Current Approaches in Toxicology*, ed. B. Ballantyne, pp. 139–157. Bristol, England: John Wright and Sons.

Balls, M., and Straughan, D.W. 1996. The three R's of Russell & Burch and the testing of biological products. In *Development of Biological Standards*, vol. 86. *Replacement, Reduction and Refinement of Animal Experiments in the Development and Control of Biological Products*, eds. F. Brown, K. Cussler, and C. Hendriksen, pp. 11–18. Basel: Karger.

Barratt, M.D. 1995a. Quantitative structure activity relationships for skin corrosivity of organic acids, bases, and phenols. *Toxicology Letters* 75:169–176.

Barratt, M. 1995b. A quantitative structure activity relationship for the eye irritation potential of neutral organic chemicals. *Toxicology Letters* 80:69–74.

Barratt, M.D., Castell, J.V., Chamberlain, M., Combes, R., et al. 1995. The integrated use of alternative approaches for predicting toxic hazard. *Alternatives to Laboratory Animals* 23:410–429.

Beasley, H., Boltralik, J.J., and Baldwin, H.A. 1975. Chloramphenicol in aqueous humor after topical application. *Archives of Ophthalmology* 93:184–185.

Beck, B.D., Calabrese, E.J., and Anderson, P.D. 1995. The use of toxicology in the regulatory process. In *Principles and Methods of Toxicology*, 3rd ed., ed. A.W. Hayes, pp. 19–58. New York: Raven Press.

Beckley, J.H. 1965. Comparative eye testing: man vs. animal. *Toxicology and Applied Pharmacology* 7(suppl):93–101.

Beckley, J.H., Russell, T.J., and Rubin, L.F. 1969. Use of the rhesus monkey for predicting human responses to eye irritants. *Toxicology and Applied Pharmacology* 15:1–9.

Bee, W.H., Korte, R., and Vogel, F. 1995. Electroretinography in the non-human primate as a standardized method in toxicology. In *Ocular Toxicology*, eds. I. Weisse, O. Hockwin, K. Green, and R.C. Tripathi, pp. 53–61. New York: Plenum Press.

Bee, W.H., Vogel, F., and Korte, R. 1997. Computer-assisted evaluation of iris color changes in primate toxicology. In *Advances in Ocular Toxicology*, eds. K. Green, H.F. Edelhauser, R.B. Hackett, D.S. Hull, D.E. Potter, and R.C. Tripathi, pp. 203–205. New York: Plenum Press.

Bell, M., Holmes, P.M., Nisbet, T.M., Uttley, M., and Van Abbe, N.J. 1979. Evaluating the potential eye irritancy of shampoos. *International Journal of Cosmetic Science* 1:123–131.

Bergstrom, T.J., Roth, M., and Martonyi, C.L. 1976. Pigmented iris angiography. *Archives of Ophthalmology* 94:1180–1182.

Beuerman, R.W., Snow, A., Thompson, H., and Stern, M. 1992. Action potential responses of the corneal nerves to irritants. *Lens and Eye Toxicity Research* 9:193–210.

Bill, A. 1974. Effects of acetazolamide and carotid occlusion on the ocular blood flow in unanesthetized rabbits. *Investigative Ophthalmology* 13:954–958.

Bito, L.Z. 1984. Species differences in the responses of the eye to irritation and trauma: a hypothesis of divergence in ocular defense mechanisms, and the choice of experimental animals for eye research. *Experimental Eye Research* 39:807–829.

Bito, L.Z., and Klein, E.M. 1981. The unique sensitivity of the rabbit eye to x-ray induced ocular inflammation. *Experimental Eye Research* 33:403–412.

Blain, L., Lachapelle, P., and Molotchnikoff, S. 1990. The effect of acute triethylene exposure on electroretinogram components. *Neurotoxicology and Teratology* 12:633–636.

Boets, E.P.M., van Best, J.A., Boot, J.P., and Oosterhuis, J.A. 1988. Corneal epithelial permeability and daily contact lens wear as determined by fluorophotometry. *Current Eye Research* 7:511–514.

Bours, J., Ahrend, M.H.J., and Hockwin, O. 1990. Crystallin profiles of calf and bovine lens in microsections stained for free sulfhydryl groups and proteins. *Lens and Eye Toxicity Research* 7:531–545.

Bours, J., Ahrend, M.H.J., Wegener, A., and Hockwin. O. 1987. Glycosylated crystallins in microsection of diabetic rat lenses. *Concepts in Toxicology* 4:350–359.

Bowman, K., and Green, K. 1982. Corneal epithelial healing rates after topical nucleotides. *Current Eye Research* 1:619–622.

Brown, G.C., Eagle, R.C., Shakin, E.P., Gruber, M., and Arbizio, V.V. 1990. Retinal toxicity of intravitreal gentamicin. *Archives of Ophthalmology* 108:1740–1744.

Bruner, L.H., Kain, D.J., Roberts, D.A., and Parker, R.D. 1991. Evaluation of seven in vitro alternatives for ocular safety testing. *Fundamental and Applied Toxicology* 17:136–149.

Burton, A.B.G. 1972. A method for the objective assessment of eye irritation. *Food and Cosmetic Toxicology* 10:209–217.

Camras, C.B., Schumer, R.A., Marsk, A., Lustgarten, J.S., Serle, J.B., Stjernschantz, J., Bito, L.Z., and Podos, S.M. 1992. Intraocular pressure reduction with PhXA34, a new prostaglandin analogue, in patients with ocular hypertension. *Archives of Ophthalmology* 110:1733–1738.

Cavanagh, H.D., Petroll, W.M., Alizadeh, H., He, Y.-G., McCulley, J.P., and Jester, J.V. 1993. Clinical and diagnostic use of in vivo confocal microscopy in patients with corneal disease. *Ophthalmology* 100:1444–1454.

Cavanagh, H.D., Petroll, W.M., and Jester, J.V. 1995. Confocal microscopy: uses in measurement of cellular structure and function. *Progress in Retinal and Eye Research* 14:527–565.

Chamberlain, M., and Barratt, M.D. 1995. Practical application of QSAR to in vitro toxicology illustrated by consideration of eye irritation. *Toxicology In Vitro* 9:543–547.

Champeau, E.J., and Edelhauser, H.F. 1986. Effect of ophthalmic preservatives on the ocular surface: conjunctival and corneal uptake and distribution of benzalkonium chloride and chlorhexidine digluconate. In *The Preocular Tear Film*, eds. F.J. Holly, D.W. Lamberts, and D.L. MacKeen, pp. 292–302. Lubbock, TX: Dry Eye Institute.

Chan, P.K., and Hayes, A.W. 1985. Assessment of chemically induced ocular toxicity: a survey of methods. In *Toxicology of the Eye, Ear and Other Special Senses*, ed. A.W. Hayes, pp. 103–143. New York: Raven Press.

Cheeks, L.T., Summerer, R.W., and Green, K. 1992. Optimal pupil diameter for Scheimpflug slit image photography of the lens in man. *Ophthalmic Research* 24:15–19.

Chiou, G.C.Y., and Yan, H.Y. 1986. Effects of antiglaucoma drugs on the blood flow in rabbit eyes. *Ophthalmic Research* 18:265–269.

Chiou, G.C.Y., Zhao, F., Shen, Z.F., and Li, B.H.P. 1990. Effects of D-timolol and L-timolol on ocular blood flow and intraocular pressure. *Journal of Ocular Pharmacology* 6:23–30.

Chrai, S.S., Makoid, M.C., Eriksen, S.P., and Robinson, J.R. 1974. Drop size and initial dosing frequency problems of topically applied ophthalmic drugs. *Journal of Pharmaceutical Sciences* 63:333–338.

Chrai, S.S., Patton, T.F., Mehta, A., and Robinson, J.R. 1973. Lacrimal and instilled fluid dynamics in rabbit eyes. *Journal of Pharmaceutical Sciences* 62:1112–1121.

Christian, M.S., and Diener, R.M. 1996. Soaps and detergents: alternatives to animal eye irritation tests. *Journal of the American College of Toxicology* 15:1–44.

Chylack, L.T., Wolfe, J.K., Singer, D.M., Leske, C., Bullimore, M.A., Bailey, I.L., Friend, J., McCurthy, D., and Wu, S.-Y., for the Longitudinal Study of Cataract Study Group. 1993. The lens opacities classification system III. *Archives of Ophthalmology* 111:831–836.

Cintron, C., Hassinger, L., Kublin, C.L., and Friend, J. 1979. A simple method for the removal of rabbit corneal epithelium utilizing n-heptanol. *Ophthalmic Research* 11:90–96.

Clayton, R.M., Green, K., Wilson, M., Zehir, A., Jack, J., and Searle, L. 1985. The penetration of detergents into adult and infant eyes: possible hazards of additives to ophthalmic preparations. *Food and Chemical Toxicology* 23:239–246.

Clerc, B., and Sayn, M.-J. 1995. ERG measurements in the dog, cat and monkey for toxicology specially type of electrode and anesthesia for ERG recordings. In *Ocular Toxicology*, eds. I. Weisse, O. Hockwin, K. Green, and R.C. Tripathi, pp. 39–51. New York: Plenum Press.

Code of Federal Regulations. 1979. Title 16, part 1500.42. Washington, DC: U.S. Government Printing Office.

Consumer Product Safety Commission. 1976. *Illustrated Guide for Grading Eye Irritation Caused by Hazardous Substances.* 16CFR 1500.

Cooper, G.P., Fox, D.A., Howell, W.E., Laurie, R.D., et al. 1980. Visual evoked responses in rats exposed to heavy metals. In *Neurotoxicity of the Visual System*, eds. W.H. Merigan and B. Weiss, pp. 203–218. New York: Raven Press.

Crosson, C., Klyce, S.D., and Beuerman, R.W. 1986. Epithelial wound closure in the rabbit cornea. *Investigative Ophthalmology and Visual Science* 27:464–473.

Csukas, S., Costarides, A., Riley, M.V., and Green, K. 1987. Hydrogen peroxide in the rabbit anterior chamber: effects on glutathione, and catalase effects on peroxide kinetics. *Current Eye Research* 6:1395–1402.

Csukas, S.C., and Green, K. 1988. Effects of intracameral hydrogen peroxide in the rabbit anterior chamber. *Investigative Ophthalmology and Visual Science* 29:335–339.

Cunha-Vaz, J.G. 1985. Vitreous fluorophotometry recording in posterior segment disease. *Graefes Archives of Clinical and Experimental Ophthalmology* 222:241–247.

D'Amico, D.J., Caspers-Velu, L., Libert, J., Shanks, E., Schrooyen, M., Hanninen, L.A., and Kenyon, K.R. 1985. Comparative toxicity of intravitreal aminoglycoside antibiotics. *American Journal of Ophthalmology* 100:264–275.

Davies, R.E., Kynoch, S.R., and Liggett, M.P. 1976. Eye irritation tests—an assessment of the maximum delay time for remedial irrigation. *Journal of the Society of Cosmetic Chemistry* 27:301–306.

De Sousa, D.J., Rouse, A.A., and Smolon, W.J. 1984. Statistical consequences of reducing the number of rabbits utilized in eye irritation testing: data on 67 petrochemicals. *Toxicology and Applied Pharmacology* 76:234–242.

Dick, E., and Miller, R.F. 1985. Extracellular K^+ activity changes related to electroretinogram components. I. Amphibian (I-type) retinas. *Journal of General Physiology* 85:885–909.

Dick, E., Miller, R.F., and Bloomfield, S. 1985. Extracellular K^+ activity changes related to electroretinogram components. II. Rabbit (E-type) retinas. *Journal of General Physiology* 85:911–931.

Dragomirescu, V., Hockwin, O., Koch, H.R., and Sasaki, K. 1978. Development of a new equipment for rotating slit image photography according to Scheimpflug's principle. In *Gerontological Aspects of Eye Research*, ed. O. Hockwin, pp. 118–130. Basel: Karger.

Draize, J.H. 1959. Dermal toxicity. In *Appraisal of the Safety of Chemicals in Foods, Drugs and Cosmetics*, pp. 44–59. Austin, TX: Association of Food and Drug Officials of the United States.

Draize, J.H., and Kelley, E.A. 1952. Toxicity to eye mucosa of certain cosmetic preparations containing surface-active agents. In *Proceedings of the Scientific Section of the Toilet Goods Association* 17:1–4.

Draize, J.H., Woodard, G., and Calvery, H.O. 1944. Methods for the study of irritation and toxicity of substances applied topically to the skin and mucus membranes. *Journal of Pharmacology and Experimental Therapeutics* 82:377–390.

Durham, R.A., Sawyer, D.C., Keller, W.F., and Wheeler, C.A. 1992. Topical ocular anesthetics in ocular irritancy testing: a review. *Laboratory Animal Sciences* 42:1–7.

Eckerskorn, U., Hockwin, O., Chen, T.T., Knowles, W., and Dobbs, R.E. 1987. Contribution of cataract epidemiological studies to the evaluation of cataractogenic risk factors. In *Drug-Induced Ocular Side Effects and Ocular Toxicology*, ed. O. Hockwin, pp. 71–78. Basel: Karger.

Eckerskorn, U., Hockwin, O., Müller-Breitenkamp, R., Chen, T.T., Knowles, W., and Dobbs, R.E. 1978. Evaluation of cataract related risk factors using detailed classification system and multivariate statistical methods. In *Cataract Epidemiology*, eds. K. Sasaki, O. Hockwin, and M.C. Leske, pp. 82–91. Basel: Karger.

Edelhauser, H.F., and Green, K. 1997. Workshop on in vitro versus in vivo models for ocular toxicity testing. In *Advances in Ocular Toxicology*, eds. K. Green, H.F. Edelhauser, R.B. Hackett, D.S. Hull, D.E. Potter, and R.C. Tripathi, pp. 207–259. New York: Plenum Press.

Edelhauser, H.F., and Ubels, J. 1992. Models and methods for testing toxicity with tear fluid, cornea, and conjunctiva. In *Manual of Oculotoxicity Testing of Drugs*, eds. O. Hockwin, K. Green, and L. Rubin, pp. 195–218. Stuttgart: G. Fischer-Verlag.

Ellingson, C.M., Schoenwald, R.D., Barfknecht, C.F., Rao, C.S., and Laban, S.L. 1992. Rapid toxicological model for use in assessing ocular drugs. *Biopharmaceutics and Drug Disposition* 13:417–436.

Farkas, S., Hull, D.S., Lazenby, F., and Green, K. 1983. Corneal endothelial cell counts in patients on chlorpromazine therapy. *Journal of Toxicology—Cutaneous and Ocular Toxicology* 2:41–45.

Fiscella, R., Peyman, G.A., Kimura, A., and Small, G. 1988. Intravitreal toxicity of cotrimoxazole. *Ophthalmic Surgery* 19:44–46.

Food and Drug Administration. 1965. *Illustrated Guide for Grading Eye Irritation by Hazardous Substances*. Washington, DC: Food and Drug Administration.

Fraunfelder, F.T. 1989. *Drug-Induced Ocular Side Effects and Drug Interactions*, 3rd ed. Philadelphia: Lea & Febiger.

Fraunfelder, F.T., and Meyer, S.M. 1985. Possible cardiovascular effects secondary to topical ophthalmic 2.5% phenylephrine. *American Journal of Ophthalmology* 99:362–363.

Fraunfelder, F.T., and Meyer, S.M. 1987. Recent advances in ocular drug toxicity. In *Drug-Induced Ocular Side Effects and Ocular Toxicology*, ed. O. Hockwin, pp. 30–39. Basel: Karger.

Fraunfelder, F.T., and Scafidi, A. 1978. Possible adverse effects from topical ocular 10% phenylephrine. *American Journal of Ophthalmology* 85:447–453.

Frazier, J.M. 1989. The joint government–industry workshop on progress towards non-animal alternatives to the Draize test: observations and recommendations. *Journal of Toxicology—Cutaneous and Ocular Toxicology* 8:141–154.

Freeberg, F.E., Griffith, J.F., Bruce, R.D., and Bay, P.H.S. 1984. Correlation of animal test methods with human experience for household products. *Journal of Toxicology—Cutaneous and Ocular Toxicology* 1:53–64.

Freeberg, F.E., Hooker, D.T., and Griffith, J.F. 1986. Correlation of animal eye test data with human experience for household products: an update. *Journal of Toxicology—Cutaneous and Ocular Toxicology* 5:115–123.

Freeberg, F.E., Nixon, G.A., Reer, P.J., Weaver, J.E., Bruce, R.D., Griffith, J.F., and Sanders, L.W., 3rd. 1986. Human and rabbit eye responses to chemical insult. *Fundamental and Applied Toxicology* 7:626–634.

Frenkel, R.E.P., Hong, Y.J., and Shin, D.H. 1988. Comparison of the Tono-Pen to the Goldmann applanation tonometer. *Archives of Ophthalmology* 106:750–753.

Friedenwald, J.S., Hughes, W.F., and Hermann, H. 1944. Acid–base tolerance of cornea. *Archives of Ophthalmology* 31:279–283.

Gad, S.C., and Changelis, C.P. 1988. Ocular irritation testing. In *Acute Toxicology Testing Perspectives and Horizons*, eds. S.C. Gad and C.P. Changelis, pp. 51–80. Caldwell, NJ: Telford Press.

Gautheron, P., Dukic, M., Alix, D., and Sina, J.F. 1992. Bovine corneal opacity and permeability test: an in vitro assay of ocular irritancy. *Fundamental and Applied Toxicology* 18:442–449.

Geller, A.M., Osborne, C.M., and Peiffer, R.L. 1995. The ERG, EOG and VEP in rats. In *Ocular Toxicology*, eds. I. Weisse, O. Hockwin, K. Green, and R.C. Tripathi, pp. 7–25. New York: Plenum Press.

Gilman, M.R., Jackson, E.M., Cerven, D.R., and Moreno, M.T. 1983. Relationship between the primary dermal irritation index and ocular irritation. *Journal of Toxicology—Cutaneous and Ocular Toxicology* 2:107–117.

Goldberg, A.M., Frazier, J.M., Brusick, D., Dickens, M.S., Flint, O., Gettings, S.D., Hill, R.N., Lipnick, R.L., Renskers, K.J., Bradlaw, J.A., Scala, R.A., Veronesi, B., Green, S., Wilcox, N.L., and Curren, R.D. 1993. Framework for validation and implementation of in vitro toxicity tests: report of the validation and technology transfer committee of the Johns Hopkins Center for Alternatives to Animal Testing. *Journal of the American College of Toxicology* 12:23–30.

Goldberg, A.M., and Silber, P.M. 1992. Status of in vitro ocular irritation testing. *Lens and Eye Toxicity Research* 9:161–192.

Gouras, P., and Gunkel, R.D. 1963. The EOG in chloroquine and other retinopathies. *Archives of Ophthalmology* 70:629–639.

Gramoni, R. 1980. Retinal function of rats exposed to organomercurials. In *Neurotoxicity of the Visual System*, eds. W.H. Merigan and B. Weiss, pp. 101–111. New York: Raven Press.

Grant, W.M., and Shuman, J.S. 1993. *Toxicology of the Eye*, 4th ed. Springfield, IL: Charles C. Thomas.

Gray, J.R., Mosier, M.A., and Ishimoto, B.M. 1985. Optimized protocol for Fluorotron Master. *Graefes Archives of Clinical and Experimental Ophthalmology* 222:225–229.

Greaves, J.L., Wilson, C.G., Galloway, N.R., Birmingham, A.T., and Olejnik, O. 1991. A comparison of the precorneal residence of an artificial tear preparation in patients with keratoconjunctivitis sicca and normal volunteer subjects using gamma scintigraphy. *Acta Ophthalmologica* 69:432–436.

Green, K. 1982. Marijuana and the eye—a review. *Journal of Toxicology—Cutaneous and Ocular Toxicology* 1:3–32.

Green, K. 1991a. Corneal endothelial structure and function under normal and toxic conditions. *Cell Biology Reviews* 25:169–207.

Green, K. 1991b. Principles and methods of ocular pharmacokinetic evaluation. In *Dermal and Ocular Toxicology. Fundamentals and Methods*, ed. D.W. Hobson, pp. 541–584. Boca Raton, FL: CRC Press.

Green, K. 1992a. History of ophthalmic toxicology. In *Ophthalmic Toxicology*, ed. G.C.Y. Chiou, pp. 1–16. New York: Raven Press.

Green, K. 1992b. Models and methods for testing toxicity with aqueous humor, iris and ciliary body. In *Manual of Oculotoxicity Testing of Drugs*, eds. O. Hockwin, K. Green, and L. Rubin, pp. 219–242. Stuttgart: G. Fischer-Verlag.

Green, K. 1992c. Models and methods for testing toxicity with intraocular pressure. In *Manual of Oculotoxicity Testing of Drugs*, eds. O. Hockwin, K. Green, and L. Rubin, pp. 243–253. Stuttgart: G. Fischer-Verlag.

Green, K. 1993. The effect of preservatives on corneal permeability of drugs. In *Biopharmaceutics of Ocular Drug Delivery*, ed. P. Edman, pp. 43–59. Boca Raton, FL: CRC Press.

Green, K. 1996. Mussel adhesive protein. In *Surgical Adhesives and Sealants: Current Technology and Applications*, eds. D.H. Sierra and R. Saltz, pp. 19–27. Lancaster, PA: Technomic Publishing Co.

Green, K., Bowman, K.A., Elijah, R.D., Mermelstein, R., and Kilpper, R.W. 1985. Dose–effect response of the rabbit eye to cetylpyridinium chloride. *Journal of Toxicology—Cutaneous and Ocular Toxicology* 4:13–26.

Green, K., and Chapman, J.M. 1986. Benzalkonium chloride kinetics in young and adult albino and pigmented rabbit eyes. *Journal of Toxicology—Cutaneous and Ocular Toxicology* 5:133–142.

Green, K., Chapman, J.M., Cheeks, L., Clayton, R.M., Wilson, M., and Zehir, A. 1987. Detergent penetration into young and adult rabbit eyes: comparative pharmacokinetics. *Journal of Toxicology—Cutaneous and Ocular Toxicology* 6:89–107.

Green, K., Cheeks, L., Slagle, T., Paul, H., and Trask, D.K. 1993a. Blood–ocular barrier permeability and electroretinogram after intravitreal silicone oils of varying composition. *Journal of Ocular Pharmacology* 9:355–363.

Green, K., Cheeks, L., Slagle, T., Stewart, D.A., and Trask, D.K. 1993b. Corneal endothelial permeability after silicone oil exposure: role of low–molecular weight components and catalyst. *Journal of Toxicology—Cutaneous and Ocular Toxicology* 12:313–321.

Green, K., Crosby, V.A., and Cheeks, L. 1990. Toxicity of intracameral thymoxamine. *Lens and Eye Toxicity Research* 7:121–132.

Green, K., Cullen, P.M., and Phillips, C.I. 1984. Aqueous humor turnover and intraocular pressure during menstruation. *British Journal of Ophthalmology* 68:736–740.

Green, K., Edelhauser, H.F., Hackett, R.B., Hull, D.S., Potter, D.E., and Tripathi, R.C., eds. 1997. *Advances in Ocular Toxicology*, pp. 1–276. New York: Plenum Press.

Green, K., and Elijah, D. 1981. Drug effects on aqueous humor formation and pseudofacility in normal rabbit eyes. *Experimental Eye Research* 33:239–245.

Green, K., Elijah, R.D., and Hampstead, D. 1986. Intraocular pressure and aqueous humor dynamics in rabbit and primate with d- and l-adrenergic compounds. *Journal of Pharmacology* 2:239–250.

Green, K., Elijah, D., and Lollis, G. 1982. Drug effects on aqueous humor formation and pseudofacility in sympathectomized rabbit eyes. *Experimental Eye Research* 34:1–6.

Green, K., Elijah, D., Lollis, G., and Mayberry, L. 1981. Beta adrenergic effects on ciliary epithelial permeability, aqueous humor formation and pseudofacility in the normal and sympathectomized rabbit eye. *Current Eye Research* 1:419–424.

Green, K., and Hatchett, T.L. 1987. Regional ocular blood flow after chronic topical glaucoma drug treatment. *Acta Ophthalmologica* 65:503–506.

Green, K., Johnson, R.E., Chapman, J.M., Nelson, E., and Cheeks, L. 1989. Surfactant effects on the rate of rabbit corneal epithelial healing. *Journal of Toxicology—Cutaneous and Ocular Toxicology* 8:253–269.

Green, K., Kim, K., Wynn, H., and Shimp, R.G. 1977. Intraocular pressure, organ weights and the chronic use of cannabinoid derivatives in rabbits for one year. *Experimental Eye Research* 25:465–471.

Green, K., Livingston, V., Bowman, K., and Hull, D.S. 1980. Chlorhexidine effects on corneal epithelium and endothelium. *Archives of Ophthalmology* 98:1273–1278.

Green, K., and MacKeen, D.L. 1976. Chloramphenicol retention on, and penetration into, the rabbit eye. *Investigative Ophthalmology* 15:220–222.

Green, K., and Padgett, D. 1979. Effect of various drugs on pseudofacility and aqueous humor formation in the rabbit eye. *Experimental Eye Research* 28:239–246.

Green, K., Paterson, C.A., Cheeks, L., Slagle, T., Jay, W.M., and Aziz, M.Z. 1990. Ocular blood flow and vascular permeability in endotoxin-induced inflammation. *Ophthalmic Research* 22:287–294.

Green, K., Paterson, C.A., and Siddiqui, A. 1985. Ocular blood flow after experimental alkali burns and prostaglandin administration. *Archives of Ophthalmology* 103:569–571.

Green, K., Phillips, C.I., Cheeks, L., and Slagle, T. 1988. Aqueous humor flow rate and intraocular pressure during and after pregnancy. *Ophthalmic Research* 20:353–357.

Green, K., Phillips, C.I., and Elijah, R.D. 1985. Decreased intraocular pressure and aqueous humor turnover rate during longitudinal ocular studies in the rabbit. *Current Eye Research* 4:155–158.

Green, K., and Schermerhorn, J. 1985. Blood flow in aphakic rabbit eyes after sub-chronic glaucoma drug treatment. *Current Eye Research* 4:667–670.

Green, K., Slagle, T., Chaknis, M.J., and Cheeks, L.T. 1992a. Intraocular silicone oil effects on rabbit blood–retinal barrier permeability. *Lens and Eye Toxicity Research* 9:139–149.

Green, K., Slagle, T., Chaknis, M.J., Cheeks, L., and Chang, S. 1993. Perfluorocarbon effects on rabbit blood–retinal barrier permeability. *Ophthalmic Research* 25:186–191.

Green, K., Slagle, T., Cheeks, L., and Norman, B.C. 1992b. The effects of intraocular gases on rabbit blood–retinal barrier permeability. *Lens and Eye Toxicity Research* 9:67–76.

Green, K., Sobel, R.E., Fineberg, E., Wynn, H.R., and Bowman, K.A. 1981. Subchronic ocular and systemic toxicity of topically applied Δ9-tetrahydrocannabinol. *Annals of Ophthalmology* 13:1219–1222.

Green, K., and Tønjum, A.M. 1971. Influence of various agents on corneal permeability. *American Journal of Ophthalmology* 72:897–905.

Green, K., Wynn, H., and Padgett, D. 1978. Effect of Δ-9-tetrahydrocannabinol on ocular blood flow and aqueous humor formation. *Experimental Eye Research* 26:65–69.

Green, S., Chambers, W.A., Gupta, K.C., Hill, R.N., Hurley, P.M., Lambert, L.A., Lee, C.C., Lee, J.K., Liu, P.T., Lowther, D.K., Roberts, C.D., Seabaugh, V.M., Springer, J.A., and Wilcox, N.L. 1993. Criteria for in vitro alternatives for the eye irritation test. *Food and Chemical Toxicology* 2:81–85.

Green, W.R., Sullivan, J.B., Hehir, R.M., Scharpf, L.G., and Dickenson, A.W. 1978. *A Systematic Comparison of Chemically Induced Eye Injury in the Albino Rabbit and Rhesus Monkey.* New York: The Soap and Detergent Association.

Griffith, J.F., Nixon, G.A., Bruce, R.D., Reer, P.J., and Bannan, E.A. 1982. Dose–response studies with chemical irritants in the albino rabbit eye as a basis for selecting optimum testing conditions for predicting hazard to the human eye. *Toxicology and Applied Pharmacology* 55:501–513.

Gupta, K.C., Chambers, W.A., Green, S., Hill, R.N., Hurley, P.M., Lambert, L.A., Liu, P.T., Lowther, D.K., Seabaugh, V.M., Springer, J.A., and Wilcox, N.L. 1993. An eye irritation test protocol and an evaluation and classification system. *Food and Chemical Toxicology* 31:117–121.

Hackett, R.B. 1990. Nonclinical study requirements for ophthalmic drugs and devices in the United States. *Lens and Eye Toxicity Research* 7:181–205.

Haddox, J.L., Pfister, R.R., and Yuille-Barr, D. 1989. The efficacy of topical citrate after alkali injury is dependent on the period of time it is administered. *Investigative Ophthalmology and Visual Science* 30:1062–1068.

Hagino, S., Igataki, H., Kato, S., Kobayashi, T., and Tanaka, M. 1991. Quantitative evaluation to predict the eye irritancy of chemicals: modification of chorioallantoic membrane test by using trypan blue. *Toxicology In Vitro* 4:301–304.

Hammond, B.R., and Bhattacherjee, P. 1984. Calibration of the Alcon applanation pneumatonograph and Perkins tonometer for use in rabbits and cats. *Current Eye Research* 3:1155–1158.

Havener, W.H. 1974. *Ocular Pharmacology,* 3rd ed. St. Louis: C.V. Mosby.

Hennekes, R., Janssen, K., Muñoz, C., and Winneke, G. 1987. Lead-induced ERG alterations in rats at high and low levels of exposure. In *Drug-Induced Ocular Side Effects and Ocular Toxicology,* ed. O. Hockwin, pp. 193–199. Basel: Karger.

Hickey, T.E., Beck, G.L., and Botta, J.A. 1973. Optimum fluorescein staining time in ocular irritation studies. *Toxicology and Applied Pharmacology* 26:571–574.

Ho, P.C., Davis, W.H., Elliot, J.H., and Cohen, S. 1974. Kinetics of corneal epithelial regeneration and epidermal growth factor. *Investigative Ophthalmology* 13:804–809.

Hockwin, O., Ahrend, M.H.J., and Bours, J. 1986. Correlation of Scheimpflug photography of the anterior eye segment with biochemical analysis of the lens. Application of a frozen-sectioning technique to investigate differences in protein distribution of single lens layers. *Graefes Archives of Clinical and Experimental Ophthalmology* 224:265–270.

Hockwin, O., Dragomirescu, V., Laser, H., Wegener, A., and Eckerskorn, U. 1987. Measuring lens transparency by Scheimpflug photography of the anterior segment. Instrumentation and application to clinical and experimental ophthalmology. *Journal of Toxicology—Cutaneous and Ocular Toxicology* 6:251–271.

Hockwin, O., Green, K., and Rubin, L.F., eds. 1992. *Manual of Oculotoxicity Testing of Drugs,* pp. 1–435. Stuttgart: G. Fischer-Verlag.

Hockwin, O., and Wegener, A. 1987. Syn- and co-cataractogenesis—a system for testing subliminal lens toxicity. In *Drug-Induced Ocular Side Effects and Ocular Toxicology,* ed. O. Hockwin, pp. 241–249. Basel: Karger.

Hockwin, O., Wegener, A., Bessems, G., Bours, J., Korte, I., Müller-Breitenkamp, U., Schmidt, J., and Schmitt, C. 1992. Models and methods for testing toxicity: lens. In *Manual of Oculotoxicity Testing of Drugs,* eds. O. Hockwin, K. Green, and L.F. Rubin, pp. 255–317. Stuttgart: G. Fischer-Verlag.

Hockwin, O., Wegener, A., Sisk, D.R., Dohrmann, B., and Kruse, M. 1984–85. Efficacy of AL-1576 in preventing naphthalene cataract in three rat strains. A slit lamp and Scheimpflug photographic study. *Lens Research* 2:321–335.

Hubert, F. 1992. The eye (rabbit/human): parameters to be measured in the field of ocular irritancy. *Alternatives to Laboratory Animals* 20:476–479.

Hull, D.S., Green, K., and Elijah, R.D. 1985. Effect of oxygen free radical products on rabbit iris vascular permeability. *Acta Ophthalmologica* 63:513–518.

Hurley, P.M., Chambers, W.A., Green, S., Gupta, K.C., Hill, R.N., Lambert, L.A., Lee, C.C., Lee, J.K., Liu, P.T., Lowther, D.K., Roberts, C.D., Seabaugh, V.M., Springer, J.A., and Wilcox, N.L. 1993. Screening procedures for eye irritation. *Food and Chemical Toxicology* 31:87–94.

Jacobi, P., Miliczek, K.-D., and Zrenner, E. 1993. Experiences with the international standard for clinical electroretinography: normative values for clinical practice, inter- and intraindividual variations. *Documenta Ophthalmologica* 85:95–114.

Jacobs, G.A., and Martens, M.A. 1989. An objective method for the evaluation of eye irritation in vivo. *Food and Chemical Toxicology* 27:255–258.

Jaeger, R.J., and Yoo, J.H.K. 1975. Analysis of drug induced changes in smooth pursuit eye movements. In *Proceedings of the 28th Annual Conference on Engineering in Medicine and Biology*, p. 321. Chevy Chase, MD: Alliance for Engineering in Medicine and Biology.

Jay, W.M., Aziz, M.Z., and Green, K. 1984. Effect of topical epinephrine and timolol on ocular and optic nerve blood flow in phakic and aphakic rabbit eyes. *Current Eye Research* 3:1199–1202.

Jester, J.V., Petroll, W.M., Feng, W., Essepian, J., and Cavanagh, H.D. 1992a. Radial keratotomy 1: the wound healing process and measurement of incisional wound gape in two animal models using in vivo, confocal microscopy. *Investigative Ophthalmology and Visual Science* 33:3255–3270.

Jester, J.V., Petroll, W.M., Garana, R.M.R., Lemp, M.A., and Cavanagh, H.D. 1992b. Comparison of in vivo and ex vivo cellular structure in rabbit eyes detected by tandem scanning confocal microscopy. *Journal of Microscopy* 165:169–181.

Jones, C.W., Cunha-Vaz, J.G., and Rusin, M.M. 1982. Vitreous fluorophotometry in the alloxan- and streptozocin-treated rat. *Archives of Ophthalmology* 100:1141–1145.

Kennah, H.E., Hignet, S., Laux, P.E., Dorko, J.D., and Barrow, C.S. 1989. An objective procedure for quantitating eye irritation based upon changes of corneal thickness. *Fundamental and Applied Toxicology* 12:258–268.

Klein, E.M., and Bito, L.Z. 1983. Species variations in the pathophysiologic responses of vertebrate eyes to a chemical irritant, nitrogen mustard. *Investigative Ophthalmology and Visual Science* 24:184–191.

Koch, H.R., Doldi, K., and Hockwin, O. 1976. Naphthalene cataracts in rats. Association of eye pigmentation and cataract development. *Documenta Ophthalmologica Proceedings Series* 8:293–303.

Kojima, M., Hockwin, O., Rao, G.S., and Garcia, J. 1990. Investigations on the presence of 3-hydroxy-3-methylglutaryl coenzyme—a reductase (HMG-CoA-reductase, E.C. 1.1.1.34) in lenses of various animal species. *Lens and Eye Toxicity Research* 7:605–623.

Kulkarni, P.S., Fleisher, L., and Srinivasan, B.D. 1984. The synthesis of cyclooxygenase products in ocular tissues of various species. *Current Eye Research* 3:447–452.

Lambert, L.A., Chambers, W.A., Green, S., Gupta, K.C., Hill, R.N., Hurley, P.M., Lee, C.C., Lee, J.K., Liu, P.T., Lowther, D.K., Roberts, C.D., Seabaugh, V.M., Springer, J.A., and Wilcox, N.L. 1993. The use of low-volume dosing in the eye irritation test. *Food and Chemical Toxicology* 31:99–103.

Lehnert, T., Grosdanoff, P., and Hockwin, O. 1987. Assessment of drug-induced oculotoxicity by animal models. In *Drug-Induced Ocular Side Effects and Ocular Toxicology*, ed. O. Hockwin, pp. 232–240. Basel: Karger.

Lehnert, T., and Ulrich, B. 1990. Requirements of preclinical examinations. *Lens and Eye Toxicity Research* 7:207–219.

Leighton, J., Nassauer, J., and Tchao, R. 1985. The chick embryo in toxicology: an alternative to the rabbit eye. *Food and Chemical Toxicology* 23:293–298.

Lerman, S. 1987. *In vivo* methods to evaluate ocular drug efficacy and side effects. In *Drug-Induced Ocular Side Effects and Ocular Toxicology*, ed. O. Hockwin, pp. 87–104. Basel: Karger.

Lerman, S. 1990. Biophysical methods to monitor lens aging and pre-cataractous changes in vivo. *Lens and Eye Toxicity Research* 7:243–249.

Lerman, S. 1992. New non-invasive methods to evaluate ocular drug efficacy and side effects. In *Manual of Oculotoxicity Testing of Drugs*, eds. O. Hockwin, K. Green, and L.F. Rubin, pp. 109–118. Stuttgart: G. Fischer-Verlag.

Levett, J., and Jaeger, R. 1980. Effects of alcohol on retinal potentials, eye movements, accommodation, and the pupillary light reflex. In *Neurotoxicity of the Visual System*, eds. W.H. Merigan and B. Weiss, pp. 87–100. New York: Raven Press.

Loget, O., and Saint-Macary, G. 1995. Determination of the effect of ketamine, thiopental and halothane on the ocular electroretinographic examination of the beagle dog to define protocols to be used in dogs, monkeys and micropigs. In *Ocular Toxicology*, eds. I. Weisse, O. Hockwin, K. Green, and R.C. Tripathi, pp. 69–77. New York: Plenum Press.

Lubek, B.M., Kubow, S., Basu, P.K., and Wells, P.G. 1990. Cataractogenicity and bioactivation of naphthalene derivatives in lens culture and in vivo. In *Ocular Toxicology*, eds. S. Lerman and R.C. Tripathi, pp. 203–209. New York: Marcel Dekker.

Marmor, M.F., Arden, G.B., Nilsson, S.E.G., and Zrenner, E. 1989. Standard for clinical electroretinography. *Archives of Ophthalmology* 107:816–819.

Maurice, D.M., and Singh, T. 1985. The absence of corneal toxicity with low-level topical anesthesia. *American Journal of Ophthalmology* 99:691–696.

McCally, A.W., Farmer, A.G., and Loomis, E.C. 1933. Corneal ulceration following use of lash-lure. *Journal of the American Medical Association* 101:1560–1561.

McCarey, B.E., and Reaves, T.A. 1997. Effect of tear lubricating solutions on in vivo corneal epithelial permeability. *Current Eye Research* 16:44–50.

McDonald, T.O., Hiddeman, J.W., Howe, W.E., and Robertson, S.M. 1987. Ocular safety evaluation: alternatives and the future. In *Dermatoxicology*, 3rd ed., eds. F.N. Marzulli and H.I. Maibach, pp. 697–710. Washington, DC: Hemisphere.

McDonald, T.O., Seabaugh, V., Shadduck, J.A., and Edelhauser, H.F. 1987. Eye irritation. In *Dermatoxicology*, 3rd ed., eds. F.N. Marzulli and H.I. Maibach, pp. 641–696. Washington, DC: Hemisphere.

McNamara, N.A., Fusaro, R.E., Brand, R.J., Polse, K.A., and Srinivas, S.P. 1997. Measurement of corneal epithelial permeability to fluorescein. A repeatability study. *Investigative Ophthalmology and Visual Science* 38:1830–1839.

Meyer, N., Hull, D.S., and Green, K. 1978. Effect of xenon arc photocoagulation on corneal endothelium. *Annals of Ophthalmology* 10:793–795.

Meyer, O. 1993. Implications of animal welfare on toxicity testing. *Human and Experimental Toxicology* 12:516–521.

Miller, R.F., and Dowling, J.E. 1970. Intracellular responses of the Müller glial cells of mudpuppy retina: their relation to b-wave of the electroretinogram. *Journal of Neurophysiology* 33:323–341.

Minsky, M. 1988. Memoir on inventing the confocal scanning microscope. *Scanning* 10:128–138.

Mishima, S., Gasset, A., Klyce, S., and Baum, J. 1966. Determination of tear volume and tear flow. *Investigative Ophthalmology* 5:264–276.

Morgan, R.L., Sorenson, S.S., and Castles, T.R. 1987. Prediction of ocular irritation by corneal pachymetry. *Food and Chemical Toxicology* 25:609–613.

Morgan, T.R., Green, K., and Bowman, K. 1981. Effects of adrenergic agonists upon regional ocular blood flow in normal and ganglionectomized rabbits. *Experimental Eye Research* 32:691–697.

Morgan, T.R., Mirate, D.J., Bowman, K., and Green, K. 1983. Topical epinephrine and regional ocular blood flow in aphakic eyes of rabbits. *Archives of Ophthalmology* 101:112–116.

NAS Committee for Revisions of NAS Publication 1138. 1978. Dermal and eye toxicity tests. In *Principles and Procedures for Evaluating the Toxicity of Household Substances*, pp. 41–54. Washington, DC: National Academy of Sciences.

Nilius, B., and Reichenbach, A. 1988. Efficient K^+ buffering by mammalian retinal glial cells is due to cooperation of specialized ion channels. *Pflügers Archives* 411:654–660.

Nilsson, S.F.E., Samuelson, M., Bill, A., and Stjernschantz, J. 1989. Increased uveoscleral outflow as a possible mechanism of ocular hypotension caused by prostaglandin $F_{2\alpha}$-1-isopropylester in the cynomolgus monkey. *Experimental Eye Research* 48:707–716.

Norman, B.C., Oliver, J., Cheeks, L., Hull, D.S., Birnbaum, D., and Green, K. 1990. Corneal endothelial permeability after anterior chamber silicone oil. *Ophthalmology* 97:1671–1677.

O'Brien, K.A.F., Dixit, M.B., McCall, J.C., Botham, P.A., and Lewis, R.W. 1992. An interlaboratory assessment of the Eyetex system. *Toxicology In Vitro* 6:549–556.

Parish, W.E. 1985. Ability of in vitro (corneal injury—eye organ—and chorioallantoic membrane) tests to represent histopathological features of acute eye inflammation. *Fundamental and Chemical Toxicology* 24:215–227.

Patton, T.F., and Robinson, J.R. 1975. Influence of topical anesthesia on tear dynamics and ocular drug bioavailability in albino rabbits. *Journal of Pharmaceutical Sciences* 64:267–271.

Patton, T.F., and Robinson, J.R. 1976. Quantitative precorneal disposition of topically applied pilocarpine nitrate in rabbit eyes. *Journal of Pharmaceutical Sciences* 65:1295–1301.

Paylor, R., Peyman, G.A., and Badri, S. 1987. Effects of intravitreal injection of fluorosilicone oil after vitrectomy in the rabbit eye. *Canadian Journal of Ophthalmology* 22:251–253.

Pfister, R.R., Haddox, J.L., and Yuille-Barr, D. 1991. The combined effect of citrate/ascorbate treatment in alkali-injured rabbit eyes. *Cornea* 10:100–104.

Pfister, R.R., Nicolaro, M.L., and Paterson, C.A. 1981. Sodium citrate reduces the incidence of corneal ulcerations and perforations in extreme alkali-burned eyes—acetylcysteine and ascorbate have no favorable effect. *Investigative Ophthalmology and Visual Science* 21:486–490.

Piatigorsky, J. 1980. Intracellular ions, protein metabolism and cataract formation. *Current Topics in Eye Research* 3:1–39.

Picciano, P.T., and Benedict, C.V. 1986a. Mussel adhesive protein: a new epithelium tissue adhesive and cell attachment factor. *Investigative Ophthalmology and Visual Science* 27(suppl):31.

Picciano, P.T., and Benedict, C.V. 1986b. Mussel adhesive protein: a new cell attachment factor. *In Vitro Cell Development and Biology* 22(suppl):24A.

Racz, P., Ruzsonyi, M.R., Nagy, Z.T., and Bito, L.Z. 1993. Maintained intraocular pressure reduction with once-a-day application of a new prostaglandin $F_{2\alpha}$ analogue (PhXA41). *Archives of Ophthalmology* 111:657–661.

Raitta, C., and Tolonen, M. 1980. Microcirculation of the eye in workers exposed to carbon disulfide. In *Neurotoxicity of the Visual System*, eds. W.H. Merigan and B. Weiss, pp. 73–86. New York: Raven Press.

Ramselaar, J.A.M., Boot, J.P., van Haeringen, N.J., van Best, J.A., and Oosterhuis, J.A. 1988. Corneal epithelial permeability after instillation of ophthalmic solutions containing local anaesthetics and preservatives. *Current Eye Research* 7:947–950.

Rasmussen, E.S. 1993. The role of in vitro experiments in animal welfare. *Human and Experimental Toxicology* 12:522–527.

Règnier, J.-F., and Imbert, C. 1992. Contributions of physicochemical properties to the evaluation of ocular irritation. *Alternatives to Laboratory Animals* 20:457–465.

Roberts, J.E., and Dillon, J. 1990. Screening for potential *in vivo* phototoxicity in the lens/retina. *Lens and Eye Toxicity Research* 7:655–666.

Robinson, F., Riva, C.E., Grunwald, J.E., Petrig, B.L., and Sinclair, S.H. 1986. Retinal blood flow autoregulation in response to an acute increase in blood pressure. *Investigative Ophthalmology and Visual Science* 27:722–726.

Rohde, B.H. 1992. In vivo eye irritation test methods. In *Ophthalmic Toxicology*, ed. G.C.Y. Chiou, pp. 83–108. New York: Raven Press.

Rougier, A., Cottin, M., de Silva, O., Roguet, R., Catroux, P., Toufic, A., and Dossou, K.G. 1992. In vitro methods: their relevance and complementary in ocular safety assessment. *Lens and Eye Toxicity Research* 9:229–245.

Rubin, L.F. 1990. Albino versus pigmented animals for ocular toxicity testing. *Lens and Eye Toxicity Research* 7:221–230.

Rubin, L.F. 1992. Current methods of eye examination in vivo. In *Manual of Oculotoxicity Testing of Drugs*, eds. O. Hockwin, K. Green, and L.F. Rubin, pp. 81–108. Stuttgart: G. Fischer-Verlag.

Santoul, C., Decrouez, E., Droit, J.Y., and Bonne, C. 1990. Use of a specular microscope with pachymeter in ocular tolerance studies of eye drops in the rabbit. Evaluation of ocular tolerance of benzalkonium chloride (BAK) in aqueous solution, 0.01% and 0.1%. *Lens and Eye Toxicity Research* 7:359–369.

Schiavo, D.M. 1992. Special topics about the use of laboratory animals in toxicology—an ophthalmoscopic assessment. In *Manual of Oculotoxicity Testing of Drugs*, eds. O. Hockwin, K. Green, and L.F. Rubin, pp. 9–20. Stuttgart: G. Fischer-Verlag.

Schmidt, J., Schmitt, C., Wegener, A., and Hockwin, O. 1987. Photographic, histologic, and biochemical investigations of the early stages of diabetic cataract in rats. In *Drug-Induced Ocular Side Effects and Ocular Toxicology*, ed. O. Hockwin, pp. 360–367. Basel: Karger.

Schmitt, C., Schmidt, J., and Hockwin, O. 1990. Ocular drug-safety study with the HMG-CoA reductase inhibitor Pravastatin. *Lens and Eye Toxicity Research* 7:631–641.

Schnieders, B. 1987. Recommendations concerning toxicity tests on medical products. State of affairs within the European Community. In *Drug-Induced Ocular Side Effects and Ocular Toxicology*, ed. O. Hockwin, pp. 1–8. Basel: Karger.

Seabaugh, V.M., Chambers, W.A., Green, S., Gupta, K.C., Hill, R.N., Hurley, P.M., Lambert, L.A., Lee, C.C., Lee, J.K., Liu, P.T., Lowther, D.K., Roberts, C.D., Springer, J.A., and Wilcox, N.L. 1993. Use of ophthalmic topical anesthetics. *Food and Chemical Toxicology* 31:95–98.

Shirao, Y., and Kawasaki, K. 1995. Retinal toxicology study using electrophysiological methods in rabbits. In *Ocular Toxicology*, eds. I. Weisse, O. Hockwin, K. Green, and R.C. Tripathi, pp. 27–37. New York: Plenum Press.

Sina, J.F., Ward, G.J., Laszek, M.A., and Gautheron, P.D. 1992. Assessment of cytotoxicity assays as predictors of ocular irritation of pharmaceuticals. *Fundamental and Applied Toxicology* 18:515–521.

Small, G.H., Peyman, G.A., Srinivasan, A., Smith, R.T., and Fiscella, R. 1987. Retinal toxicity of combination antiviral drugs in an animal model. *Canadian Journal of Ophthalmology* 22:300–303.

Sparrow, J.M., Bron, A.J., Brown, N.A.P., Ayliffe, W., and Hill, A.R. 1986. The Oxford clinical cataract classification system. *International Ophthalmology* 9:207–225.

Spielmann, H., Kalweit, S., Liebsch, M., Wirnsberger, T., Gerner, I., Bertram-Neis, E., Krauser, K., Kreiling, R., Miltenburger, H.G., Pape, W., and Steiling, W. 1993. Validation study of alternatives to the Draize eye irritation test in Germany: cytotoxicity testing and HET-CAM test with 136 industrial chemicals. *Toxicology In Vitro* 7:505–510.

Springer, J.A., Chambers, W.A., Green, S., Gupta, K.C., Hill, R.N., Hurley, P.M., Lambert, L.A., Lee, C.C., Lee, J.K., Liu, P.T., Lowther, D.K., Roberts, C.D., Seabaugh, V.M., and Wilcox, N.L. 1993. Number of animals for sequential testing. *Food and Chemical Toxicology* 31:105–109.

Stjernschantz, J., and Astin, M. 1993. Anatomy and physiology of the eye. Physiological aspects of ocular drug therapy. In *Biopharmaceutics of Ocular Drug Delivery*, ed. P. Edman, pp. 1–25. Boca Raton, FL: CRC Press.

Stolwijk, T.R., van Best, J.A., Boot, J.P., Lemkes, H.P.J., and Oosterhuis, J.A. 1990. Corneal epithelial barrier function after oxybuprocaine provocation in diabetes. *Investigative Ophthalmology and Visual Science* 31:436–439.

Sugai, S., Murata, K., Kitagaki, T., and Tomita, I. 1990. Studies on eye irritation caused by chemicals in rabbits. I. A quantitative structure–activity relationship approach to primary eye irritation of chemicals in rabbits. *Journal of Toxicology Science* 15:245–262.

Swamy-Mruthinti, S., Green, K., and Abraham, E.C. 1996a. Scheimpflug densitometric analysis of cataracts in diabetic rats: correlation with glycation. *Ophthalmic Research* 28:230–236.

Swamy-Mruthinti, S., Green, K., and Abraham, E.C. 1996b. Inhibition of cataracts in moderately diabetic rats by aminoguanidine. *Experimental Eye Research* 62:505–510.

Swanston, D.W. 1983. Eye irritancy testing. In *Animals and Alternatives in Toxicity Testing*, eds. M. Balls, R.J. Riddell, and A.N. Worden, pp. 337–366. New York: Academic Press.

Talsma, D.M., Leach, C.L., Hatoum, N.S., Gibbons, R.D., Roger, J.C., and Garvin, P.J. 1988. Reducing the number of rabbits in the Draize eye irritancy test: a statistical analysis of 155 studies conducted over 6 years. *Fundamental and Applied Toxicology* 10:146–153.

Toris, C.B., Camras, C.B., and Yablonski, M.E. 1993. Effects of PhXA41, a new prostaglandin analog, on aqueous humor dynamics in human eyes. *Ophthalmology* 100:1297–1304.

Tuffs, A., Wegener, A., and Hockwin, O. 1987. Pilot study on cataractogenesis by UV irradiation. In *Drug-Induced Ocular Side Effects and Ocular Toxicology*, ed. O. Hockwin, pp. 276–284. Basel: Karger.

Van Buskirk, E.M. 1980. Adverse reactions from timolol administration. *Ophthalmology* 87:447–450.

Van Buskirk, E.M., and Fraunfelder, F.T. 1984. Ocular beta-blockers and systemic effects. *American Journal of Ophthalmology* 98:623–624.

Van Nerom, P.R., Rosenthal, A.R., Jacobson, D.R., Pieper, I., Schwartz, H., and Grieder, B.W. 1981. Iris angiography and aqueous photofluorometry in normal subjects. *Archives of Ophthalmology* 99:489–493.

Walker, R.E., and Litovitch, T.L. 1972. An experimental and theoretical study of the pneumatic tonometer. *Experimental Eye Research* 13:14–23.

Ward, D.A., Ferguson, D.C., Kaswan, R.L., and Green, K. 1992a. Leukotrienes and sensory innervation in blood–aqueous barrier disruption in the dog. *Journal of Ocular Pharmacology* 8:69–76.

Ward, D.A., Ferguson, D.C., Kaswan, R.L., Green, K., and Bellhorn, R.W. 1991. Fluorophotometric evaluation of experimental blood–aqueous barrier disruption in dogs. *American Journal of Veterinary Research* 52:1433–1437.

Ward, D.A., Ferguson, D.C., Ward, S.L., Green, K., and Kaswan, R.L. 1992b. Comparison of the blood–aqueous barrier stabilizing effects of steroidal and non-steroidal anti-inflammatory agents in the dog. *Progress in Veterinary and Comparative Ophthalmology* 2:117–124.

Ward, S.L., Walker, T.L., and Dimitrijevich, S.D. 1997. Evaluation of chemically induced toxicity using an in vitro model of human corneal epithelium. *Toxicology In Vitro* 11:121–139.

Watson, P., Stjernschantz, J., and The Scandinavian Latanoprost Study Group. 1996. A six-month, randomized, double-masked study comparing latanoprost with timolol in open-angle glaucoma and ocular hypertension. *Ophthalmology* 103:126–137.

Wegener, A., and Hockwin, O. 1987. Animal models as a tool to detect the subliminal cocataractogenic potential of drugs. In *Drug-Induced Ocular Side Effects and Ocular Toxicology*, ed. O. Hockwin, pp. 250–262. Basel: Karger.

Wegener, A., Laser, H., and Hockwin, O. 1987. Measurement of lens transparency changes in animals. Comparison of the Topcon SL-45 combined with linear microdensitometry and the Zeiss SLC system. In *Drug-Induced Ocular Side Effects and Ocular Toxicology*, ed. O. Hockwin, pp. 263–275. Basel: Karger.

Weil, C.A., and Scala, R.A. 1971. Study of the intra-laboratory and inter-laboratory variability in the results of rabbit eye and skin irritation tests. *Toxicology and Applied Pharmacology* 19:276–360.

Weisse, I., Hockwin, O., Green, K., and Tripathi, R.C., eds. 1995. *Ocular Toxicology*. New York: Plenum Press.

Weisse, I., Loosen, H., and Peil, H. 1990. Age-related retinal changes—a comparison between albino and pigmented rabbits. *Lens and Eye Toxicity Research* 7:717–739.

Weltman, A.S., Sparber, S.B., and Jurtshuk, T. 1965. Comparative evaluation and the influence of various factors on eye-irritation scores. *Toxicology and Applied Pharmacology* 7:308–319.

Wilcox, D.K., and Bruner, L.H. 1990. In vitro alternatives: their development and role in ocular safety assessment. *Alternatives to Laboratory Animals* 18:117–128.

Wilcox, N.L. 1992. The status of eye irritancy testing: a regulatory perspective. *Lens and Eye Toxicity Research* 9:259–271.

Williams, S.J. 1984. Prediction of ocular irritancy potential from dermal irritation test results. *Food and Chemical Toxicology* 22:157–161.

Yan, H.Y., and Chiou, G.C.Y. 1987. Effects of L-timolol, D-timolol, haloperidol and domperidone on rabbit retinal blood flow measured with laser doppler method. *Ophthalmic Research* 19:45–48.

Yousufzai, S.Y.K., Chen, A.L., and Abdel-Latif, A.A. 1988. Species differences in the effects of prostaglandins on inositol triphosphate accumulation, phosphatidic acid formation, myosin light chain phosphorylation and contraction in iris sphincter of the mammalian eye: interaction with the cyclic AMP system. *Journal of Pharmacology and Experimental Therapeutics* 247:1064–1072.

Zbinden, G. 1991. Predictive value of animal studies in toxicology. *Regulatory Toxicology and Pharmacology* 14:167–177.

Zlioba, A., Peyman, G.A., and Nikoleit, J. 1988. Retinal toxicity study of intravitreal carboplatin and iproplatin. *Annals of Ophthalmology* 20:71–72.

Zrenner, E. 1992. Tests of retinal function in drug toxicity. In *Manual of Oculotoxicity Testing of Drugs*, eds. O. Hockwin, K. Green, and L.F. Rubin, pp. 331–361. Stuttgart: G. Fischer-Verlag.

Ophthalmic Toxicology
Edited by George C. Y. Chiou
Copyright © 1999 Taylor & Francis

6

In Vitro Methods in Ophthalmic Toxicology

George C. Y. Chiou, Bo Xuan, and Brooks Rohde

Institute of Ocular Pharmacology and Department of Medical Pharmacology and Toxicology, Texas A&M University College of Medicine, College Station, Texas, USA

- **Isolated Rabbit Eye**
  - Method
  - Examples
- **Isolated Chicken Eye**
  - Method
  - Examples
- **Isolated Corneal Preparations**
  - Eytex Method
  - Opacity of Isolated Cornea
  - Corneal Cup Method
  - Cornea Fluorescent Probe Method
- **Isolated Lens Preparation**
  - MRS and MRI
  - Fluorescence Spectroscopy
  - Scanning Lens Monitor
  - Lens Metabolism and Enzyme Activities
  - Calcium Accumulation
  - Special Ca^{2+},K^+ Channels
  - Distribution of Cholesterol, Phospholipid, and Protein
- **Isolated Retina Preparations**
  - Example
- **Alternatives To Eye Tissues**
  - Chicken Egg Test
  - Vaginal Mucous Membrane
  - Ileum Contractility
- **Cell Cultures**
  - Cytotoxicity Tests
  - Conjunctiva Cell Culture
  - Corneal Cell Culture
  - Lens Cell Cultures
  - Fibroblast Cultures
  - Peritoneal Cell Cultures

- HeLa Cell Cultures
- Madin–Darby Canine Kidney Cell Culture
- RBC Hemolysis
- Cell Viability Assayed in Terms of Type I Collagen Gel Configuration
- **Toxicity Prediction**
- **References**

Although in vivo modified Draize eye irritation test is still the official model for eye irritation and toxicology studies (Wilcox, 1992; Chu and Toft, 1993; Booman et al., 1988), it has major problems, including (a) the lack of objective and accurate quantitation for the grading system and (b) opposition by animal welfare groups and many other individuals, primarily because of the pain involved (Green, 1998). To solve these problems, numerous, new sophisticated methods have been developed to accurately measure the changes that occur by instillation of test materials onto the eyes or the responses induced by systemic chemicals.

Furthermore, various steps have been taken to reduce the number of animals used and to avoid irritation and pain induced by test materials. These steps include the study of physicochemistry of the test materials, skin tests on rodents, and in vitro methods to exclude irritating and toxic materials before they are instilled onto the test eyes. Therefore, only one to three animals are needed for the Draize test to prove the safety of test materials rather than to show their irritation and toxicities.

Thus, tremendous efforts have been made to develop in vitro methods to replace in vivo methods, although it is still far from successful because no single in vitro method can be used as a complete alternative to the rabbit eye irritation test; the eye in vivo is a complex system capable of producing a wide variety of actions due to injurious stimuli and insults. Reactions may vary because of chemical irritation, direct physical irritation, damage to corneal or conjunctival cells, release of histamine or prostaglandins, and even because of prior medication of the animals. In vitro methods are, in general, capable of evoking and measuring a single aspect of eye irritation rather than replicating the multiple aspects of eye irritation produced in vivo. Therefore, the safety of certain groups of chemicals must be evaluated with several in vitro methods to obtain a semicomplete and relatively accurate picture of their irritation potential in living animal eyes.

There are both advantages and disadvantages to in vitro methods. The advantages include the following: (a) they allow a large number of observations to be measured quantitatively; (b) they are easily controllable and reproducible, and are particularly suitable for studies on dose–response relationships and pharmacokinetics; (c) they can be carried out in a relatively short period of time compared with in vivo methods; (d) they are painless and devoid of the variability among animals; (e) they are, in general, less expensive than in vivo methods; and (f) some methods involve the use of no living animals. Disadvantages include the following: (a) they are unable to produce the complete irritation reaction produced by in vivo methods; (b) they are unable to mimic the tearing and pain that are common phenomena in human eye irritation; (c) they are still in the developmental stage and are not widely accepted by regulatory agencies; (d) they lack a large database for comparison; and (e) they are devoid of the recovery or healing stages found in in vivo eye irritation experiments. In addition, in many instances it is difficult to extrapolate the in vitro data to in vivo eye irritation, even if the tissues and cells used are obtained from the same species, because in vitro systems represent only a small aspect of the complicated in vivo eye system and function. It is even more difficult to extrapolate in vitro data obtained from animal tissues or cells to the living human eye system. Furthermore, effective concentrations obtained from in vitro experiments are hard to relate to the effective irritation doses in in vivo systems, as the slope of the dose–response relationship in these two systems can be quite different. Most in vitro assays measure acute irritation and are not suitable models for evaluating the long-term toxicity and carcinogenicity effects of potential eye irritants.

Despite these difficulties, the development of in vitro alternative methods to in vivo eye irritation test methods is urgently needed. Increasing numbers of chemicals that are developed for ocular and cosmetic uses require eye irritation tests. In vitro methods will provide a workable way to meet the large demand in a humane way.

It is most important that a valid relationship between an in vitro method and the in vivo Draize test be established. In some instances, the relationship might be valid only for testing certain classes of chemicals; in these cases, the limitation of the in vitro method ought to be clearly indicated. Although a false positive result obtained with an in vitro method is unacceptable, a false negative obtained with an in vitro method is even worse, indicating that an unsafe product is safe. To minimize these problems, the dose–response relationship must be promptly established for all in vitro method experiments.

To establish fully the relationship between in vitro and in vivo tests, large numbers of chemicals of various classes must be tested in vitro and the results compared with the known data from Draize rabbit ocular irritation tests. The ranking of these chemicals established by in vitro testing should match as closely as possible the Draize ocular irritancy test in rabbit eyes.

ISOLATED RABBIT EYE

To mimic the in vivo Draize test, rabbit eyes are enucleated immediately after death and placed in a temperature-controlled chamber where they are superfused with normal saline solution (Burton et al., 1981; York, 1983). Test substances are applied topically to the eyes, and the effects are observed with a slit-lamp biomicroscope.

This method has a number of advantages over other possible in vitro systems: (a) The system will identify materials that have the potential to be extremely irritant to the in vivo eye. Such materials cause direct, clearly visible damage to the in vitro cornea following a very short period of contact. (b) The system investigates the effect of the products or chemicals in the form in which they might enter the human eye. The system does not need to rely on dilution or solubilization of the material to ascertain whether the product is particularly toxic to cells. (c) As materials are applied directly onto the cornea, the system can be used for a very wide range of irritants, from corrosive materials to totally nonirritating materials. The test's versatility across this wide range of irritants is of considerable advantage; it is doubtful whether other in vitro systems would be able to cope adequately with products that differ so widely in their irritation potentials. An example to illustrate this advantage is sodium hydroxide. It must be present at a misleadingly high concentration in cell culture to cause a toxic effect; therefore, it appears to be less of a hazard than itactually is in vivo (York, 1983).

Method

This method was developed mainly by Burton and co-workers (Burton et al., 1981). The eyes of rabbits were examined using a slit-lamp biomicroscope, and the initial corneal thickness was measured with depth measurement attachment #1 for the slit lamp. The rabbits were then killed by an overdose of pentobarbital sodium. Immediately after death, each animal was laid on its side, and one drop of isotonic NaCl was applied to the surface of the eye to prevent drying during dissection. The eyeball was enucleated carefully to avoid touching the surface of the cornea or cutting the optic nerve too close to the eyeball.

Any eye that had abnormalities or had been damaged during dissection was discarded. Eye viability was determined by application of 2% fluorescein sodium dye to the corneal surface for a few seconds followed by rinsing with isotonic NaCl solution. Eyes that were significantly swollen after dissection, that stained with fluorescein dye, or that showed any other signs of damage were rejected.

Enucleated eyes were mounted in a Perspex clamp with the cornea positioned vertically and placed in a temperature-controlled ($32°C \pm 1°C$) superfusion chamber (Burton et al., 1981; York, 1983). Normal saline solution was pumped into the chamber through a stainless-steel tube at a rate of 0.10–0.15 ml/min. It dripped onto the cornea at the limbus and flowed down over the corneal surface. The chamber was enclosed in a water jacket through which water was pumped at approximately 4 l/min from a temperature-controlled water bath. The saline was passed through tubing within the water jacket so that it was warmed to the correct temperature before entering the chamber. The chamber wall was made of black Perspex, providing a suitable background for slit-lamp observation. Readers are referred to the original reports (Burton et al., 1981; York, 1983) for more details and illustrations of the superfusion chamber.

Enucleated eyes were reexamined using the slit-lamp to ensure that they had not been damaged during dissection. The corneal thickness was also measured. Enucleated eyes were left in the chambers for 45–75 min to equilibrate. The saline superfusion was then stopped. Test substances (2 drops or 50 μl) were applied to the eye so that the cornea was continuously bathed with the test substances for 10 sec. The corneal solution was then rinsed thoroughly with warm isotonic saline solution

(20 ml) and the saline superfusion immediately restarted. Solids were tested by applying 50 mg for 10 sec and then rinsing as before.

The eyes were reexamined at intervals for up to 4 hr after the application of the test substances, and any changes in the normal appearance of the cornea were carefully noted. The corneal thickness was also measured, either in terms of instrument units (1 unit = 0.8 mm) or as corneal swelling, which was expressed as

$$\left(\frac{\text{corneal thickness at time } t}{\text{corneal thickness before treatment}} - 1 \right) \times 100\%.$$

Examples

Sodium Hydroxide

The examples chosen were compounds known to cause dose-dependent ocular irritation and corneal damage as determined by the Draize test and by most other tests. Sodium hydroxide caused rapidly developing and intense opacity of the anterior stroma of the cornea. The areas of opacity had well-defined margins. The epithelium remained relatively clear but was permeable to fluorescein. The corneal thickness was increased by 50% in 4 hr.

Ethanol

Ethanol caused opacity in the epithelium and increased permeability to fluorescein. Areas of the epithelium became detached from the cornea. Stromal opacity and edema developed gradually. The increase in corneal thickness after 4 hr was 65%.

Acetone

Acetone caused slight opacity of the epithelium, probably representing the loss of some of the surface layers of cells, and increased permeability to fluorescein. There was little stromal opacity. Corneal thickness after 4 hr increased by 20%.

ISOLATED CHICKEN EYE

The isolated rabbit eye test still needs laboratory animals as eye donors. Therefore, slaughter animals as possible eye donors were searched among the cow, pig, and chicken. From these donors, the chicken was selected as the best candidate (Prinsen, 1996; Prinsen and Koeter, 1993).

To be a valuable alternative to the in vivo Draize test, chicken eyes were enucleated within 2 hr of death and placed in a temperature-controlled superfusion apparatus with normal saline solution. Corneal swelling, corneal opacity, and fluorescein retention were used as parameters to detect possible adverse eye effects. The test compound was applied topically to the eyes, and the eyes were observed with a slit-lamp biomicroscope.

This method has a couple of advantages: (a) This system does not need laboratory animals as eye donors. In view of the numerous chickens killed daily, the chicken eye can be obtained easily with cornea suitable for testing. (b) Compared with the European Community (EC) classification based on in vivo studies, the isolated chicken eye test correctly classified all irritating compounds tested in this comparative study. It seems that this in vitro test system is reliable and accurate in the evaluation of eye irritation potential of the test compounds.

Method

The chicken heads were obtained from the slaughter house, and the eyeballs were enucleated and placed in a superfusion apparatus for further treatment and examination within 2 hr after death.

Before enucleation, the chicken eyes were examined with a slit-lamp microscope to ensure that there was no corneal damage. If undamaged, the eyeball was removed from the orbit carefully to avoid touching the cornea or cutting the optical nerve too short. The enucleated eye was mounted in a stainless-steel clamp with the cornea positioned vertically, then placed in the temperature-controlled ($32°C \pm 1°C$) chambers of the superfusion apparatus. The entire cornea was perfused with normal saline through a stainless-steel tube at a rate of 0.10–0.15 ml/min. After six eyes had been mounted in the superfusion apparatus, the eyes were reexamined with the slit-lamp microscope to make sure they were not damaged during the procedure. The corneal thickness was determined with depth measuring attachment # II for the Haag–Streit slit-lamp microscope and expressed in instrument units. Eyes that showed any signs of damage or that had a corneal thickness deviating by more than 10% of the average corneal thickness of the six eyes were discarded and replaced. After 40–60 min equilibration, the corneal thickness was determined again as the zero reference value. Immediately after zero reference measurement ($t = 0$), the test substance was administered to the eye. For this reason, the eye was placed on a paper tissue with the cornea facing upward. The standard dosing volume of 0.1 ml or 0.1 g of the test substance was reduced to 0.03 ml or 0.03 g since the surface area of the chicken cornea is only one-third that of the rabbit cornea. Liquid and solid materials were used in such a way that the entire surface of the cornea was bathed with the test substance for 10 sec, then the corneal surface was rinsed thoroughly with 20 ml normal saline, and the eye in the holder was returned to its chamber. Each test compound was tested on five out of the six eyes; the sixth eye was treated in the same way with normal saline and served as a control. The eyes were reexamined at 30, 75, 120, 180, and 240 min after treatment. The parameters used to describe the changes in the appearance of the cornea were as follows:

1. Corneal swelling. The corneal swelling was expressed as

$$\left(\frac{\text{corneal thickness at time } t}{\text{corneal thickness before treatment}} - 1 \right) \times 100\%$$

2. Corneal opacity. The following criteria were used to score the corneal opacity at each of the observation time points: 0 = no opacity; 1 = scattered or diffuse areas, details of iris clearly visible; 2 = easily discernible translucent area, details of iris slightly obscured; 3 = severe corneal opacity, no details of iris visible, size of pupil barely discernible; 4 = complete corneal opacity, iris invisible.
3. Fluorescein retention. The fluorescein retention was scored from 0 to 3 at 30 min only: 0 = no fluorescein retention; 1 = small number of cells retaining fluorescein; 2 = individual cells and areas of the cornea retaining fluorescein; 3 = large areas of the cornea retaining fluorescein.
4. Morphological effects. There are some morphological changes, including "pitting" of corneal epithelial cells, "loosening" of epithelium, "roughening" of the corneal surface, and "sticking" of the test compound to the cornea.
5. Assessment of in vitro irritancy grades. According to the degree of corneal swelling, opacity, and fluorescein retention, a category score from I to IV was assigned. There are four grades as follows: not, slightly, moderately, or severely irritating. These grades are the combination of category scores as given for corneal swelling, opacity, and fluorescein retention: not irritating = at most one category score of II; slightly irritating = at least two category scores of II or, at most, one category of III; moderately irritating = at least two category scores of III or, at most, one category of IV; and severely irritating = at least two category scores of IV.

Examples

Acetic Acid

Acetic acid caused corneal swelling III, opacity IV, and fluorescein retention and was classified as a severely irritating compound, which matches the EC classification.

Sodium Dodecyl Sulfate

Sodium dodecyl sulfate (SDS) would be classified as a moderately irritating substance based on corneal swelling (III), opacity (II), and fluorescein retention (II). However, it was considered to upgrade the classification to severely irritating because of loosening of the epithelium, which still matches the EC classification.

ISOLATED CORNEAL PREPARATIONS

The cornea is the part of the eyeball that is in direct contact with chemicals that enter the eye topically and is directly exposed to toxic radiation. Therefore, in vitro methods to determine toxic responses induced by chemicals, pollutants, and radiation on the cornea ought to be developed in order to reduce or eliminate the need for the in vivo Draize test. There are at least four methods of in vitro corneal preparations that have been developed, including the Eytex method, corneal opacity method, corneal cup method, and corneal fluorescent probe method.

Eytex Method

The Eytex method (Gordon and Kelly, 1989a,b) was developed by the National Testing Corporation and can reduce or eliminate the need for the Draize test. This method is a corneal opacification assay to predict ocular irritation of chemicals and formulations based on alterations in a protein matrix reagent. There is a high degree of correlation between results from the in vitro Eytex method and the in vivo Draize method. The Eytex method is quantitative and reproducible, and may allow more uniform testing results. This method, however, measures only chemical irritancy; facts of in vivo irritation, such as abrasion, allergy, and sensitization, or the ability to heal after irritation, must be measured by other means.

The Eytex method can rapidly identify irritants, which can be eliminated from further testing by in vivo methods. This method can identify increased ocular irritancy and can follow product stability by monitoring breakdown products. It can also identify and quantitate anti-irritants in personal care products.

Method

The protein matrix is extracted from jack bean powder and does not require the sacrifice of any animal or sampling of any animal tissue. Finely ground jack bean meal is soaked in saline solution with acetate buffer and ethylenediaminetetraacetic acid (EDTA) added. The mixture is filtered and pH adjusted to 8.0 with sodium borate. The mixture is again filtered and the filtrate, or protein matrix, is analyzed for composition and then lyophilized. A prototype method has been used to establish a relationship between ocular irritants and their ability to produce opacity in vitro. Additional studies have been conducted to establish a direct relationship between ocular irritation of known irritants and their ability to cause aggregation or denaturation of certain proteins in vitro.

An Eytex kit consists of the protein matrix reagent, six calibrators, a dilution buffer, distilled water, and special 1-ml cuvette. Equipment needed includes a colorimeter, cuvette rack, and dispensing pipettes; this represents a much smaller investment than most methods and certainly much smaller than is needed for the Draize test. Samples of soluble test solutions (30, 50, or 100 μl) or soluble solids (30, 50, or 100 mg) are added directly to the Eytex reagent. The membrane partition assay (MPA) protocol is used for insoluble chemicals; samples are placed in a membrane cut that is permeable to molecules of 16,000 daltons or less and that separates the sample from the reaction chamber with the Eytex reagent. The standard and MPA vessels are incubated at 25°C for 1 hr or 24 hr. A set of calibrators defines the relationship of the optical density produced in the Eytex reagent with the Draize score, and three known controls are assayed for internal assay control. Optical density after incubation is converted to Eytex/Draize equivalents (Eytex score), and the substance is classified as an irritant or nonirritant.

Examples

The scientific validation of the Eytex method has been pursued by the National Testing Corporation in many ways. A study presented at the 1987 Center for Alternatives to Animal Testing (CAAT) symposium showed Eytex results to have a 96% correlation with in vivo Draize test results.

   In 1987, studies of the Eytex method were conducted in 12 industrial, military, university, and independent laboratories. Each lab chose between 5 and 60 materials for testing. The in vitro results exhibited an overall substantial equivalence of 89% to the in vivo test results. It was determined that the ability of the assay to discriminate between irritants and nonirritants was 99% (Gordon and Bergman, 1989).

   A two-lab, double-masked study of 70 products (including furniture polish, laundry detergent, air freshener, insect repellent, shampoos, and first-aid creams) was conducted by S.C. Johnson and Son. A 93% predictive value of the Eytex method was demonstrated (Griffith, 1980).

   In 12% of the samples in these studies the Eytex method overpredicted irritancy. A new rapid membrane assay (RMA), used together with the Eytex method, estimates the irritancy of compounds, such as highly ethoxylated surfactants, correctly (Muir, 1984); the earlier MPA underestimated their irritancy. In these studies, advantages observed of the Eytex method included lower costs, reduction in animal use, and an increased capability to test undiluted products.

Opacity of Isolated Cornea

The opacitometer (Muir, 1984) was designed and constructed to monitor corneal opacity development. Readers are directed to the original reference (Muir, 1984) for an illustration and detailed description of the opacitometer. The Perspex corneal holders allow the cornea to be firmly clamped with 5 ml of solution in contact with the front (epithelial) and 5 ml with the rear (endothelial) part. The opacitometer allows a beam of white light to be directed through the cornea in its holder to a photocell. The instrument is first calibrated by shining the light beam through an empty holder. The voltage recorded is set at 25 V before each reading by adjusting the variable register. To eliminate reflections and scatter, all surfaces of the opacitometer are mat black. Dark current is small with this system; a voltage of below 0.005 V is recorded with the lamp off. With a cornea in place, development of opacity is indicated by a drop in the voltage measured. All incubations are carried out at 32°C, the cornea being bathed in Tyrode solution with or without surfactant on both sides.

Method

The corneas were removed from fresh whole bovine eyes and washed with Tyrode solution (Igarashi, 1986). For some preparations, the epithelium was scraped off gently before the cornea was removed from the eyeball; in other preparations, the endothelium and Descemet's membrane were scraped off after first removing the rear of the eyeball, removing the lens, and everting the cornea over a second eyeball. Some corneas were used with both epithelium and Descemet's membrane removed. Holders, designed to allow contact of either or both surfaces with Tyrode solution or sodium lauryl sulfate (NaLS) solutions of various concentrations, were filled with Tyrode solution and placed in a Muir opacitometer. The voltage was adjusted to 2.5 V. The Tyrode solution was discarded and a cornea fixed in the chamber. Tyrode solution or NaLS solution was then placed on one or both sides of the cornea. The holder, with cornea and solutions, was placed again in the opacitometer and the voltage recorded (V1). Corneas were then incubated for 4.5 hr. The solutions on both sides of the cornea were then replaced with fresh Tyrode's solution and the voltage recorded again (V2). Since a drop in voltage indicates the development of opacity in the cornea, the results were expressed as percent opacity:

$$\left(\frac{V1 - V2}{V1} \right) \times 100\%$$

where $V1 - V2 = 0$ represents zero opacity and $V1 - V2 = 2.5$ represents 100% opacity.

Examples

In one study (Muir, 1984), control corneas showed no opacity for 8 hr and then became more opaque over 24 hr. Care had to be taken to use fresh Tyrode solution as solutions became turbid with time. Sodium dodecyl sulfate (NaDS) at 1 mM caused almost complete opacity by 8 to 12 hr, whereas sodium lauryl sulfate (NaLS) at 1 mM caused opacity to fall more slowly, leveling off at 0.5 at 20 hr. Opacity with both surfactants was concentration-dependent, with NaDS much more potent as an irritant; this contrasts to its lower toxicity to cultured cells (Scaife, 1982).

Another study of isolated corneas exposed to NaLS (Igarashi, 1986) showed that opacity developed primarily in the stroma, in a concentration-dependent manner, and was greatest when epithelium and endothelium were removed. Igarashi (1986) thought that opacity was due to a reaction of NaLS with stromal proteins.

Corneal Cup Method

Leukocyte Chemotactic Factor Production

Corneas are prepared from fresh bovine eyes as illustrated in Fig. 1 (Elgebaly, Gillies, et al., 1985; Elgebaly, Downes, et al., 1987). The attached lens and most of the iris

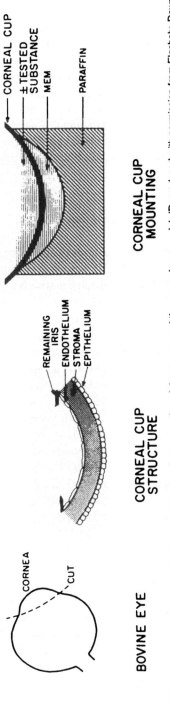

BOVINE EYE

CORNEAL CUP
STRUCTURE

CORNEAL CUP
MOUNTING

FIG. 1. Diagrammatic representation of the isolation and preparation of the cornea and the corneal cup model. (Reproduced with permission from Elgebaly, Downes, et al., 1987 and Oxford University Press.)

175

are removed and the resulting "corneal cup" is then washed twice in saline and maintained in cold minimal essential medium (MEM) until used. The cup is mounted in a paraffin well with the epithelial surface facing upward and covered by tissue culture MEM. Using the corneal cup model, the capability of corneal tissues t , produce leukocyte chemotactic factor (LCF) in response to inflammatory chemicals and/or leukocyte-mediated injury to corneal epithelium can be evaluated. The production of LCF is a response of cells to irritation and damage, and is proportional to the degree of cell damage. The migration of leukocytes in response to supernatants containing released LCF provides a method of quantitating this damage. It is a valuable model because cells in the epithelium of the corneal cup, like cells in vivo, may produce LCF for some time after very brief exposure to an irritating chemical or physical insult.

Leukocyte Production

The epithelial surfaces of isolated bovine corneal cups were treated with 1 N NaOH for 35 sec at room temperature. The NaOH was then removed, and the epithelial surfaces were washed once with MEM and incubated with fresh serum-free MEM for 1, 2, 4, and 6 hr at 37°C in a 5% CO_2 atmosphere. At various time points, experimental and control supernatants from the epithelial surfaces were removed and assayed for chemotactic activity using a modified Boyden chamber (Elgebaly, Downes, et al., 1987; Kreutzer et al., 1978). This protocol imitated the effects of an alkali burn followed by eye washing; the formation of LCF is a measure of cell damage and cell repair. A Boyden chamber is a small cylinder divided into two parts by a micropore membrane. In this study, the pores were 5 μm in diameter. Substances that will or will not attract leukocytes are placed in the bottom compartment while a leukocyte suspension is placed in the top compartment. If the cells are attracted to the bottom compartment, they attempt to cross the membrane and are caught in the pores. After incubating for a fixed time (1 hr for neutrophils, 5 hr for mononuclear cells) the filter is removed, fixed in pure isopropyl alcohol, and stained with hematoxylin, and cells are counted on a glass slide using a microscope with an Optomax image analyzer.

Unfractionated leukocytes were isolated from fresh bovine blood by a modified procedure of Boyum (Boyum, 1974; Elgebaly, Forouhar, et al., 1984). Sodium citrate-dehydrate was used as an anticoagulant. Methylcellulose was mixed with citrated blood, and the blood was centrifuged. The white, buffy leukocyte layer on the pellet of erythrocytes was pipetted off, and the contaminating erythrocytes were lysed. Isolated leukocytes were washed twice by resuspension in isotonic saline followed by recentrifugation. The unfractionated leukocytes were then suspended in sterile saline and layered over 3 ml of Ficoll/Hypaque mixture in a tube and centrifuged at 800 × g at room temperature. Mononuclear cells were found on top of the separation fluid, whereas neutrophils were sedimented at the bottom of the tube. The isolated leukocytes were resuspended in serum-free MEM for leukocyte chemotactic activity assay using modified Boyden chambers (Elgebaly, Herbert, et al., 1987).

Cell migration in response to the putative chemoattractants was expressed as

$$\text{maximum chemotactic response} = \left(\frac{\text{CI}_{\text{experimental}} - \text{CI}_{\text{HBSS}}}{\text{CI}_{\text{C5fragment}} - \text{CI}_{\text{HBSS}}} \right) \times 100\%$$

where CI is the chemotactic index (distance traveled on the filter × cell number), C5 fragment is the positive control for 100% chemotactic response, and HBSS is Hank's balanced salt solution (a blank with no attractant property).

Example

The effects of supernatants obtained from NaOH-treated bovine corneas on the migration of neutrophils or mononuclear cells in vitro are shown in Fig. 2. After 2 hr of incubation, significant levels of chemotactic activity for both cell types were detected. Less activity, however, was found in supernatants of corneas incubated for 4 or 6 hr. The observed decline in the chemotactic activity is probably due to the release of LCF deactivators and/or inhibitors (Elgebaly, Downes, et al., 1987).

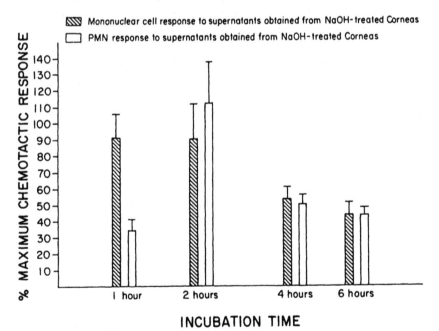

FIG. 2. Mononuclear cell and neutrophil chemotactic activity present in supernatants of bovine corneas exposed to 1 N NaOH for 35 sec, washed once with MEM, and then incubated with MEM for 1, 2, 4, and 6 hr. The figure represents the mean of four experiments ± standard deviation: ▨ mononuclear cell response to supernatants obtained from NaOH-treated corneas; ▢ PMN response to supernatants obtained from NaOH-treated corneas. (MEM-treated corneas produced low levels of LCF of maximum activity of 10%.) (Reproduced with permission from Elgebaly, Downes, et al., 1987 and Oxford University Press.)

Epithelial–Leukocyte Interactions

Not only will irritated cells release LCF, but leukocytes attracted to the epithelium will adhere, penetrate, and damage the corneal epithelium. The corneal cup can be used to model this kind of irritation and damage (Elgebaly, Gillies, et al., 1985). The isolated bovine leukocytes and leukocyte lysates, both prepared in MEM, were added separately to the epithelial surfaces of isolated bovine corneal cups. The cups were incubated and at time intervals of 5, 10, 20, 60, 120, and 180 min samples were taken for light and ultrastructural evaluations to assess the status of corneal epithelial cells.

Example

Histological and ultrastructural evaluation had indicated that leukocyte-epithelial cell interactions are characterized by five successive stages (Elgebaly, Gillies, et al., 1985):

Stage 1: Brief interactions of leukocytes with epithelial cells (0–20 min) demonstrated tight adhesion of leukocytes to the epithelial surface, but no significant alteration of the corneal epithelial cell structure was observed.

Stage 2: As the duration of leukocyte contact with epithelial cells increased (20–60 min), leukocytes penetrated beneath the superficial layer of epithelium.

Stage 3: In this period, leukocyte penetration beneath the epithelial layer induced mild to severe injury to corneal epithelial cells and caused detachment of several superficial layers.

Stage 4: Phagocytosis of dead epithelial cells by leukocytes was observed following 20- to 60-min exposures.

Stage 5: After 2–3 hr of postleukocyte exposure, significant damage to the entire epithelial layer was observed.

The damage to the epithelial cell layer was proportional to the concentration of leukocytes applied. Intact leukocytes are necessary to induce epithelial cell injury; lysates were ineffective. Direct leukocyte–epithelial contact plays a role in stimulating the synthesis and release of effector inflammatory mediators.

Cornea Fluorescent Probe Method

Increases in permeability of the epithelium of living rabbit cornea to [24]Na parallel inflammatory response (Maurice, 1955) suggests that permeability might be used as a measure of corneal injury. Permeability can be measured using a fluorescent probe.

Method

Two fluorescent dyes, fluorescein and sulforhodamine B (SRB), were investigated in the first experiments. The dyes were dissolved in saline at neutral pH to make 10%

solutions. Adult pigmented mice were killed using T61 euthanasia solution (American Hoechst Corp., Somerville, NJ) (Maurice and Singh, 1986). Immediately after death, the eyes of the mice were pushed forward by pulling down the skin below the ears and clamping it beneath the neck. The test substance was placed on one eye so as to cover the cornea. After 1 min, it was washed off with saline. A drop of fluorescent dye solution was then applied to both corneas and then washed off after 1 min. With a slit-lamp fluorophotometer, measurements of the fluorescence of the corneas were made at four points around a circle imagined halfway between the apex and periphery. The measurements were averaged. This averaged out regional differences in fluorescent dye uptake. Six animals were used for each substance tested. Each animal was scored as the ratio of the average fluorescent measurement from the control cornea to that from the test (drug-treated) cornea. To evaluate the method, a variety of substances were tested, including NaOH, benzalkonium chloride, Tween-20, Tween-80, propacaine, and water. Tween-20 increases permeability to fluorescein, whereas Tween-80 does not. This method may be promising as a cheap and rapid screening test for substances with acute ocular toxicity. It does require the sacrifice of mice but does not involve the application of irritants to the eyes of a live animal. A simple fluorometric device was reported to be under development in 1986, which would make it unnecessary to acquire an expensive slit-lamp fluorophotometer (Maurice and Singh, 1986).

ISOLATED LENS PREPARATION

Numerous chemicals and physical stimuli can cause cataracts. Frequently, biochemical changes in the lens occur long before cloudiness of the lens can be diagnosed with the naked eye. Therefore, new technologies have been developed to detect the biochemical changes that occur in the lens after eye irritation. Methods include nuclear magnetic resonance spectroscopy (MRS), nuclear magnetic resonance imaging (MRI), scanning lens monitor, and fluorescence spectroscopy. In vitro, lens metabolism and enzyme activities can also be analyzed for detection of biochemical abnormalities caused by eye irritation.

MRS and MRI

Nuclear magnetic resonance spectroscopy (MRS) and imaging (MRI) have received attention as both in vivo and in vitro methods for monitoring lens metabolism, hydration, and T_1 and T_2 pulse relaxation (Schleich et al., 1985; Lerman and Moran, 1989; Lerman et al., 1982). Nuclear magnetic resonance techniques were developed from the observation that nuclei of certain isotopes (including protium, ^{13}C, and ^{31}P) absorb energy from a magnetic field at discrete wavelengths. The wavelength of energy perturbation is constant under a constant environment and shifts reproducibly with changes in the environment, revealing the environment of the atoms absorbing energy and something of the structure of the molecule to which they belong. The time that certain molecules take to release energy after absorbing distinct quanta of energy from a magnetic pulse (T_1 and T_2 pulse relaxation times) are sensitive to changes in the environments of these molecules and provide a reproducible means of assessing changes in environment. MRS and MRI are superior over traditional observation with a slit-lamp microscope in many aspects, including (a) objective data generated, (b) speed of getting data, and (c) various aspects of the studies allowed depending on the nuclei used. Nuclear magnetic resonance (NMR) has the advantage of being usable noninvasively; it can measure quantitatively otherwise unobservable parameters pertinent to lens integrity, such as the small subtle alterations in protein structure in the lens with changes in the interaction of proteins with the surrounding water, or lens hydration (Lerman and Moran, 1989). Low molecular weight phosphorus compounds have very sharp ^{31}P-NMR spectra, whereas phosphorus atoms bound to high molecular weight compounds have broad diffuse spectra (Schleich et al., 1985), so levels of inorganic phosphate (Pi) and adenosine triphosphate (ATP) can be monitored through NMR.

^{31}P-MRS Study

^{31}P-MRS was used to monitor lenticular organophosphate metabolism and the ability to maintain lens viability in vitro (Schleich et al., 1985; Lerman and Moran, 1989). Enucleated bovine globes were rendered aphakic by intracapsular lens extraction. A large ($160°$–$180°$) limbal incision was made superiorly, the zonular fibers cut, and the lens removed using forceps. Following lens extraction, a thin-walled glass phantom, approximately the geometry and size of the lens, filled with 120 mM NaCl, was inserted into the lens cavity. The phantom, filled with only saline or with phosphate solutions, would be used to calibrate the instrument and determine optimum experimental conditions. Corneal tissue was excised from the globe through an incision that extended circumferentially at the limbus. The iris was removed by way of the incision made for the lens extraction. The limbal incision was then closed with silk sutures.

Method

A Nicolet Magnetics NT-200 spectrometer, equipped with a 4.7-cm wide-bore Oxford superconducting magnet interfaced with a Nicolet 1180 computer system, was used. In a typical experiment, a globe covered with Saran wrap to retard tissue dehydration was mounted in the probe of the instrument with the anterior pole proximal to the surface coil. Position was assessed by the use of thin feeler gauges and the graduated scale of the globe holder. The probe was positioned in the magnet, and air at 5°C was blown over the globe to stabilize ocular tissue metabolite levels. The probe was carefully tuned to 80.96 MHz for each tissue sample. Shimming was accomplished using the water proton resonance in the tissue. Water line widths of 20–40 Hz were usually attained. This is a standard procedure for setting up the instrument prior to making a spectrum of an unknown sample. A 20- or 30-Hz exponential line-broadening factor was employed. Chemical shift values are expressed in parts per million (ppm) relative to internal tissue glycerolphosphorylcholine (GPC) (+0.49 ppm). This was accomplished by using the tissue water proton resonance as an intermediate standard. GPC is an internal standard for this procedure; the instrument is able to take the spectrum of the naturally occurring [31]P.

Titration curves relating the chemical shift of phosphorus-containing metabolites to pH were obtained using lens homogenates diluted by the addition of a small amount of 120 mM NaCl to reduce solution viscosity, followed by adjustment to the desired pH. Titration measurements were made at 80.96 MHz using a conventional saddle-coil probe. Typical spectrometer parameters are the following: pulse width, variable; 2,000 data points per free induction decay; sweep width, ±4000 Hz; and repetition time, 0.378 sec.

Example

A bovine globe phantom containing 10 mM inorganic phosphate (Pi) and 120 mM NaCl in the lens compartment, and with both the anterior and posterior compartments filled with 120 mM NaCl, was used to obtain an initial kRF pulse duration

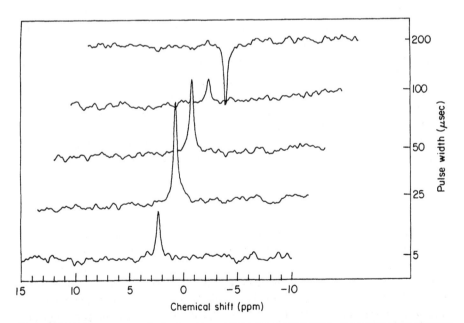

FIG. 3. ^{31}P NMR spectra, acquired using different RF pulse duration times, of a bovine globe phantom containing 10 mM P_i and 120 mM NaCl (plus a trace amount of $MnCl_2$ to reduce the sample T_1 to ca. 1 sec) in the lens compartment; the anterior and posterior compartments contained 120 mM NaCl. The surface coil diameter was 3.8 cm. All other spectral acquisition parameters are described in Method. (Reproduced with permission from Schleich et al., 1985.)

with maximized signal-to-noise ratio for the lens compartment when used with a 3.8-cm-diameter surface coil (Fig. 3). It was possible to "focus" the coil on the lens compartment of the eye (Schleich et al., 1985) and subtract the signal from an aphakic globe, which represents other parts of the eye. Sharply defined signals of lens Pi, and alpha, beta, and gamma phosphate moieties of ATP could be determined. Interestingly, the iris contains almost no detectable phosphates of any kind.

^{13}C-MRS Study

It has been found (Lerman et al., 1982) that there is a direct correlation between the relative concentration of gamma-crystallin fraction in the lens and the degree of acrylamide incorporation and its ability to affect the cold cataract phenomenon. Localized alterations in the density of packing of lens proteins leads to changes in transparency. A classic example of this is the cold cataract phenomenon, which can be reversed by warming. It is known that certain reagents, such as acrylamide, can prevent the cold cataract phenomenon.

Carbon-13 is an isotope that occurs naturally; however, the concentrations are not high enough to be used for MRS analysis. Therefore, exogenous carbon-13, such as ^{13}C-glucose has to be added. To study lens protein packing by MRS, lenses were placed in sample tubes and ^{13}C and ^{1}H-MRS were obtained at 75 and 46 MHz. Lenses were incubated in a medium of balanced salt solution with a bicarbonate buffer containing 7 mM glucose, 0.75 mM L-glutamine, 2 mg/dl potassium penicillin G, and 2 mg/dl streptomycin sulfate. The medium was gassed with 95% oxygen–5% CO_2 to maintain oxygen tension and regulate pH. The incubations were maintained at controlled temperatures; to prevent the cold cataract, 5% acrylamide was added. For deuterated experiments, the components of the incubation media were added to deuterium oxide (D_2O) solutions. The pH was maintained at preincubation levels. Deuterium has no MRS spectrum, so peaks due to solvent water or protons exchangeable with solvent water will disappear. Buffering is important because deuterium oxide is not equivalent to water in its acidity behavior.

Method

Water-proton transverse relaxation rates were measured on lenses to which 1.3 mM dextran-magnetite had been added to the solution outside the lens. The transverse magnetization decay was obtained by signal averaging the output from a Spin-lock CPS-2 pulsed spectrometer, employing the CPMG pulse sequence and sampling echo maxima. Data analysis was performed on a DEC system-10 computer, and temperature was controlled at ±1.0°C by a YSI Model 72 Proportional Temperature Controller employing thermally regulated nitrogen gas. Control of temperature is important because heat can alter protein–solvent interactions and even denature some proteins, and the probes generate heat. The amount of acrylamide in the lenses was estimated with ^{13}C-MRS to measure the loss of acrylamide from the incubating solution by using dioxane as a reference and by measuring area ratios.

Example

For diabetic cataract studies, the lenses were incubated in 35.5 mM glucose for 48 hr. The ^{13}C-sorbitol peaks grow taller and taller over the time period; growth of the peaks can be blocked by certain aldose reductase inhibitors, such as flavonoids.

MRI

MRI is an established tool in clinical imaging, but has been largely limited to whole-body imaging (Lauterbur, 1973; Weisman et al., 1972). Aguayo and co-workers (Aguayo et al., 1986) were able to use the technique for ova of frogs and on a mouse eye, obtaining a clear image of the interior of an intact eye without invading the eye in any way.

Fluorescence Spectroscopy

Tryptophan (TRP) in lens proteins can be made to produce fluorescence that can be detected with fluorescence spectroscopy. This fluorescence allows the study of the lens proteins, their structural integrity, and their relationship with their solvent medium, and is particularly useful in studying phenomena like cold cataract. Acrylamide is a neutral quencher of TRP fluorescence in the interior of proteins, whereas iodide does not significantly quench TRP fluorescence in native proteins due to surface charges. Prevention of cold cataract with acrylamide can be studied with TRP fluorescence in lenses incubated with either acrylamide or iodide. MRS of ^{13}C-labeled acrylamide is used to monitor which crystallins are most affected, using the techniques presented in the previous section.

Method

Fresh human lenses of various ages were used in the study presented here. Five percent acrylamide (20% of which is ^{13}C-labeled) was added to Earle's media containing 5.5 mM glucose. A similar amount of iodide was used in a parallel study. The lenses remained clear during the 2-hr incubation (37°C). The effects of exposing one lens to low-level broadband UV radiation were compared with the contralateral lens incubated in the dark. Both fluorescence and NMR spectra were recorded (Lerman and Moran, 1988). After incubation, the lenses were scanned with a Farand MKII spectrometer. The lenses were dialyzed against Earle's media overnight at 37°C, and the fluorescence and NMR spectra were repeated. One percent acrylamide or iodide was used for the fluorescence-quenching studies, after which the proteins were extracted and separated.

Example

In lenses incubated with acrylamide in the dark, there was a marked diminution in the TRP fluorescence intensity compared with its preincubation levels. TRP fluorescence returned to at least 75% of its preincubation level after overnight dialysis, indicating the acrylamide was not covalently bound to proteins. In contrast, when the lens was exposed to UV radiation there was marked quenching, and the lens never recovered its preincubation fluorescence, even after overnight dialysis, indicating the acrylamide was covalently bound. UV light alone, without acrylamide, had no effect on fluorescence. It was also observed that the degree of acrylamide photobinding decreased progressively with age as did the extent of acrylamide incorporated in the dark. NMR also showed the most acrylamide binding in young lenses. Iodide had no quenching effect in the intact lens but had a little effect on extracted alpha and beta crystallins, which do have some exposed tryptophan residues (Lerman and Moran, 1988).

Scanning Lens Monitor

Lenses can develop opacities due to exposure to various chemicals, including high glucose concentrations. The opacities can be detected with the scanning lens monitor (Mitton et al., 1990). Results correlate well with the development of the sorbitol peak in the lens detected with ^{13}C-MRS as described previously.

Lenses isolated from freshly enucleated rat eyes were quickly rinsed with sterile phosphate buffered saline (PBS) solution and placed in normal medium (M199 containing 10% fetal calf serum and 0.1% glutamine). Lenses were then transferred to sterile clear-plastic culture tubes containing 3 ml of normal glucose medium (5.5 mM glucose) or high glucose medium (55 mM glucose) and incubated at 37°C in a water-jacketed incubator with 5% carbon dioxide.

Lenses were examined after 21 hr of culturing using the scanning lens monitor. Kevex hardware–software was also used to analyze the intensity distributions of lens light projections. Wide-beam white light from a tungsten light source was projected through rat lenses onto an opaque white plastic screen. On the opposite side of this screen, an RCA video camera was focused on the light image and fed into a Colorado Video unit. The video signal was modulated and calibrated by the Colorado unit and the same setup conditions were held for imaging of lenses.

After 21 hr of incubation, lenses in normal medium were clear, whereas lenses in high glucose medium had developed opacities. A scanning lens monitor generated plots of focal length as a function of distance from the optical center. Kevex imaging of lens light projections revealed differences in intensity distributions between 5.5-mM and 55-mM glucose lenses. The system allowed the lens opacities produced by culturing in high glucose medium to be detected not only qualitatively but also quantitatively.

Lens Metabolism and Enzyme Activities

Lens metabolism and lens enzyme activities can be changed by eye irritation. Therefore, detection of these changes can measure eye irritation and intoxication.

Each lens of one pair (bovine or porcine) was laid into an Erlenmeyer flask containing a culture medium (Korte et al., 1987). The compound to be tested was added to the medium of one lens of the pair; the other lens was not treated and served as the control. After 20–24 hr of incubation (this may be prolonged even to 96 hr) at 37°C, lenses were taken out of the medium and were prepared for analysis.

Numerous parameters might be analyzed in a single lens, provided that the lens extract was divided in a proper way. In a deproteinized extract, energy-rich compounds such as the free adenine nucleotides, carbohydrates, intermediates of glycolysis, glutathione, and the coenzymes nicotinamide-adenine dinucleotide, reduced (NADH), and nicotinamide-adenine dinucleotide phosphate, reduced (NADPH), in both their oxidized and reduced states might be determined. In the aqueous extract, most enzymes catalyzing the breakdown of carbohydrates are found; their catalytic activities, kinetic properties, and heat labilities might be measured. Not all of the above parameters can be determined in a single lens. Frequently, only a few of the parameters are altered by an experimental compound and will need to be tested further.

Many enzyme activities can be determined in lens homogenates, allowing a detailed picture of normal lens metabolism and perturbations of metabolism by specific compounds to be obtained (Muller et al., 1987). In one protocol, lenses were dissected from the eye, weighed, and frozen at −28°C. Samples of the different layers were obtained using a newly constructed slicing instrument. With this technique, layers down to 0.25 mm can be obtained. The layers were weighed and worked up into a 10% homogenate. This was centrifuged at 11,630 × g for 30 min, and the supernatants were taken for the determination of enzyme activities and protein concentrations. The authors determined the activities of key enzymes of several metabolic pathways: aldose reductase (AR) and sorbitol dehydrogenase (SDH) for the sorbitol pathway, phosphofructokinase (PFK) and aldolase (ALD) for glycolysis, and glutathione reductase (GR) and glutathione peroxidase (GPX) as representatives for the protection of the lens against oxidative stress. The enzyme activities were expressed as specific activities (mU/mg water-soluble protein).

Some results using incubated lenses have been negative (Korte et al., 1987). Many eye drops contain potassium iodide (KI), which is said to protect protein-SH groups from oxidation and to reduce disulfides produced by oxidation. However, KI had no effect on the distribution and numbers of any oxidized or reduced-SH groups in bovine lenses after incubation.

Another study using cultured lenses dealt with aldose reductase inhibitors (Muller et al., 1987). Aldose reductase catalyzes the first step in the conversion of glucose to sorbitol, which in turn is converted to fructose. An excess of glucose (as in diabetes) produces an excess of sorbitol, which disturbs the lens's osmotic balance and leads to sugar cataracts. It was possible to study the levels of glucose and fructose, of ATP and adenosine monophosphate (AMP), and of glutathione in its oxidized and reduced states in lenses and determine that different aldose reductase inhibitors may have very different effects on these ratios.

Calcium Accumulation

Human cataracts do not necessarily have high calcium accumulations; however, high and low calcium levels in vitro are cataractogenic to cultured lenses (Kuck and Kuck, 1989). These authors showed that calcium accumulation is often a secondary change in human cataractogenesis. Lens calcium levels are not elevated prior to the first appearance of cataract, but are greatly elevated in severe cataracts. It is hoped that studies of lens calcium accumulation will give a greater understanding of cataractogenesis.

Method

Emory mice are used in many cataract studies because they develop cataracts spontaneously. Lenses were removed from the enucleated eyes of Emory mice and were cleaned and weighed under conditions chosen to minimize contamination with extraneous calcium. A lens pair was treated with 0.8 N KOH in a microcentrifuge tube. The lenses were dissolved with occasional vigorous vortex-mixing at room temperature over several days. More 0.8 N KOH was added, and the solution was mixed well. The resulting lens extract was suitable for direct calcium determination.

The total protein was determined by a bicinchoninic acid (BCA) procedure (Smith et al., 1985). Calcium was determined by a modified calcium fluorometry procedure (Wallach and Steck, 1963). An aliquot of the initial lens extract was diluted with KOH to give suitable calcium concentrations for fluorometry. The tubes for the procedure had been carefully cleaned by soaking in a special cleaning solution (nitric acid and sodium bichromate) followed by rinsing with distilled water. This removed most extraneous calcium. The tubes were read in a Turner model 111 fluorometer, and a calibration curve was constructed for each batch of calcium stock solution.

Example

There was no age-dependent increase in calcium in the normal mouse lens (cataract-resistant strain). Since cataractous changes precede the first detectable increases in calcium, calcium accumulation was thought to be a secondary event. It would still be useful to demonstrate that calcium accumulation is secondary to cataract formation with an animal model. Calcium levels went up as cataracts developed in Emory mice, but did not go up significantly in mice with late-forming cataracts until the cataracts actually developed. In addition, mercaptopropionylglycine, a calcium chelating agent, failed to prevent development of cataracts in Emory mice (Kuck and Kuck, 1989) and could not remove the calcium from old cataracts. The data all confirmed that calcium accumulation in cataracts is secondary to the development of the cataract and is due in part to tight binding of calcium to proteins.

Special Ca^{2+},K^+ Channels

The apical membrane of the chick lens epithelial cell has been shown to contain several varieties of K^+ selective channels, including a large conductance channel activated by internal Ca^{2+} and depolarization (the Ca^{2+},K^+ channel). Rae and Cooper (1989) have examined the changes in these channels with maturation. Their technique shows the possibility of using not only chicks but chick embryos as model systems for studying the lens.

Two different types of preparations were used. For 5- to 7-day chick embryos, explants were used. Capsule–epithelial preparations were attached to 35-mm petri dishes by making four cuts through the epithelia with a scalpel blade. For embryos older than 7 days and for chicks after hatching, the lens was excised from its ciliary body attachments. The dissections were done in a sodium aspartate Ringer solution because this resulted in many viable cells. The lens was decapsulated, and the capsule and epithelium were pinned with stainless-steel insect pins to a Sylgard cylinder. This was fitted into an acrylic chamber for visualization under a compound microscope. Single-channel currents were recorded, and the data was digitized into a pulse code modulated videocassette recorder or into an INDEC computer interface.

Example

From day 5 of the embryo until hatching, the apical membrane of the lens epithelium contained primarily large conductance Ca^{2+},K^+ channels. A new maxi-K^+ channel appeared about the same time the Ca^{2+},K^+ channels disappeared. The function of these channels in vivo proved something of a mystery to Rae and Cooper (1989). They speculated that one channel is somehow converted into another; if so, this would suggest that the interconversion of channels is a model for studying lens maturation and a site at which potential ocular teratogens could be tested. Beebe and Feagans (1981) suggested that changes in potassium ion permeability might be important for the differentiation of fiber cells from epithelial cells even in adult lenses; therefore, the effect of potential ocular toxins on this receptor could provide a measure of their potency in inhibiting lens repair after injury.

Distribution of Cholesterol, Phospholipid, and Protein

The lens tissue normally has a cholesterol to phospholipid molar ratio of 3.5:1.0. It has been found that if this ratio is reduced or elevated, cataracts result (Jain, 1977). In this study (Borchman et al., 1989), the regional distribution of cholesterol, phospholipid, and protein content were determined in human and bovine lenses.

Human lenses were excised from eyes obtained 4 hr postmortem and were frozen in liquid nitrogen. A 5.5-mm-diameter thin-walled trephine was placed in a hand drill and used to remove a core sample from the frozen lens (warmed to $-20°C$ in a freezer prior to taking the sample). This sample was divided into four sections.

Core sections and surrounding tissue from lenses of about the same age were pooled. Lipid was extracted at 0°C under a stream of argon. Buffer B contained urea and dithiothreitol buffered with tris/HCl (pH 7.4). Ice-cold buffer B was added to each of the pooled lens sections and was homogenized with a Teflon grounder jacketed in ice. Lipid was extracted with cold chloroform/methanol, mixed, and centrifuged. The lower phase was removed and evaporated under argon. This dried extract was rectified to remove any denatured lipoprotein with ice-cold chloroform and KCl. The bottom phase was then removed and assayed for phospholipid and cholesterol.

Protein was determined by the Peterson modification of the Lowry assay (Peterson, 1977). Two standard curves were made consisting of aliquots of bovine diluted lens homogenate. The protein concentration was determined by dividing the slope of the sample curve by the slope of the standard curve. This was necessary as differences in protein composition may alter the apparent protein concentrations measured by the ordinary Lowry method.

Lipid phosphorus was determined using a modified Bartlett assay (Bartlett, 1959). Two standard curves were made with inorganic phosphorus. Aliquots of lipid extract were dried under argon before assaying.

Cholesterol was determined by a modification of the Huang et al. assay (Huang et al., 1961). Aliquots of lipid extract were dried under argon before assay. Cholesterol detection reagent was added to the dried samples and sonicated for 5 min.

ISOLATED RETINA PREPARATIONS

Although chemicals that contact the eye topically do not penetrate well enough into the eyeball to reach the retina in the back of the eye, photostimulation from the frontal part of the eye (which can lead to phototoxicity) and retinal toxicity caused by systemic drugs are rather common occurrences. Therefore, the isolated perfused bovine eye can be used as a model for the study of acute retinal toxicity.

Electroretinography (ERG) is a measurement of the total neuronal activity of retinal cells and is said to measure "the objective and functional response of the retina" to light (Doly et al., 1990). It follows that any inflammatory mediator that can alter the ERG "may be a messenger between ocular inflammatory impairments and visual function".

Bovine eyes were enucleated immediately following exsanguination (Doly et al., 1990; Tseng et al., 1990). A branch of the ophthalmociliary artery feeding the retina was identified and cannulated with a 22-gauge needle. The cannula was secured with a small clamp and the residual blood flushed with Hank's balanced salt solution containing heparin. Subsequently, the eyes were attached to a peristaltic pump set at a rate of 1.2–1.3 ml/min.

The cannulated eye was placed in a stand equipped with an overhead Grass flash unit before a recording electrode was implanted through its cornea. One reference electrode was placed midway down the globe, and a ground electrode was connected to the stump of the severed optic nerve. The eyes were continuously perfused and dark adapted before further experimentation. For the determination of the stability of the preparation, electronic flashes were given at 15-min intervals and ERG responses recorded until expiration of the preparation. The responses to changing oxygen tension were tested by stopping the perfusion. Photic flashes were administered at 1-min intervals until extinction of the ERG; at this time, an additional 20 min of ischemia was maintained. The effects of reperfusion were determined by recording ERG responses to photic stimuli at 1-min intervals.

At the conclusion of each experiment, the eye was perfusion fixed through the attached cannula for 5 min. Retinas from these eyes were carefully dissected and immersion fixed for 2 hr in 2% paraformaldehyde-glutaraldehyde solution. Small rectangular pieces were carefully dissected, placed in specimen vials, washed overnight in cacodylate buffer, postfixed in osmium tetroxide, and dehydrated in ascending concentrations of ethanol before being embedded in Araldite 502. The polymerized blocks were sectioned at 1-μm or 800-nm thickness and stained for light or electron microscopy, respectively.

Isolated retinas could be kept viable for several hours and reproducible ERGs recorded. The primary response of the cells monitored is the b-wave generated by the Müller cells. Introduction of hydroxyl radicals with Fe^{2+} and ascorbate considerably shortened the life of the retinas, as measured by loss of the b-wave. This effect was reduced by the addition of free radical scavengers.

Example

Leukotriene B_4 (LTB$_4$) perfused into the isolated retina reduced the ERG amplitude in a dose-dependent manner; LTC$_4$ and LTD$_4$ had a similar effect. They may increase Na^+ membrane permeability and have an opposite effect to light on rod outer segment membranes. Platelet activating factor (PAF) and derivatives also were toxic to the ERG; PAF binds to a specific retinal receptor and stimulates phosphatidylinositol breakdown, mobilizing intracellular calcium. The data suggested a role for PAF in visual function.

ALTERNATIVES TO EYE TISSUES

Chemicals that irritate eye tissues will also irritate other sensitive tissues such as egg chorioallantoic membrane, vaginal mucous membrane, and ileum (which alters ileum contractility). Therefore, these tissues can also be used as alternatives to eye irritation studies.

Chicken Egg Test

Huhner–Embryonen Test

The Huhner–Embryonen test (HET) can be used to give information on embryo lethality, embryonic development and growth, teratogenicity, and systemic toxicity, including immunopathology and metabolic pathways (Luepke, 1985). Testing with incubated hen's egg is a borderline case between in vivo and in vitro systems. The HET has now been extended to include chorioallantoic membrane (CAM) testing as a mucous-membrane irritation test.

Chorioallantoic Membrane Test

Eggs to be treated were first candled to discard those that were defective; only fresh, fertile eggs were used. Eggs weighing less than 50 g or more than 60 g were rejected. For CAM testing according to Leighton and co-workers, eggs were incubated at 37.5°C ± 0.5°C and a relative humidity of 62.5% ± 7.5% (Leighton et al., 1983). The eggs were candled on day 5 of incubation and every day thereafter; eggs with nonviable embryos were removed. On day 10 of incubation, the egg shell was scratched around the air cell with a dentist's rotary saw and then pared off. After careful removal of the inner egg membranes, the vascular CAM was exposed. The test substance, dissolved or suspended, was dropped onto the membrane. Solid test

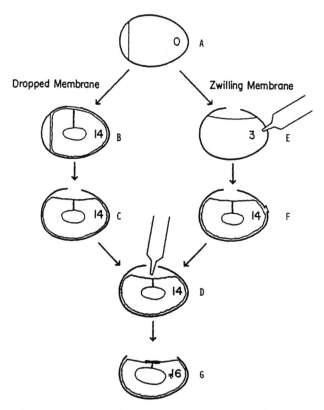

FIG. 4. Two procedures for preparing chicken egg chorioallantoic membrane (CAM). (Reproduced with permission from Leighton et al., 1983.)

materials were applied directly on the vascular chorioallantois and irrigated with warm water. In every case, a series of four eggs was used; two eggs treated with vehicle only served as controls. The CAM, the blood vessels, including the capillary system, and the albumin were examined and scored for irritant effects (hyperemia, hemorrhages, coagulation) at 0.5, 2, and 5 min after treatment.

The CAM can also be used to test for irritation and damage that develop over the course of days rather than minutes. There are two basic procedures for preparing the CAM (Fig. 4). In one procedure, a fertile egg is incubated for a week or more, at which time a window is cut in the shell and a small tear is made in the shell membrane. A small hole is made over the natural airspace at the blunt end of the egg so that the chorioallantoic membrane is dropped below the window. The chemical being tested is applied to the dropped CAM through the window, and the aperture is then closed with adhesive tape.

Another procedure for preparing the CAM was developed by Zwilling (1959). In the 2- or 3-day-old embryo egg, 2 ml of albumin is removed from the egg near the pointed end, and a window is cut through the shell. In the course of the preparation the airspace shifts; the "floor" of the chamber created now consists of the upper aspect of the liquid contents of the egg. The window is closed with tape and the egg returned to the incubator. The chorioallantois becomes the floor of the chamber. With either technique, a test substance is applied to the CAM, and the opening is retaped; 2 or 3 days after application, the tape is removed from the window and the adjacent shell removed to enlarge the window and provide a clear macroscopic view of the site of injury on the CAM.

Example

In preliminary experiments with the classically dropped CAM (Figs. 5–7), graded concentrations of a strong acid and strong base were applied to the 14-day-old membrane, with the reaction to injury observed 3 days later (Leighton et al., 1983). The data showed the surface areas of lesions in square millimeters, measured as a product of the length of the axes. There was an overall (mean) decrease in size of lesion with decrease in concentration of the acid ($p < 0.001$). A similar correlation of irritant concentration and lesion area was found for NaOH. There was a decrease in the size of the lesion as the concentration of base was lowered ($p < 0.001$).

In other experiments, two substances were used; solution A, which was strongly positive by the Draize test, and solution B, which was negative in the same assay procedure (Leighton et al., 1983). Each solution was diluted 1:40 with normal saline and then applied to Zwilling membranes. There was a clearly significant difference between A and B, despite a fairly large degree of variation between eggs. In these experiments, the numerical time-dependent scores for hyperemia, hemorrhage, and coagulation were summed to give a single numerical value indicating the irritation potential of the test substance on a scale with a maximum value of 21.

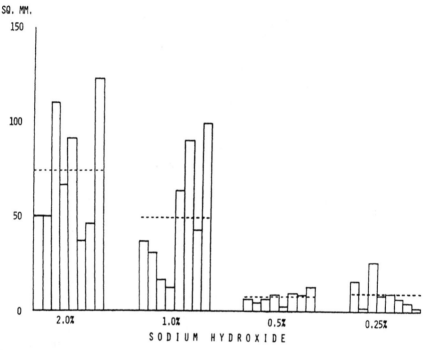

FIG. 5. Acid lesioning of chicken egg chorioallantoic membrane (CAM). (Each bar represents one egg.) (Reproduced with permission from Leighton et al., 1983.)

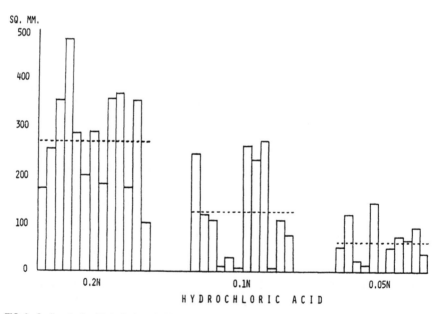

FIG. 6. Sodium hydroxide lesioning of chicken egg chorioallantoic membrane (CAM). (Each bar represents one egg.) (Reproduced with permission from Leighton et al., 1983.)

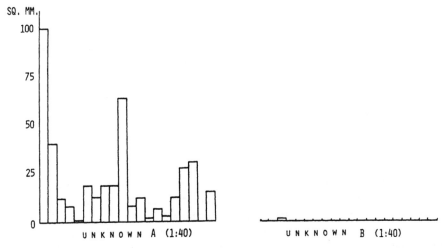

FIG. 7. Lesion of chicken egg chorioallantoic membrane (CAM) with two unknowns, A and B. Unknown A is known to be corrosive to the eyes of rabbits; unknown B is not. (Each bar represents one egg.) (Reproduced with permission from Leighton et al., 1983.)

Vaginal Mucous Membrane

The vagina and cervix have mucous membranes that are susceptible to a variety of irritants. A general indicator of inflammation and cellular toxicity in these tissues is the release of prostanoids by the affected tissues. Prostanoids are products of arachidonic acid or fatty acid metabolism, released to activate various protective mechanisms for the tissue under attack by noxious stimuli. The type of prostanoid produced depends on the particular cell activated.

Method

Female rats were followed daily with vaginal smears to establish estrus cycles. When cytotoxicity was to be determined using a rat (Dubkin et al., 1984), it was anesthetized with pentobarbital and exsanguinated. The reproductive tract was isolated and trimmed of fat and connective tissue. The vagina was divided longitudinally into two or four segments, which were placed in wells containing Krebs' bicarbonate buffer at room temperature. The tissue was then transferred to wells containing either irritant solutions or buffer, which served as a control. After 45 sec, the tissues were rinsed with buffer and replaced in wells containing only buffer. The tray containing tissues was placed in a shaking water bath (37°C) in a 95% O_2–5% CO_2 atmosphere. After incubation for 30 min, the medium over the tissue, containing the released prostanoids, was frozen at −70°C and stored until assayed for prostanoids by radioimmunoassay methods.

Example

The concentrations of various prostanoids found in the media of control vaginal tissue were compared to tissues exposed to 70% ethanol. The amounts of PGE_2 produced during different stages of the estrus cycle are slightly different, with the highest production occurring during the estrus. The PGE_2 release is a function of the concentration of ethanol used.

Ileum Contractility

Various surfactants have been shown to inhibit spontaneous drug-induced or electrically induced muscle contractions. When applied to an intact tissue, a surfactant has to penetrate the outer surface layers before reaching the contractile cells. The penetration of superficial cell layers and ability to deactivate contractile fibers determine the overall effect of a surfactant on a muscle preparation; such a preparation might serve as an experimental indicator for ocular irritation. Surfactants are common in household and laboratory products and are common causes of eye irritation. A study (Muir et al., 1983) has been done to compare the ability of surfactants to hemolyze bovine erythrocytes (chosen as a single cytotoxicity model) and to block spontaneous contractions of mouse and rabbit ileum with the effect of the same surfactant on the rabbit eye in vivo.

Methods

Sections of terminal ileum were set up under a resting tension of 0.7 g for mouse and 1.0 g for rabbit in organ baths containing Tyrode–Ringer solution at 35°C and were bubbled with atmospheric air. Spontaneous contractions were recorded via isotonic displacement transducers on Washington 400MD oscillographs. The tissues were allowed 25 min to equilibrate before addition of any surfactant. Surfactants were added at 10-min intervals, so the concentration grew progressively greater. If > 50% block of spontaneous activity had not been achieved after six additions the tissue was discarded. Concentration–effect curves were constructed enabling the calculation of the concentration required to produce 50% block of spontaneous activity for mouse ileum (EC_{50} mouse) and rabbit ileum (EC_{50} rabbit).

Examples

The most potent hemolytic action, as previously determined (Scaife, 1982), was generally achieved with the longer alkyl chain surfactant. The C-12 (triethanolamine lauryl sulfate, sodium lauryl sulfate) and C-14 (triethanolamine myristyl sulfate) anionics showed greater hemolytic potency than the corresponding C-12 (lauryl trimethyl ammonium bromide) and C-14 (myristyl trimethyl ammonium bromide) cationics. These results are at variance with the in vivo results in rabbits, where the cationics were more irritant than the corresponding anionics. Order of potency for EC_{50} mouse or EC_{50} rabbit also differed from the order for EC_{50} hemolysis. There is an apparent trend from EC_{50} hemolysis, in which long alkyl chains were most potent, through EC_{50} mouse to EC_{50} rabbit and finally to in vivo, where short chains are most potent. Correlation between EC_{50} rabbit and both corneal and conjunctival irritancy scores in vivo is good.

CELL CULTURES

In addition to isolated tissues, cell cultures can also be used as alternatives to the in vivo Draize test. Cell cultures are more convenient than isolated tissues and in most cases do not require the sacrifice of animals. Some cell lines are of human origin, eliminating any interspecies differences and the inherent complications these produce in toxicology. However, in vitro tests generally have to be used for individual classes of chemicals and to represent a single aspect of the in vivo Draize test; this is partly because of the great variation in physicochemical properties and biological activities of the many classes of potentially irritating chemicals. The acceptable cell culture methods must give results that correlate well with human experiences. It is hoped that cell culture in vitro methods will eventually replace the Draize test so that eye irritancy tests can be done by more humane methods.

Cytotoxicity Tests

More than a dozen methods are available for the measurement of the cytotoxicity of cell cultures. These methods are applicable to all cell cultures regardless if they are eye cells or non eye cells. Therefore, they will be presented here first before dealing with individual cell cultures.

Cytotoxicity Assayed in Terms of DNA Synthesis

For example, confluent cultures of rabbit corneal epithelium were grown in complete medium: minimal essential medium with D-valine supplemented with 10% heat-inactivated fetal calf serum, 10 μg/ml crystalline insulin, 20 ng/ml epidermal growth factor, and 0.1 ng/ml cholera toxin (North-Root et al., 1982; Shopsis et al., 1984; Lazarus et al., 1990). Cultures were inspected daily, and the culture medium was changed every 48 hr. After 7–12 days, confluent cultures from the master primary culture plates were reseeded into 24-well Primaria polystyrene tissue culture plates. After 48 hr culture to allow the cells to reattach, the complete medium was removed and fresh complete medium added, either with the drug to be tested in it or with no additions (control). Drugs tested included ophthalmic preservatives, antiviral, and aminoglycoside drugs.

After 5, 30, or 60 min, the medium containing the drug (or the control medium) was removed, and the culture plates were twice washed with Dulbecco's phosphate buffered saline without calcium or magnesium. Cytotoxicity was determined by measuring DNA synthesis. One-half milliliter of complete medium, containing 1 μCi of sterile ^{3}H-thymidine (specific activity 6.7 mCi/mmol) was added to each well. After 8–12 hr of incubation, DNA was extracted. Samples were solubilized in Aquasol and counted in a liquid scintillation counter. Data were expressed as the percentage inhibition of ^{3}H-thymidine incorporation compared with the control.

Example

Increased doses of a variety of cytotoxic agents (Lazarus et al., 1990) caused progressive inhibition of ^{3}H-thymidine incorporation. Cytosine arabinoside produced significant inhibition of ^{3}H-thymidine incorporation at 10^{-7} M. Concentrations of methotrexate of 1 mM were required for significant inhibition of ^{3}H-thymidine incorporation. Melphalan, 5-fluorouracil, and thiotepa significantly inhibited ^{3}H-thymidine incorporation at 10^{-8}, 10^{-6}, and 10^{-4} M, respectively. These are antineoplastic drugs to which growing cells are especially sensitive. It is not surprising they were toxic to corneal epithelial cells.

Cytotoxicity Assayed in Terms of RNA Synthesis

This toxicity system measures the ability of xenobiotics to inhibit the uptake of uridine into cultured cells (Shopsis et al., 1984; Shopsis and Sathe, 1984). Uridine uptake is a much more sensitive indicator of the toxic action of compounds than that of the cell death. The concentration of the test substance required to produce a 50% inhibition in uridine uptake (UI_{50}) provides a measure of toxicity. The uridine uptake inhibition test is also readily applicable to the assessment of toxicity of mixtures of compounds. Cells treated simultaneously with irritants bearing different chemical functional groups may show additive uridine uptake inhibition effects. In addition, because this procedure can quantitatively indicate nonlethal cytotoxicity, it can be used to determine the ability of cells to recover from toxic insult.

Balb/c 3T3 mouse fibroblasts were plated into 35-mm dishes at 50,000 cells/dish. After 8 hr, the medium was removed and replaced with fresh growth medium (for control dishes) or medium containing various concentrations of test agents. Freshly plated cells will be rapidly growing and multiplying and synthesizing DNA and RNA. After 4 hr of incubation, the media were removed, the cells were washed with buffered saline, allowed to take up ^{3}H-uridine for 15 min, and then were dissolved in 0.5 N NaOH. Aliquots were taken for the determination of cell protein per dish and uridine uptake. Changes in cell protein per dish (an indication of cell death) and in uridine uptake relative to control cultures were plotted against the concentration of toxicant.

Examples

Screening of groups of compounds previously ranked for toxicity in vivo indicated that UI_{50} values formed an excellent rank correlation with published Draize test results. Cells treated simultaneously with irritants bearing different chemical functional groups showed additive uridine uptake inhibition effects. This effect is very relevant to human eye irritation; humans are as likely to come into contact with preparations that are combinations of many substances as they are to encounter a pure irritant substance. The effects were generally reversible: cultures treated with levels of irritants that reduced uridine uptake capacity by 40–80% were able to recover most of their uridine uptake capacity within 20 hr.

Cytotoxicity Assayed in Terms of Protein Synthesis

For viability studies, SIRC cells, a stable fibroblast cell line derived from rabbit cornea, were cultured in 6-cm dishes for 24 hr in the absence of interleukin-1 blockers. The compounds and vehicle were then added to the dishes. At the end of 24, 48, or 72 hr, five dishes were triturated for cell counts using a hemocytometer, and cell viability was determined with the trypan blue exclusion method. Other dishes were given [^{3}H]Leucine (0.5 μCi/ml, 121 Ci/mmol). Cells were incubated for 6 hr with the isotopes. The cell medium was drained off; the cells adhering to the dish were washed with cold phosphate-buffered saline (PBS) three times and were solubilized with 1 ml of hyamine hydroxide solubilizer to release the incorporated radioactivity. A 0.2-ml aliquot of dissolved cells was transferred to 5 ml ScintiVerse II counting solution, and the radioactivity was counted with a Beckman LS 5000 CE Beta counter (Chen et al., 1996). [^{35}S]-Methionine incorporation can also be used to determine the biosynthesis of protein in the cell.

Plasminogen Activation Measurement

The enzyme plasminogen activator (PA) is produced and released by a number of cell types in culture; release is correlated with the growth state of the cells. Production and release of PA are also subject to modulations such as hormonal regulation, malignant transformation, mitogenic stimulation, and cellular injury. Chemical injury to cells usually causes them to express lower levels of the enzyme. Therefore, the levels of PA released by cells exposed to chemicals, relative to cells exposed to saline, can be used as an index of chemical injury. Chan (1985) used a sensitive photometric method to measure PA in cultured rabbit corneal epithelial cells, and published an initial evaluation of the test's predictability of chemical hazard to the human eye using eight standard toxic chemicals.

Method

Enucleated eyes of rabbits were placed in 0.1 M phosphate-buffered saline at pH 7.3. Sterile saline was injected intrastromally until the whole cornea appeared opaque and swollen. The cornea was dissected along the limbus and separated into anterior and posterior portions. The anterior half, containing epithelium and stroma, was cut into 1-mm squares and treated with Dipase II in serum-free culture medium at room temperature for about 1 hr. The intact epithelium could then be peeled away from the stroma with fine forceps. The epithelial cells were washed twice with serum-free culture medium, minced, and treated with 0.25% trypsin in Puck's saline containing no calcium or magnesium ion. The epithelial cells were dissociated by repeated passage through a hypodermic needle. The cells were washed and collected by centrifugation.

The dissociated epithelial cells were plated in multiwell or microtest plates (Falcon). The cells were maintained as monolayer cultures in Dulbecco's modified Eagle medium supplemented with 2% fetal calf serum and trace substances at 37°C in a humidified atmosphere of 2% CO_2–98% air. Culture in multiwell plates was used to study PA release under normal conditions.

Coleman and Green's (1981) two-step coupled assay was used to quantify PA secreted by the cultured corneal epithelial cells. Plasminogen was first activated to plasmin by PA, and the resulting plasmin was allowed to react with thiobenzyl benzoxycarbonyl-L-lysinate to form Z-lysin and benzyl mercaptan. Benzyl mercaptan reacts instantly and nonenzymatically with 5,5'-dithiobis (2-nitrobenzoic acid) (DTNB) to form mixed disulfide and colored thiophenolate anion. The resulting color reaction is read at 412 nm using a spectrophotometer. PA was measured by the esterolytic unit (E.U.). One E.U. is equivalent to approximately 5×10^{-4} Ploug units. In the tests, the percentage inhibition of plasminogen activation (PIPA) was used as an index of the extent of chemical injury.

$$\text{PIPA} = \left(1 - \frac{\text{PA level of culture exposed to chemical}}{\text{PA level of culture exposed to saline}} \right) \times 100\%.$$

Example

Cultures in microtest plates were used for the corneal epithelium plasminogen activator (CEPA) test. The cells were rinsed in normal saline and exposed briefly to a test chemical. Initially, household bleach containing 5% sodium hypochlorite (NaClO) was used to test the response of cells to chemical injury. Eight test chemicals were then used: benzalkonium chloride, triethanolamine, acetic acid, isopropyl alcohol, NaClO, sodium lauryl sulfate, formaldehyde, and sodium hydroxide. Control cultures were exposed to saline alone. After treatment, the cells were rinsed in serum-free culture medium and were maintained through a recovery period in which the modulation of PA secretion was initiated. At the end of the recovery period, the culture medium was removed for PA assay. The eight chemicals listed were divided into nonirritant (first four compounds) and irritant (last four compounds) groups. This method has the advantages of requiring only cell culture facilities and a colorimeter, without the need for expensive equipment or hazardous procedures.

To predict chemical hazards to the human eye, CEPA scores can be correlated with the Draize scores. When this was done in this study, only the bleach and the sodium lauryl sulfate were overscored (predicted to be more irritating than they were), and no substance was underscored. The results suggest strongly that the CEPA test can be used to distinguish irritants from nonirritants and will be an effective alternative to the Draize rabbit eye irritancy test.

^{51}Cr-Release Method

The isotopic chromium ^{51}Cr-release assay has been widely used to quantitate toxicity in corneal endothelial cell culture systems (Shadduck et al., 1985; Douglas and Spilman, 1983; Stewart-Dettaan et al., 1990). In the present study, the Descemet's membrane and endothelial cells of freshly harvested corneas were cut into 2-mm^2 fragments and placed in 60-mm plastic tissue culture dishes. The explant cultures were maintained in 3 ml of RPMI 1640 tissue culture medium plus 10% calf serum. When the outgrowth extended 10 mm around the explants, the cells were harvested with 0.1% trypsin and 0.1% EDTA, pelleted by centrifugation, and used in toxicity tests. The cells were preincubated with 0.5 μCi/ml medium with ^{51}Cr (as sodium chromate) for 1 hr during which time the cells took up 60,000–200,000 disintegrations per minute (dpm) of the isotope per well. Each monolayer was washed three times to remove unincorporated chromate. When cells are killed, the isotope is released into the culture medium. The isotope in the medium may be measured in a gamma counter or in a liquid scintillation counter.

Three types of cytotoxicity assays have been performed with the ^{51}Cr-release method: (a) a range-finding experiment to identify a maximum no-effect dose of the test substance and a minimum dose resulting in 100% ^{51}Cr release; (b) one assay determining the time course of ^{51}Cr release (indicating how rapidly acting a substance is and defining an appropriate incubation time); and (c) a dose–response study performed by incubating endothelial cells with a range of test substances. From these studies, an estimated dose resulting in 50% maximal toxicity (ED$_{50}$) was derived. The ED$_{50}$s of different substances allowed these toxins to be ranked or grouped in vitro, and the order of potency was compared to in vivo results.

^{51}Cr-release assays could take several forms. In the ^{51}Cr-release assay, both the amount of the isotope released into the medium and that remaining in the monolayers of cells (^{51}Cr-retention assay) could be measured. Another variation was treating the cells with the test substance first and then measuring the ^{51}Cr uptake of the cells. This latter method was advantageous for long durations of exposure to the test substances.

The assays were conducted in 96-well tissue culture microtiter plates; each well was equivalent to one rabbit. In one typical experiment, adherent cells were labeled for 18–24 hr with 1 mCi/1 $\times$ 10^7 cells. The same concentration of ^{51}Cr was used to label suspended cells (for 2 hr). The cells were washed and used for toxicity assay. Using Dulbecco's modified Eagle medium (DMEM) tissue culture buffer, serial 10-fold dilutions of test compounds were prepared for preliminary screening. For routine testing, serial twofold dilutions were used.

The radiolabeled cells in microtiter plates were exposed to test compounds for between 0.5 and 4 hr. The plates were then centrifuged, and samples of the supernatants were collected and counted in a gamma counter. The 50% cytotoxic dose (CD$_{50}$) was calculated by subtracting the number of counts in the supernatants of cells held in control (drug-free) medium from the test results. The results were then calculated as a percentage of the maximum.

Example

For the corresponding Draize test, the low-volume eye irritation test described by Griffith et al. (1980) was used. Using 0.5 M concentrations of compounds, irritation scores were reported as sums of all scores from the first day when irritation was detected to the last day of irritation. Five of the six surfactants could be ranked, but polysorbate 20 was never ranked correctly in any test. Cytotoxicity data in vitro suggested that this compound should rank fifth or sixth in irritancy; the in vitro results always suggested the compound was more irritative than the actual in vivo tests demonstrated. Despite some variability seen in the cells, data were otherwise quite consistent, and the results were reproducible. Some of the variability may have resulted from difficulty in radiolabeling the cells uniformly. The results still suggested that the determination of CD_{50} using these cells yields data appropriate for ranking the relative irritative potential of materials in vivo without recourse to the Draize test. The results also indicate that irritating materials are not likely to be classified as nonirritating using this cytotoxicity method.

Cytotoxicity Assayed in Terms of Cell Death

Fibroblasts are nonocular cells, but they can be used to assess cytotoxicity of a great variety of substances, including most substances that are potentially toxic to the eyes. They offer several advantages: (a) there is extensive literature on growth, growth inhibition, and cytotoxicity of compounds to these cells; (b) they are easy to culture, being a naturally proliferative culture; (c) toxicity can be measured in terms of cell death, cell morphology, cell function, and cell detachment, so nonlethal damage can be studied; and (d) they do not require the death of any new animals. Indeed, some lines of fibroblast are of human origin, and potential interspecies differences are eliminated from the analysis of the results of the experiments.

At least three cytotoxicity assays are available for fibroblast assays (Reinhardt et al., 1985; Kennah et al., 1989): (a) the cell detachment assay using detachment of cells after a 4-hr incubation; (b) the growth inhibition assay using a 2-day logarithmic growth period with the test compound present or absent; and (c) cloning efficiency during a 7-day growth and exposure period. In the studies cited here, three types of fibroblasts were used: (a) baby hamster kidney fibroblasts (BHK-21/C13), (b) early (Keller) passage human fibroblasts, and (c) "late late" (MRC-5) passage human fibroblasts.

Method

Solvents used for test compounds were water, Hank's balanced salt solution (HBSS), dimethyl sulfoxide (DMSO), minimal essential medium (MEM), and absolute ethanol. The test compound solutions were filter-sterilized and diluted with MEM immediately before use so that the final concentration of solvent in the medium was 1% for controls and 1% or less for the dilution series. Five concentrations of test compound and one control were placed in a single 24-well dish. Phenol red color changes indicated changes in the pH of the test solutions. BHK-21/C13 cells were cultured in MEM, whereas human Keller and MRC-5 cells were cultured in Dulbecco's MEM under 5% O_2 and 8% CO_2.

Cell Detachment

In the cell detachment assay, BHK cells were placed in 24-well plates, allowed 24 hr to settle and attach, and were exposed to the test substance for 4 hr. Some cells were trypsinized and electrically counted before adding the test substance to get an initial titer. In solvent controls, a maximum of 5% of total cells were detached. The lowest concentration of the compound that induced a significant toxic effect (CD_{low}) was determined by measuring the number of detached BHK cells.

Growth Inhibition

Growth inhibition was determined under subconfluent culture conditions. Twenty-four-well plates were seeded with 4,000 cells per well, 24 hr prior to incubation with test substances. Under these conditions, the cells will be rapidly dividing after 24 hr. The cells were then exposed to diluted series of test substances in full medium for 48 hr. Cells were briefly checked for morphological changes and contaminations. The medium was discarded, and the cells were washed with phosphate-buffered saline and trypsinized with 0.25% trypsin for 5–15 min. The cells were resuspended with fresh medium and electronically counted. The data were expressed as percentage of the initial cell number.

Cloning Efficiency

The cloning efficiency of the BHK cells was determined in 24-well plates. The cells were exposed to test solutions or solvent under conditions identical to the detachment assay cited above. One hundred BHK cells were put into each well with medium and the test compound or solvent. The cells were exposed to test compound for 7 days and then were fixed and stained with Giemsa. This is a test for long-term toxicity (North-Root et al., 1982; Shopsis et al., 1984; Lazarus et al., 1989).

Example

The ranking order of chemicals tested was similar for all three assays, although the cell detachment assay was up to three orders of magnitude more sensitive than the other two assays. The growth inhibition assay proved to be more reliable than the cloning efficiency assay. The ranking order resulting from the in vitro data correlated better with threshold limit values for human workroom air (TLV/TWA) than with LD_{50} values. A crude classification was made of the CD_{low} values into three groups: (a) nonirritant, (b) mild to moderate irritant, and (c) strong irritant or corrosive. When compared with the known irritation potential for skin and mucous membranes derived from human exposure data for the test compounds, the in vitro data were more than 80% predictive of the in vivo classifications (Reinhardt et al., 1985). Unfortunately, many of the errors indicated substances were less toxic in vitro than they have proven in vivo; a bad example is sodium hydroxide. It was hoped that using different thresholds for different classes of chemicals would improve correlation between in vitro and in vivo results.

Cell Viability Assayed in Terms of Metabolism and Permeability

LS cells derived from NCTC L929 mouse fibroblasts were used in this study (Kemp et al.,1983). Cells were stored under liquid nitrogen in reserve, and then were thawed and grown in 1-liter round-bottomed flasks and maintained in suspension at 37°C with a Vibromixer, which utilizes the Bernoulli effect. The culture medium was Eagle's modified MEM (Flow) with 5% (vol/vol) fetal calf serum, 0.859 g/l sodium bicarbonate, 2 mM glutamine, plus penicillin and streptomycin.

Cells were used when the stock culture had reached 1 million cells/ml. Aliquots of 4.9 ml were transferred to 25-ml Erlenmeyer flasks, and 0.1 ml of test compounds in the same medium was added. Test compounds in the study cited were detergent-based products labeled by code, diluted from a stock solution of 100 mg/ml. The flasks were gassed with 5% carbon dioxide in air and placed in a shaker at 37°C for 4 hr. The internal standard used to assess the health of the cells was sodium lauryl sulfate, Analar grade (60 mg/ml), which consistently gave a CD_{50} figure of 1.00 ± 0.03 mg/ml.

Viability after 4 hr was assessed in terms of metabolism and permeability, after mixing a combination of the fluorescent dyes, fluorescein diacetate, and ethidium bromide in Eagle's modified MEM with the cell suspension. Esterase activity in living cells causes the formation of fluorescein, whereas the breakdown of the cell permeability barrier of the membrane allows the rapid accumulation of ethidium bromide in dead cells, primarily in the nucleus. Live (green fluorescence) and dead (red fluorescence) cells were counted in a silver-backed modified Fuchs–Rosenthal hemocytometer under a Zeiss fluorescence microscope with epifluorescence condenser.

Cell Viability Assayed in Terms of Intracellular ATP

A sensitive and automated technique was used in this study (Kemp et al., 1985) to estimate the levels of intracellular ATP. ATP is the primary energy donor in the cell and is considered a good indicator of cellular health.

Method

LS cells derived from NCTC L929 mouse fibroblasts were cultured in Eagle's modified MEM with 5% (vol/vol) fetal calf serum (Kemp et al., 1983). Cells were grown as above in Erlenmeyer flasks in "spinner" culture. Substances truly soluble in culture medium were made up as stock solutions, whereas insoluble and immiscible materials were weighed directly into the Erlenmeyer flasks used for culture; then volumes of medium were added before cells were seeded to give an appropriate range of concentrations. The flasks were gassed with 5% CO_2 in air and incubated in the shaker at 37°C for 24 hr. At the end of the period, the material in the flask was centrifuged to separate phases, and the aqueous phase ("extract") was removed. Cells from stock cultures were counted using a silver-backed Fuchs-Rosenthal hemocytometer and placed in centrifuge tubes, 5 million cells per tube, for pelleting by centrifugation. The growth medium was then discarded, and the pelleted cells were resuspended in the extracts. Toxicity was determined by the method described below (Kemp et al., 1983), with a 4-hr incubation period.

In a second variation of the procedure, a weighed amount of test material was added to a known volume of growth medium; the concentration of test substance was at least double the approximate CD_{50} from a standard run. The appropriate-sized Erlenmeyer flask was then gassed with 5% CO_2 in air and incubated at 37°C on an orbital shaker for 24 hr. The flask's contents were centrifuged, and the aqueous layer (extract) was removed and tested for toxicity.

To check for complete extraction of immiscible organics, sufficient medium was added to an amount of test substance fivefold greater than its CD_{50} to give a total volume of 5 ml. The flask was gassed and shaken to achieve further extraction. The flask contents were centrifuged, the aqueous phase removed, and the oily (nonaqueous) layer resuspended in fresh culture medium. Cells were pelleted as above (5 million cells) and resuspended in the oily medium. The normal protocol described above was used to determine cytotoxicity, using fluorescein diacetate and ethidium bromide.

The assay fo⁻ ATP utilized the firefly luciferase bioluminescent reaction measured in a Packard Auto Picolite Luminometer charged with Packard luminescence materials, ATP extraction (Picoex B), and luciferase-luciferin (Picozyme F) reagents. Samples from the culture flasks were placed in monitoring tubes that were loaded into the luminometer. The internal standard for which the instrument was programmed was 50 μl of 10^{-7} M ATP (Picochec) in tris-magnesium sulfate buffer, pH 7.75. An ATP standard curve revealed a linear relationship from 10^{-10} to 10^{-14} mol ATP in a 19-μl sample.

Example

A lotion formulation was studied by this technique. The complete lotion formulation gave a much higher CD_{50} in the standard test than did the internal standard, sodium lauryl sulfate. The CD_{50} value for lotion obtained using the preincubation technique with variable volumes differed only slightly from that found by the standard method, but there was a marked improvement in standard deviation.

The concentration lowering cellular ATP by 50% (ATP_{50}) value itself did not always give a clear indication of the increased sensitivity of the ATP estimation when compared with the viability dyes technique. Compounds might kill cells without lowering the ATP concentration of the flask proportionally. In no case, however, was the ATP_{50} higher than the CD_{50}.

Cell Viability Assayed in Terms of the Uptake of Neutral Red and Others

The neutral red (NR) assay developed by Borenfreund and Puerner (Borenfreund and Puerner, 1984) is based on the inability of dead and damaged mouse fibroblast 3T3 cells to take up the dye neutral red. If dye-treated cells are lysed, the color is released and can be measured photometrically. Toxic effects of test substances are manifested as a reduction in the intensity of the extracted color compared with the untreated controls. Applying this assay to monolayer cultures is particularly advantageous. The test consists of two parts: (a) screening of cells under an inverted phase contrast microscope for the detection of morphological alterations, and (b) a quantitative spectrophotometric procedure, based on the incorporation of neutral red, a supravital dye, into the lysosomes of viable cells (Borenfreund and Puerner, 1984; Hockley and Baxter, 1986). Both of these assays were carried out, in the study cited, in the same culture in a 96-well test plate.

Cell Culture

Mouse embryo fibroblast 3T3 cells were grown in Dulbecco's modified Eagle medium (DMEM) containing calf serum and antibiotics. To subculture, the growth medium was discarded, and the cells were rinsed with trypsin in serum-free DMEM and incubated until the cells became rounded and could be detached from the plastic surface. The cells were resuspended in fresh growth medium and dispensed into tissue culture flasks.

Assay Procedure

The 3T3 cells were harvested from 75%-confluent cultures by trypsin treatment and were resuspended in fresh growth medium and incubated for 6 hr to allow the cells to become firmly attached to the plastic. A constant plate format was maintained for all assays using eight replicates for each treatment as follows: column 1, blanks (no compound or NR); columns 2 and 12, controls (NR only); columns 3–11, dilutions of test substances. Test substances were diluted in growth medium. The original growth medium was decanted from plated cells and replaced with control DMEM or with medium containing the diluted test substance. The plates were returned to the incubator for 17 hr. The medium was then removed, each well was rinsed, and growth medium containing NR was added to all except the blank wells. After 3-hr incubation, the NR medium was removed, and the wells were rinsed. Plates were inverted and allowed to drain before the addition of extraction medium. After 30-min extraction, plates were shaken briefly, and the optical density of the solutions in the wells was determined using a Kontro SL/T210 automatic plate reader. The more dye present, the healthier the cells were in that well.

This method is a rapid, reliable, inexpensive, and reproducible in vitro assay for screening potentially toxic agents. If it is adopted, the number of animals used to determine ocular toxicity could be greatly reduced.

Other Uptake Markers

The cytotoxicity of a variety of cell lines of different origin can be determined by examining the marker's inclusion–exclusion–leakage as indices of membrane integrity (Ecobichon, 1997). For example, fluorescein diacetate enters only viable cells just like neutral red, becoming localized there or leaking back out through a damaged cell membrane. On the other hand, propidium iodide and ethidium bromide are larger molecules than neutral red and fluorescein and are excluded from viable cells but can enter damaged cells to stain DNA. Similarly, trypan blue penetrates only damaged cell membranes to stain proteins in the nonviable cells.

The major problem of using these marker uptake systems is that, although they can produce excellent correlations between cytotoxicity endpoints and Draize irritation within a single class of chemicals, the overall correlations are poor when comparisons are made across different chemical classes (Sina and Gautheron, 1994; Sina et al., 1995). Therefore, these methods are used only for screening toxic agents rather than for assuring safety of test materials.

Cytotoxicity Assay in Terms of Decreased MTT Vital Dye Metabolism

MTT (3-[4,5-dimethylthiazol-2-yl] 2,5-diphenyltetrazolium bromide) is a yellow dye which can be metabolized to a purple formazan dye by mitochondrial succinate dehydrogenase in viable cells (Mossman, 1983; Carmichael et al., 1987; Triglia et al., 1991; Osborne et al., 1995). When the cells were killed, the metabolism reduced, and the color changes also decreased. This method is more sensitive than the neutral red uptake method described above.

Method

Cell cultures which were exposed to test material for up to 30 min and washed were immersed in MTT reagent solution (0.5 mg/ml assay medium, 1 ml/culture) for 3 hr at 37°C on a rotating–shaking platform. The purple formazan product was extracted from cells with isopropanol (2 ml/culture) for 2 hr at room temperature on a rotating–shaking platform. The aliquots of isopropanol extract containing purple formazan product were measured on a BioTek 312 96-well plate reader at 540 nm.

Cytotoxicity was calculated from the plot of A_{450} unit at each exposure time as percentage reduction of A_{450} unit versus time matched control values (assay medium alone). The t_{50} value was defined as the time required (in min) for a 50% reduction of MTT metabolism in treated cells, and was calculated by interpolation at the 50% level along a straight line between two points spanning above and below the 50% response level. Responses to test materials were determined in at least duplicated cultures at each time point in each time course experiment. Independent time course experiments were conducted 2–4 times with each test material (Osborne et al., 1995).

Cytotoxicity Assay in Terms of Glutathione Content

Glutathione is present in most cells in high concentrations to protect cells against oxidation and damage by a large number of toxicomponents (Reed, 1990). Cellular glutathione exists in two forms: reduced and oxidized. The total glutathione was measured using a modified method of cycling assay of Liu and Miller (1992).

Method

The sf-1-Ep (CCL 68) rabbit skin epithelial cell line, SIRC rabbit corneal (CCL 60) fibroblast cell lines, and 3T3 mouse embryo (CCL 92) fibroblast cell lines were obtained from American Type Culture Collection and used. Cells collected were spun down by centrifugation for 3 min at 3000 rpm (Eppendorf, Model 5415C). The supernatant was removed, and 200 μl of solution containing 10% trichloroacetic acid and 5 mM EDTA in water was added. Cells were then broken by sonication for 8 sec using a sonicator with a microtip (Heat Systems). The cell homogenate was centrifuged at 14,000 rpm for 3 min, and the supernatant was assayed for glutathione.

Sample or glutathione standard was mixed with assay solution in individual wells of a 96-well plate. The assay solution contained DTNB (5,5'-dithio-bis (2-nitrobenzoic acid) 0.3 mg/ml, 50 μl), NADPH (0.15 mg/ml, 0.8 ml), and glutathioreductase (8.3 units/ml, 0.8 ml) in 5.6 ml phosphate buffer (0.5 M sodium phosphate plus 5 mM EDTA at pH 7.5). The absorbance at 405 nm was measured each minute using automated microplate reader (Perkin-Elmer). The rate of absorbance change is proportional to the level of glutathione. The reduction in glutathione content of the cells is a measure of cytotoxicity of the cells (Pasternak and Miller, 1995).

Conjunctiva Cell Culture

Determination of CDT_{50} (50% Cell Damage Time)

Chang's human conjunctival cells were cultured in Eagle's minimal essential medium (pH 7.2) with 10% fetal bovine serum. A sheet of 10 million cells was grown for 3–4 days in an incubator at 37°C, trypsinized with 0.25% trypsin and 0.02% ethylenediaminetetraacetic acid (EDTA, pH 7.2), and then suspended in 40–50 ml of medium. Two milliliters of cell suspension was transferred to each of 16–20 small glass flasks with a counted inoculum cell population of 2–3×10^5/ml (Takahashi and Ikowa, 1990; Takahashi et al., 1987).

The cultures were sealed and incubated at 37°C for 48 hr to obtain a confluent cell sheet. After decanting of the media from the cultures, a monolayer of cells was exposed to a test solution of 0.5 ml during a given period of time. Controls were exposed to a phosphate buffer solution (PBS). Following exposure to the test agents, the medium was replaced with 2 ml of fresh medium, and cells were incubated another 24 hr at 37°C. The sheets of cells were separated by trypsinization and suspended in 2 ml of medium for cell counting. All topical drugs in this study contained benzalkonium chloride (BAC) as a preservative.

Example

The CDT_{50} values of an aminoglycoside preparation with BAC were 3 min 56 sec in micromycin sulfate, 9 min 26 sec in dibekacin sulfate, 17 min 35 sec in sisomycin sulfate, 24 min 24 sec in tobracin, and 77 min 49 sec in amikacin sulfate. Aminoglycosides without BAC, with the exception of micromycin, showed no cytotoxicity. The CDT_{50} of micromycin without BAC was 13 min 20 sec.

Morphological Study

Light Microscopy. After a confluent cell sheet was formed, cells were exposed to test drugs for 30 sec and immediately washed by PBS to completely eliminate the test drug from the medium (Takahashi and Ikowa, 1990). Cells were examined under the microscope with Giemsa stain. To know whether the cells had been restored to their normal appearance, they were examined again under the microscope 48 hr after the passage of cells exposed to 5-fluorouracil (5-FU), a compound causing cell degeneration by interfering with DNA replication.

Scanning Electron Microscope. After the cells had been exposed to test solutions for 30 sec, they were washed with PBS and fixed with 2.5% glutaraldehyde for 30 min at 4°C. After being washed with PBS, they were fixed with 1% osmium tetroxide and then dehydrated in graded series of ethanol. They were treated in a carbon dioxide critical point drying, coated with gold palladium, and examined under the scanning electron microscope.

Example. When the cells were exposed to 5-FU at concentrations greater than 0.01% for 30 sec, clear signs of cell damage were found. Scanning electron microscopy revealed reduction of microvilli and filopodia.

Corneal Cell Culture

Morphology of Human Corneal Epithelium

This part of the book has aimed at presenting a sensitive in vitro corneal cell culture model to assess ocular toxicology. Corneal cells are the cells most directly exposed to environmental toxins, and are the cells most affected by the Draize test. It is hoped that corneal cells in culture will replace the Draize test, which has been criticized on several counts (Green, 1998).

The stratified squamous epithelium, characterized by apical tight junctions and superficial microvilli and microplicae, is the primary barrier to penetration of toxic or irritative substances into the eye. Jumblatt and Neufeld (1985) have developed a tissue culture system for obtaining sheets of pure rabbit corneal epithelium with morphological features similar to cells in vivo. These cultures have been used for corneal wound closure in rabbits. This technique was then applied to human corneal epithelium.

Human corneas with normal epithelium were obtained from donor eyes judged unsuitable for transplantation. The eyes were rinsed with Earle's balanced salt solution (EBSS) containing Garamycin sulfate. The full-thickness cornea was removed to a dish containing EBSS for initiation of tissue culture. Donor human corneal rims were also placed in EBSS containing Garamycin. The scleral portions were trimmed, and the full-thickness corneal rim obtained was 2–3 mm in width.

The endothelium was removed from the full-thickness corneas and corneal rims of humans or of rabbits by blunt dissection with forceps, and the stromal–epithelial tissue was used to initiate explant cultures or pure cultures of isolated corneal epithelium. For explant cultures, the posterior lamellae of the stroma were peeled off. The remaining epithelium was minced, drained, placed in a well tissue culture plate, dried for 5 min, and incubated at 37°C in air/CO_2. Pure epithelial cultures were dried for 5 min, and incubated at 37°C in air/CO_2. Pure epithelial cultures were established using cell sheets isolated from the stroma that had undergone digestion with Dipase II. The Descemet's membrane and corneal endothelium were stripped, and remaining cornea was placed in Dipase II in calcium- and magnesium-free Hank's balanced salt solution at 37°C. Cell sheets were peeled and used to initiate cell cultures. The cultures were maintained in medium consisting of equal parts of Dulbecco's modified Eagle medium and Ham's F-12 supplemented with 5% fetal bovine serum, epidermal growth factor, insulin, and cholera toxin.

Using a phase contrast microscope, all cultures were examined for epithelial cell growth. Cultures were fixed using Karnovsky's fixative and processed for microscopy. In the initial cultures in which Dipase II was used to free epithelial cells from the underlying stroma, cultures never grew to confluency. From epithelial–stromal explants, however, extensive epithelial outgrowths could be obtained. Scanning electron microscopy revealed typical epithelial specialization with microvilli and microplicae on the epithelial surface.

Following treatment with Dipase II to digest the proteins anchoring the cells to the culture vessel surface, the cell layers could be released as sheets. These sheets contained columnar basal cells, squamous superficial cells, desmosomes, apical villi, and keratin bundles. Human corneal cell culture was not as successful as rabbit cell culture; human cells treated with Dipase II either failed to attach or, if attached, failed to grow. This lack of success may be due to a difference in enzymatic susceptibility of rabbit and human epithelial–stromal adhesion complexes.

Cytotoxicity

Cytotoxicity of corneal cell cultures can be measured with all methods described above. In particular, plasminogen activation measurement and ^{51}Cr-release method are widely used (Chan, 1985; Coleman and Green, 1981; Shadduck et al., 1985; Douglas and Spilman, 1983; Griffith et al., 1980).

Lens Cell Cultures

Morphology and Cytotoxicity of Lens Epithelial Cells

Lens epithelial cells derived from 6-day-old rat lenses or from bovine lenses were cultured in medium T 199 (Morgan's medium) supplemented with 20% fetal bovine serum (Rink et al., 1986). Cells were trypsinized weekly, inoculated in fresh petri dishes or cell culture flasks (T-27, T-75), and grown in an incubator under 5% CO_2 at 37.6°C. One day after an inoculation, the drugs to be tested were applied at different concentrations in medium. After incubation for specific times, living cells were counted in Fuchs–Rosenthal chambers after trypan blue staining.

Dose–effect curves were established for several compounds by counting viable cells. Three experimental protocols were followed: (a) adding the compound to the cells 1 day after inoculation in order to test the effect of the compound on the proliferation ability of growing cells; (b) adding the compound to densely grown monolayers of cells to study the effect on an already existing (and nonproliferative) monolayer of cells; and (c) adding a compound to cells at each cell transfer over a period of 4–6 weeks to detect the effects of long-term treatment.

For detection of cytological alterations, the morphological appearance of cells, after Giemsa staining, was documented by light microscopy using an invertoscope with photographic equipment. Proteins of cells exposed to distinct concentrations of the compounds in question were analyzed by isoelectric focusing on polyacrylamide gels. (These methods are similar to those presented in the section on corneal cell cultures.)

In one study, Rink showed that an organic antioxidant was less toxic than an inorganic one. Antioxidants were tested for safety because they may be useful in preventing cataracts. In another study (Rink et al., 1986), dexamethasone proved much more toxic than the nonsteroidal anti-inflammatory compound indomethacin.

Endocytosis

Endocytosis is believed to play an important role in the transport of macromolecules from the extracellular environment into the cytoplasm of cells. Lo and Zhang (1989) studied the vesicular transport (endocytosis) of the protein tracer, horseradish peroxidase (HRP) into the lens epithelium and fiber cells of guinea pig and rabbit.

Freshly isolated adult guinea pig lenses and rabbit lenses were incubated at 34°C in closed vials containing 0.3% horseradish peroxidase (HRP) in TC-199 medium from 5 to 240 min.

All lenses were fixed after incubation in 2.5% glutaraldehyde in 0.1 M cacodylate buffer (pH 7.4) containing 1% tannic acid. Thick tissue slices were cut with a vibrotome for cytochemical demonstration of HRP activity. Thin-section electron microscopy (EM) was also done. Electron micrographs were taken, and quantitative analysis on the number of tracer-carrying endocytic vesicles and secondary lysosomes was done, with a computerized digitizer, on the electron micrographs. Freeze-fracture EM of lens epithelial cells was done only with rabbit cells.

As shown by thin-section EM, the many endocytic vesicles along the lateral membranes of epithelial cells became filled with the tracer, HRP, after incubation. Endocytosis was found to occur primarily in the lens epithelial cells, elongating young fiber cells where metabolic activity was the highest. Endocytosis is quite sensitive to ocular toxins, which can abolish endocytosis before causing cytolysis.

Aldose Reductase Activity

The enzyme aldose reductase converts glucose to sorbitol in the lens. When glucose levels are high, as with diabetes, more glucose is reduced to sorbitol. This may lead to development of a sugar cataract. Aldose reductase (AR) inhibition would be advantageous to prevent this. The aldose reductase inhibitors, sorbinil, verapamil, AL-1567, and AL-1576, were tested on lenses in culture (Hockwin et al., 1984).

Bovine lenses were extracted and placed in TC-199. To imitate metabolic conditions found with diabetes, the culture medium was enriched with glucose. HEPES (N-2-hydroxyethylpiperazine-N'-2-ethane sulfonic acid) buffer was used with all incubations except verapamil, when sodium bicarbonate was used. One lens of each pair served as control. Lenses were incubated for 8 hr at 37°C, rinsed and dabbed dry, and prepared for analysis. For verapamil, lenses were incubated for 5 hr at 37°C in a pure Ringer solution. Lenses were then placed for 7 hr in TC-199 at 37°C with a higher level of glucose.

After homogenization of lenses in 6% $NaClO_4$ and centrifugation, the substrates were determined in the deproteinized neutralized supernatant. Reduced glutathione (GSH) and oxidized glutathione (GSSG) were measured, and free adenine nucleotides and the metabolites of glycolysis were also analyzed. This work showed how many things could be measured in a lens in vitro.

With longer incubation times in glucose, the lenses had elevated levels of the phosphorylated products of glucose and fructose. Verapamil caused a decrease in glucose and fructose concentrations. In fact, verapamil was found to be a relatively poor aldose reductase inhibitor, which impaired lens metabolism to a certain extent. ATP was depleted, whereas AMP rose, and glutathione was oxidized to GSSG from GSH. Sorbinil, AL-1567, and AL-1576 all were efficient aldose reductase inhibitors, raising glucose and lowering fructose, and also increasing the ratio of ATP/AMP and GSH/GSSG. AL-1576 was found to be the most effective AR inhibitor among the four compounds studied.

Cell Elongation and Potassium Efflux

Lens fiber cell differentiation is important for lens growth and is often defective in human cataracts. The most prominent morphological feature of this process is extensive cell elongation. Beebe and Cerrelli (1989) studied the mechanism by which cytochalasin D prevents cell elongation.

Explants of chick embryo lenses were cultured in Ham's F-10 medium. Vitreous humor extract was prepared from 15-day-old chicken embryo eyes. Three subprotocols were followed. The vitreous group (a control) was incubated in vitreous humor extract only. The experimental group was incubated with cytochalasin D in vitreous humor for the entire incubation period (up to 6 hr). The reversal group was incubated in the experimental medium for the first 1.5 hr and then rinsed twice with Ham's F-10 medium and incubated in vitreous humor for the remainder of the experiment. Cell lengths for the vitreous and reversal groups were measured at 1.5, 3.0, 4.5, and 6.0 hr using an inverted microscope. The experimental groups were also observed at earlier points. Cell length was measured.

In another protocol, six central epithelial explants from 6-day-old chicken embryo lenses were prepared, and the tissues were treated with chicken vitreous humor or Ham's F-10 medium, with or without cytochalasin D, for 1 hr, and then changed to Ham's F-10 medium for 30 min. Cells were examined as above.

Rubidium-86 was used as a radioactive tracer to follow potassium movement in and out of cells. ^{3}H-labeled mannitol was used to estimate extracellular space of the tissues. Cytochalasin D was prepared in dimethyl sulfoxide (DMSO); control media contained an equivalent amount of DMSO. Eight central lens epithelia were explanted in a 35-mm culture dish, exposed for 30 min to either vitreous extract or Ham's F-10 medium, and later to medium containing rubidium-86 and ^{3}H-mannitol. The tissues were then rinsed three times with Ham's medium and placed in an orbital rotator at 10 rpm. The medium was sampled in 100-μl aliquots every minute for 10 min. The tissues were then solubilized with 1% sodium dodecyl sulfate and counted.

Cytochalasin D prevented lens epithelial cell elongation, which normally occurs when 6-day-old lens epithelial cells are exposed to vitreous humor. These epithelial cells remained short for 3 hr. Cytochalasin D also increased the rate of potassium efflux from both vitreous-stimulated and -unstimulated lens epithelia.

Oxidative Stress

Hydrogen peroxide concentrations were assayed using the dianisidine method (Trevithick and Metzenberg, 1964) using horseradish peroxidase in sodium phosphate buffer at pH 7.0. At the end of the experiment, the solution was acidified with two drops 6 M HCl and the concentration of colored product estimated at 420 nm with a Beckman spectrophotometer.

When the cells were exposed to 10 mM hydrogen peroxide, the phase contrast micrograph showed globules on the surface of the cells that were much more obvious in the scanning electron micrograph. When labeled control chick lenses were incubated for 24 hr in M199, 63% of the radioactivity was released into the medium. This was increased by hydrogen peroxide. The presence of vitamin C prevented the peroxide-induced increase in ^{51}Cr-release.

Fibroblast Cultures

Cytotoxicity

Fibroblasts are nonocular cells, but they can be used to assess cytotoxicity of a great variety of substances, including most substances that are potentially toxic to the eyes. They offer several advantages: (a) there is extensive literature on growth, growth inhibition, and cytotoxicity of compounds to these cells; (b) they are easy to culture, being a naturally proliferative culture; (c) toxicity can be measured in terms of cell death, cell morphology, cell function, and cell detachment, so nonlethal damage can be studied; and (d) they do not require the death of any new animals. Indeed, some lines of fibroblast are of human origin, and potential interspecies differences are eliminated from the analysis of the results of the experiments.

Fibroblasts are widely present in all tissues, and their cytotoxicity is measured in all methods presented in the section of cytotoxicity tests. Commonly used methods include cell death assay, cell metabolism and permeability, intracellular ATP assay, neutral red uptake, DNA synthesis, RNA synthesis, and protein synthesis.

Peritoneal Cell Cultures

Measurement of Serotonin (5-HT) Release

Peritoneal mast cells can be harvested and cultured; they are another model system for studying cytotoxicity. Rat peritoneal mast cells release serotonin (5-HT) under certain conditions. This release can be affected by toxic compounds. An in vitro experimental system for measuring cytotoxicity by measuring 5-HT release was developed by Chasin and co-workers (Chasin et al., 1979). This assay was distinguished by the cells needing to be exposed to hormones. It was found that low concentrations (1 μg/ml) of an active compound, compound 48/80, consistently produced a six- to eightfold increase in serotonin release. Disodium chromoglycate (DSCG), a standard inhibitor of histamine release, effectively inhibited compound 48/80-stimulated serotonin release.

Method

Rat peritoneal mast cells were obtained from female Sprague–Dawley rats (180–250 g). After sacrificing by carbon dioxide inhalation, 10–15 ml of Tyrode's buffer and heparin were injected i.p. followed by 25–30 ml more of Tyrode's buffer. After massaging 1 min, a midline incision was made in the abdominal wall, and the fluid was removed with a Pasteur pipette. Cell washings, containing about 10% mast cells, were pooled. The cells were washed by centrifugation and then incubated to preload them with radioactive 5-hydroxytryptophan (the precursor of 5-HT) for 3 hr in a Gyrotary water-bath shaker at 37°C. The cells were then washed three times by centrifugation followed by suspension in fresh medium. The final pellet of cells was reconstituted so that each assay tube held about 4 million cells/ml. The assay was run in triplicate in disposable 12 × 75-mm plastic test tubes. Drugs were added in 100-μl aliquots to the tubes before the addition of cells. After cells were added, the tubes were incubated at 37°C in a shaking water bath, then tubes were cooled and the cells and supernatant were separated by centrifugation at 4°C. Supernatant fractions were decanted into Aquasol (scintillation counting fluid) and counted by a liquid scintillation counter. Cell pellets were resuspended, boiled to release radioactivity, and decanted into Aquasol.

Example

It was found that significant [^{3}H]-serotonin release could be stimulated by only 1 μg/ml of compound 48/80; these cells are sensitive to toxicants. DSCG inhibited the release of serotonin effectively.

The major limitation of the serotonin release assay is that only peritoneal mast cells that release serotonin can be used. Human mast cells produce little or no serotonin, so human systems cannot be studied.

Measurement of Histamine Release

Peritoneal mast cells also may release histamine; this property has been used in an in vitro alternative to in vivo tests (Prottey and Ferguson, 1976; Jacaruso et al., 1985). Using mixed rat peritoneal cells, a technique was developed to assess the ability of test substances to cause histamine release, which was determined fluorometrically. The assay allowed test materials to be ranked in terms of irritation potential (ocular and dermal). Histamine is an important mediator of primary-irritant-type responses through its ability to increase vascular permeability, thereby allowing edema and inflammatory cell infiltration. It is reasonable to assume that materials promoting membrane permeability could result in nonspecific histamine release and thereby elicit a primary irritant response.

Method

Male Wistar rats (400–500 g) were used as a source of mast cells. Cells were collected, pooled, washed in Hank's balanced salt solution containing 1% bovine serum albumin (HBSS-BSA), and resuspended in HBSS-BSA. The final suspension contained 4–6% mast cells. The rest consisted mostly of macrophages, leukocytes, and erythrocytes.

Cells were exposed to test materials for 10 min at 37°C. Exposures were terminated by the addition of ice-cold saline, and cells were collected by centrifugation. The supernatant was decanted and stored at −15°C until assayed.

Spontaneous release of histamine was assessed using the method of Shore et al. (Shore et al., 1959). The supernatants from the test aliquots were compared to aliquots of cell suspensions exposed only to HBSS-BSA. The pellets obtained were resuspended in saline and incubated for 5 min at 100°C to release all histamine. The total histamine release was expressed as a percentage of the average total histamine content of similar aliquots of pooled cells. Acid was added to stop the condensation reaction between fluorophore and histamine; albumin was included to minimize spontaneous degradation. Reacted samples were also centrifuged prior to detection of condensation product fluorescence at 450 nm.

Example

The observations recorded agree with in vivo studies and with data assessing the effects of materials upon membrane integrity of cultured rabbit corneal cells. Three materials tested were propylene glycol, triethanolamine, and triethanolamine lauryl sulfate. The histamine release was dependent upon the concentrations of these substances. The order of potency was based upon determinations of the lowest concentration causing significant histamine release.

Chemotaxis of Macrophages

Chemotaxis is a specific characteristic of the inflammation reaction. Agents released from cells at the site of inflammation or irritation cause macrophages to migrate to the inflamed area. A Boyden chemotactic chamber can be used to measure the movement of macrophages toward an area of inflammation (Stark et al., 1983).

Method

The Boyden chemotactic chamber is a Perspex chamber that consists essentially of two compartments that are separated during the course of an experiment by a Millipore filter membrane. Mouse peritoneal macrophages placed on one side of a permeable membrane are attracted to fibroblast-conditioned medium obtained from cultured cells that have been exposed to an irritant (Stark et al., 1983). The movement of the macrophages from their source on one side of the membrane toward the other side can be easily quantitated by staining and counting a specified area of the membrane after 4 hr of chemotaxis.

Measurement of Lysosomal Enzyme Release

The release of lysosomal enzyme in vivo is widely believed to be a contributing factor to inflammation; thus it might be expected that primary cutaneous inflammation caused by surfactants involves lysosomal membrane damage. This study was undertaken to examine the major structural factors influencing lysosomal lysis by surfactants (Gibson, 1980).

Method

Rabbits were injected intraperitoneally with 200 ml of 0.1% glycogen in pyrogen-free saline. Four hours later, 100 ml of heparinized saline were introduced into the peritoneal cavity, and exudate was withdrawn by gravity drainage. The peritoneal exudate was centrifuged and the supernatant discarded. The cell pellet was washed by resuspension in isotonic saline containing 50 IU heparin/ml, and was again centrifuged. The washed pellet was then resuspended in ice-cold 0.34 M sucrose to yield a suitable cell concentration. The cells were homogenized by forcing the suspension through a Millipore filter grid, and the homogenate was centrifuged. The opaque supernatant (granule-rich suspension) was decanted and the pellet taken up in a small volume of ice-cold sucrose and rehomogenized. This suspension was diluted and recentrifuged. The supernatant from this step was combined with that obtained from the first centrifugation, and the pooled fraction constituted the granule-rich suspension used in the lysis test.

Example

The lysis of granules by surfactants was measured by the Lowe–Turner method (Lowe and Turner, 1973). The granule-rich suspension was diluted with 0.34 M sucrose to an optical density (OD) of about 0.5. One-half milliliter of the suspension was incubated in a semimicro glass cuvette in a Unicam SP 800 photometer (Pye-Unicam, Cambridge, England), and the OD at 400 nm was recorded for 1 min. Surfactant solution (0.01–0.05 ml) was then mixed in, and the decrease in OD over 20 sec was measured. The maximum decrease in OD possible was determined by adding the detergent Triton X-100.

A variety of detergents were tested. The ranking of detergents was found to be independent of concentration, so a standard concentration of 0.5 mM was used. It was found that detergents were more potent at cell lysis in proportion to the polarity of the head group, and activity increased with carbon chain length. Unlike Prottey and Ferguson (1976), Gibson (1980) reported that nonionic detergents were less potent than anionic ones. Although there was some correlation between irritancy of detergents and their ability to lyse membranes, there were some noted exceptions, particularly sodium lauryl isothionate, which is very mild in vivo and very potent on the lysis test.

HeLa Cell Cultures

Cytotoxicity

HeLa cells are another kind of cell that can be cultured in vitro and used to test for cytotoxicity (Ernst and Arditti, 1980; Selling and Erwall, 1985). HeLa cells were continuously subcultured in Sani glass flasks nourished by Parker 199 medium with 10% (vol/vol) calf serum. Before use in tests, cells were harvested by using Versene (0.2 mg EDTA/liter PBS; SBL, Solna, Sweden) and then made round by suspension in a spinner culture for 2 hr. The cells were counted by the Buerker technique and the cell density of the spinner culture adjusted to 100,000 cells/ml. Compounds were dissolved in sterile saline or directly in the medium. Test solutions were diluted in steps of 1:5 in the test areas of 5×8 cups of a 96-cup flat-bottomed microtiter tray. Each test area thus consisted of five identical dilution series. The cups were then inoculated with cells from the spinner culture, so each cup contained 50,000 cells/ml in 0.2 ml Parker's medium 199, including 5% (vol/vol) calf serum, 3 mg/ml glucose, 20 mg/ml phenol red, 200 IU benzylpenicillin/ml, 0.1 mg/ml streptomycin sulfate, and a varying concentration of the test substance. Cultures were sealed with sterile liquid paraffin and plastic film and incubated at 37°C for 7 days. This system is a model for long-term toxicity.

After 24 hr, and at later time points, cell viability was determined by microscopy on an inverted microscope. Cultures with the same percentage of spindle-shaped and fusiform cells as reference cultures were considered not inhibited, whereas cultures with 100% round cells, like the original inoculum, were considered totally inhibited. Partially inhibited cultures, with less outgrowth of fusiform cells, could also be recognized. After 7 days, the pH of each culture was determined with the color indicator phenol red. Violet cultures (pH 8.0) were considered totally inhibited, whereas orange-yellow cultures (pH 6.0–6.5) were considered fully viable; the fall in pH was produced by acid metabolites of the cells. Red cultures were judged to be partially inhibited. Approximated IC_{50} (50% inhibitory concentration) values could be calculated from the geometric mean value between the minimal total inhibitory and the maximal noninhibitory concentrations. Inhibition of DNA, RNA, and protein synthesis is also commonly used for cytotoxicity assay.

Madin–Darby Canine Kidney Cell Culture

An initial physiological event in the development of eye irritancy may be a change in the permeability of the corneal epithelium; an increase in permeability allows the irritant access to the underlying stroma. Normally, there are tight junctions and desmosomes between corneal epithelial cells. A cell line in culture that also develops tight junctions between cells is the Madin–Darby canine kidney (MDCK) cell line (Shaw et al., 1990). These cells have been used as a model system for determining ocular irritancy and compared with in vivo irritancy potential for series of chemicals.

Cells were cultured in Dulbecco's modified Eagle medium combined with Ham's F-12 medium containing 10% fetal calf serum, and supplemented with antibiotics. The cells were subcultured into 96-well flat-bottomed plates for the FRAME neutral red release (NRR) assay and onto Anocell 10 porous tissue culture plate inserts in multiwell plates for fluorescein leakage testing (Shaw et al., 1990). For cytotoxicity assay, neutral red release and fluorescein leakage are commonly used in this cell culture.

RBC Hemolysis

A modification of the Stefanski–Ruppel procedure (Stefanski and Ruppel, 1991; Rohde et al., 1994) was used. Three buffers were prepared: veronal buffered saline (VBS), containing 5 mM veronal, 150 mM NaCl, 0.15 mM $CaCl_2$, 1 mM $MgCl_2$, and 1 g/l Knox gelatin, pH 7.3; VBS glucose (VBSG), which was VBS but with 170 mM glucose and 60 mM NaCl, pH 7.3; and veronal-EDTA (VBS-EDTA), which contained 4 mM veronal, 120 mM NaCl, 20 mM EDTA, and 1 g/l gelatin, pH 7.5.

Freshly obtained erythrocytes were washed three times with 20 volumes of VBS-EDTA and centrifuged in a clinical centrifuge (80 g for 3–5 min) to pellet the cells. The supernatant was aspirated. The rabbit antibovine red cell antibody stock solution was thawed. The aliquots of cells were divided into 5-ml batches. A 50-μl aliquot of the stock antired cell antibody was added to each tube of bovine red cells and vortexed. The cells were then incubated in VBS-EDTA at 37°C for 15 min at a cell density of about 10^9 cells/ml. Cells were washed again with VBS-EDTA, then VBS, and finally twice with VBSG. The pelleted cells were stored for up to 5 days at 4°C. Cells were washed three times with VBSG and diluted to about 2.5×10^8 cells/ml prior to use.

An aliquot of rabbit whole blood (2 ml) was collected from normal New Zealand White rabbits from an ear vein and mixed with 0.5 ml heparinized saline (50 U/ml). The blood sample was centrifuged (80 g) for 5 min, and a 1-ml aliquot of serum was taken for serial dilutions. The stock dilutions ranged from 1:4 to 1:64 in VBSG. Rabbit blood was used on the same day it was drawn. Blanks used VBSG without any serum added.

The drug to be studied was usually mixed freshly with VBSG. Three concentrations of the drug were prepared by 1:10 serial dilutions. In some cases, the drugs were dissolved in 10% DMSO, then the DMSO was diluted with VBSG.

Tubes were made up with 0.2 ml of the diluted serum stock solutions, 0.05 ml VBSG, 0.2 ml of either VBSG (controls) or of the drug solution, and finally 0.05 ml of the erythrocyte suspension. Tubes were immediately vortexed and incubated at 37°C for 45 min. Another 0.5 ml VBSG was then added to the tubes, and they were centrifuged (80 g) for 3 min to pellet cells. The supernatant was decanted into disposable microcuvettes, and the absorbance at 412 nm was read using a Gilford model 260 spectrophotometer. Drug concentrations ranged from 0.5 to 0.001 mg/ml. The solvent used for dissolution of the drugs was tested by itself also. In the case of colored compounds, the absorbance of the drug solution diluted in VBSG, with no serum or erythrocytes, was determined and subtracted from the sample values. Values from four to six separate determinations were averaged and SEM determined for each plasma dilution and each drug concentration.

Cell Viability Assayed in Terms of Type I Collagen Gel Configuration

In vivo cells are tightly associated in three-dimensional extracellular matrix (ECM) composed of glucoprotein, proteoglycans, and other biomolecules. The growth, attachment, morphology, and function of cells cultured in ECM extracts or components may be altered compared with cultures on plastic. The responses of cells on plastic were compared with those cultured on the surface or embedded within gel of type I collagen, which is a major stromal ECM component (Pasternak and Miller, 1995).

Method

Collagen gels were prepared using a modified method of Parkhurst and Saltzman (1992). Fresh rat tails were stored in 70% ethanol at 4°C until collagen extraction (48 hr after animal decapitation). Collagen fibrils were removed from the tails with forceps, washed three times in PBS, and sterilized in 70% ethanol. The collagen was then dissolved in 0.1% acetic acid at 4°C with stirring for at least 48 hr. The resulting viscous solution was centrifuged at 16,000 rcf for 90 min. The supernatant was diluted with 0.1% acetic acid to form a stock collagen solution at 3 mg/ml concentration. Collagen gel was prepared by mixing stock collagen solution, concentrated medium (10× without supplements) and sodium bicarbonate solution (pH 7.4) at volume ratios of 7:1:2. The gel solution was poured quickly and then placed in an incubator at 37°C. The gels formed in 10 min. For collagen gels containing embedded fibroblasts, a small amount of concentrated cell suspension was mixed into the collagen gel solution by inverting the mixture several times before pouring (Pasternak and Miller, 1995). The effects of collagen gel and gel configuration were described in detail, with photos, by Pasternak and Miller (1995).

TOXICITY PREDICTION

Eye irritation potential can be estimated by using the TOPKAT QSAR model on a personal computer version of the program leased from Health Designs Inc. (Rochester, NY) (Sina et al., 1995). After the new molecular structure was entered, the TOPKAT QSAR model compared the new unknown molecule with the existing database of chemicals with known in vivo data. Substructures on the new molecule were compared with those in the database that are believed to contribute the agent's irritating properties. Other parameters which enter the calculation include shape of the molecule and distribution of electrons. After analysis of structure–activity relationship, the compound can be classified into four categories: severe, moderate, mild, and none of these. After computer analysis, the estimate can be validated with suitable in vitro and then in vivo methods. Those agents that are classified as severe or moderate are not studied further.

Drug efficacy and safety are two parameters that have to be studied before the Food and Drug Administration (FDA) can approve the human clinical trial with investigative new drugs (IND). Reasonable prediction of drug toxicity in humans has to be made depending on the laboratory data obtained from animal experiments. Prediction from laboratory animal data to humans in the real world, however, has always been controversial and dangerous because of species and environmental differences between animals in the controlled lab and humans in the noncontrolled environment (Tamura, 1983). Extrapolation of in vitro data to in vivo systems does not necessarily deal with metabolism, excretion, compartmentalization, and blood circulation, which are common factors needed to be considered in in vivo experiments.

Traditionally, prediction of drug toxicity from in vitro to in vivo or from animal data to human systems was done using a straight-line predictive technique and discarding insignificant parameters. Obviously, this method is too simplistic and unreasonable. The real world is much more complicated and requires alternative non-straight-line predictive techniques.

The alternative nonlinear predictive technique is designed to cope with random events that occur mostly in the real world. Therefore, it should be able to incorporate historically stored data, to take input from diversified scientific disciplines, and to consider simultaneously the host factors, external influences, and physicochemical characteristics of the chemical in question.

The chemical toxicity can be considered as a particulate entity traversing through time and space in a random order driven by internal and external forces. Therefore, the Brownian equation could be used to describe its random movement through time and space. With this equation, various parameters can be fed into the equation, including molecular weights of the chemicals, eye irritation of chemicals in man, external factors of the chemicals in functional systems, and so forth.

Another major problem in predicting toxicity is in the use of animal experimental data on humans. The difficulty could be due largely to the lack of continuity in time and space of animal and human data. Historical data are based to some degree on a posteriori data and are required to make a priori probability judgments on a future phase. Bayes' equation could be used properly to deal with these two entities.

The denominator of Bayes' equation defines historical data experiments, case reports, and data banks. It also includes the long-term memory of reports in physiochemistry, toxicology, and medical practice of agents. The numerator represents the projection and prediction of Brownian motion by the intuitive force of experts in the field. With Bayes' equation, an extremely large number of parameters can be dealt with simultaneously, including interactions of organisms, tissue cultures, toxic chemicals, and so forth. The data bank in our expert's long-term memory is equivalent to the denominator of Bayes' equation and is complementary to the data banks of a computerized information system. The short-term memory of the expert is equal to the numerator in Bayes' equation but is far superior to the computerized information because the expert's speed of using recent information to weigh probabilities is almost instantaneous compared with batching operations.

A nonlinear approach to predicting chemical toxicity is now workable. It allows a multidisciplinary approach to incorporate a large number of inputs for simultaneous assessment. With the assistance of a computer, it can predict chemical toxicity in humans efficiently. Most important, the prediction can be accomplished without dependence solely on animal data but on the large mass of historical data, tissue-culture data, invertebrate data, exposure data, and long-and short-term memories of man. For more details, the readers are advised to read Tamura's article in *Product Safety Evaluation* (Tamura, 1983).

REFERENCES

Aguayo, J.B., Blackband, S.J., Schoenigar, J., Mattingly, M.A., and Hintermann, M. 1986. Nuclear magnetic resonance imaging of a single cell. *Nature* 322:190–191.

Bartlett, G.R. 1959. Phosphorus assay in column chromatography. *Journal of Biological Chemistry* 234:446.

Beebe, D.C., and Cerrelli, S. 1989. Cytochalasin prevents cell elongation and increases potassium efflux from embryonic lens epithelial cells: implications for the mechanism of lens fiber cell elongation. *Lens Eye Toxicity Research* 6:589–601.

Beebe, D., and Feagans, D. 1981. A tissue culture system for studying lens cell differentiation. *Vision Research* 21:113–118.

Booman, K.A., Cascieri, T.M., Demetrulius, J., Driedyer, A., Griffith, J.F., Grochoski, G.T., Kong, B., McCormick, W.C., North-Root, H., Rozen, M.G., and Sedlak, R.I. 1988. In vitro methods for estimating eye irritancy of cleaning products. Phase 1: preliminary assessment. *Journal of Toxicology—Cutaneous and Ocular Toxicology* 7:173–185.

Borchman, D., Delamere, N.A., McCauley, L.A., and Paterson, C.A. 1989. Studies on the distribution of cholesterol phospholipid and protein in the human and bovine lens. *Lens Eye Toxicity Research* 6:703–724.

Borenfreund, E., and Puerner, J.A. 1984. A simple quantitative procedure using monolayer cultures for cytotoxicity assays (HTD/NR-90). *Journal of Tissue Culture Methods* 9:7–9.

Boyum, A. 1974. Separation of blood leucocytes, granulocytes and lymphocytes. *Tissue Antigens* 4:269–274.

Burton, A.B.G., York, M., and Laurence, R.S. 1981. The in vitro assessment of severe eye irritants. *Food and Cosmetic Toxicology* 19:471–480.

Carmichael, J., Degraff, W.G., Gazdar, A.F., Minna, J.D., and Michell, J.B. 1987. Evaluation of a tetrazolium-based semiautomated colorimetric assay: assessment of chemosensitivity testing. *Cancer Research* 47:936–942.

Chan, K.Y. 1985. An in vitro alternative to the Draize test. In *Alternative Methods in Toxicology, In Vitro Toxicology*, vol. III, ed. A.M. Goldberg, pp. 43–83. New York: Mary Ann Liebert.

Chasin, M., Scott, C., Shaw, C., and Persico, F. 1979. A new assay for the measurement of mediator release from rat peritoneal mast cells. *International Archive of Allergy Applied Immunology* 58:1–10.

Chen, Z., Liu, S.X.L., and Chiou, G.C.Y. 1996. Inhibitory effects of interleukin-1 blockers on corneal fibroblast proliferation. *Journal of Ocular Pharmacology and Therapeutics* 12:169–182.

Chu, I.H., and Toft, P. 1993. Recent progress in the eye irritation test. *Toxicology Industrial Health* 9:1017–1025.

Coleman, P.L., and Green, G.D.J. 1981. A sensitive coupled assay for plasminogen activator using a thiol ester substrate for plasmin. *Annals of the New York Academy of Sciences* 370:617.

Doly, M., Gaillard, G., and Braquent, P. 1990. Electroretinogram and mediators of inflammation. In *Lipid Mediators in Eye Inflammation*, ed. N.G. Bazan, pp. 149–167. Basel: Karger.

Douglas, H.J., and Spilman, S.D. 1983. In vitro ocular irritancy testing. In *Alternative Methods in Toxicology: Product Safety Evaluations*, vol. I, ed. A.M. Goldberg, pp. 205–230. New York: Mary Ann Liebert.

Dubkin, N.H., DiBlasi, M.C., Thomas, C.L., and Wolff, M.C. 1984. Development of an in vitro test for cytotoxicity in vaginal tissues: effect of ethanol on prostanoid release. In *Alternative Methods in Toxicology: Acute Toxicity Testing: Alternative Approaches*, vol. II, ed. A.M. Goldberg, pp. 127–138. New York: Mary Ann Liebert.

Ecobichon, D.J. 1997. Acute toxicity studies. In *The Basis of Toxicity Testing*, pp. 43–86. Boca Raton, FL: CRC Press.

Elgebaly, S.A., Downes, R.T., Bohr, M., Forouhar, F., O'Rourke, J., and Kreutzer, D.L. 1987. Inflammatory mediators in alkali-burned corneas; preliminary characterization. *Current Eye Research* 6:1263–1273.

Elgebaly, S.A., Forouhar, F., Gillies, C., Williams, S., O'Rourke, J., and Kreutzer, D.L. 1984. Leucocyte-mediated injury to corneal endothelial cells: a mode of tissue injury. *American Journal of Pathology* 116:407–416.

Elgebaly, S.A., Gillies, C., Forouhar, F., Hashem, M., Baddour, M., O'Rourke, J., and Kreutzer, D.L. 1985. An in vitro model of leucocyte mediated injury to the corneal epithelium. *Current Eye Research* 4:31–41.

Elgebaly, S.A., Herbert, N., O'Rourke, J., and Kreutzer, D.L. 1987. Characterization of neutrophil and monocyte-specific chemotactic factors derived from the cornea in response to hydrogen peroxide injury. *American Journal of Pathology* 126:22–32.

Ernst, R., and Arditti, J. 1980. Biological effects of surfactants. IV. Effects of non-ionics and amphoterics on HeLa cells. *Toxicology* 15:233–242.

Gibson, W.T. 1980. Lysis of rabbit polymorphonuclear leucocyte granules by surfactants of differing structure and irritancy. *Food and Cosmetic Toxicology* 88:511–515.

Gordon, V.A., and Bergman, H.C. 1989. External evaluation of the Eytex system in twelve labs to determine the correlation of results with in vivo results. In *Progress in In Vitro Toxicology*, ed. A.M. Goldberg, pp. 99–112. New York: Mary Ann Liebert.

Gordon, V.C., and Kelly, C.P. 1989a. An in vitro method for determining ocular irritation. *Cosmetics and Toiletries* 104:69–73.

Gordon, V.C., and Kelly, C.P. 1989b. Validation of an in vitro method for determining ocular irritation of cosmetic ingredients and products. *Cosmetics and Toiletries* 104:67–69.

Green, K. 1998. In vivo eye irritation test methods. In *Ophthalmic Toxicology*, 2nd ed., ed. G.C.Y. Chiou, pp. 115–163. Washington, DC: Taylor & Francis.

Griffith, J.F. 1980. Dose–response studies with chemical irritants for predicting hazards to the human eye. *Toxicology and Applied Pharmacology* 55:501.

Griffith, J.F., Nixon, G.A., Bruce, R.D., Reer, P.J., and Bannan, E.A. 1980. Dose–response studies with chemical irritants in the albino rabbit eye as a basis for selecting optimum testing conditions for predicting hazard to the human eye. *Toxicology and Applied Pharmacology* 55:501–513.

Hockley, K., and Baxter, D. 1986. In vitro: use of the 3T3 cell—neutral red uptake assay for irritants. *Food and Chemical Toxicology* 24:473–475.

Hockwin, O., Korte, I., Noll, E., and Schwarz, B. 1984. The effect of aldose reductase inhibitors on bovine lens metabolism in vitro. *Lens Research* 2:243–262.

Huang, T.C., Chen, C.P., Wefler, V., and Raftery, A. 1961. A stable reagent for the Liebermann–Bruchaud reaction. Application to rapid serum cholesterol determination. *Analytical Chemistry* 33:1405.

Igarashi, H. 1986. In vitro—opacity of the isolated cornea produced by NaLS. *Toxicology Letter* 32:249.

Jacaruso, R.B., Barletta, M.A., Carson, S., and Trombetta, L.D. 1985. Release of histamine from rat peritoneal cells in vitro as an index of irritation potential. *Journal of Toxicology—Cutaneous and Ocular Toxicology* 4:39–48.

Jain, M.K. 1977. Role of cholesterol in biomembranes and related systems. In *Membranes and Transport*, ed. A. Kleinyeller, pp. 1–77. New York: Academic Press.

Jumblatt, M.M., and Neufeld, A.H. 1985. A tissue culture model of the human corneal epithelium. In *Alternative Methods in Toxicology: In vitro Toxicology*, vol. III, ed. A.M. Goldberg, pp. 393–404. New York: Mary Ann Liebert.

Kemp, R.B., Meredith, R.W.J., Gamble, S., and Frost, M. 1983. A rapid cell culture technique for assessing the toxicity of detergent-based products in vitro as a possible screen for eye irritancy in vivo. *Cytobios* 36:153–159.

Kemp, R.B., Meredith, R.W.J., and Gamble, S.H. 1985. Toxicity of commercial products on cells in suspension culture: a possible screen for the Draize eye irritation test. *Food and Chemical Toxicology* 23:267–270.

Kennah, H.E., Albulesen, D., Hignet, S., and Barrow, C.S. 1989. A critical evaluation of predicting ocular irritancy potential from an in vitro cytotoxicity assay. *Fundamental Applications in Toxicology* 12:281–290.

Korte, I., Ohrloff, C., and Hockwin, O. 1987. Influence of drugs on lens metabolism in vitro. *Concepts of Toxicology* 4:326–332.

Kreutzer, D.L., O'Flaherty, J.T., Orr, W., Showell, H.J., Ward, P.A., and Becker, E.L. 1978. Quantitative comparison of various biological responses of neutrophils to different active and inactive chemotactic factors. *Immunopharmacology* 1:39–49.

Kuck, J.F.R., and Kuck, K.D. 1988. The Emory mouse cataract: the effects on cataractogenesis of alpha-tocopherol, penicillamine, triethylenetetramine and mercaptopropionylglycine. *Journal of Ocular Pharmacology* 4:243.

Kuck, J.F.R., and Kuck, K.D. 1989. In vitro—the Emory mouse cataract: increased accumulation of calcium during cataractogenesis. *Lens Eye Toxicity Research* 6:853–862.

Lauterbur, P.C. 1973. Image formation by induced local interactions: examples employing nuclear magnetic resonance. *Nature* 242:190–191.

Lazarus, H.M., Imperia, P.S., Botti, R.E., Mack, R.J., and Lass, J.H. 1990. An in vitro method which assesses corneal epithelial toxicity due to antineoplastic and antimicrobial agents. In *Ocular Toxicology*, eds. S. Lerman and R.C. Tripathi, pp. 59–85. New York: Marcel Dekker.

Lazarus, H.M., Imperia, P.S., Botti, R.E., Mack, R.J., and Lass, J.H. 1989. An in vitro method which assesses corneal epithelial toxicity due to antineoplastic, preservative and antimicrobial agents. *Lens Eye Toxicity Research* 6:59–85.

Leighton, J., Nassauer, J., Tchao, R., and Verdone, J. 1983. Development of a procedure using the chick egg as an alternative to the Draize rabbit test. In *Alternative Methods in Toxicology: Product Safety Evaluation*, vol. I, ed. A.M. Goldberg, pp. 163–177. New York: Mary Ann Liebert.

Lerman, S., Ashley, D.L., Long, R.C., Goldstein, J.H., Megaw, J.M., and Gardner, K. 1982. Nuclear magnetic resonance analyses of the cold cataract: whole lens studies. *Investigative Ophthalmology and Visual Science* 23:218–226.

Lerman, S., and Moran, M. 1988. Acrylamide and iodide fluorescence quenching studies on whole human lenses and their protein extracts. *Current Eye Research* 7:403–410.

Lerman, S., and Moran, M. 1989. NMR pulse relaxation studies on the normal aging and cataractous lens. *Experimental Eye Research* 48:451–459.

Liu, A.A., and Miller, W.M. 1992. Modulation of glutathione level in CHO cells. *Annals of the New York Academy of Sciences* 665:117–126.

Lo, W.K., and Zhang, W. 1989. In vitro. Endocytosis of macromolecules in the lenses of guinea pig and rabbit. *Lens Eye Toxicity Research* 6:603–612.

Lowe, J.S., and Turner, E.H. 1973. The effect of adjuvant arthritis and drugs on the ability of rat plasma to inhibit the Triton X-100-induced lysis of rabbit polymorphonuclear leucocyte granules. *Biochemical Pharmacology* 22:2069.

Luepke, N.P. 1985. Hen's egg chorioallantoic membrane test for irritation potential. *Food Chemical Toxicology* 23:287–291.

Maurice, D.M. 1955. Influence on corneal permeability of bathing with solutions of different reaction and tonicity. *British Journal of Ophthalmology* 39:463–473.

Maurice, D.M., and Singh, T. 1986. A permeability test for acute corneal toxicity. *Toxicology Letter* 31:125–130.

Mitton, K.P., Dzialoszynski, T., Weerheim, J., Trevithick, J.R., and Sivak, J.G. 1990. Modeling cortical cataractogenesis. X. Evaluation of lens optical function by computer based image analysis using in vitro rat lens elevated glucose model. In *Ocular Toxicology*, ed. S. Lerman and R.C. Tripathi, pp. 211–228. New York: Marcel Dekker.

Mossman, T. 1983. Rapid colorimetric assay for cellular growth and survival: application to proliferation and cytotoxicity assays. *Journal of Immunology Methods* 65:55–63.

Muir, C.K. 1984. A simple method to assess surfactant-induced bovine corneal opacity in vitro: preliminary findings. *Toxicology Letter* 22:199.

Muir, C.K., Flower, C., and Van Abbe, N.J. 1983. A novel approach to the search for in vitro alternatives to in vivo eye irritancy testing. *Toxicology Letter* 18:1–5.

Muller, A., Moller, B., Dragomirescu, V., and Hockwin, O. 1987. Profiles of enzyme activities in bovine lenses. *Concepts of Toxicology* 4:343–349.

North-Root, H., Yackowvich, F., Demetrulius, J., Gacula, M., and Heinz, J.E. 1982. Evaluation of an in vitro cell toxicity test using rabbit corneal cells to predict the eye irritation potential of surfactants. *Toxicology Letter* 14:207–212.

Osborne, R., Perkins, M.A., and Roberts, D.A. 1995. Development and intralaboratory evaluation of an in vitro human cell-based test to aid ocular irritancy assessments. *Fundamental and Applied Toxicology* 28:139–153.

Parkhurst, M.R., and Saltzman, W.M. 1992. Quantification of human neutrophil motility in three-dimensional collagen gels: effect of collagen concentration. *Biophysics Journal* 61:306–315.

Pasternak, A.S., and Miller, W.M. 1995. First-order toxicity assays of eye irritation using cell lines: parameters that affect in vitro evaluation. *Fundamental and Applied Toxicology* 25:253–263.

Peterson, G.L. 1977. A simplification of the protein assay method of Lowry et al. which is more generally applicable. *Annals of Biochemistry* 83:346.

Prinsen, M.K. 1996. The chicken enucleated eye test (CEET): a practical (pre)screen for the assessment of eye irritation/corrosion potential of test materials. *Food and Chemical Toxicology* 34:291–396.

Prinsen, M.K., and Koeter, H.B.M.W. 1993. Justification of the enucleated eye test with eyes of slaughterhouse animals as an alternative to the Draize eye irritation test with rabbits. *Food and Chemical Toxicology* 31:69–76.

Prottey, C., and Ferguson, T.F.M. 1976. The effect of surfactants upon rat peritoneal mast cell in vitro. *Food and Cosmetic Toxicology* 14:425–430.

Rae, J.L., and Cooper, K.E. 1989. Potassium channels in chick lens epithelium change with maturation. *Lens Eye Toxicity Research* 6:833–843.

Reed, D.J. 1990. Glutathione: toxicological implications. *Annual Review of Pharmacology and Toxicology* 30:605–631.

Reinhardt, C.A., Pelli, D.A., and Zbinden, G. 1985. Interpretation of cell toxicity data for the estimation of potential irritation. *Food and Chemical Toxicology* 23:247–257.

Rink, H., Seifert, R., and Bauer, K. 1986. Effects of hydrocortisone, dexamethasone and indomethacin in lens epithelial cells growing in vitro. *Concepts of Toxicology* 4:397–406.

Rohde, B.H., Okawara, T., Varma, R.S., and Chiou, G.C.Y. 1994. Effect of some phytogenic agents and synthetic compounds on complement cascade-mediated hemolysis. *Ophthalmic Research* 26:116–123.

Scaife, M.C. 1982. An investigation of detergent action on cells in vitro and possible correlation with in vivo data. *International Journal of Cosmetic Science* 4:179.

Schleich, T., Matson, G.B., Willis, J.A., Acosta, G., Serdahl, C., Campbell, P., and Garwood, M. 1985. Surface coil phosphorus-31 nmr studies of the intact eye. *Experimental Eye Research* 40:343–355.

Selling, J., and Erwall, B. 1985. Screening for eye irritancy using cultured HeLa cells. *Xenobiotica* 15:713–717.

Shadduck, J.A., Everitt, J., and Bay, P. 1985. Use of in vitro cytotoxicity to rank ocular irritation of six surfactants. In *Alternative Methods in Toxicology: In Vitro Toxicology*, vol. III, ed. A.M. Goldberg, pp. 643–649. New York: Mary Ann Liebert.

Shaw, A.J., Clothier, R.H., and Balls, M. 1990. Loss of trans-epithelial impermeability of a confluent monolayer of Madin–Darby canine kidney (MDCD) cells as a determinant of ocular irritancy potential. *Alternative to Laboratory Animals* 18:145–151.

Shopsis, C., and Sathe, S. 1984. In vitro uridine uptake inhibition as a cytotoxicity test. *Toxicology* 29:195–206.

Shopsis, C., Borenfreund, E., Walberg, J., and Stark, D.M. 1984. In vitro cytotoxicity assays: a potential alternative to the Draize ocular irritancy test. In *Alternative Methods in Toxicology: Acute Toxicity Testing: Alternative Approaches*, vol. II, ed. A.M. Goldberg, pp. 101–114. New York: Mary Ann Liebert.

Shore, P.A., Burkhalter, A., and Cohn, V.H. 1959. A method for the fluorometric assay of histamine in tissues. *Journal of Pharmacology and Experimental Therapeutics* 127:182–186.

Sina, J.F., Galer, D.M., Sussman, R.G., Gautheron, P.D., Sargent, E.V., Leong, B., Shah, P.V., Curren, R.D., and Miller, K.V. 1995. A collaborative evaluation of seven alternatives to the Draize eye irritation test using pharmaceutical intermediates. *Fundamental and Applied Toxicology* 26:20–31.

Sina, J.F., and Gautheron, P. 1994. Ocular toxicity assessment in vitro. In *In vitro Toxicology*, ed. S.C. God, pp. 21–46. New York: Raven Press.

Smith, P.K., Krohn, R.I., Hermanson, G.T., et al. 1985. Measurement of protein using bicinchoninic acid. *Analytical Biochemistry* 150:76.

Stefanski, V., and Ruppel, H.G. 1991. A new quantitative assay for the determination of complement activity. *Immunology Letter* 30:1–6.

Stark, D.M., Shopsis, C., Borenfreund, E., and Walberg, J. 1983. Alternative approaches to the Draize assay: chemotaxis, cytology, differentiation and membrane transport studies. In *Alternative Methods in Toxicology: Product Safety Evaluation*, vol. I, ed. A.M. Goldberg, pp. 179–203. New York: Mary Ann Liebert.

Stewart-Dettaan, P.J., Sanval, M., Creighton, M.O., Inch, W.R., and Trevithick, J.R. 1990. [51]Cr release and oxidative stress in the lens. In *Ocular Toxicity*, eds. S. Lerman and R.C. Tripathi, pp. 183–202. New York: Marcel Dekker.

Takahashi, N., and Ikowa, N. 1990. The cytotoxic effect of 5-FU on cultured human conjunctival cells. In *Ocular Toxicology*, eds. S. Lerman and R.C. Tripathi, pp. 315–330. New York: Marcel Dekker.

Takahashi, N., Mukai, Y., Nakaizumi, H., and Sasaki, K. 1987. An evaluation of the cytotoxicity of ophthalmic solutions on cell culture: aminoglycosides and dexamethasone sodium phosphate. *Concepts of Toxicology* 4:383–389.

Tamura, R.M. 1983. A model for toxicological prediction. In *Alternative Methods in Toxicology, Product Safety Evaluation*, vol. 1. ed. A.M. Goldberg, pp. 315–330. New York: Mary Ann Liebert.

Trevithick, J.R., and Metzenberg, R.L. 1964. Kinetics of the inhibition of *Neurospora* invertase by products and oxidative stress. *Archives of Biochemistry and Biophysics* 107:260.

Triglia, D., Sherard Braa, S., Yonan, C., and Naughton, G.K. 1991. Cytotoxicity testing using neutral red and MTT assays on a three-dimensional human skin substrate. *Toxicology In Vitro* 5:573–578.

Tseng, M.T., Liu, K.N., and Radtke, N.D. 1990. Isolated perfused bovine eye—a model for acute retinal toxicity screening. In *Ocular Toxicology*, eds. S. Lerman and R.C. Tripathi, pp. 369–371. New York: Marcel Dekker.

Wallach, J.F.R., and Steck, T.L. 1963. Properties of the metal derivatives of calcein: determination of aluminum, alkaline earths, cobalt, copper, nickel and zinc. *Analytical Chemistry* 35:1035.

Weisman, I.O., Bennett, L.H., Maxwell, L.R., Sr., Woods, M.W., and Burk, D. 1972. Recognition of cancer in vivo by nuclear magnetic resonance. *Science* 178:1288–1290.

Wilcox, N.L. 1992. The status of eye irritancy testing: a regulatory perspective. *Lens Eye Toxicity Research* 9:259–271.

York, M. 1983. An isolated rabbit eye technique. In *Animals and Alternatives in Toxicology Testing*, eds. M. Balls, P. Riddell, and J. Worden, pp. 309–371. New York: Academic Press.

Zwilling, E. 1959. A modified chorioallantoic grafting procedure. *Transplant Bulletin* 6:115–116.

Ophthalmic Toxicology
Edited by George C. Y. Chiou
Copyright © 1999 Taylor & Francis

7

Ophthalmic Toxicity by Systemic Drugs

Jimmy D. Bartlett

Department of Optometry, School of Optometry, University of Alabama at Birmingham, Birmingham, Alabama, USA

- **Anticholinergic Drugs**
  - Ocular Manifestations
  - Patient Management
- **Antiadrenergic Drugs**
  - Pathogenesis
  - Ocular Manifestations
  - Patient Management
- **Cardiovascular Drugs**
  - Pathogenesis
  - Ocular Manifestations
  - Patient Management
- **Antipsychotic Agents and Ethanol**
  - Pathogenesis
  - Ocular Manifestations
  - Patient Management
- **Chemotherapeutic Agents**
  - Ocular Manifestations
  - Pathogenesis
  - Patient Management
- **Antituberculosis Drugs**
  - Pathogenesis
  - Ocular Manifestations
  - Patient Management
- **Antimalarial Compounds**
  - Pathogenesis
  - Ocular Manifestations
  - Patient Management
- **Antineoplastics**
  - Pathogenesis
  - Ocular Manifestations
  - Patient Management

- **Isotretinoin**
  - Pathogenesis
  - Ocular Manifestations
  - Patient Management
- **Corticosteroids**
  - Pathogenesis
  - Ocular Manifestations
  - Patient Management
- **Nonsteroidal Anti-Inflammatory Drugs**
  - Pathogenesis
  - Ocular Manifestations
  - Patient Management
- **Gold Compounds**
  - Pathogenesis
  - Ocular Manifestations
  - Patient Management
- **Oral Contraceptives**
  - Pathogenesis
  - Ocular Manifestations
  - Patient Management
- **Photosensitizing Drugs**
  - Pathogenesis
  - Ocular Manifestations
  - Patient Management
- **Talc**
  - Pathogenesis
  - Ocular Manifestations
  - Patient Management
- **References**

During the past several decades considerable attention has been devoted to how systemic drug therapy can affect ocular tissues or visual functions. Various monographs and major reviews have addressed this subject (Fraunfelder, 1982; Jaanus et al., 1995), and mechanisms have been devised that encourage reporting of possible cause-and-effect relationships between systemic drug use and ocular effects (Fraunfelder and Meyer, 1982). By encouraging the reporting of such relationships, it is hoped that our understanding of ocular toxicity associated with systemic drugs will be improved and that, ultimately, patient care will be enhanced by preventing such adverse reactions or by finding better methods of treating such effects once they occur.

The eye has an extremely rich blood supply but a relatively small total mass, and thus exhibits an unusually high susceptibility to toxic substances. Drug molecules present in systemic circulation can reach the ocular structures by way of the uveal or retinal vasculatures. Once they reach the eye, systemic drugs can be deposited in several locations acting as drug depots, such as the cornea, crystalline lens, and retina. Moreover, systemic medications can affect numerous ocular and visual functions, including pupil size and reactivity, accommodation, intraocular pressure, and lid position. Thus, many systemically administered drugs have the potential to cause adverse ocular effects, and nearly all ocular structures can be vulnerable. This picture is complicated even more by the fact that multiple drug therapy can influence the eye through mechanisms that are currently not well understood (Koneru et al., 1986).

This chapter considers the clinically important ocular or visual responses attributable to systemic drug therapy. Innumerable anecdotal reports exist in the literature describing the presumed ocular effects of various systemic medications or dosage formulations. This chapter, however, emphasizes only those ocular manifestations of systemic drug toxicity that, over time, have become well documented, and only the most common drugs that affect the eye are considered. The ocular toxicity associated with each drug class is considered in terms of it pathogenesis, specific ocular manifestations, and appropriate patient management strategies.

ANTICHOLINERGIC DRUGS

Drugs with anticholinergic properties can commonly affect the eye by inhibiting the cholinergic innervation to lacrimal gland tissues, iris sphincter muscle, or ciliary muscle. Clinically important effects can be induced in the lacrimal system, pupil, intraocular pressure, or accommodation. Among the most important drugs capable of causing clinically significant ocular effects include atropine, ipratropium, scopolamine, antihistamines, anxiolytic agents, and antidepressants.

Ocular Manifestations

Atropine and related drugs inhibit glandular secretions in a dose-dependent manner. Thus, dryness of mucous membranes, including dry eye, is a common side effect of anticholinergic drug use (Peters, 1989; Mader and Stulting, 1991). In one study (Balik, 1958) oral administration of atropine caused tear secretion to fall from 15 μl/min to 3 μl/min. A similar dose of atropine given subcutaneously gave a nearly 50% reduction in lacrimal secretion (Erickson, 1960). Scopolamine 1–2 mg orally caused a reduction in tear secretion from 5 μl/min to 0.8 μl/min (Balik, 1958).

In addition to their receptor-blocking effects, H_1 antihistamines have varying degrees of atropine-like actions, including the ability to alter tear film integrity (Erickson, 1960; Crandall and Leopold, 1979; Miller, 1973). Both aqueous and mucin production have been reported to decrease with antihistamine use (Balik, 1958). Koeffler and Lemp (1980) administered 4 mg/day of chlorpheniramine maleate to a 20-year-old age group of volunteers. Tear secretion was measured using Schirmer's test. A significant reduction in tear flow was observed on the days when chlorpheniramine was taken.

Drugs with anticholinergic effects, such as atropine or related compounds, can cause mydriasis. Systemic administration of 2 mg or more of atropine can cause clinically significant mydriasis and cycloplegia (Leopold and Comroe, 1948). Since patients with extremely narrow anterior chamber angles are at risk for the development of angle-closure glaucoma, drugs that can potentially dilate the pupil, such as atropine, may induce acute or subacute angle-closure glaucoma (Ahmad, 1990; Lieberman and Stoudemiere, 1987; Mandak et al., 1996). These drugs include any medication with anticholinergic or strong adrenergic agonist properties (Frucht et al., 1984). Angle-closure glaucoma has been reported to be induced by fluoxetine and paroxetine, selective serotonin reuptake inhibitors with weak anticholinergic and adrenergic activity (Eke and Bates, 1997; Kirwan et al., 1997; Ahmad, 1991), and by ipratropium bromide given by nebulization or metered-dose inhalation (Hall, 1994). Hiatt and associates (Hiatt et al., 1970) have shown, however, that the risk of elevating intraocular pressure or inducing angle-closure glaucoma with systemically administered anticholinergic agents is small, even in patients with narrow angles.

Patient Management

In most instances these drug-induced effects on the eye are self-limited once the anticholinergic medication is reduced or discontinued. Symptoms of dry eye, dilated pupil, or cycloplegia may be annoying but are rarely incapacitating. During drug therapy annoying symptoms can be relieved using appropriate artificial tear formulations or ocular lubricants for dry eye, or by employing appropriate reading lenses for symptoms induced by cycloplegia. In rare cases of angle-closure glaucoma induced by anticholinergic medications, treatment should be instituted following the usual clinical guidelines.

Before administering systemic medications that have anticholinergic properties, it is advisable to screen patients for narrow anterior chamber angles. This procedure may include careful questioning regarding a history of transient blurred vision, ocular pain, or redness, or other signs or symptoms of angle-closure glaucoma. The risk of angle-closure glaucoma is greatest in older patients with cataract or hyperopia. Children with asthma appear to have little ocular risk when administered nebulized ipratropium (Watson et al., 1994).

ANTIADRENERGIC DRUGS

Drugs classified as β-adrenergic receptor antagonists have become the mainstay in the treatment of systemic hypertension, ischemic heart disease, cardiac arrhythmias, and migraine headache. When systemically administered, these drugs can cause dry-eye syndrome and can reduce intraocular pressure.

Pathogenesis

The mechanism responsible for reduced aqueous tear secretion is unknown. It has been documented, however, that β-adrenergic antagonists reduce tear lysozyme levels, with a reduction of IgA (Mackie et al., 1977; Almog et al., 1983).

Most studies (Yablonski et al., 1978; Coakes and Brubaker, 1978; Neufeld, 1979) indicate that β-antagonists exert their primary ocular hypotensive action by inhibiting aqueous formation. Of the commercially available β-antagonists, timolol is the most widely investigated ocular hypotensive agent, but all β-antagonists may act by a similar mechanism. Neufeld (1979) has postulated that timolol can act on secretion, ultrafiltration, or both. Since aqueous formation depends on blood flow and perfusion pressure within the ciliary vasculature, timolol may induce a net vasoconstriction by preventing β-receptor-mediated vasodilation of the afferent vessels in the ciliary processes. This vascular action of timolol, however, has not been confirmed experimentally. It has also been suggested (Neufeld, 1979) that timolol reduces aqueous formation through a direct action on the ciliary epithelium. The molecular and intracellular mechanisms of β-receptor blockade are still unclear, but it has been speculated that β-blockers either affect active transport at the nonpigmented ciliary epithelium or alter ultrafiltration of blood in the ciliary body (Juzych and Zimmerman, 1997).

Ocular Manifestations

Reduced aqueous tear secretion is a reported side effect of orally administered β-adrenergic antagonists. Although most of the reported cases deal with practolol (Felix et al., 1975), other β-blockers, such as propranolol and timolol, have also been implicated in dry eye syndrome (Mackie et al., 1977; Scott, 1977). Ocular side effects of practolol have been described as an oculomucocutaneous syndrome, in which patients suffer from symptomatic lesions of the conjunctival and lid tissues (Felix et al., 1975). Atenolol, metoprolol, oxyprenolol, and pindolol have all been implicated in patients with dry-eye symptoms and in reduction of tear lysozyme levels (Mackie et al., 1977; Almog et al., 1983).

Systemically administered β-adrenergic antagonists are well known to reduce intraocular pressure (Smith et al., 1979; Borthne, 1976; Rennie and Smerdon, 1985). This occurs in patients with normal pressure as well as in those with glaucoma. The ocular hypotensive action observed after systemic administration may be beneficial in patients with ocular hypertension or in the glaucoma patient controlled with antiglaucoma drugs other than epinephrine. The reduction of intraocular pressure induced by systemic β-receptor antagonists ranges from 20% to 41%. Intraocular pressure decreases following systemic administration of atenolol (MacDonald et al., 1976), metroprolol (Heel et al., 1979), nadolol (Duff, 1987), propranolol (Wettrell and Pandolfi, 1975), or timolol (Ohrstrom, 1982).

Patient Management

Patients who exhibit dry-eye syndrome associated with systemically administered β-adrenergic antagonists should be treated symptomatically using artificial tear solutions and ointment formulations as required. Reduction of intraocular pressure associated with systemic β-adrenergic antagonists may actually prove beneficial if the patient has ocular hypertension or glaucoma. However, since systemic β-blockers also reduce blood pressure, this route of administration may be detrimental in certain glaucomatous patients. The reduction of perfusion pressure to the optic nerve produced by decreased systemic blood pressure may offset the benefit derived form reducing intraocular pressure. Conversely, when the systemic β-blocker is discontinued, intraocular pressure may increase to levels that increase the risk of optic nerve damage and visual field loss associated with glaucoma. Thus, patients should be monitored carefully if systemic β-blocker therapy is discontinued.

CARDIOVASCULAR DRUGS

A benzofuran derivative, amiodarone, has been used for several decades to treat a variety of cardiac abnormalities. This drug is highly effective in the treatment of atrial and ventricular arrhythmias as well as in the treatment of Wolff–Parkinson–White syndrome (Chew et al., 1982). Following its introduction into clinical practice, however, amiodarone was observed to cause keratopathy early in the course of treatment, and ultrastructural changes can also occur in the conjunctiva and eyelids.

Digitoxin and digoxin have been widely used for the treatment of congestive heart disease and certain cardiac arrhythmias. Visual symptoms associated with digitalis have been recognized for several centuries and include symptoms of dimness of vision, flickering or flashing scotomas, as well as disturbances of color vision.

Pathogenesis

Amiodarone belongs to a group of drugs having the physical and chemical properties of cationic amphiphilia (Gittinger and Asdourian, 1987). Amphiphilic drugs bind to polar lipids and accumulate within lysosomes. Several investigators (Chew et al., 1981; Ghosh and McCulloch, 1984; Haug and Friedman, 1991) have performed electron microscopy on ocular tissues of patients who had taken amiodarone, and these studies have consistently revealed intracytoplasmic membrane-bound lamellar bodies similar to myelin. These changes not only have been noted in the corneal epithelium, conjunctiva, and crystalline lens, but also have been found in the corneal endothelium, the iris, ciliary body, choroid, and retina (Chew et al., 1981; Ghosh and McCulloch, 1984). The presence of such complex lipid deposits within these tissues has led recent investigators to conclude that amiodarone keratopathy is probably a drug-induced lipid storage disease. The whorl-like pattern of the keratopathy may result from an effect at the limbus on the epithelial cells that are migrating centripetally (Bron, 1973). Exposure to light may have an important role since the lenticular changes are largely limited to the pupillary aperture (Flach and Dolan, 1990).

The retina, rather than optic nerve, appears to be the site of digitalis toxicity (Madreperla et al., 1994). Binnion and Frazer (1980) have demonstrated in dogs that the highest concentrations of digoxin are found in the choroid and retina, and electrodiagnostic studies have confirmed reversible rod and cone dysfunction in patients with digitalis intoxication (Weleber and Shults, 1981; Madreperla et al., 1994). The precise mechanism underlying digoxin's toxicity may involve inhibition of photoreceptor Na^+-K^+-activated adenosine triphosphatase (ATPase), an enzyme that plays an important role in the maintenance of normal photoreceptor function (Madreperla et al., 1994).

Ocular Manifestations

Keratopathy occurs as early as 6 days following initial amiodarone therapy (Orlando et al., 1984), but it more commonly appears after 1–3 months of treatment (Dolan et al., 1985). Virtually all patients will demonstrate corneal changes after 3 months of therapy (Orlando et al., 1984; Ingram et al., 1982). These corneal deposits are bilateral, but are often asymmetric, and they are easily observed with the slit lamp. The keratopathy can be divided into several stages (Orlando et al., 1984; Dolan et al., 1985). In grade I, a faint horizontal line, similar to a Hudson–Stähli line, appears in the interpalpebral fissure at the junction of the middle and lower third of the cornea. It consists of golden-brown microdeposits in the epithelium just anterior to Bowman's layer. Transition to grade II occurs by 6 months, during which the deposits become aligned in a more linear pattern and extend toward the limbus. The grade-II pattern does not necessarily proceed to grade III, but in grade III the deposits increase in number and density, and the lines extend superiorly to produce a whorl-like pattern within the visual axis. Grade-IV keratopathy is characterized by irregular, round clumps of deposits. The development of the first three stages of keratopathy is shown in Fig. 1, and a clinical representation of amiodarone keratopathy is shown in Fig. 2. Upon discontinuing drug therapy, the keratopathy gradually resolves within 6–18 months (Dolan et al., 1985).

The severity of the keratopathy appears to be significantly correlated with total drug dosage as well as with duration of treatment (Kaplan and Cappaert, 1982; Nielsen et al., 1983). It is possible, however, for patients taking lower doses of amiodarone to demonstrate marked keratopathy, whereas other patients taking high doses of drug show minimal corneal changes (Ghosh and McCulloch, 1984). In gen-

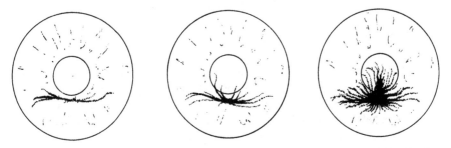

FIG. 1. Stages of amiodarone keratopathy: *left*, grade I; *center*, grade II; *right*, grade III. (Modified from Kingele et al., 1984.)

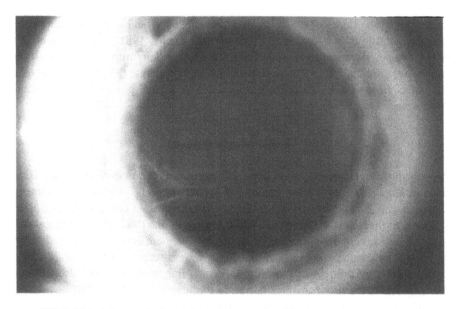

FIG. 2. Clinical photograph of grade-III amiodarone keratopathy. (From Jaanus et al., 1995.)

eral, patients taking low dosages of drug (100–200 mg daily) retain clear corneas or demonstrate only mild keratopathy regardless of duration of treatment or cumulative dosage. Patients taking higher dosages (400–1,400 mg daily) demonstrate more advanced keratopathy depending on the duration of treatment (Kaplan and Cappaert, 1982). Once the keratopathy becomes fully developed, it remains relatively stationary until the drug dosage is reduced or discontinued (Ghosh and McCulloch, 1984).

Amiodarone-induced lenticular opacities have also been reported (Dolan et al., 1985; Flach et al., 1983). Fine anterior subcapsular lens deposits occur in about half of patients taking amiodarone in moderate to high doses (600–800 mg daily) (Flach et al., 1983) after a duration of treatment of 6–18 months. The deposits first appear as small, golden-brown or white-yellow punctate opacities located just below the anterior lens capsule. They are loosely packed and cover an area greater than 2 mm in diameter within the pupillary aperture (Flach et al., 1983). Unlike the lenticular deposits associated with chlorpromazine therapy, which develop prior to corneal changes, the lens opacities associated with amiodarone may develop in the presence of marked keratopathy.

Symptoms associated with amiodarone-induced corneal and lenticular changes are minimal or absent (Dolan et al., 1985). Lenticular opacities generally cause no visual symptoms, but moderate to severe keratopathy can lead to complaints of blurred vision, glare, halos around lights, or light sensitivity. Visual acuity is usually normal but may be slightly decreased if the keratopathy is severe.

Although chronic administration of this antiarrhythmic agent has produced no visible biomicroscopic changes in the conjunctiva, electron microscopic studies of

TABLE 1. *Visual symptoms in cardiac glycoside intoxication*

Dyschromatopsia
Flickering or flashes of light
Colored spots
Snowy vision
Disturbances of visual acuity
Dimming of vision
Glare sensitivity

human material have indicated that some ultrastructural changes may occur during therapy (Ghosh and McCulloch, 1984; D'Amico and Kenyon, 1981). Intracytoplasmic membrane-bound deposits similar to myelin have been demonstrated in the cytoplasm of nearly all ocular structures, including the conjunctival epithelium (D'Amico and Kenyon, 1981). Amiodarone has also been reported to concentrate within a chalazion that developed in a patient who had been taking the drug for 2 years (Reifler et al., 1987).

The most common symptoms induced by the cardiac glycosides are changes in color vision and various visual phenomena (Table 1). These symptoms often precede cardiac abnormalities as the earliest symptoms of digitoxin intoxication (Sykowski, 1949). A common symptom is snowy vision, wherein objects of regard appear to be covered with frost or snow (Weleber and Shults, 1981; Robertson et al., 1966). Elevated dark adaptation thresholds have been reported, which gradually return to normal within 2–3 weeks after digitalis is discontinued (Robertson et al., 1966, p. 852).

Complaints of color vision disturbances are common with both digoxin and digitoxin, but color vision impairment can often be detected even in patients without symptoms (Rietbrock and Alken, 1980). Both the incidence and severity of color vision impairment tend to correlate with the plasma glycoside level (Rietbrock and Alken, 1980). About 80% of patients with digoxin intoxication will demonstrate generalized color vision deficiencies, but detectable color vision impairment occurs even at therapeutic drug levels. In contrast, patients treated with digitoxin in therapeutic concentrations (i.e., 0.1 mg daily) usually show no significant color vision abnormality (Haustein et al., 1982). At such concentrations, the pattern electroretinogram and visual evoked potential are normal, but slight increases in the total error score of the Farnsworth–Munsell 100-hue test can be demonstrated (Duncker et al., 1994).

The onset of visual symptoms following drug administration may be as soon as 1 day but is often within 2 weeks of initial therapy. Occasionally ocular toxicity is not shown until several years of treatment (Robertson et al., 1966). Digitalis-induced visual disturbances other than chromatopsia or disturbances of color vision may occur in elderly patients who have no other clinical manifestation of digitalis intoxication even if the serum glycoside level is within or below the therapeutic range (Butler et al., 1995). Once digitalis therapy is discontinued, visual symptoms usually subside within several weeks.

Patient Management

Since the corneal and lenticular changes associated with amiodarone therapy are benign, special follow-up of affected patients is not required unless the opacities have caused visual symptoms. In the rare cases in which visual symptoms are annoying or incapacitating, reducing or discontinuing drug therapy usually results in resolution of the corneal findings. It is unusual for ocular side effects to necessitate discontinuation of drug therapy, but occasionally treatment must be discontinued because of drug intolerance or other side effects such as diarrhea, vomiting, pulmonary fibrosis, or liver damage (Ghosh and McCulloch, 1984; Dolan et al., 1985). Because the early stages of amiodarone keratopathy can mimic a Hudson–Stähli line, a careful drug history relative to amiodarone use should be carefully elicited. More advanced stages of amiodarone keratopathy may resemble the corneal changes of Fabry's disease or chloroquine toxicity. Because of the systemic implications of Fabry's disease, patients with no history of having taken medications known to induce verticillate keratopathy, such as amiodarone or chloroquine, should be evaluated by an internist.

Patients taking cardiac glycosides should be monitored carefully for visual symptoms, including color vision changes, chromatopsia, flashing or flickering lights, and other entoptic phenomena. Color vision evaluation, especially during the first several weeks of therapy, can be especially helpful in detecting signs of early intoxication. Periodic color vision testing should be performed as long as the patient continues taking the medication. Detectable changes in color vision, or the onset of visual disturbances not explained by the clinical examination, should warrant consultation with the prescribing physician with regard to potential digitalis intoxication.

ANTIPSYCHOTIC AGENTS AND ETHANOL

Chlorpromazine and thioridazine, both phenothiazine derivatives, are used for their antipsychotic effects. Often high, prolonged dosages are required, and these have led to well-documented pigmentary changes in the cornea, crystalline lens, and retina. It is now generally accepted that chlorpromazine is the only phenothiazine to cause toxic changes in the cornea and lens, and it is recognized that only thioridazine produces retinal toxicity. Although most of the current literature describes the toxic effects on the cornea, lens, and retina, phenothiazines have also been reported to affect the conjunctiva, sclera, eyelids, pupils, and lacrimal system, and to have the potential to induce cycloplegia.

The use of lithium in bipolar affective disorder and recurrent depression has been associated with increased sensitivity to light and with various neurologic symptoms, including nystagmus.

Ethyl alcohol is widely consumed in the form of beer, whiskey, and other alcoholic beverages. This drug can lower intraocular pressure, induce changes in extraocular muscle motility, and may influence the risk of cataract development.

Pathogenesis

The precise nature of chlorpromazine-induced pigmentary granules observed in the cornea and crystalline lens is unknown. A common hypothesis, however, is that the pigmentary changes are a result of drug interaction with ultraviolet radiation as it passes through the cornea and lens, causing exposed proteins to denature, opacify, and accumulate in the anterior subcapsular region of the lens as well as in corneal stroma (Deluise and Flynn, 1981).

It is known that the phenothiazines bind to melanin in the uveal tract, especially the choroid (Davidorf, 1973; Potts, 1962; Salazar-Bookaman et al., 1994). Drug uptake by the choroid occurs even in patients whose serum levels of thioridazine are in the nontoxic range (Kimbrough and Campbell, 1981). It has been proposed that such drug binding is retinotoxic by damaging the choriocapillaris, thus leading to changes in the retinal pigment epithelium (Davidorf, 1973; Miller et al., 1982). It is also possible that thioridazine may alter retinal enzyme kinetics, inhibiting the oxidation of retinol. Alterations in the enzyme systems of Müller cells and photoreceptors may lead to atrophy and disorganization of the rods and cones as one of the initial degenerative changes, followed later by loss of the retinal pigment epithelium and choriocapillaries (Miller et al., 1982).

The effect of the phenothiazines on pupil size, the lacrimal system, and accommodation is related to the anticholinergic properties of these drugs. The phenothiazines can cause pupillary dilation, cycloplegia, and dry-eye associated with decreased aqueous tear secretion.

Ethyl alcohol (ethanol) is distributed in total body water and penetrates the eye very rapidly. However, penetration of the vitreous is somewhat slower than penetration of the aqueous. This lag results in a sufficient osmotic gradient between plasma and vitreous to draw fluid from the eye (Krupin et al., 1967). Ethyl alcohol also inhibits secretion of antidiuretic hormone (ADH) (Houle and Grant, 1967). A hypotonic diuresis is produced following administration of ethanol, and it has been suggested that the diuresis also contributes to the increase of serum osmolality induced by ethyl alcohol.

The mechanism by which light to moderate consumption of ethanol protects against cataract may relate to an antioxidant property of the drug. With high consumption, however, ethanol may be cataractogenic either directly or through other, metabolic mechanisms (Phillips et al., 1996).

Ocular Manifestations

Both corneal and lenticular changes are associated with chlorpromazine therapy. Thaler and associates (Thaler et al., 1985) have divided the lenticular pigmentation into five stages. The earliest sign of lenticular toxicity (grade I) is fine dotlike opacities on the anterior lens surface. At this stage the pigmentary deposits are small and tend to assume a disciform distribution within the pupillary area. Grade-II lenticular changes consist of dotlike opacities that are more opaque and denser than in grade I.

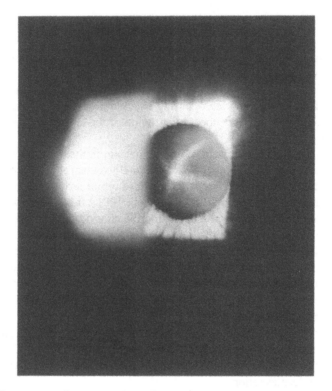

FIG. 3. Stellate pattern of anterior subcapsular cataract associated with chlorpromazine. (From Jaanus et al., 1995.)

The pigmentary granules may begin to assume a stellate pattern. As the condition progresses, grade-III changes are characterized by larger granules of pigment within an anterior subcapsular stellate pattern that is easily recognized. At this stage the opacity can range in color from white to yellow to tan. The stellate pattern has a dense central area with radiating branches (Fig. 3). A readily visible stellate pattern with three to nine star points characterizes grade-IV lenticular pigmentation. The lens changes at this stage can be recognized with a penlight, and diagnosis does not necessarily require slit lamp examination. Grade-V lenticular changes are characterized by a central, lightly pigmented, opaque mass surrounded by smaller clumps of pigment.

Corneal pigmentary changes invariably occur only in patients who have concomitant lens opacities in the higher grades (Thaler et al., 1985; Prin et al., 1970). There is often little or no corneal involvement with lens grades I and II, but grades III and higher have detectable corneal pigmentation ranging from light to heavy (Thaler et al., 1985). The pigmentation is white, yellow-white, brown, or black, and occurs at the level of the endothelium and Descemet's membrane primarily in the interpalpebral fissure (Fig. 4). Specular endothelial microscopy has failed to detect any

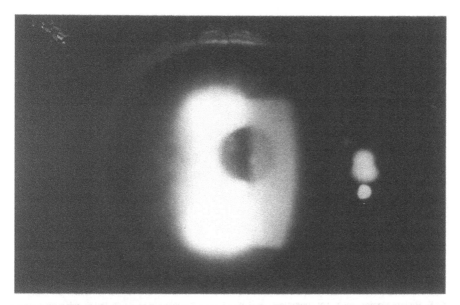

FIG. 4. Heavy pigment deposits on corneal endothelium associated with chlorpromazine. (From Jaanus et al., 1995.)

associated morphometric abnormalities of the corneal endothelium (Yasuhara et al., 1996).

Although patients may occasionally report glare, halos around lights, or hazy vision, both the corneal and lenticular changes only rarely reduce visual acuity. The keratopathy and lenticular pigmentary changes usually progress to a point beyond which no further changes are observed (Rasmussen et al., 1976). Upon reducing or discontinuing drug therapy, the pigmentary deposits are generally irreversible (Mathalone, 1968; Prin et al., 1970; Rasmussen et al., 1976). This observation is not surprising given that the deposits associated with chlorpromazine are located in avascular tissues. In rare instances the lenticular pigmentation can begin after chlorpromazine therapy is discontinued (Siddall, 1968).

The corneal and lenticular changes associated with chlorpromazine are dose-related. Lenticular pigmentation is rarely observed when the total dosage is less than 500 g, and the prevalence of pigmentary changes increases with total dosages between 1,000 and 2,000 g, until 90% of patients demonstrate pigmentation when the total dosage exceeds 2,500 g (Thaler et al., 1985; Alexander et al., 1985). Since some psychiatric conditions may require daily dosages exceeding 800 mg, lenticular pigmentation can appear as early as 14–20 months of therapy (Thaler et al., 1985). Dosages consisting of 200 mg daily have been reported to cause lenticular changes in as early as 6 months of therapy (Prin et al., 1970). Corneal toxicity has been reported to occur within 6 months of therapy in 12% of patients receiving 2,000 mg of chlorpromazine daily but in only 1% of patients receiving 300 mg of chlorpromazine daily (Prin et al., 1970).

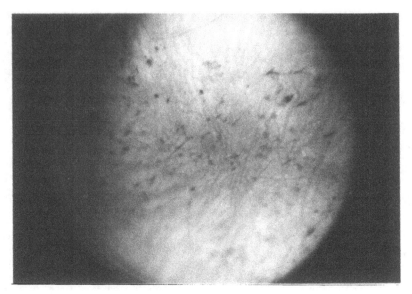

FIG. 5. Retinal pigment epithelial hyperplasia and atrophy in a 33-year-old man with thioridazine retinopathy. (From Jaanus et al., 1995.)

Thioridazine can cause significant retinal toxicity, leading to reduced visual acuity, changes in color vision, and disturbances of dark adaptation. These symptoms typically occur 30–90 days after treatment is begun (Miller et al., 1982; Kjaer, 1968). Visual field changes consist of concentric contractions or irregular paracentral or ring scotomas (Miller et al., 1982). The fundus appearance is often normal during the early stages of symptoms, but within several weeks or months a pigmentary retinopathy develops, characterized by fine clumps of pigment developing first in the periphery and progressing toward the posterior pole (Fig. 5) (Davidorf, 1973; Kjaer, 1968). In milder cases the pigment remains fine and peppery, but in more severe cases the pigment can form plaquelike lesions with multiple confluent areas of hypopigmentation and choroidal atrophy (Miller et al., 1982). Retinal edema can also occur (Kjaer, 1968), but the optic discs and retinal vasculature are usually normal.

The electroretinogram (ERG) and electrooculogram (EOG) are often normal during the early stages of toxicity, but as the retinal pigmented epithelium (RPE) becomes diffusely abnormal, the EOG becomes attenuated (Meredith et al., 1978). The amplitude of the oscillatory potential of the ERG decreases in proportion to the daily dosage of thioridazine, but the a- and b-waves as well as the latencies are normal (Miyata et al., 1980). Godel and associates (Godel et al., 1990) have suggested that the ERG will be diminished to red stimuli in the initial stages of retinal toxicity.

The primary clinical factor associated with thioridazine retinopathy is the daily drug dosage (Davidorf, 1973). Before the dose-related retinal toxicity was recognized, dosages exceeding 1,600 mg per day were commonly used. Few cases of pigmentary retinopathy have been reported, however, with daily dosages of less than

800 mg (Neves et al., 1990, Tekell et al., 1996). Thus, thioridazine therapy appears to be nonretinotoxic as long as daily dosages of less than 800 mg are employed (Davidorf, 1973; Siddall, 1968; Cameron et al., 1972).

Although it is possible for thioridazine retinopathy to resolve despite continued drug therapy, resolution usually occurs only in patients taking low dosages (Kjaer, 1968). If significant resolution is to occur, drug therapy must generally be reduced or discontinued. Depending on the severity of toxicity, retinal function can return to normal, but the pigmentary changes are often permanent. In severe cases there may be permanent impairment of visual acuity, visual field, and dark adaptation (Davidorf, 1973; Siddall, 1968). The pigmentary retinopathy may even progress after thioridazine therapy has been discontinued (Marmor, 1990), and some cases of progressive retinopathy can have a late onset, occurring from 4 to 10 years following discontinuation of thioridazine (Davidorf, 1973; Meredith et al., 1978).

Discoloration of the conjunctiva, sclera, and exposed skin of the eyelid has been reported with administration of phenothiazine derivatives. The skin of the face and lids can be equally pigmented, whereas the palpebral folds contain an area of non-pigmented skin deep within the creases. The discoloration is usually slate-blue. Melanin-like granules have been observed in the superficial dermis of the skin (Hays et al., 1964; Cairns et al., 1965). This oculodermatologic syndrome is usually associated with pigmentary deposits in the exposed interpalpebral area of the bulbar conjunctiva, especially near the limbus. The palpebral conjunctiva does not appear to be involved. Patients exposed to dosages of chlorpromazine ranging from 500 to 3,000 mg per day for 1–6 years may develop discoloration of the exposed skin, lids, and bulbar conjunctiva (Siddall, 1965; McClanahan et al., 1966). There have been sporadic reports of allergic conjunctivitis and edema of the eyelids associated with phenothiazine use (Editorial, 1969).

Transient disturbances of accommodation often occur in patients taking chlorpromazine and other phenothiazines (Alkemade, 1968). These effects are most likely due to the anticholinergic properties of the medication and are most pronounced when benztropine is administered along with the phenothiazine (Thaler, 1979, 1982). The visual symptoms may also be ascribed to reduced tearing and drying of the cornea, causing blurred vision. In patients with narrow anterior chamber angles, acute or subacute angle-closure glaucoma secondary to dilated pupils could also contribute to symptoms of blurred vision (Durkee and Bryant, 1978).

Although many clinical studies have failed to demonstrate any consistent ocular effect of lithium treatment, changes in retinal light sensitivity and drug-induced nystagmus have been reported with some frequency. Chronic lithium treatment has been implicated in causing decreased retinal sensitivity as demonstrated on automated perimetry (Wirz-Justice et al., 1997), but there is no clinical or electrophysiologic evidence of retinal toxicity with long-term lithium treatment (Wirz-Justice et al., 1997; Lam et al., 1997). Cases of lithium-induced photophobia have also been reported in association with lithium intoxication as well as normal therapeutic doses of the drug (Pridmore et al., 1996).

Patients with lithium-induced nystagmus usually present with complaints of blurred vision, particularly in lateral gaze (Williams et al., 1988; Halmagyi et al., 1989). Electrooculogram (EOG) recordings show a linear waveform jerk nystagmus, present in both primary position and in downgaze. The nystagmus is usually unaffected by head position, head velocity, or convergence. Saccadic eye movements are clinically normal (Halmagyi et al., 1989), serum chemistry analysis is usually normal, and serum lithium levels are within the normal therapeutic ranges. The nystagmus may not resolve with reduction of drug dosage or cessation of drug use. Prolonged drug abstinence, up to 6 months or even years, may be necessary to produce improvement (Williams et al., 1988).

Oral administration of ethyl alcohol can reduce intraocular pressure in both normal and glaucomatous eyes (Krupin et al., 1967; Peczon and Grant, 1965). Normal individuals demonstrate only a minimal reduction of pressure following consumption of 50 ml of 43% ethyl alcohol in the form of whiskey (Bartlett et al., 1995). Patients with open-angle glaucoma, however, have a much greater reduction of pressure lasting for 3–5 hr. Although the ocular hypotensive effect is slower in onset than with other commercially available hyperosmotic agents, the maximum effect occurs in 1–2 hr (Krupin et al., 1967).

Alcohol is well documented to affect eye movement ability (Bittencourt et al., 1980, Wilson and Mitchell, 1983; Rosenberg, 1983). Both smooth pursuits and saccades are impaired when blood ethanol concentrations reach the range of 60–100 mg/dl. Bittencourt and associates (Bittencourt et al., 1980) have reported a direct linear relationship between blood alcohol concentration and reduction in smooth pursuit velocity. Their results indicate that at a blood ethanol concentration of 80 mg/dl, the capacity of the eyes to track objects moving across the visual field is impaired by 25%.

Although some studies have found no association between ethanol consumption and cataract (Taylor, 1980), Phillips and associates (Phillips et al., 1996) have demonstrated that both total abstention from alcohol and high consumption are associated with increased risk of cataract development. Moderate or occasional consumption of alcohol seems to have a protective effect. Alcohol use has been associated with all types of age-related cataract, including nuclear sclerotic, cortical, and posterior subcapsular opacities (Phillips et al., 1996).

Patient Management

Patients receiving high-dosage or long-term, low-dosage chlorpromazine therapy should be monitored annually by careful slit-lamp examination. Since lenticular pigmentation is the most frequent ocular change observed, slit-lamp examination of the lens with the pupil dilated is the most direct method for detecting early chlorpromazine toxicity. It may be possible to delay ocular pigmentary changes by avoiding long-term, high-dosage therapy, or by employing intervals of treatment with non-phenothiazine drugs such as haloperidol (Mathalone, 1968; Prin et al., 1970). If the corneal and lenticular changes occur but visual acuity is not affected and the patient is asymptomatic, the drug dosage can generally be continued without modification. If the patient becomes symptomatic, however, the dosage should be reduced or therapy should be changed to a different drug.

Since the danger of retinal toxicity with thioridazine is significantly correlated with daily dosage, patients should generally be placed on dosages less than 800 mg per day (Miller et al., 1982). Regardless of dosage, patients should receive careful fundus examinations before treatment is initiated, during the first 2–4 months of therapy, and every 6 months thereafter (Tekell et al., 1996). Electrodiagnostic tests such as the ERG and EOG may be of limited value in detecting early retinopathy (Godel et al., 1990; Henkes, 1967). If symptoms or objective signs of retinal toxicity are observed, the medication should be discontinued to improve the chances of resolution. Since the pigmentary retinopathy may be progressive even after thioridazine has been discontinued, patients should receive follow-up examinations on an annual basis.

Management of drug-induced cycloplegia entails the use of appropriate spectacle lenses to correct for accommodative insufficiency, and the use of artificial tears and lubricants for the relief of symptoms associated with dry-eye. These management strategies are usually sufficient without modifying the drug therapy.

Since downbeat nystagmus has neurologic significance and may be related to a variety of metabolic or drug-related causes, a careful medical history and communication with the prescribing physician are essential in patients suspected to have lithium-induced ocular motility disturbances. Patients on chronic lithium therapy should have at least yearly ocular examinations. Baseline exophthalmometry measurements may also be considered.

It is important for the practitioner to be cognizant of the ability of ethyl alcohol to reduce intraocular pressure. Patients presenting for routine eye examination following consumption of ethyl alcohol may be found to have "borderline normal" intraocular pressures that may increase once the effects of the alcohol have subsided. These patients perhaps should be monitored for development of glaucomatous optic nerve damage and visual field loss.

The fact that alcohol can affect eye movement ability has been employed to devise a test known as the alcohol gaze nystagmus test. This procedure was developed to augment the traditional field evaluation of suspected drunk drivers by law enforcement officials. The test involves the observation of ocular version movements, endpoint nystagmus, and angle of lateral deviation at which the nystagmoid movements begin. When properly administered and evaluated, the test can help to correctly identify about 80% of drivers with blood alcohol levels of 0.10% or higher (Halperin and Yolton, 1986; Tiffany, 1986).

CHEMOTHERAPEUTIC AGENTS

Systemically administered antimicrobial agents usually present no risk to the eye or vision. Some of these drugs, however, can cause a variety of ocular complications, ranging from discoloration of the sclera or contact lenses to transient myopia or optic neuropathy.

Ocular Manifestations

Drug penetration into tears has been reported with certain antimicrobial agents. Sulfonamides, tetracyclines, erythromycin, and rifampin have been assayed in tears of human subjects (Melon and Register, 1976). Ampicillin and penicillin penetrate into the tears very poorly, but in contrast, erythromycin levels in tears have been found to be higher than the serum concentration, implying active transport of this antibiotic into tears following systemic administration (Melon and Register, 1976). Following its oral administration, 36–88% of the daily erythromycin dosage is present in tears. An interesting observation is that the preocular tear film can become discolored after the use of systemic rifampin (Fraunfelder, 1980). The tears usually become orange but may also be pink or red. Contact lenses may become stained, leading to the recommendation that soft contact lens wear be discontinued during rifampin therapy (Lyons, 1979).

Blue-grey discoloration of the sclera can occur following the oral administration of minocycline. Although rare, scleral pigmentation seems to occur only in individuals who encounter generalized cutaneous pigmentation (Sabroe et al., 1996; Fraunfelder and Randall, 1997). Pigmentation of the sclera characteristically occurs in a band 3–5 mm in width near the limbus but can appear temporally as well (Fraunfelder and Randall, 1997). In most cases oral minocycline therapy lasting several years is required to produce the pigmentary changes in the sclera, but scleral pigmentation has occurred with 100–200 mg daily dosage for as little as 4 months (Fraunfelder and Randall, 1997). The pigmentation may resolve over a course of several years, or it may be permanent.

Eyelid edema, conjunctivitis, and chemosis have been reported with high-dose administration of sulfanilamide (Alvaro, 1943). These reactions appear to be analogous to systemic hypersensitivity reactions such as urticaria and edema seen in some patients who are allergic to sulfonamides. Tilden and associates (Tilden et al., 1990) reported bilateral anterior uveitis associated with systemic administration of sulfamethoxazole.

A modest number of cases have been described of transient myopia associated with oral sulfonamides in which there was reduced accommodation, shallow or closed anterior chamber angles, and moderate mydriasis (Mattsson, 1952; Postel et al., 1996; Kreig and Schipper, 1996). Vaginal absorption of sulfonamides can also lead to myopia. Chirls and Norris (1984) reported a patient with myopia following use of a vaginal sulfonamide suppository, and Maddallena (1984) described a patient with 7 D of induced myopia following use of sulfonamide vaginal cream.

Conjunctival deposits similar to those seen in epinephrine-treated glaucoma patients have been observed in patients treated orally with tetracyclines (Brothers and Hidayat, 1981; Messmer et al., 1983). Dosages range from 250 to 1,500 mg per day of tetracycline and at least 100 mg per day of minocycline. The deposits appear as dark brown to black granules in the palpebral conjunctiva (Brothers and Hidayat, 1981). The granules vary in size and are located in conjunctival cysts, surrounded by minute, gray-white, noncrystalline soft spots. Under ultraviolet light microscopy the brown pigmented concentrations give a yellow fluorescence characteristic of tetracycline (Messmer et al., 1983).

Optic neuropathy as a consequence of chloramphenicol therapy is well known, especially when the drug is used to treat cystic fibrosis in children. This drug causes both optic neuritis and retrobulbar neuritis (Huang et al., 1966). Severe, bilateral reduction of visual acuity accompanied by dense central scotomas is characteristic of most cases (Huang et al., 1966; Harley et al., 1970; Godel et al., 1980). Although there may be no fundus changes, the optic discs are usually edematous and hyperemic, the retinal veins are engorged and tortuous, and hemorrhages are often seen in the parapapillary area (Lieberman, 1968). Optic atrophy is a late sign. Peripheral neuritis characterized by numbness and cramping of the feet often precedes the visual complaints by 1–2 weeks and may therefore serve as an early warning sign of impending ocular toxicity (Huang et al., 1966).

Visual impairment associated with chloramphenicol therapy usually recovers after the drug is discontinued, but pretreatment visual acuity is often not regained and visual field defects may persist (Lieberman, 1968). Some patients may tolerate further prolonged treatment with chloramphenicol without recurrent optic neuritis, and occasionally patients can demonstrate improvement of visual function despite continued treatment. Most cases of optic neuritis associated with chloramphenicol therapy have occurred in children with cystic fibrosis who were treated with large daily dosages of drug, 1–6 g daily. Although the onset of visual symptoms can be as early as 10 days after therapy has begun, ocular toxicity commonly occurs after several months or years of treatment (Harley et al., 1970; Walker, 1961). Harley and associates (Harley et al., 1970) have reported a dosage-dependent relationship between chloramphenicol therapy and optic neuritis. The incidence of optic neuritis varies from 5% of patients treated with a daily dosage of 10–25 mg/kg body weight, to 38% of patients treated with a daily dosage exceeding 50 mg/kg body weight. There is typically no vision loss among patients treated for less than 3 months, but the incidence of optic neuritis increases to 16% in patients treated longer than 12 months.

Pathogenesis

Transient myopia caused by systemically administered drugs may be produced by ciliary body edema, resulting in relaxation of the zonules, which causes thickening and anterior movement of the crystalline lens (Hook et al., 1986). Drug-induced myopia associated with sulfonamides has been documented by ultrasonographic A-scan measurements and refraction to be due to edema of the ciliary body (Bovino and Marcus, 1982). The ciliary body edema, occasionally associated with retinal edema, has led to the speculation that sulfonamide-induced myopia may be related to hypersensitivity reactions (Mattsson, 1952). It has been speculated that the drug-induced ciliary body edema may be associated with a disturbance in eicosanoid metabolism

(Kreig and Schipper, 1996). Alternatively, ultrasound biomicroscopy has demonstrated the presence of choroidal effusion causing forward displacement of the lens–iris diaphragm, producing the clinical manifestations of increased myopia, anterior chamber shallowing, and angle-closure glaucoma (Postel et al., 1996).

It has been hypothesized that either tetracycline or its metabolite forms an insoluble chelation complex that results in pigmentation of the palpebral conjunctiva (Messmer et al., 1983). In the case of scleral pigmentation associated with oral minocycline therapy, the type of scleral deposit is unknown since biopsies have not been performed (Fraunfelder and Randall, 1997).

The precise mechanism by which chloramphenicol produces optic neuritis is unknown, but visual evoked potentials have confirmed optic nerve involvement in patients taking chloramphenicol (Spaide et al., 1987). Although not substantiated, several authors have proposed that chloramphenicol may induce optic neuropathy by causing a vitamin deficiency (Keith, 1964). Genetic factors may be involved, and it has also been suggested that chloramphenicol may be metabolized to degradation products that are potentially toxic to the optic nerve (Lieberman, 1968). Histopathologic studies have found bilateral optic atrophy with primary involvement of the papillomacular bundle, loss of the retinal ganglion cells, and gliosis of the nerve fiber layer (Harley et al., 1970). The presence of peripheral visual field defects in some patients is evidence that there is also involvement of the peripheral portion of the visual pathway.

Patient Management

Most of the ocular effects of systemically administered antimicrobial agents are benign and will usually subside quickly once drug therapy is reduced or discontinued. Before starting long-term minocycline therapy, patients should be advised of the possibility of scleral pigmentary changes. If skin or scleral pigmentation occurs, the drug should be withdrawn immediately to improve the likelihood of resolution (Fraunfelder and Randall, 1997).

Patients who are to receive long-term chloramphenicol therapy should undergo a comprehensive baseline examination consisting of visual acuity, visual fields, color vision, and fundus examination. The risk of optic neuropathy is minimized if the daily dosage of drug is limited to 25 mg/kg body weight or less for a period of time not exceeding 3 months (Harley et al., 1970). Patients or their parents should be encouraged to be alert to the development of peripheral neuritis, which might indicate impending vision loss. Once signs or symptoms of optic neuropathy are detected, drug therapy should be promptly discontinued.

ANTITUBERCULOSIS DRUGS

Ethambutol was introduced in, 1961 for the treatment of tuberculosis. Severe toxic side effects were initially reported, but these were linked to use of the racemic mixture of the drug. The dextroisomer was consequently selected as the most therapeutically useful and has been found to have a lower incidence of ocular toxicity than the racemic form (Roberts, 1974).

Pathogenesis

Although the mechanism by which ethambutol causes retrobulbar neuritis is largely unknown, van Dijk and Spekreijse (1983) and Kakisu and associates (Kakisu et al., 1988) have suggested that ethambutol may affect the amacrine and bipolar cells of the retina since color vision can be affected without altering visual acuity. It has also been proposed that ethambutol may chelate zinc, subsequently causing zinc deficiency. Patients with preexisting zinc deficiency may thus be at greater risk for developing drug-induced toxicity (Russo and Chaglasian, 1994).

Ocular Manifestations

Ethambutol is well documented to cause ocular symptoms of reduced visual acuity, changes in color vision, and visual field loss (Carr and Henkind, 1962). Signs of ocular toxicity can appear as early as several weeks following initial therapy, but the onset of ocular complications usually occurs several months after therapy is begun (Addington, 1979; Trusiewicz, 1975). Although various forms of optic neuritis have been described, the primary ocular manifestation of ethambutol toxicity is retrobulbar neuritis. This condition commonly occurs in several forms (Table 2): (a) The most common form involves the loss of visual acuity associated with a central or pericentral scotoma along with color vision disturbances. This type is caused by compromise of the central optic nerve fibers. (b) Less commonly, ethambutol can affect the peripheral optic nerve fibers, causing defects in the peripheral visual field. (c) In rare cases, ethambutol can cause visible retinal manifestations, including hyperemia and swelling of the optic discs, flame-shaped hemorrhages on the optic disc and in the retina, and macular edema. After several weeks, these signs can be followed by primary optic atrophy (Kuming and Braude, 1979).

Color vision disturbances are probably the most sensitive indicator of early ethambutol optic neuropathy (Polak et al., 1985). When the patient is examined with a sensitive test such as the Farnsworth–Munsell 100-Hue or desaturated Panel D-15,

TABLE 2. *Characteristics of ethambutol optic neuropathy*

Characteristic	Central (axial)	Peripheral
Toxic dosage	Low	High
Visual acuity	Reduced	Normal
Visual field	Central scotoma	Peripheral constriction
Color vision	Red–green deficiency	Normal

Modified from Garrett (1985).

both red–green or blue–yellow defects may be observed in early stages of toxicity. These changes in color vision can occur even before visual acuity and visual fields are affected.

Contrast sensitivity function can also be affected, in some cases before visual acuity or color vision become impaired. Salmon and associates (Salmon et al., 1987) have suggested that testing using Arden contrast sensitivity plates may be effective in detecting subclinical toxic optic neuropathy associated with ethambutol.

Once changes have occurred in visual acuity, visual field, or color vision, these functional disturbances may continue to deteriorate even after ethambutol has been discontinued. More often, however, there is recovery of pretreatment visual acuity within 3–4 months following discontinuation of drug treatment (Carr and Henkind, 1962; Woung et al., 1995). The degree of recovery depends largely on the extent to which ethambutol has compromised optic nerve function. If the ocular toxicity is not recognized early, the drug can cause permanent loss of vision (Yiannikas et al., 1983; Russo and Chaglasian, 1994) or compromise visual function, even if visual acuity has completely recovered (Woung et al., 1995).

There is considerable evidence that ocular toxicity associated with ethambutol therapy is dose-related. It is now recognized that ethambutol rarely causes ocular changes at a dosage of 15–20 mg/kg body weight/day (Trusiewicz, 1975), and this has led to the current recommendation that ethambutol dosages should not generally exceed 15 mg/kg body weight/day. Many clinicians employ the drug in dosages of 25 mg/kg/day for a period of time not exceeding 2 months, followed by a maintenance dose of 15 mg/kg/day, and this regimen has been shown to cause virtually no ocular complications (Addington, 1979; Barron et al., 1974; Russo and Chaglasian, 1994).

Patient Management

Patients beginning treatment with ethambutol should have baseline examinations and frequent monitoring of visual acuity, visual fields, color vision, and fundus appearance. Patients should be instructed to report promptly any changes in visual acuity or color perception. Since it is rare for ocular toxicity to occur with dosages as low as 15 mg/kg/day, patients taking such dosages can be monitored every 3–6 months (Polak et al., 1985). Patients with renal insufficiency, however, have impaired ability to excrete the drug and therefore may be at greater risk for developing ocular changes. Verifying renal and liver functions is an important precaution prior to initiating ethambutol therapy, and patients with renal disease should be monitored on a monthly basis (Kuming and Braude, 1979; DeVita et al., 1987). Patients with low plasma zinc levels should also be monitored more carefully (DePalma et al., 1989). Periodic evaluations must include color vision, static threshold visual fields, visual acuity, and ophthalmoscopy. Use of the desaturated Panel D-15 test or the Farnsworth–Munsell 100-Hue is effective for the detection of subtle color vision changes associated with early ethambutol toxicity (Polak et al., 1985). Visual evoked potentials have been recommended for the routine monitoring of patients to detect subclinical optic nerve disease that can precede changes in visual acuity and color vision.

Ethambutol therapy must be discontinued in patients who develop reduced visual acuity, color vision deficiency, or visual field defects characteristic of optic neuropathy (Citron and Thomas, 1986). If discontinuation of drug therapy alone does not result in improvement of visual function, consideration can be given to treatment with parenteral hydroxycobalamin. Guerra and Casu (1981) have reported recovery of visual acuity in four patients treated with hydroxycobalamin several months after the discontinuation of ethambutol had failed to improve visual acuity. Although the mechanism of action of hydroxycobalamin in the treatment of ethambutol-induced optic neuropathy is uncertain, this vitamin may act by neutralizing the chelating action of ethambutol on the optic nerve. Supplemental zinc therapy has also been suggested, but this treatment has not been demonstrated to restore visual function, nor is it useful for advanced optic atrophy (Russo and Chaglasian, 1994).

ANTIMALARIAL COMPOUNDS

Chloroquine and hydroxychloroquine are used for the treatment of malaria, rheumatoid arthritis, discoid and systemic lupus erythematosus, and other collagen diseases. These quinoline drugs have been employed for these purposes since the early, 1950s. These drugs are well known to cause changes in the cornea and retina, and to induce clinically significant cycloplegia.

Quinine has been employed for the treatment of malaria, but it is now used primarily for the management of leg cramps, myotonia congenita, and eyelid myokymia. Quinine toxicity has been recognized for many years, and overdosage of quinine is still encountered in patients who attempt abortion or suicide. Accidental ingestion of quinine can also lead to serious side effects. Acute vision loss is one of the most significant reactions associated with quinine use.

Pathogenesis

The origin of chloroquine-induced corneal opacities is somewhat obscure but appears to represent reversible binding of the drug to intracellular nucleoproteins (Bernstein, 1967). The changes induced by the quinolines are limited to the corneal epithelium, which the drug may reach by deposition in the tear film or by the limbal vasculature (Beebe et al., 1986). Individual susceptibility probably plays an important role in the development of chloroquine keratopathy since, at lower dosages (e.g., 250 mg chloroquine or 200 mg hydroxychloroquine daily), there appears to be no relationship between the occurrence of keratopathy and total dosage and duration of therapy (Cullen and Chou, 1986). Patients receiving chloroquine doses exceeding 750 mg daily or hydroxychloroquine doses exceeding 800 mg daily appear to develop keratopathy earlier in the course of treatment (Calkins, 1958).

Although the precise mechanism by which chloroquine and hydroxychloroquine cause retinal toxicity is unknown, it is widely recognized that these drugs bind tenaciously to melanin within the eye (Rosenthal et al., 1978; Bernstein and Ginsberg, 1964). It is understood, moreover, that the pigmented tissues of the eye will continue to hold the drug for prolonged periods of time after drug therapy is discontinued (Rosenthal et al., 1978). This can lead to degenerative changes of the retinal pigmented epithelium (RPE). Rosenthal and associates (Rosenthal et al., 1978), however, have shown that chloroquine also accumulates in the retina itself, suggesting that the neurosensory retina may also have the ability to bind the drug. Investigations in monkeys have shown that chloroquine initially causes degenerative effects in the ganglion cells, followed by disruption of the photoreceptors and finally of the RPE and choroid (Rosenthal et al., 1978). Ramsey and Fine (1972) have confirmed in humans that the initial pathologic change occurs in the ganglion cells and that the changes within the RPE and photoreceptors occur late in the disease process. The destructive process within the RPE leads to migration of pigment-laden cells from the RPE to the outer nuclear and outer plexiform layers (Bernstein, 1967; Wetterholm and Winter, 1964). There is frequently sparing of the foveal cones, which explains the ophthalmoscopic appearance seen in cases of "bull's-eye" maculopathy (Bernstein and Ginsberg, 1964).

The precise mechanism underlying the cycloplegic effect of chloroquine is unknown. However, the fact that the accommodative insufficiency is rapid in both its onset and reversibility suggests that the effect is related to melanin binding (Bernstein, 1967). The change in amplitude of accommodation might also be explained by a drug effect on the central nervous system (Rubin and Thomas, 1970).

Our current understanding of the pathogenesis of quinine ocular toxicity is largely derived from various electrodiagnostic studies demonstrating that quinine has a direct toxic effect on the retinal photoreceptors and ganglion cells (Yospaiboon et al., 1984; Brinton et al., 1980; Dyson et al., 1985–86). There is also damage to the RPE (Brinton et al., 1980). Visual evoked potentials confirm the conduction abnormality in the nerve fiber layer associated with secondary optic atrophy (Gangitano and Keltner, 1980).

Ocular Manifestations

The pattern of chloroquine keratopathy can be divided into three stages (Hobbs et al., 1961). In the early stage diffuse punctate deposits appear in the corneal epithelium. Later the deposits aggregate into curved lines that converge and coalesce just below the central cornea. Finally, green-yellow pigmented lines appear in the center of the cornea as a whorl-like opacity.

Less than half of affected patients with corneal changes have visual symptoms (Bernstein, 1970), but the most common complaints relate to halos around lights, glare, and photophobia. Visual acuity usually remains unchanged (Bernstein, 1970). Upon discontinuation of drug therapy, both subjective symptoms and objective corneal signs invariably disappear (Goldhammer and Smith, 1974; Petrohelos, 1974; Mantyjarvi, 1985).

Keratopathy occurs in 30–75% of patients treated with either chloroquine or hydroxychloroquine (Lozier and Friedlaender, 1989), but the corneal changes are much less frequently observed in patients treated with hydroxychloroquine (Petrohelos, 1974). Although Calkins (1958) reported that the corneal findings are related to total (cumulative) drug dosage or duration of therapy, other studies (Cullen and Chou, 1986; Marks and Power, 1979) have found no correlation between severity of keratopathy and the dosage or duration of drug therapy (Calkins, 1958; Bernstein, 1970), and there is no relationship between the development of corneal deposits and the occurrence of retinopathy (Marks and Power, 1979). In about half of patients treated with chloroquine there is decreased or absent corneal sensitivity unrelated to the development of corneal opacities (Bernstein, 1967).

Hydroxychloroquine is now the preferred quinoline for the treatment of collagen disease because of fewer side effects, and its ocular toxicity is considerably less than that of chloroquine (Shearer and Dubois, 1967; Mantyjarvi, 1985). Tobin and associates (Tobin et al., 1982) monitored 99 patients treated with hydroxychloroquine during a 7-year period. All patients received the drug for at least 1 year, and most patients received a daily dosage of 400 mg. No keratopathy was observed in any patient. At higher dosage levels, however, a higher incidence of keratopathy occurs (Shearer and Dubois, 1967). In a group of patients receiving an average daily dosage of 800 mg, 6% developed keratopathy within 6 months of beginning therapy, and the incidence increased to 32% during the second 6 months. Corneal changes were present in all patients after 4 years of hydroxychloroquine treatment. Shearer and Dubois (1967) have reported a rapid rise in the incidence of keratopathy when the total drug dosage exceeds 150 g. Upon reducing or discontinuing drug therapy, the corneal opacities decreased or disappeared during an average of 8 months.

The first visible evidence of chloroquine retinopathy is a fine, pigmentary mottling within the macular area with or without loss of the foveal reflex (Cruess et al., 1985; Henkind et al., 1964). However, even before visible ophthalmoscopic changes are detectable, a "premaculopathy" state can exist in which the drug interferes with metabolism of the macular tissues, causing subtle relative visual field defects in patients with ophthalmoscopically normal maculas (Percival and Behrman, 1969). As the macular pigmentary change progresses, a classic pattern develops consisting of a granular hyperpigmentation surrounded by a zone of depigmentation, which, in turn, is surrounded by another ring of pigment. Although this clinical picture can vary in intensity, it is pathognomonic of chloroquine retinopathy and is referred to as a "bull's-eye" lesion (Fig. 6) (Bernstein, 1967; Cruess et al., 1985; Henkind et al., 1964). Variations of retinal pigment epithelial disturbances can occur and are commonly observed as a well-circumscribed area of RPE atrophy in the macular area, which can resemble a macular hole (Fig. 7) (Cruess et al., 1985). In moderate to advanced cases of retinal toxicity, the arterioles may become attenuated, and the optic disc can become pale (Bernstein, 1967; Carberg, 1966; Martin et al., 1978). Occa-

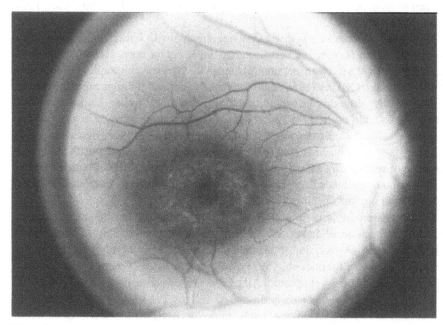

FIG. 6. Characteristic "bull's-eye" maculopathy associated with chloroquine toxicity. (From Jaanus et al., 1995.)

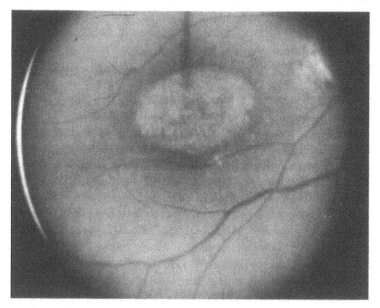

FIG. 7. Retinal pigment epithelial atrophy in macular area as a consequence of chloroquine therapy. (From Jaanus et al., 1995.)

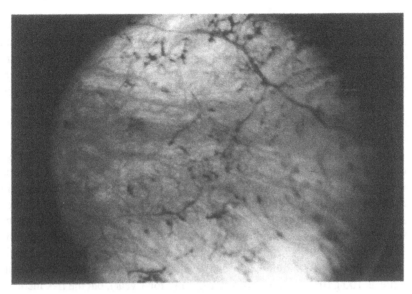

FIG. 8. Peripheral retinal pigment epithelial hyperplasia characteristic of pseudoretinitis pigmentosa in a 42-year-old man with chloroquine toxicity. (From Jaanus et al., 1995.)

sionally there may be signs of macular edema (Bernstein, 1967). There usually is a high degree of bilateral symmetry between the eyes, but occasionally the toxicity can affect one eye more than the other.

Some patients with chloroquine retinopathy may have retinal changes that resemble retinitis pigmentosa (Bernstein, 1967; Brinkley et al., 1979). Peripheral RPE hyperplasia can occur, but in contrast to retinitis pigmentosa, the pigment does not tend to accumulate around the retinal veins (Nylander, 1966). These peripheral lesions can occur with or without simultaneous macular involvement (Fig. 8). Other changes include attenuated retinal vessels, optic atrophy, peripheral visual field loss, and a subnormal electroretinogram. The fact that the dark adaptation threshold is normal or only minimally abnormal further differentiates this condition from true retinitis pigmentosa.

Although the visual fields may be normal even in the presence of definite macular pigmentary changes (Marks and Power, 1979), visual field loss generally correlates well with the degree of retinal damage. The typical visual field defects in chloroquine retinopathy consist of central, paracentral, or pericentral scotomas (Goldhammer and Smith, 1974; Banks, 1987). The paracentral scotomas may be confluent and form a complete ring scotoma.

In the early stages of retinopathy electrodiagnostic studies are usually of little value in detecting early chloroquine toxicity (Bernstein, 1967). Both the ERG and EOG can be normal or abnormal. Advanced cases of chloroquine retinopathy, however, are generally characterized by markedly abnormal or even extinguished ERGs (Banks, 1987). This is especially true in cases involving the retinal periphery.

Although it is possible for patients with chloroquine maculopathy to be asymptomatic, extensive macular damage will often lead to symptoms of decreased visual acuity, metamorphopsia, and visual field disturbances (Bernstein, 1967). Paracentral ring scotomas can cause reading difficulty. Although color vision is normal in the early stages of chloroquine toxicity, more extensive macular damage can lead to severe impairment of color vision. Dark adaptation is typically normal, an important feature distinguishing the drug-induced peripheral retinal changes from those seen in retinitis pigmentosa (Bernstein, 1967).

Risk factors for the development of chloroquine retinopathy include daily dosage, duration of treatment, serum drug levels, and patient age. The incidence of retinopathy increases with patient age, and in older patients retinal toxicity appears to correlate with total drug dosage (Finbloom et al., 1985; Ehrenfeld et al., 1986). Ehrenfeld and associates (Ehrenfeld et al., 1986) contend that daily dosage is the most critical risk factor. Most cases of chloroquine retinopathy occur in patients taking 500 mg daily, but dosages as low as 250 mg or less daily can also be retinotoxic (Bernstein, 1967; Easterbrook, 1987). Retinopathy can develop when the total cumulative dosage is as little as 100 g (the equivalent of 250 mg daily for 1 year), but the risk increases significantly when the total dosage exceeds 300 g (Lozier and Friedlaender, 1989). The duration of therapy required to produce chloroquine retinopathy can be as little as 6 months, but most patients require 2–4 years of therapy before retinal changes develop (Cullen and Chou, 1986).

Chloroquine retinopathy tends to remain stable once therapy is discontinued (Brinkley et al., 1979). Some patients, however, may demonstrate regression of macular changes if the retinal involvement is mild and if the visual acuity is normal (Brinkley et al., 1979). Although some patients with the classic "bull's-eye" maculopathy may have reversible macular changes (Marks and Power, 1979), patients with moderately advanced retinopathy may show progression even after drug therapy is discontinued (Easterbrook, 1988). Progressive impairment of visual acuity can occur for up to 5 years following discontinuation of chloroquine therapy (Ogawa et al., 1979). Duncker and Bredehorn (1996) have demonstrated in rats that retinal photoreceptors can continue to degenerate after chloroquine has been withdrawn.

The risk of retinopathy associated with hydroxychloroquine appears to be considerably less than that associated with chloroquine (Terrell et al., 1988). Tobin and associates (Tobin et al., 1982) reported retinal toxicity in only 4 of 99 patients receiving hydroxychloroquine in a daily dosage of 400 mg for at least 1 year. No patient, however, sustained significant vision loss, and the abnormalities were reversible after the medication was discontinued. In some cases the macular changes may be reversible without recurrence even if the medication is reinstituted (Rynes et al., 1979). In other cases the retinal lesions may be irreversible (Mavrikakis et al., 1996). As little as 73 g of hydroxychloroquine taken over 6 months has been reported to cause retinopathy (Rynes et al., 1979), and the incidence of retinopathy may be as high as 30% if the cumulative dosage exceeds 800 g (Mills et al., 1981). Several investigators (Tobin et al., 1982; Johnson and Vine, 1987), however, have discounted the role of cumulative dosage and believe that the risk of maculopathy associated with hydroxychloroquine therapy is more closely related to daily dosage. Johnson and Vine (1987) found no evidence of retinopathy in nine patients treated with massive total dosages of hydroxychloroquine ranging from 1,054 to 3,922 g. These authors suggest that patients who take prudent daily dosages of hydroxychloroquine (400 mg/day or 6.5 mg/kg body weight/day, whichever is less) are at little risk for developing retinopathy even when therapy is prolonged.

Accommodative insufficiency, with its associated reading difficulty, is a common side effect of long-term chloroquine therapy (Bernstein, 1967; Rubin and Thomas, 1970).This usually begins within several weeks after treatment is begun, and the effect appears to be dose-related. As many as 40% of patients taking 500–750 mg daily will have impairment of accommodation (Howell, 1957). The accommodative insufficiency is often rapid in onset but is quickly reversible upon reduction or discontinuation of drug therapy (Bernstein, 1967).

Mild toxic reactions from quinine are characterized by slight reduction of visual acuity or "flickering" of vision. In more severe cases symptoms consist of sudden complete loss of vision, dizziness, and even deafness. Patients with acute quinine overdose frequently have no light perception in both eyes, and pupils are often dilated and nonreactive (Yospaiboon et al., 1984; Brinton et al., 1980). Patients may complain of impairment of night vision, but color vision is usually normal. The visual fields usually demonstrate concentric contraction, and improvement of visual fields following the acute episode may require days or months, but the field loss may show no recovery and become permanent (Gangitano and Keltner, 1980).

Ophthalmoscopic examination of the fundus soon after acute quinine overdose may reveal a normal fundus (Brinton et al., 1980), but constriction of the arterioles, optic disc pallor, venous dilation, or retinal edema can also be observed.

The visual prognosis for patients with acute quinine toxicity is guarded. Visual acuity can improve from no light perception to 20/20 within days to several weeks (Brinton et al., 1980). Sometimes vision does not improve to normal for several months. As vision recovers there is progressive constriction of the retinal vessels, and the optic disc becomes pale. Although central visual acuity often returns to normal levels, the visual fields can remain constricted (Gangitano and Keltner, 1980).

Patient Management

Patients taking chloroquine or hydroxychloroquine should receive careful baseline and periodic slit-lamp examinations. Early identification of the corneal changes is facilitated by using retroillumination (Calkins, 1958). It is important for the ophthalmic practitioner to distinguish early chloroquine keratopathy from the normal development of Hudson–Stähli lines, which it can resemble. Fabry's keratopathy is another important condition in the differential diagnosis. The verticillate corneal findings are similar to those induced by chloroquine, but the systemic implications in Fabry's disease warrant consultation with an internist. Since the drug-induced corneal condition is relatively benign and only rarely results in significant visual symptoms, the development of chloroquine keratopathy does not contraindicate continued use of the medication (Bernstein, 1970; Petrohelos, 1974). If, however, symptoms of glare, halos, or reduced vision are bothersome to the patient, consideration can be given to decreasing or changing drug therapy.

Since early chloroquine or hydroxychloroquine retinopathy is frequently reversible if drug dosage is reduced or discontinued, patients should be monitored carefully after receiving baseline evaluations. Baseline examinations of the fundus and using Amsler charts are especially important since chloroquine and hydroxychloroquine maculopathy can resemble age-related macular disease. Once drug treatment has started, it is prudent to monitor patients every 6 months, especially if the patient is over 65 years of age (Silman and Shipley, 1997; Mazzuca et al., 1994). Frequent and meticulous follow-up appears to be unnecessary during the first several years because toxicity rarely develops in the early years of therapy (Mavrikakis et al., 1996). Elderly patients should be monitored more carefully since chloroquine and hydroxychloroquine are detoxified and eliminated from the body by the liver and kidney, respectively, which might be impaired in these patients (Mantyjarvi, 1985).

As the patient is monitored over time, careful ophthalmoscopic examination of the fundus, including retinal periphery, is one of the most sensitive indicators of early retinopathy (Mills et al., 1981; Fleck et al., 1985). Testing of contrast sensitivity function is also useful to detect early macular dysfunction (Bishara and Matamoros, 1989). Visual field assessment using static threshold techniques is of value in detecting the early stages of visual field loss (Hart et al., 1984). Patients should be encouraged to self-evaluate using the Amsler charts every 2 weeks (Easterbrook, 1987). Electrodiagnostic testing, however, as well as fluorescein angiography are less sensitive than routine ophthalmoscopy or color photography in the detection of early retinal toxicity (Easterbrook, 1990). Since the clinical signs and symptoms of retinal toxicity may not appear until after drug therapy is discontinued, it is important to monitor patients for several years after drug therapy has been stopped, especially for patients who have received at least 300 g of chloroquine or the equivalent of hydroxychloroquine (Ehrenfeld et al., 1986).

Because the cycloplegic effects of chloroquine are transient and are related to drug dosage, symptoms of accommodative insufficiency can be managed by prescribing appropriate reading lenses during long-term drug therapy, or drug dosage may be reduced or discontinued. The cycloplegic effects of chloroquine will often abate when the dosage is reduced, and accommodation will completely return to pretreatment levels after drug therapy is discontinued (Rubin and Thomas, 1970).

The maximum daily dosage of quinine should generally not exceed 2 g, and quinine toxicity is common in dosages over 4 g (Brinton et al., 1980). Toxic reactions to relatively small doses of quinine are probably idiosyncratic in nature but can result in a clinical picture similar to that caused by higher doses (Horgan and Williams, 1995). Since central vision tends to recover spontaneously even without treatment, patients with acute quinine toxicity should be managed by immediate gastric emptying, administration of activated charcoal, and other supportive measures. Following the acute episode, patients should be monitored carefully for improvement in visual acuity, visual fields, and fundus appearance.

ANTINEOPLASTICS

The use of aggressive anticancer drug regimens, and the recent development of new agents and drug combination protocols, has led to an increase in reported cases of chemotherapy-induced ocular side effects (Al-Tweigeri et al., 1996) (Table 3).

Of the commonly used antineoplastic agents, tamoxifen citrate and carmustine (BCNU) are most likely to cause adverse ocular effects. Tamoxifen is an orally administered nonsteroidal antiestrogen and is one of the most effective antitumor agents for the palliative treatment of metastatic breast carcinoma in postmenopausal women. This drug has been in clinical use since, 1970 and is used both alone and in combination with other agents, usually without serious side effects. Carmustine is used for the treatment of various malignant neoplasms, including metastatic malignant melanoma, malignant gliomas of the central nervous system, metastatic breast cancer, and leukemia.

Pathogenesis

The first clinicopathologic correlation of tamoxifen retinopathy was provided by Kaiser-Kupfer and associates (Kaiser-Kupfer et al., 1982). These investigators have shown that high-dosage tamoxifen treatment causes widespread axonal degeneration, primarily in the perimacular area. The yellow-white lesions seen on fundus examination appear to represent products of the axonal degeneration. They are 3–10 μm in diameter in the perimacular area, and they are confined to the nerve fiber and inner plexiform layers.

The retinal toxicity resulting from intracarotid infusion of carmustine is probably related to the increased flow of drug into the ophthalmic artery. The precise mechanism whereby carmustine causes retinal toxicity is unknown, but several investigators (Shingleton et al., 1982; Miller et al., 1985) have suggested that the drug may be toxic to the retinal and choroidal vasculature, causing segmental intraretinal vasculitis with or without vascular obstructions. This process leads to nerve fiber infarcts and retinal hemorrhage.

Ocular Manifestations

Tamoxifen retinopathy has been well documented, and the retinal findings include white or yellow refractile opacities in the macular or perimacular area, with or without macular edema (Fig. 9) (Kaiser-Kupfer and Lippman, 1978; McKeown et al., 1981). Although the lesions are usually more numerous in the macular area, they can also extend to the ora. The lesions occur in the sensory retina, and many appear superficial to the retinal vessels. The affected patient may experience a reduction of visual acuity associated with the macular lesions, and the visual fields can show abnormalities corresponding to the retinal lesions. At normal dosage levels tamoxifen rarely causes retinal toxicity (Longstaff et al., 1989; Nayfield and Gorin, 1996;

TABLE 3. *Reported cases of ocular toxicity associated with systemic anticancer drugs*

Agent	Conjunctiva	Cornea	Retina	Optic nerve	Other side effects
Mechlorethamine (intracarotid)			Necrotizing uveitis, vasculitis of the choroid		
Chlorambucil			Hemorrhagic papilledema	Papilledema	
Cyclophosphamide	Conjunctivitis	Keratitis			Reversible blurred vision,
Ifosfamide	Conjunctivitis	Keratitis			Reversible blurred vision
Busulfan	Conjunctivitis	Keratitis			Cataract
					Blurred vision
					Sicca syndrome
Carmustine (intracarotid)		Corneal edema	Exudates and hemorrhage	Optic neuritis	Blurred vision, ocular pain, glaucoma
Cisplatin				Optic neuritis, papilledema, color blindness	Blurred vision, cortical blindness
Carboplatin			Maculopathy	Optic neuritis	Blurred vision, ocular pain, cortical blindness
Cytosine arabinoside (high dose)	Conjunctivitis	Keratitis			Ocular pain, blurred vision, photophobia
Cytosine arabinoside ara-C (intrathecal)				Optic neuropathy	
5-fluorouracil	Conjunctivitis	Keratitis		Optic neuropathy	Blurred vision photophobia, excessive lacrimation, circumorbital edema, cicatricial ectropion, punctal-canalicular stenosis
Methotrexate	Conjunctivitis				Blurred vision, eye pain, photophobia, blepharitis, decreased tears
Methotrexate (intrathecal)				Optic neuropathy	Internuclear ophthalmoplegia

Drug					
Deoxycoformycin Vinca alkaloids	Conjunctivitis	Keratitis		Optic neuropathy, optic atrophy	Ptosis, cranial nerve palsy, cortical blindness, night blindness
Paclitaxel				Ischemic optic neuropathy	Photopsia, decreased acuity
Doxorubicin	Conjunctivitis				Excessive lacrimation
Mitomycin C (intravenous)					Blurred vision
Tamoxifen		Keratopathy	Retinal hemorrhage, retinopathy, macular edema	Optic neuritis	
Corticosteroids	Corneal ulcers	Fungal keratitis	Hemorrhage; glaucoma, pseudotumor cerebri, candida endophthalmitis cytomegalovirus retinitis, retinal toxoplasmosis		Cataract, acute myopia, myopathic extraocular muscle palsy, exophthalmos, scleral thinning
Retinoids	Conjunctivitis	Corneal opacities	Pseudotumor cerebri, papilledema		Night blindness
Interferon-α			Hemorrhage, cotton wool spots, papilledema		Oculomotor nerve palsy, ocular pain, exophthalmos, ptosis
Cyclosporine				Optic disc edema	Retinopathy, cottonwool spots, proliferative retinopathy

Modified from Al-Tweigeri et al., 1996, Ocular toxicity and cancer chemotherapy. A review. *Cancer* 78:1359–1373. Copyright 1996, American Cancer Society. Reprinted by permission of Wiley-Liss, Inc., a subsidiary of John Wiley & Sons, Inc.

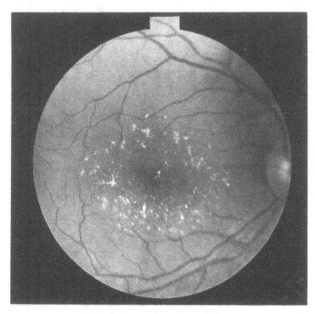

FIG. 9. Tamoxifen maculopathy in a 66-year-old woman administered 120 mg of tamoxifen twice daily for 2 years. Note macular edema with yellow-white crystalline deposition. (From Jaanus et al., 1995.)

Pavlidis et al., 1992; Heier et al., 1994), but when taken in high dosages (e.g., 90–100 mg twice daily) the toxic effects can be observed within 17–27 months as the total cumulative dosage exceeds 90 g (Kaiser-Kupfer et al., 1982; McKeown et al., 1981). In rare cases, however, tamoxifen can be retinotoxic in low dosages. Griffiths (1987) reported a patient with tamoxifen retinopathy who had received less than 8 g of drug. Once tamoxifen therapy is discontinued, the number and size of the retinal lesions generally remain unchanged, and the degenerative changes appear to be irreversible (Kaiser-Kupfer et al., 1982; Pavlidis et al., 1992). Visual acuity, however, can improve upon discontinuation of tamoxifen (Nayfield and Gorin, 1996). Both the development of ocular toxicity and the potential improvement in visual acuity may be related to total cumulative drug dosage (Nayfield and Gorin, 1996).

Retinal toxicity associated with carmustine usually begins within 2–14 weeks following intraarterial infusion of the drug (Shingleton et al., 1982). Approximately 65% of patients develop retinal complications, consisting of retinal infarction, periarteritis, periphlebitis, nerve fiber layer hemorrhage, or macular edema (Miller et al., 1985). Loss of vision commonly occurs, and visual acuity can be reduced to 20/60 to light perception, or even no light perception (Shingleton et al., 1982). Qualitative and quantitative tear film abnormalities (Cruciani et al., 1994) and ischemic optic neuropathy (Pickrell and Purvin, 1987) have also been reported. Although a definite relationship between dosage of carmustine and retinopathy has not been established, retinal complications can be avoided using intracarotid administration by passing the infusion catheter beyond the origin of the ophthalmic artery (Chrousos et al., 1986).

Patient Management

Since tamoxifen retinopathy can occur at relatively low total dosages of drug, it is important to obtain a baseline examination before therapy is begun. This should include best corrected visual acuity, visual fields, Amsler chart evaluation, and fundus photography. Subsequently, the patient should be monitored periodically during therapy since macular compromise can result in irreversible vision loss. Annual examinations are sufficient if normal drug dosages are administered (Heier et al., 1994). Patients receiving higher than normal doses, however, should be monitored every 6 months. When drug-induced ocular changes occur, tamoxifen should be discontinued to prevent further progression and irreversible visual impairment (Mihm and Barton, 1994).

The retinotoxic effects of intracarotid carmustine can be minimized or avoided by employing an infusion catheter that is advanced beyond the origin of the ophthalmic artery (Chrousos et al., 1986; Kupersmith et al., 1988).

ISOTRETINOIN

An analogue of vitamin A, 13-*cis*-retinoic acid is used to treat severe recalcitrant cystic acne and other keratinizing dermatoses. Oral administration of 1–2 mg/kg body weight/day causes suppression of sebaceous gland activity and inhibition of keratinization. Ocular complications include blepharoconjunctivitis, dry–eye symptoms, contact lens intolerance, and subepithelial corneal opacities. Impairment of dark adaptation can also occur (Bigby and Stern, 1988).

Pathogenesis

The meibomian glands are important modified subaceous glands of the eyelids, and when meibomian gland activity is suppressed by isotretinoin, the normal lipid layer of the preocular tear film becomes deficient. This deficiency promotes evaporation of the underlying aqueous layer, leading to dry-eye or blepharoconjunctivitis secondary to increased tear osmolarity (Mathers et al., 1991). In rabbits, degenerative changes in the meibomian gland acini have been demonstrated (Kremer et al., 1994). These changes lead to cell necrosis and a reduction of basaloid cells lining the acini walls.

Although the precise mechanism explaining isotretinoin's effect on dark adaptation is unclear, it has been suggested that the drug may become incorporated into the rod photoreceptor elements during the process of outer disk shedding and renewal. Weleber and associates (Weleber et al., 1986) have hypothesized that isotretinoin may compete for normal retinol binding sites on cell surfaces or transport molecules, accounting for the reduction in retinal sensitivity.

Ocular Manifestations

Milson and associates (Milson et al., 1982) observed a dose-dependent relationship between isotretinoin therapy and blepharoconjunctivitis. Dosages of 2 mg/kg body weight/day of isotretinoin resulted in blepharoconjunctivitis in 43% of patients, whereas dosages of 1 mg/kg body weight/day showed a 20% incidence of blepharoconjunctivitis. A retrospective study (Fraunfelder et al., 1985) of 237 patients showed the most common ocular side effect was blepharoconjunctivitis, occurring in 37% of patients.

The incidence of dry–eye symptoms has been estimated to be as high as 20%, with about 8% of patients experiencing contact lens intolerance (Fraunfelder et al., 1985). Isotretinoin has been observed to decrease tear breakup time (Fraunfelder et al., 1985; Ensink and VanVoorst Vader, 1983). Analysis of lacrimal gland fluid of rabbits and human tears of subjects treated with isotretinoin has shown the presence of this compound in tears. Thus, the actual presence of isotretinoin in tear fluid could decrease stability of the lipid layer of the tear film, which would enhance tear film rupture and the formation of dry spots. This effect could be responsible, in turn, for the dry-eye symptoms, contact lens intolerance, and conjunctival irritation accompanying isotretinoin therapy (Ubels and MacRae, 1984).

Impairment of dark adaptation with or without excessive glare sensitivity has been reported with isotretinoin therapy in dosages of 1 mg/kg body weight/day (Weleber et al., 1986). These complaints may be associated with an abnormal ERG or EOG. Once therapy is discontinued, both the abnormal dark adaptation and abnormal ERG usually resolve within several months.

Patient Management

Decreasing the dosage or discontinuing the drug will usually alleviate the side effects, although several months may be required in some patients before significant relief is obtained. In the meantime, treatment of dry-eye symptoms or blepharoconjunctivitis using artificial tear preparations and ocular lubricants is usually satisfactory. Symptoms of contact-lens intolerance can be managed with artificial tear preparations or reduction of wearing schedules (Gold et al., 1989).

Patients taking isotretinoin should be monitored for changes in night vision. Reports of night vision impairment should suggest more definitive evaluation procedures such as visual fields, dark adaptometry, and electroretinography. If retinal function is documented to be abnormal, the drug should be withdrawn. Once drug therapy has been discontinued, retinal function should be monitored for improvement.

CORTICOSTEROIDS

Corticosteroids are sometimes used to treat collagen diseases such as rheumatoid arthritis and systemic lupus, and they are also used for the treatment of sarcoidosis. However, because of their potential for systemic side effects, steroids are limited to conditions for which less conservative therapy is inadequate. The association between steroid use and cataracts has been well known for several decades, but direct interpretation of published reports of patients with steroid-induced cataracts is often subject to error because of variations in duration or dosages of steroids used. In, 1960, Black and associates (Black et al., 1960) were the first to suggest that systemic steroid therapy could lead to posterior subcapsular (PSC) cataracts. They had observed PSC cataracts in 39% of a group of patients with rheumatoid arthritis who had undergone prolonged systemic steroid therapy. Although several authors subsequently refuted the relationship between systemic steroids and PSC cataracts, it is now widely accepted that under certain circumstances oral steroid therapy can induce cataract formation.

PSC cataracts are also associated with use of nasal or inhalation steroids (Fraunfelder and Meyer, 1990). In a population-based, cross-sectional study of over 3,000 people, Cumming and associates (Cumming et al., 1997) demonstrated that use of inhaled steroids is associated with the development of both PSC and nuclear cataracts. In addition, steroids are widely known to elevate intraocular pressure in patients with open anterior chamber angles.

Pathogenesis

Although the precise mechanism whereby steroids lead to cataract formation is unknown, Urban and Cotlier (1986) have proposed that steroids gain entry into the fiber cells of the crystalline lens and then react with specific amino groups of the lens crystallins. This alteration frees protein sulfhydryl groups to form disulfide bonds, which subsequently lead to protein aggregation and, ultimately, to complexes that refract light. Other mechanisms have also been proposed (Mayan et al., 1979; Bucala et al., 1982).

The pathogenesis of steroid-induced pressure elevation is less well understood. As with topically applied steroids, steroids administered systemically may reduce aqueous outflow facility in susceptible patients (Feiler-Ofry et al., 1972), but there is substantial evidence that systemically administered steroids may also increase aqueous formation, leading to elevated pressure (Lindholm et al., 1965; Godel et al., 1972a,b). Diotallevi and Bocci (1965) have shown that systemically administered steroids can increase aqueous production without elevating intraocular pressure, implying a concomitant increase in aqueous outflow. Compared with topical steroids, systemic steroids may evoke different changes in the ocular fluid dynamics because of the distinctly different routes of administration (Godel et al., 1972a). Patients on long-term systemic steroids may accumulate excessive amounts of mucopolysaccharide in the trabecular meshwork, causing obstruction of aqueous outflow by hydrating the trabeculum (Spaeth et al., 1977).

Ocular Manifestations

Systemic steroids can produce PSC cataracts (Fig. 10) that are clinically indistinguishable from complicated cataract and cataracts caused by exposure to ionizing radiation (Black et al., 1960). They often cannot be distinguished from age-related PSC cataracts except that the latter frequently have other associated findings such as anterior capsular or subcapsular vacuoles, cortical opacities, or nuclear sclerosis. Even if the steroid dosage is reduced or discontinued, the cataract usually remains unchanged and will neither progress in size nor become smaller or less dense (Kobayashi et al., 1974; Furst et al., 1966). On rare occasions, however, the size of the opacity may decrease following reduction of steroid therapy. It has been suggested that spontaneous regression of steroid-induced PSC cataract might occur in cases associated with relatively low doses of steroid or when the duration of treatment is less than 2 years (Kobayashi et al., 1974). In other cases, progressive changes may occasionally occur when the steroid dosage is reduced or discontinued.

Several of the earliest studies on the relationship between systemic steroids and cataracts suggested that the dosage or duration of treatment was significantly correlated with the development of cataract (Furst et al., 1966; Oglesby et al., 1961). Furst and associates (Furst et al., 1966), however, proposed that it is possible for patients to develop steroid-induced cataract even when taking very low doses of steroid. In, 1961, Oglesby and associates (Oglesby et al., 1961) provided data to suggest that no patient taking steroids for less than 1 year would develop lens opacities. The relationship of dosage and duration of therapy was further defined by Crews (1963),

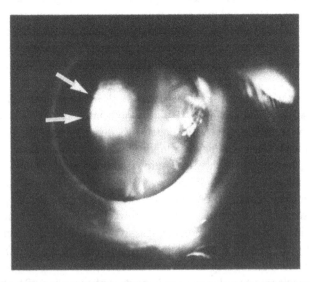

FIG. 10. Posterior subcapsular (PSC) cataract (*arrows*) in a 48-year-old man who had taken oral prednisone 7.5 mg daily for 13 years for treatment of rheumatoid arthritis. Visual acuity was 20/30 (6/9). (From Jaanus and Lesher, 1995.)

who suggested that steroids could cause cataracts with short-term therapy only if the dosage was extremely high.

Because of considerable variation in the numbers of patients studied, dosage and duration of treatment, criteria for cataract diagnosis, route of drug administration, and the underlying disease process itself, attention has focused more recently on the possibility that PSC cataract formation may be related more to factors of individual susceptibility than to drug-related factors of dosage or duration of therapy (Kristensen, 1968; Limaye et al., 1988). Skalka and Prchal (1980) found no statistically significant correlation between PSC opacities and total steroid dosage, weekly dosage, duration of therapy, or patient age. There may also be special susceptibility among various ethnic groups. Hispanics are apparently more predisposed to steroid-induced PSC cataracts than are either Caucasians or blacks (Loredo et al., 1972; Rooklin et al., 1979).

It has been suggested that children are more susceptible than adults to the development of steroid-induced cataracts (Kobayashi et al., 1974), developing them at a lower dosage and in a shorter period of time than do adult patients (Furst et al., 1966). This can be attributed to the relatively massive doses of steroid, in relation to body weight, sometimes prescribed in children (Urban and Cotlier, 1986).

Visual impairment is rare in patients with steroid-induced PSC cataracts (Urban and Cotlier, 1986; Limaye et al., 1988). Astle and Ellis (1974) reported that 88% of a group of patients with steroid-induced cataracts had visual acuity of 20/40 or better in each eye. Although severe reduction in visual acuity is uncommon, patients may nevertheless report light sensitivity, frank photophobia, reading difficulty, or glare.

In addition to their systemic effects, steroids administered orally can cause elevated intraocular pressure, although the prevalence of elevated pressure is less than that occurring with topical steroids. This reduced prevalence is probably due to the lower concentration of steroid within the anterior chamber when steroids are administered systemically. Nevertheless, it is possible for systemic steroids to elevate pressure enough to cause glaucomatous damage to the optic disc and visual fields (Covell, 1958).

The long-term administration of systemic steroid typically produces a relatively small increase in pressure (Astle and Ellis, 1974), and the elevated pressure is self-limiting as the drug therapy is reduced or discontinued. In one study (Godel et al., 1972a), about 34% of the patients on systemic steroids had ocular pressures of 29 mm Hg or higher, whereas only 6% of the control group had similar pressure elevations.

As with topically applied steroids, the degree of response to systemic steroids is not related to dosage or duration of treatment, but is due, instead, to factors of individual susceptibility or responsiveness to the effects of steroids (Godel et al., 1972a,b). In patients who are steroid responders, pressure elevations with systemic steroids average about 60% of those produced by topically applied steroids (Feiler-Ofry et al., 1972). Thus, patients with glaucoma would be expected to be particularly sensitive to the pressure-elevating effects of systemic steroids.

Patient Management

Patients taking systemic steroids should have careful slit-lamp examinations performed through a dilated pupil every 6 months. Since it is possible for patients to develop cataracts even when taking very low doses of steroid (Bluming and Zeegen, 1986), every patient, regardless of dosage or duration of treatment, must be carefully evaluated for the presence of drug-induced cataracts. When drug-induced cataracts are discovered, the prescribing practitioner should be notified so that the dosage can be reduced, if possible, to the minimum that will control the disease process. Alternatively, alternate-day therapy can be considered, or a nonsteroidal anti-inflammatory drug may be substituted. Episodes of renal transplant rejection can often be equally well controlled by lower doses of steroid, and these reduced dosages may help to prevent cataracts following transplantation (Pavlin et al., 1977).

Ocular hypertension or open-angle glaucoma associated with systemic steroid therapy should be managed according to the usual guidelines governing treatment of these conditions. A reduction of steroid dosage, if possible, almost always results in reduction of intraocular pressure. If continuation of steroid therapy is deemed necessary, the ocular pressure can often be controlled with topical antiglaucoma therapy despite continuation of systemic steroids (Wilson et al., 1973).

NONSTEROIDAL ANTI-INFLAMMATORY DRUGS

Nonsteroidal anti-inflammatory agents are commonly used for their analgesic, anti-inflammatory, and antipyretic actions in the treatment of arthritis, musculoskeletal disorders, dysmenorrhea, and acute gout. Although these drugs are widely used and are often employed for prolonged periods of time, ocular side effects rarely occur (Henkes et al., 1972). These drugs can occasionally be toxic to the cornea or retina.

Pathogenesis

Controlled, prospective clinical trials are needed to further establish and clarify the association between nonsteroidal anti-inflammatory agents and corneal opacities. The mechanism of such ocular changes is unknown. With regard to retinal effects, most investigators have speculated that indomethacin may have a direct or indirect effect on the retinal pigment epithelium, but the precise mechanism has not been established (Henkes et al., 1972; Palimeris et al., 1972; Burns, 1968). Localization of the retinotoxic effect to the retinal pigment epithelium is supported by changes observed in the ERG and EOG in patients with indomethacin retinopathy (Henkes et al., 1972). In newborn piglets indomethacin and diclofenac do not alter the ERG. In contrast, propionic acid derivatives such as ibuprofen, naproxen, and flurbiprofen affect both the amplitude and implicit time of the ERG under photopic and scotopic conditions, suggesting generalized disturbances in both the rods and cones (Hanna et al., 1995).

Ocular Manifestations

The incidence of corneal toxicity associated with indomethacin therapy has been reported to be 11–16% (Palimeris et al., 1972; Burns, 1968). The corneal lesions appear either as fine stromal, speckled opacities or have a whorl-like distribution resembling that seen in chloroquine keratopathy. The corneal changes diminish or disappear within 6 months of discontinuing indomethacin therapy. Although no definite relationship has been established between dosage of drug and corneal changes, Palimeris and associates (Palimeris et al., 1972) found corneal opacities in patients who had taken indomethacin for 12–18 months with daily dosage ranging from 75 to 200 mg and the total dosage ranging from 20 to 70 g. Symptoms associated with the corneal opacities can include mild light sensitivity or even photophobia. Corneal sensitivity, however, is normal (Palimeris et al., 1972).

Salicylates are well known for their anticoagulant properties, and in high dosages or prolonged use these drugs can cause subconjunctival or retinal hemorrhage (Mortada and Abboud, 1973; Werblin and Peiffer, 1987; Kingham et al., 1988). Most of the reported cases of retinopathy associated with nonsteroidal anti-inflammatory agents have involved indomethacin therapy. Although there have been no prospective, controlled clinical trials investigating the relationship between indomethacin and retinopathy, there is evidence that the drug can induce pigmentary changes of the macula and other retinal areas (Graham and Blach, 1988). The lesions usually consist of discrete pigment scattering of the retinal pigment epithelium perifoveally as well as fine areas of depigmentation around the macula. In some cases the pigmentary changes can be more marked in the periphery of the retina (Henkes et al., 1972). Depending on the amount of retinal involvement, the ERG and EOG can be normal or abnormal (Burns, 1968). Likewise, the amount of retinopathy will dictate whether or not changes occur in visual acuity, dark adaptation, and visual fields. Acquired color vision deficiencies of the blue-yellow type have been reported (Palimeris et al., 1972; Koliopoulos and Palimeris, 1972). No definite relationship has been established between the dosage of indomethacin and retinal toxicity. When drug therapy is discontinued, however, most of the functional disturbances associated with the retinopathy will usually improve although the pigmentary changes of the retina are generally irreversible (Henkes et al., 1972; Burns, 1968). Significant improvement of color vision, visual acuity, dark adaptation, and visual fields may require at least 6–12 months following discontinuation of drug therapy.

Patient Management

Since the corneal opacities associated with nonsteroidal anti-inflammatory drugs are benign and represent no significant threat to vision, patients taking these drugs can be monitored annually or biannually for evidence of corneal toxicity. Patients who develop evidence of keratotoxicity should be reassured regarding the benign nature of these changes. The benign corneal opacities do not warrant reducing or discontinuing drug therapy except in unusual circumstances in which severe corneal changes cause visual symptoms that are annoying or incapacitating.

Patients taking high or prolonged doses of salicylates or indomethacin should be monitored carefully for evidence of retinal hemorrhage or pigmentary changes, especially in the macular area. Evaluation of color vision may be helpful to identify patients with early retinotoxic effects associated with indomethacin (Koliopoulos and Palimeris, 1972). Consideration should also be given to other functional disturbances, and these can be monitored by performing serial visual acuity, visual fields, and dark adaptation. Once retinal toxicity is documented, the prognosis for improved retinal function is good provided indomethacin therapy is decreased or discontinued.

GOLD COMPOUNDS

Both parenteral and oral gold salts are used in the treatment of rheumatoid arthritis. After prolonged administration, gold can be deposited in various tissues of the body, a condition known as chrysiasis. Ocular chrysiasis can involve the conjunctiva, cornea, crystalline lens, and eyelids.

Pathogenesis

The available evidence suggests that the gold is deposited in the cornea and crystalline lens by circulation in the aqueous fluid in the anterior chamber (McCormick et al., 1985). The mechanism of gold deposition in the conjunctiva and eyelids has not been established but presumably occurs by direct transfer from systemic circulation.

Ocular Manifestations

Corneal chrysiasis consists of numerous, minute gold particles appearing as yellowish-brown to violet or red particles distributed irregularly in the stroma (McCormick et al., 1985; Gottlieb and Major, 1978). The deposition of gold generally spares the peripheral 1–3 mm as well as the superior one-fourth to one-half of the cornea, and the deposits tend to localize to the posterior one-third of the stroma (McCormick et al., 1985). There is typically no involvement of the epithelium, Descemet's membrane, or endothelium. Figure 11 shows the general distribution of gold deposits in a typical case of corneal chrysiasis.

Corneal chrysiasis is a common finding in patients on long-term maintenance gold therapy for rheumatoid arthritis. McCormick and associates (McCormick et al., 1985) found gold deposits in 97% of patients receiving continuous gold therapy consisting of a cumulative dosage of at least 1,000 mg. Gottlieb and Major (1978) reported corneal chrysiasis in 45% of patients who had received a mean cumulative dosage greater than 7 g during a mean 6-year period. Although no correlation exists

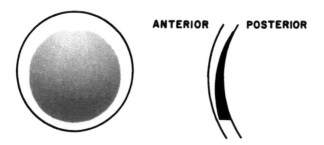

FIG. 11. Distribution of gold deposits in corneal chrysiasis. The deposits spare the peripheral and superior cornea and are more dense inferiorly. (Modified from McCormick et al., 1985.)

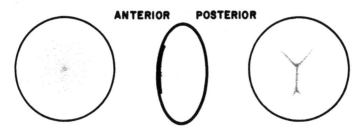

FIG. 12. Lenticular chrysiasis. Gold deposits can diffusely involve the anterior capsule and concentrate within the axial region, or can involve the anterior suture line. (Modified from McCormick et al., 1985.)

between the density of corneal deposits and the cumulative dose, there is a positive correlation between the duration of gold therapy and the density of corneal deposits (McCormick et al., 1985).

Lenticular chrysiasis appears as fine, dustlike, yellowish, glistening deposits in the anterior capsule or in the anterior suture lines (Gottlieb and Major, 1978). Deposition of oral auranofin occurs in the anterior subcapsular region (Fig. 12) (Weidle, 1987).

Various studies (McCormick et al., 1985; Gottlieb and Major, 1978) have established the prevalence of lenticular chrysiasis from parenteral gold to be from 36% to 55%. Although there is no correlation between the dosage of gold and the presence of lenticular deposits (Gottlieb and Major, 1978), the deposition of gold in the lens generally requires at least 3 years of parenteral chrysotherapy (McCormick et al., 1985). The lowest cumulative dosage to produce such lenticular deposits is about 2,500 mg (McCormick et al., 1985). Weidle (1987) reported lenticular chrysiasis in a 72-year-old woman who had received 960 mg of oral auranofin during a 5-month period.

There is no significant correlation between corneal chrysiasis and lenticular chrysiasis, and there is no evidence that gold therapy leads to true cataract formation (Gottlieb and Major, 1978). Deposits of gold in the cornea or lens do not cause visual disturbances or other symptoms.

Patient Management

Since ocular chrysiasis does not lead to visual impairment, inflammation, or corneal endothelial changes, gold therapy does not need to be reduced or discontinued (Mc-Cormick et al., 1985). This benign process requires only routine monitoring. The deposits often disappear within 3–6 months following cessation of therapy, but they may occasionally be found years after chrysotherapy has been discontinued.

ORAL CONTRACEPTIVES

Although ocular side effects have been widely reported with oral contraceptive use, most of these effects have been based primarily on isolated, anecdotal case reports. Animal studies as well as prospective clinical trials in humans have failed to document any significant relationship between use of oral contraceptives and ocular side effects (Wood, 1977). Various authors have speculated that oral contraceptives may influence contact lens wear or cause cataracts, but there is no firm evidence to suggest that such a relationship actually exists (Koetting, 1966; Ruben, 1966; Varga, 1976; Connell and Kelman, 1968; Drill et al., 1975; Faust and Tyler, 1966).

Nevertheless, there is circumstantial evidence that retinal vascular disease may have an association with oral contraceptives because patients have been reported with retinal lesions that disappeared when the drug was discontinued, promptly reappearing when the drug was resumed, and then regressing when treatment was again discontinued (Smith and Krieger, 1970; Goren, 1967). Furthermore, the retinal vascular disturbances occur at an unusually young age when vascular damage associated with arteriosclerosis is rare.

Pathogenesis

The mechanism underlying retinal vascular complications associated with oral contraceptives is unknown. Schenker and associates (Schenker et al., 1972) have shown that oral contraceptives may cause changes in the retinal microvasculature. Fluorescein angiography was used to demonstrate narrowing of the capillary arterioles and postcapillary venules. Women who complained of headache while taking oral contraceptives demonstrated dilation of perimacular vessels several weeks after the drug was discontinued. Retinal vascular occlusive episodes might also occur as a consequence of marked intimal proliferation, or as a result of contraceptive-enhanced platelet adhesiveness. Fibrinogen and clotting factors may also be increased (Wood, 1977; Stowe et al., 1978).

Ocular Manifestations

The most common retinal findings reportedly associated with oral contraceptive use are retinal vascular occlusions. These may present as typical branch or central retinal vein occlusion (Ruskiewicz, 1983), as branch or central retinal artery occlusion

TABLE 4. *Retinotoxic effects reported with oral contraceptives*

Central or branch retinal vein occlusion
Central or branch retinal artery occlusion
Perivasculitis
Impending central retinal vein occlusion
Retinal artery attenuation
Macular hemorrhage
Retinal edema

TABLE 5. *Risk factors for vascular complications associated with oral contraceptives*

Migraine headache
Phlebitis
Inclination to varicosity
Systemic hypertension
Hyperlipidemia or hypercholesterolemia
Diabetes
Cigarette smoking
Obesity

(McGrand and Cory, 1969), or may involve atypical presentations such as tortuosity of the perimacular venules (Gombos et al., 1975) or combined central retinal artery and vein occlusion (Stowe et al., 1978). Acquired color vision deficiencies have also been reported. Marre and associates (Marre et al., 1974) found acquired tritanomaly in 28% of women using oral contraceptives when tested with the Panel D-15 test. Table 4 lists other retinotoxic effects reported with use of oral contraceptives (Smith and Kreiger, 1970; Radnot and Follmann, 1973).

Patient Management

The risk of retinal vascular disease associated with oral contraceptive use in women of childbearing age is generally considered to be minimal. Certain predisposing factors, however, may increase the risks of retinal vascular episodes. Women who experience migraine headache, phlebitis, or diabetes, or who are obese may be at increased risk for vascular complications (Wood, 1977; Radnot and Follmann, 1973). Other risk factors are listed in Table 5. These patients should therefore be monitored more carefully for evidence of retinal disease. If the patient develops retinal vascular complications that are suspected of being associated with oral contraceptive use, consideration can be given to changing the mode of contraception.

PHOTOSENSITIZING DRUGS

Photosensitizing drugs are compounds that absorb optical radiation (ultraviolet [UV] and visible) and undergo a photochemical reaction resulting in chemical modifications in nearby molecules of the tissue (Lerman et al., 1982). The psoralen compounds are photosensitizing drugs widely used by dermatologists to treat disorders such as psoriasis and vitiligo. This treatment is commonly referred to as PUVA therapy and involves the administration of 8-methoxypsoralen (8-MOP) or related compounds, followed by exposure to UVA radiation (320–400 nm) for short periods of time (Lerman, 1986). The most common photosensitizing reactions involve the skin and eye. Cataract formation is well documented in patients undergoing PUVA therapy.

Pathogenesis

The eye and the skin are the only tissues of the body that are particularly susceptible to damage from nonionizing wavelengths of optical radiation (280–1,400 nm) (Lerman, 1986). The crystalline lens has the ability to absorb varying amounts of UV radiation and thus photobind susceptible drugs present in that tissue. Most ocular damage from photosensitizing drugs occurs on exposure to UV radiation (Lerman et al., 1982). Because the adult crystalline lens effectively filters most UV radiation, there is minimal risk of photobinding susceptible drugs in the retina. UV radiation, however, can penetrate to the retina in aphakic individuals and in young eyes, thus causing potential photosensitizing damage to the retina (Lerman, 1986; British Photodermatology Group, 1994).

Ocular Manifestations

Lerman and associates (Lerman et al., 1980) have demonstrated psoralens in the crystalline lens following oral administration and have further shown that the psoralens may photobind to lens protein if subsequently exposed to UVA radiation. Stern and associates (Stern et al., 1985) have shown that there is a slightly greater prevalence of nuclear sclerosis and PSC opacities, but without decreased visual acuity, in patients treated on over 100 occasions than in patients treated on fewer occasions. The incidence of symptomatic cataract, however, is not significantly increased if patients wear UVA-blocking lenses following each treatment.

Patient Management

If the eye is protected from UV radiation during PUVA therapy, free 8-MOP can be found in the lens for only 12–24 hr (Lerman et al., 1982). Thus, to prevent permanent photobinding of this drug, dermatologists usually provide specially manufactured UVA filtering goggles to patients undergoing PUVA therapy. The patient should wear the lenses for at least 24 hr beginning when the drug is first taken. Twenty-four-hour protection is especially important for children, patients with preexisting cataract, and patients with atopic dermatitis (British Photodermatology Group, 1994). These filters must be worn indoors as well as outdoors since there is sufficient UV radiation in ordinary fluorescent lighting to photobind the 8-MOP (Lerman et al., 1982). These measures are generally effective in preventing development of cataracts associated with PUVA therapy (Stern et al., 1985; Cox et al., 1987).

TALC

Tablets of medication intended for oral use contain inert filler materials such as talc (magnesium silicate), corn starch, cotton fibers, and other substances (Michelson et al., 1979). Chronic drug abusers are known to prepare a suspension of medication for injection by dissolving in water the crushed tablets of cocaine, heroin, or other narcotic. They then boil the solution and filter it through a crude cigarette or cotton filter prior to injecting the solution. The talc particles eventually embolize to the retinal circulation and produce a characteristic retinopathy.

Pathogenesis

As the talc, corn starch, and other insoluble tablet fillers embolize to the lungs, they become trapped within the pulmonary tissues and eventually cause pulmonary hypertension. This leads to the development of collateral vessels that allow part of the venous return to bypass the lungs and enter the left side of the heart, where the particles are allowed to further embolize to the eye (Tse and Ober, 1980). The presence of talc particles in the eye is an indication that substantial foreign body damage has occurred in the lungs (Atlee, 1972).

The particles lodge in the walls of the precapillary arterioles and capillaries, producing focal occlusion of these vessels in the retina and choroid. The occlusions are caused primarily by the cellular reaction to the emboli (Kaga et al., 1982). The neovascular lesions of the talc retinopathy are thought to be associated with peripheral arteriolar nonperfusion, which leads to retinal ischemia and secondary neovascularization (Tse and Ober, 1980).

Ocular Manifestations

Fundus examination reveals multiple, tiny, yellow-white, glistening particles scattered throughout the posterior pole, but they are more numerous in the capillary bed and small arterioles of the perimacular area (Fig. 13) (Atlee, 1972). Some patients can also have macular edema, dotlike and flame-shaped hemorrhages, as well as arterial occlusion.

Retinal neovascularization can appear in the retinal periphery as neovascular tufts in the shape of sea fans at the junction of the perfused and nonperfused retina. This is a potentially serious complication of talc injection because it can lead to retinal detachment, vitreal hemorrhage, and optic disc neovascularization (Bluth and Hanscom, 1981).

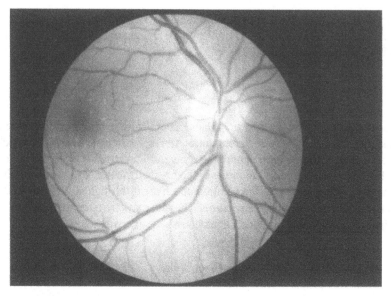

FIG. 13. Talc retinopathy characterized by numerous yellow-white intraarteriolar particles scattered throughout the perimacular area. (From Jaanus et al., 1995.)

Most patients have no significant visual symptoms (Bluth and Hanscom, 1981). Some patients, however, may report blurred vision, blind spots in the visual fields, and occasionally may have severe reduction of vision.

Patient Management

Because of the psychological and emotional implications involved in the diagnosis, the practitioner must rule out other conditions that may have a similar clinical appearance. The differential diagnosis includes Gunn's dots, multiple cholesterol emboli, drusen, and Stargardt's disease. Once the diagnosis has been established, appropriate drug abuse counseling should be offered to prevent further risk of severe pulmonary or ocular complications. Consideration should also be given to pulmonary consultation since patients with eye findings usually have acute or chronic impairment of pulmonary function (Paré et al., 1979). Proliferative retinopathy can be treated with the use of laser photocoagulation, and vitreal hemorrhage may require vitrectomy (Tse and Ober, 1980).

REFERENCES

Abel, A., and Leopold, I.H., 1980. Ocular diseases. In *Drug Treatment*, ed. J.S. Avery, Chap. 12. New York: Adis Press.

Addington, W.W., 1979. The side effects and interactions of anti-tuberculosis drugs. *Chest* 76(suppl):782–784.

Ahmad, S., 1990. Disopyramide: pulmonary complications and glaucoma. *Mayo Clinic Proceedings* 65:1030–1031.

Alexander, L.J., Bowerman, L., and Thompson, L.R., 1985. The prevalence of the ocular side effects of chlorpromazine in the Tuscaloosa Veterans Administration patient population. *Journal of the American Optometric Association* 56:872–876.

Alkemade, P.P.H., 1968. Phenothiazine retinopathy. *Ophthalmologica* 155:70–76.

Almog, Y., Monselise, M., Almog, C.H., et al., 1983. The effect of oral treatment with beta blockers on tear secretion. *Metabolic Pediatric Systemic Ophthalmology* 6:343–345.

AL-Tweigeri, T., Nabholtz, J.-M., and Mackey, J.R., 1996. Ocular toxicity and cancer chemotherapy. A review. *Cancer* 78:1359–1373.

Alvaro, M.E., 1943. Effects other than antiinfections of sulfonamide compounds on eye. *Archives of Ophthalmology* 29:615–632.

Astle, J.N., and Ellis, P.P., 1974. Ocular complications in renal transplant patients. *Annals of Ophthalmology* 6:1269–1274.

Atlee, W.E., 1972. Talc and cornstarch emboli in eyes of drug abusers. *Journal of the American Medical Association* 219:49–51.

Balik, J., 1958. Effect of atropine and pilocarpine on the secretion of chloride ion into the tears. *Ceskia Ophthalmology* 14:28–33.

Banks, C.N., 1987. Melanin: blackguard or red herring? Another look at chloroquine retinopathy. *Australian and New Zealand Journal of Ophthalmology* 15:365–370.

Barron, G.J., Tepper, L., and Iovine, G., 1974. Ocular toxicity from ethambutol. *American Journal of Ophthalmology* 77:256–260.

Bartlett, J.D., and Jaanus, S.D., 1989. Ocular effects of systemic drugs. In *Clinical Ocular Pharmacology*, eds. J.D. Bartlett and S.D. Jaanus, pp. 801–842. Stoneham, MA: Butterworth.

Bartlett, J.D., Novack, G.D., Hiett, J.A., et al., 1995. Antiglaucoma drugs. In *Clinical Ocular Pharmacology*, 3rd ed, eds. J.D. Bartlett and S.D. Jaanus, pp. 183–248. Boston: Butterworth-Heinemann.

Beebe, W.E., Abbott, R.L., and Fund, W.E., 1986. Hydroxychloroquine crystals in the tear film of a patient with rheumatoid arthritis. *American Journal of Ophthalmology* 101:377–378.

Bernstein, H.N., 1967. Chloroquine ocular toxicity. *Survey of Ophthalmology* 12:415–447.

Bernstein, H.N., and Ginsberg, J., 1964. The pathology of chloroquine retinopathy. *Archives of Ophthalmology* 71:238–245.

Bernstein, N.H., 1970. Some iatrogenic ocular diseases from systemically administered drugs. *International Ophthalmology Clinics* 10:553–619.

Bigby, M., and Stern, R.S., 1988. Adverse reactions to isotretinoin. A report from the adverse drug reaction reporting system. *Journal of the American Academy of Dermatology* 18:543–552.

Binnion, P.F., and Frazer, G., 1980. [3]H digoxin in the optic tract in digoxin intoxication. *Journal of Cardiovascular Pharmacology* 2:699–706.

Bishara, S.A., and Matamoros, N., 1989. Evaluation of several tests in screening for chloroquine maculopathy. *Eye* 3:777–782.

Bittencourt, P., Wade, P., Richens, A., et al., 1980. Blood alcohol and eye movements. *The Lancet* 16:981.

Black, R.L., Oglesby, R.B., vonSallmann, L., et al., 1960. Posterior subcapsular cataracts induced by corticosteroids in patients with rheumatoid arthritis. *Journal of the American Medical Association* 174:166–171.

Bluming, A.Z., and Zeegen, P., 1986. Cataracts induced by intermittent Decadron used as an antiemetic. *Journal of Clinical Oncology* 4:221–223.

Bluth, L.L., and Hanscom, T.A., 1981. Retinal detachment and vitreous hemorrhage due to talc emboli. *Journal of the American Medical Association* 246:980–981.

Borthne, A., 1976. The treatment of glaucoma with propranolol (Inderal). A clinical trial. *Acta Ophthalmologica* 54:291–300.

Bovino, J.A., and Marcus, D.F., 1982. The mechanism of transient myopia induced by sulfonamide therapy. *American Journal of Ophthalmology* 94:999.

Brinkley, J.R., Dubois, E.L., and Ryan, S.J., 1979. Long-term course of chloroquine retinopathy after cessation of medication. *American Journal of Ophthalmology* 88:1–11.

Brinton, G.S., Norton, E.W.D., Zahn, J.R., et al., 1980. Ocular quinine toxicity. *American Journal of Ophthalmology* 90:403–410.

British Photodermatology Group., 1994. British Photodermatology Group guidelines for PUVA. *British Journal of Dermatology* 130:246–255.

Bron, A.J., 1973. Vortex patterns of the corneal epithelium. *Transactions of the Ophthalmology Society United Kingdom* 43:455–472.

Brothers, D.M., and Hidayat, A.A., 1981. Conjunctival pigmentation associated with tetracycline medication. *Ophthalmology* 88:1212–1215.

Bucala, R., Fishman, J., and Cerami, A., 1982. Formation of covalent adducts between cortisol and 16 α-hydroxyesterone and protein: possible role in the pathogenesis of cortisol toxicity and systemic lupus erythematosus. *Proceedings of the National Academy of Science USA* 79:3320–3324.

Burns, C.A., 1968. Indomethacin, reduced retinal sensitivity, and corneal deposits. *American Journal of Ophthalmology* 66:825–835.

Butler, V.P., Odel, J.G., Rath, E., et al., 1995. Digitalis-induced visual disturbances with therapeutic serum digitalis concentrations. *Annals of Internal Medicine* 123:676–680.

Cairns, R.H., Capoore, H.S., and Gregory, J.D.R., 1965. Oculocutaneous changes after years of high doses of chlorpromazine. *The Lancet* 1:239–241.

Calkins, L.L., 1958. Corneal epithelial changes occurring during chloroquine (Aralen) therapy. *Archives of Ophthalmology* 60:981–988.

Cameron, M.E., Lawrence, J.M., and Olrich, J.G., 1972. Thioridazine (Mellaril) retinopathy. *British Journal of Ophthalmology* 56:131–134.

Carberg, O., 1966. Three cases of chloroquine retinopathy. A follow-up investigation. *Acta Ophthalmologica* 44:367–374.

Carr, R.E., and Henkind, P., 1962. Ocular manifestations of ethambutol. Toxic amblyopia after administration of an experimental anti-tuberculosis drug. *Archives of Ophthalmology* 67:50–55.

Chew, E., Ghosh, M., and McCulloch, C., 1982. Amiodarone-induced corneal verticillate. *Canadian Journal of Ophthalmology* 17:96–99.

Chirls, I.A., and Norris, J.W., 1984. Transient myopia associated with vaginal sulfanilamide suppositories. *American Journal of Ophthalmology* 98:120–121.

Chrousos, G.A., Oldfield, E.H., Doppman, J.L., et al., 1986. Prevention of ocular toxicity of carmustine (BCNU) with supraophthalmic intracarotid infusion. *Ophthalmology* 93:1471–1475.

Citron, K.M., and Thomas, G.O., 1986. Ocular toxicity from ethambutol. *Thorax* 41:737–739.

Coakes, R.L., and Brubaker, R.F., 1978. The mechanism of timolol in lowering intraocular pressure in the normal eye. *Archives of Ophthalmology* 96:2045–2048.

Connell, E.B., and Kelman, C.D., 1968. Ophthalmologic findings with oral contraceptives. *Obstetrics and Gynecology* 17:1–6.

Covell, L.L., 1958. Glaucoma induced by systemic steroid therapy. *American Journal of Ophthalmology* 45:108–109.

Cox, N.H., Jones, S.K., Downey, D.J., et al., 1987. Cutaneous and ocular side effects of oral photochemotherapy: results of an 8-year follow-up study. *British Journal of Dermatology* 116:145–152.

Crandall, D.C., and Leopold, I.H., 1979. The influence of systemic drugs on tear constituents. *Ophthalmology* 86:115–125.

Crews, S.J., 1963. Posterior subcapsular lens opacities in patients on long-term corticosteroid therapy. *British Medical Journal* 1:1644–1647.

Cruciani, F., Tamanti, N., Abdolrahimzadeh, S., et al., 1994. Ocular toxicity of systemic chemotherapy with megadoses of carmustine and mitomycin. *Annals of Ophthalmology* 26:97–100.

Cruess, A.F., Schachat, A.P., Nicholl, J., et al., 1985. Chloroquine retinopathy. Is fluorescein angiography necessary? *Ophthalmology* 92:1127–1129.

Cullen, A.P., and Chou, B.R., 1986. Keratopathy with low dose chloroquine therapy. *Journal of the American Optometric Association* 57:368–372.

Cumming, R.G., Mitchell, P., and Leeder, S.R., 1997. Use of inhaled corticosteroids and the risk of cataracts. *New England Journal of Medicine* 337:8–14.

D'Amico, D.S., and Kenyon, R.R., 1981. Drug-induced lipidoses in the cornea and conjunctiva. *International Ophthalmology* 4:67–76.

Davidorf, F.H., 1973. Thioridazine pigmentary retinopathy. *Archives of Ophthalmology* 90:251–255.

Deluise, V.P., and Flynn, J.T., 1981. Asymmetric anterior segment changes induced by chloropromazine. *Annals of Ophthalmology* 13:953–955.

DePalma, P., Franco, F., Bragliani, G., et al., 1989. The incidence of optic neuropathy in 84 patients treated with ethambutol. *Metabolic Pediatric Systemic Ophthalmology* 12:80–82.

DeVita, E.G., Miao, M., and Sadun, A.A., 1987. Optic neuropathy in ethambutol-treated renal tuberculosis. *Journal of Clinical Neuro Ophthalmology* 7:77–83.

Diotallevi, M., and Bocci, N., 1965. Effect of systemically administered corticosteroids on intraocular pressure and fluid dynamics. *Acta Ophthalmologica* 43:524–527.

Dolan, B.J., Flach, A.J., and Peterson, J.S., 1985. Amiodarone keratopathy and lens opacities. *Journal of the American Optometric Association* 56:468–470.

Drill, V.A., Rao, K.S., McConnell, R.G., et al., 1975. Ocular effects of oral contraceptives. I. Studies in the dog. *Fertility and Sterility* 26:908–913.

Duff, G.R., 1987. The effect of twice daily nadolol on intraocular pressure. *American Journal of Ophthalmology* 104:343–345.

Duncker, G., and Bredehorn, T., 1996. Chloroquine-induced lipidosis in the rat retina: functional and morphological changes after withdrawal of the drug. *Graefe's Archives of Clinical and Experimental Ophthalmology* 234:378–381.

Duncker, G.I.W., Kisters, G., and Grille, W., 1994. Prospective, randomized, placebo-controlled, double-blind testing of colour vision and electroretinogram at therapeutic and subtherapeutic digitoxin serum levels. *Ophthalmologica* 208:259–261.

Durkee, D.P., and Bryant, B.G., 1978. Drug therapy reviews: drug therapy of glaucoma. *American Journal of Hospital Pharmacists* 35:682–690.

Dyson, E.H., Proudfoot, A.T., and Bateman, D.N., 1985–86. Quinine amblyopia: is current management appropriate? *Clinical Toxicology* 23:571–578.

Easterbrook, M., 1987. Dose relationships in patients with early chloroquine retinopathy. *Journal of Rheumatology* 14:472–475.

Easterbrook, M., 1988. Ocular effects and safety of antimalarial agents. *American Journal of Medicine* 85:23–29.

Easterbrook, M., 1990. Is corneal deposition of antimalarial any indication of retinal toxicity? *Canadian Journal of Ophthalmology* 25:249–251.

Editorial., 1969. Iatrogenic symptoms in ophthalmology. *British Medical Journal* 2:199–200.

Ehrenfeld, M., Mesher, R., and Merin, S., 1986. Delayed-onset chloroquine retinopathy. *British Journal of Ophthalmology* 70:281–283.

Eke, T., and Bates, A.K., 1997. Acute angle-closure glaucoma associated with paroxetine. *British Medical Journal* 314:1387.

Ensink, B.W., and VanVoorst Vader, P.C., 1983. Ophthalmological side effects of 13-cis-retinoic therapy. *British Journal of Dermatology* 108:637–641.

Erickson, O.F., 1960. Drug influences on lacrimal lysozyme production. *Stanford Medical Bulletin* 18:34–49.

Faust, J.M., and Tyler, E.T., 1966. Ophthalmologic findings in patients using oral contraception. *Fertility and Sterility* 17:1–6.

Feiler-Ofry, V., Godel, V., and Stein, R., 1972. Systemic steroids and ocular fluid dynamics. III. The genetic nature of the ocular response and its different levels. *Acta Ophthalmologica* 50:699–706.

Felix, F.H., Ive, F.A., and Dahl, M.G.C., 1975. Cutaneous and ocular reactions with practolol administration. Oculomucocutaneous syndrome. *British Medical Journal* 1:595–598.

Finbloom, D.S., Silver, K., Newsome, D.A., et al., 1985. Comparison of hydroxychloroquine and chloroquine use and the development of retinal toxicity. *Journal of Rheumatology* 12:692–694.

Flach, A.J., Dolan, B.J., Sudduth, B., et al., 1983. Amiodarone-induced lens opacities. *Archives of Ophthalmology* 101:1554–1556.

Flach, A.J., and Dolan, B.J., 1990. Amiodarone-induced lens opacities: an eight-year follow-up study. *Archives of Ophthalmology* 108:1668–1669.

Fleck, B.W., Bell, A.L., Mitchell, J.D., et al., 1985. Screening for antimalarial maculopathy in rheumatology clinics. *British Medical Journal* 291:782–784.

Fraunfelder, F.T., 1980. Orange tears. *American Journal of Ophthalmology* 89:752.

Fraunfelder, F.T., 1982. *Drug-Induced Ocular Side Effects and Drug Interactions*, 2nd ed. Philadelphia: Lea and Febiger.

Fraunfelder, F.T., Baico, J.M., and Meyer, S.M., 1985. Adverse ocular reactions possibly associated with isotretinoin. *American Journal of Ophthalmology* 100:534–537.

Fraunfelder, F.T., and Meyer, S.M., 1982. The national registry of drug-included ocular side effects. *Journal of Toxicology and Cutaneous Ocular Toxicology* 1:65–70.

Fraunfelder, F.T., and Meyer, S.M., 1990. Posterior subcapsular cataracts associated with nasal or inhalation corticosteroids. *American Journal of Ophthalmology* 109:489–490.

Fraunfelder, F.T., and Randall, J.A., 1997. Minocycline-induced scleral pigmentation. *Ophthalmology* 104:936–938.

Frucht, J., Freimann, I., and Merin, S., 1984. Ocular side effects of disopyramide. *British Journal of Ophthalmology* 68:890–891.

Furst, C., Smiley, W.K., and Ansell, B.M., 1966. Steroid cataract. *Annals of Rheumatology Diseases* 25:364–368.

Gangitano, J.L., and Keltner, J.L., 1980. Abnormalities of the pupil and visual-evoked potential in quinine amblyopia. *American Journal of Ophthalmology* 89:425–430.

Garrett, C.R., 1985. Optic neuritis in a patient on ethambutol and isoniazid evaluated by visual evoked potentials: case report. *Military Medicine* 150:43–46.

Ghosh, M., and McCulloch, C., 1984. Amiodarone-induced ultrastructural changes in human eyes. *Canadian Journal of Ophthalmology*, 19:178–186.

Gittinger, J.W., and Asdourian, G.K., 1987. Papillopathy caused by amiodarone. *Archives of Ophthalmology* 105:349–351.

Godel, V., Feiler-Ofry, V., and Stein, R., 1972a. Systemic steroids and ocular fluid dynamics. I. Analysis of the sample as a whole. Influence of dosage and duration of therapy. *Acta Ophthalmologica* 50:655–663.

Godel, V., Feiler-Ofry, V., and Stein, R., 1972b. Systemic steroids and ocular fluid dynamics. II. Systemic vs. Topical steroids. *Acta Ophthalmologica* 50:664–676.

Godel, V., Loewenstein, A., and Lazar, M., 1990. Spectral electroretinography in thioridazine toxicity. *Annals of Ophthalmology* 22:293–296.

Godel, V., Nemet, P., and Lazar, M., 1980. Chloramphenicol optic neuropathy. *Archives of Ophthalmology* 98:1417–1421.

Gold, J.A., Shupack, J.L., and Nemec, M.A., 1989. Ocular side effects of the retinoids. *International Journal of Dermatology* 28:218–225.

Goldhammer, Y., and Smith, J.L., 1974. Bitemporal hemianopia in chloroquine retinopathy. *Neurology* 24:1135–1138.

Gombos, G.M., Moreno, D.A., and Bedrossian, P.B., 1975. Retinal vascular occlusion induced by oral contraceptives. *Annals of Ophthalmology* 7:215–217.

Goren, S.B., 1967. Retinal edema secondary to oral contraceptives. *American Journal of Ophthalmology* 64:447–449.

Gottlieb, N.L., and Major, J.C., 1978. Ocular chrysiasis correlated with gold concentrations in the crystalline lens during chrysotherapy. *Arthritis and Rheumatology* 21:704–708.

Graham, C.M., and Blach, R.K., 1988. Indomethacin retinopathy: case report and review. *British Journal of Ophthalmology* 72:434–438.

Griffiths, M.F.P., 1987. Tamoxifen retinopathy at low dosage. *American Journal of Ophthalmology* 104:185–186.

Guerra, R., and Casu, L., 1981. Hydroxycobalamin for ethambutol-induced optic neuropathy. *The Lancet* 2:1176.

Hall, S.K., 1994. Acute angle-closure glaucoma as a complication of combined β-agonist and ipratropium bromide therapy in the emergency department. *Annals of Emergency Medicine* 23:884–887.

Halmagyi, G.M., Lessell, I., Curthoys, I.S., et al., 1989. Lithium-induced downbeat nystagmus. *American Journal of Ophthalmology* 107:664–670.

Halperin, E., and Yolton, R.L., 1986. Is the driver drunk? Oculomotor sobriety testing. *Journal of the American Optometric Association* 57:654–657.

Hanna, N., Lachapelle, P., Roy, M.-S., et al., 1995. Alterations in the electroretinogram of newborn piglets by propionic acid-derivative nonsteroidal anti-inflammatory drugs but not by indomethacin and diclofenac. *Pediatric Research* 37:81–85.

Harley, R.D., Huang, N.N., Macri, C.H., et al., 1970. Optic neuritis and optic atrophy following chloramphenicol in cystic fibrosis patients. *Transactions of the American Academy of Ophthalmology and Otolaryngology* 74:1011–1031.

Hart, W.M., Burde, R.M., Johnston, G.P., et al., 1984. Static perimetry in chloroquine retinopathy. Perifoveal patterns of visual field depression. *Archives of Ophthalmology* 102:377–380.

Haug, S.J., and Friedman, A.H., 1991. Identification of amiodarone in corneal deposits. *American Journal of Ophthalmology* 111:518–520.

Haustein, K.-O., Oltmanns, G., Rietbrock, N., et al., 1982. Differences in color vision impairment caused by digoxin, digitoxin, or pengitoxin. *Journal of Cardiovascular Pharmacology* 4:536–541.

Hays, G.B., Lyle, C.B., and Wheeler, C.E., 1964. Slate gray color in patients receiving chlorpromazine. *Archives of Dermatology* 90:471–476.

Heel, R.C., Brogden, R.N., Speight, T.M., and Avery, G.S., 1979. Atenolol: A review of its pharmacological properties and therapeutic efficacy in angina pectoris and hypertension. *Drugs* 17:425–460.

Heier, J.S., Dragoo, R.A., Enzenauer, R.W., et al., 1994. Screening for ocular toxicity in asymptomatic patients treated with tamoxifen. *American Journal of Ophthalmology* 117:772–775.

Henkes, H.E., 1967. Electro-oculography as a diagnostic aide in phenothiazine retinopathy. *Transactions of the Ophthalmology Society United Kingdom* 87:285–287.

Henkes, H.E., vanLith, G.H.M., and Canta, L.R., 1972. Indomethacin retinopathy. *American Journal of Ophthalmology* 73:846–856.

Henkind, P., Parr, R.E., and Siegel I.M., 1964. Early chloroquine retinopathy: clinical and functional findings. *Archives of Ophthalmology* 71:157–165.

Hiatt, R.L., Fuller, I.B., Smith, L., et al., 1970. Systemically administered anticholinergic drugs and intraocular pressure. *Archives of Ophthalmology* 84:735–740.

Hobbs, H.E., Eadie, S.P., and Somerville, F., 1961. Ocular lesions after treatment with chloroquine. *British Journal of Ophthalmology* 45:284–298.

Hook, S.R., Holladay, J.T., Prager, T.C., et al., 1986. Transient myopia induced by sulfonamides. *American Journal of Ophthalmology* 101:495–496.

Horgan, S.E., and Williams, R.W., 1995. Chronic retinal toxicity due to quinine in Indian tonic water. *Eye* 9:637–638.

Houle, R.E., and Grant, W.M., 1967. Alcohol, vasopressin and intraocular pressure. *Investigative Ophthalmology* 6:145–154.

Howell, R., 1957. Treatment of discoid lupus erythematosus. *St John's Hospital Dermatology Society* 39:48.

Huang, N.N., Harley, R.D., Promadhattavedi, V., et al., 1966. Visual disturbances in cystic fibrosis following chloramphenicol administration. *Journal of Pediatrics* 68:32–44.

Ingram, D.V., Jaggarao, N.S.V., and Chamberlain, D.A., 1982. Ocular changes resulting from therapy with amiodarone. *British Journal of Ophthalmology* 66:676–679.

Jaanus, S.D., Lesher, G.A., 1995. Anti-inflammatory drugs. In *Clinical Ocular Pharmacology*, 3rd ed., eds. J.D. Bartlett and S.D. Jaanus, pp. 303–335. Boston: Butterworth-Heinemann.

Jaanus, S.D., Bartlett, J.D., and Hiett, J.A., 1995. Ocular effects of systemic drugs. In *Clinical Ocular Pharmacology*, 3rd ed., eds. J.D. Bartlett and S.D. Jaanus, pp. 957–1006. Boston: Butterworth-Heinemann.

Johnson, M.W., and Vine, A.K., 1987. Hydroxychloroquine therapy in massive total doses without retinal toxicity. *American Journal of Ophthalmology* 104:139–144.

Juzych, M.S., and Zimmerman, T.J., 1997. Beta-blockers. In *Textbook of Ocular Pharmacology*, ed. T.J. Zimmerman, pp. 261–275. Philadelphia: Lippincott-Raven.

Kaga, N., Tso, M.O.M., and Jampol, L.M., 1982. Talc retinopathy in primates: a model of ischemic retinopathy. III. An electron microscopic study. *Archives of Ophthalmology* 100:1649–1657.

Kaiser-Kupfer, M.I., Kupfer, C., and Rodriques, M.M., 1982. Tamoxifen retinopathy. A clinicopathologic report. *Ophthalmology* 100:1766–1772.

Kaiser-Kupfer, M.I., and Lippman, M.E., 1978. Tamoxifen retinopathy. *Cancer Treatment Report* 62:315–320.

Kakisu, Y., Adachi-Usami, E., and Mizota, A., 1988. Pattern electroretinogram and visual evoked cortical potential in ethambutol optic neuropathy. *Documenta Ophthalmologica* 67:327–334.

Kaplan, L.J., and Cappaert, W.E., 1982. Amiodarone keratopathy. Correlation to dosage and duration. *Archives of Ophthalmology* 100:601–602.

Keith, C.G., 1964. Optic atrophy induced by chloramphenicol. *British Journal of Ophthalmology* 48:567–570.

Kimbrough, B.O., and Campbell, R.J., 1981. Thioridazine levels in the human eye. *Archives of Ophthalmology* 99:2188–2189.

Kingham, J.D., Chen, M.C., and Levy, M.H., 1988. Macular hemorrhage in the aging eye: the effects of anticoagulants. *New England Journal of Medicine* 318:1126–1127.

Kingele, T.G., Alves, L.E., and Rose, E.P., 1984. Amiodarone keratopathy. *Annals of Ophthalmology* 16:1172–1176.

Kirwan, J.F., Subak-Sharpe, I., and Teimory, M., 1997. Bilateral acute angle-closure glaucoma after administration of paroxetine. *British Journal of Ophthalmology* 81:252.

Kjaer, G.C.D., 1968. Retinopathy associated with phenothiazine administration. *Diseases of the Nervous System* 29:316–319.

Kobayashi, Y., Akaishi, K., Nishio, T., et al., 1974. Posterior subcapsular cataract in nephrotic children receiving steroid therapy. *American Journal of Diseaser in Children* 128:671–673.

Koeffler, B.H., and Lemp, M.A., 1980. The effect of an antihistamine (chlorpheniramine maleate) on tear production in human. *American Journal of Ophthalmology* 12:217–219.

Koetting, R.A., 1966. The influence of oral contraceptives on contact lens wear. *American Journal of Optometry and Archives of the American Academy of Optometry* 43:268–274.

Kolb, H., 1965. Electro-oculogram findings in patients treated with antimalarial drugs. *British Journal of Ophthalmology* 49:573–589.

Koliopoulos, J., and Palimeris, G., 1972. On acquired colour vision disturbances during treatment with ethambutol and indomethacin. *Modern Problems in Ophthalmology* 11:178–184.

Koneru, P.B., Lien, E.J., and Koda, R.T., 1986. Oculotoxicities of systemically administered drugs. *Journal of Ocular Pharmacology* 2:385–404.

Kreig, P.H., and Schipper, I., 1996. Drug-induced ciliary body oedema: a new theory. *Eye* 10:121–126.

Kremer, I., Gaton, D.D., David, M., et al., 1994. Toxic effects of systemic retinoids on meibomian glands. *Ophthalmic Research* 26:124–128.

Krill, A.E., Potts, A.M., and Johanson, C.E., 1976. Chloroquine retinopathy. Investigation of discrepancy between dark adaptation and electroretinographic findings in advanced stages. *American Journal of Ophthalmology* 54:819–826.

Kristensen, P., 1968. Posterior subcapsular cataract (PSC) and systemic steroid therapy. *Acta Ophthalmologica* 46:1025–1032.

Krupin, T., Kolker, A.E., and Becker, B., 1967. Alcohol and intraocular pressure. *Investigative Ophthalmology* 6:559–560.

Kuming, B.S., and Braude, L., 1979. Anterior optic neuritis caused by ethambutol toxicity. *South African Medical Journal* 55:4.

Kupersmith, M.J., Frohman, L.P., Choi, I.S., et al., 1988. Visual system toxicity following intra-arterial chemotherapy. *Neurology* 38:284–289.

Lam, R.W., Allain, S., Sullivan, K., et al., 1997. Effects of chronic lithium treatment on electrophysiologic function. *Biological Psychiatry* 41:737–742.

Leopold, I.H., and Comroe, J.H., 1948. Effect of intramuscular administration of morphine, atropine, scopolamine and neostigmine on the human eye. *Archives of Ophthalmology* 40:285–290.

Lerman, S., Megaw, J., and Willis, I., 1980. The photoreactions of 8-methoxypsoralen with tryptophan and lens proteins. *Photochemistry and Photobiology* 31:235.

Lerman, S., 1986. Photosensitizing drugs and their possible role in enhancing ocular toxicity. *Ophthalmology* 93:304–313.

Lerman, S., Megaw, J., and Garner, K., 1982. Psoralens. Long-wave ultraviolet therapy and human cataractogenesis. *Investigative Ophthalmology and Visual Science* 23:801.

Lieberman, E., and Stoudemiere, A., 1987. Use of tricyclic antidepressants in patients with glaucoma. Assessment and appropriate precautions. *Psychosomatics* 28:145–148.

Lieberman, T.W., 1968. Ocular effects of prolonged systemic drug administration corticosteroids, chloramphenicol, and anovulatory agents). *Diseases of the Nervous System* 29:44–50.

Limaye, S.R., Pillai, S., and Tina, L.U., 1988. Relationship of steroid dose to degree of posterior subcapsular cataracts in nephrotic syndrome. *Annals of Ophthalmology* 20:225–227.

Lindholm, B., Linner, E., and Tengroth, B., 1965. Effects of long-term systemic steroids on cataract formation and on aqueous humor dynamics. *Acta Ophthalmologica* 43:120–127.

Longstaff, S., Sigurdsson, H., O'Keeffe, M., et al., 1989. A controlled study of the ocular effects of tamoxifen in conventional dosage in the treatment of breast carcinoma. *European Journal of Cancer and Clinical Oncology* 25:1805–1808.

Loredo, A., Rodriguez, R.S., and Murillo, L., 1972. Cataracts after short-term corticosteroid treatment. *New England Journal of Medicine* 286:160.

Lozier, J.R., and Friedlaender, M.H., 1989. Complications of antimalarial therapy. *International Ophthalmology Clinics* 29:172–178.

Lyons, R.W., 1979. Orange contact lenses from rifampin. *New England Journal of Medicine* 300:372.

Macdonald, M.J., Cullen, P.M., and Phillips, C.I., 1976. Atenolol vs. Propranolol. *British Journal of Ophthalmology* 60:789–791.

Mackie, I.A., Seal, D.V., and Pescod, J.M., 1977. Beta-adrenergic receptor blocking drugs: tear lysozyme and immunological screening for adverse reactions. *British Journal of Ophthalmology* 61:354–359.

Maddallena, M.A., 1984. Transient myopia associated with acute glaucoma and retinal edema. *Archives of Ophthalmology* 98:120–121.

Mader, T.H., and Stulting, R.D., 1991. Keratoconjunctivitis sicca caused by diphenoxylate hydrochloride with atropine sulfate (Lomotil). *American Journal of Ophthalmology* 111:377–378.

Madreperla, S.A., Johnson, M.A., and Nakatani, K., 1994. Electrophysiologic and electroretinographic evidence for photoreceptor dysfunction as a toxic effect of digoxin. *Archives of Ophthalmology* 112:807–812.

Mandak, J.S., Minerva, P., Wilson, T.W., et al., 1996. Angle-closure glaucoma complicating systemic atropine use in the cardiac catheterization laboratory. *Catheterization and Cardiovascular Diagnosis* 39:262–264.

Mantyjarvi, M., 1985. Hydroxychloroquine treatment in the eye. *Scandinavian Journal of Rheumatology* 14:171–174.

Marks, J.S., and Power, B.J., 1979. Is chloroquine obsolete in treatment of rheumatic disease? *The Lancet* 1:171–173.

Marmor, M.F., 1990. Is thioridazine retinopathy progressive? Relationship of pigmentary changes to visual function. *British Journal of Ophthalmology* 74:739–742.

Marre, M., Neubauer, O., and Nemetz, U., 1974. Colour vision and the "pill." *Modern Problems in Ophthalmology* 13:345–348.

Martin, L.J., Bergen, R.L., and Dobrow, H.R., 1978. Delayed onset chloroquine retinopathy: case report. *Annals of Ophthalmology* 10:723–726.

Mathalone, M.B.R., 1968. Ocular effects of phenothiazine derivatives and reversibility. *Diseases of the Nervous System* 29:29–35.

Mathers, W.D., Shields, W.J., Sachdev, M.S., et al., 1991. Meibomian gland morphology and tear osmolarity: changes with Accutane therapy. *Cornea* 10:286–290.

Mattsson, R., 1952. Transient myopia following the use of sulphonamides. *Acta Ophthalmologica* 30:385–398.

Mavrikakis, M., Papazoglou, S., Sfikakis, P.P., et al., 1996. Retinal toxicity in long-term hydroxychloroquine treatment. *Annals of Rheumatology Diseases* 55:187–189.

Mayan, C.I., Miller, D., and Tigerina, M.L., 1979. In vitro production of steroid cataract in bovine lens: II. Measurement of sodium-potassium adenosine triphosphatase activity. *Acta Ophthalmologica* 57:1107–1116.

Mazzuca, S.A., Yung, R., Brandt, K.D., et al., 1994. Current practices for monitoring ocular toxicity related to hydroxychloroquine (Plaquenil) therapy. *Journal of Rheumatology* 21:59–63.

McClanahan, W.S., Harris, J.E., Knobloch, W.H., et al., 1966. Ocular manifestations of chronic phenothiazine derivative administration. *Archives of Ophthalmology* 75:319–325.

McCormick, S.A., DiBartolomeo, G., Raju, V.K., et al., 1985. Ocular chrysiasis. *Ophthalmology* 92:1432–1435.

McGrand, J.C., and Cory, C.C., 1969. Ophthalmic disease and the pill. *British Medical Journal* 2:187.

McKeown, C.A., Swartz, M., Blom, J., et al., 1981. Tamoxifen retinopathy. *British Journal of Ophthalmology* 65:177–179.

Melon, J., and Register, M., 1976. Passage into normal salivary, lacrimal and nasal secretions of ampicillin and erythromycin administered intramuscularly. *Acta Otorhinolaryngology Belgium* 30:643–651.

Meredith, T.A., Aaberg, T.M., and Willerson, D., 1978. Progressive chorioretinopathy after receiving thioridazine. *Archives of Ophthalmology* 96:1172–1176.

Messmer, E., Font, R.L., Sheldon, G., et al., 1983. Pigmented conjunctival cysts following tetracycline/minocycline therapy. *Ophthalmology* 90:1462–1468.

Michelson, J.B., Whitcher, J.P., Wilson, S., et al., 1979. Possible foreign body granuloma of the retina associated with intravenous cocaine addiction. *American Journal of Ophthalmology* 87:278–280.

Mihm, L.M., and Barton, T.L., 1994. Tamoxifen-induced ocular toxicity. *Annals of Pharmacotherapy* 28:740–742.

Miller, D., 1973. Role of the tear film in contact lens wear. *International Ophthalmology Clinics* 13:247–262.

Miller, D.F., Bay, J.W., Lederman, R.J., et al., 1985. Ocular and orbital toxicity following intracarotid injection of BCNU (carmustine) and cisplatinum for malignant gliomas. *Ophthalmology* 92:402–406.

Miller, F.S., Bunt-Milam, A.H., and Kalina, R.E., 1982. Clinical ultrastructural study of thioridazine retinopathy. *Ophthalmology* 89:1478–1488.

Mills, P.V., Beck, M., and Tower, B.J., 1981. Assessment of the retinal toxicity of hydroxychloroquine. *Transactions of the Ophthalmology Society United Kingdom* 101:109–113.

Milson, J., Jones, D.H., and King, K., 1982. Ophthalmological effects of 13-*cis*-retinoic acid therapy for acne vulgaris. *British Journal of Dermatology* 107:491–495.

Miyata, M., Imai, H., Ishikawa, S., et al., 1980. Change in human electroretinography associated with thioridazine administration. *Ophthalmologica* 181:175–180.

Mortada, A., and Abboud, I., 1973. Retinal hemorrhages after prolonged use of salicylates. *British Journal of Ophthalmology* 57:199–200.

Nayfield, S.G., and Gorin, M.B., 1996. Tamoxifen-associated eye disease: a review. *Journal of Clinical Oncology* 14:1018–1026.

Neufeld, A.H., 1979. Experimental studies on the mechanism of action of timolol. *Survey of Ophthalmology* 23:363–370.

Neves, M.S., Jordan, K., and Dragt, H., 1990. Extensive chorioretinopathy associated with very low dose thioridazine. *Eye* 4:767–770.

Nielsen, C.E., Andreasen, F., and Bjerregaard, P., 1983. Amiodarone-induced corneal verticillata. *Acta Ophthalmologica* 61:474–480.

Nylander, U., 1966. Ocular damage in chloroquine therapy. *Acta Ophthalmologica* 44:335–348.

Ogawa, S., Kurumatani, N., Shibaike, N., et al., 1979. Progression of retinopathy long after cessation of chloroquine therapy. *The Lancet* 1:1408.

Oglesby, R.B., Black, R.L., vonSallmann, L., et al., 1961. Cataracts in patients with rheumatic diseases treated with corticosteroids. Further observations. *Archives of Ophthalmology* 66:625–630.

Ohrstrom, A., 1982. Dose response of oral timolol combined with adrenaline. *British Journal of Ophthalmology* 66:242–246.

Orlando, R.G., Dangel, M.E., and Schaal, S.F., 1984. Clinical experience and grading of amiodarone keratopathy. *Ophthalmology* 91:1184–1187.

Palimeris, G., Kolipoulis, J., and Velissaropoulos, P., 1972. Ocular side effects of indomethacin. *Ophthalmologica* 164:339–353.

Paré, J.A.P., Fraser, R.G., Hogg, J.C., et al., 1979. Pulmonary "mainline" granulomatosis: talcosis of intravenous methadone abuse. *Medicine* 58:229–239.

Pavlidis, N.A., Petris, C., Briassoulis, E., et al., 1992. Clear evidence that long-term, low-dose tamoxifen treatment can induce ocular toxicity. A prospective study of 63 patients. *Cancer* 69:2961–2964.

Pavlin, C.R., deVeber, G.A., Cook, G.T., et al., 1977. Ocular complications in renal transplant recipients. *Canadian Medical Association Journal* 117:360–362.

Peczon, J.D., and Grant, W.M., 1965. Glaucoma, alcohol, and intraocular pressure. *Archives of Ophthalmology* 73:495–501.

Percival, S.P.B., and Behrman, P., 1969. *Ophthalmological* safety of chloroquine. *British Journal of Ophthalmology* 53:101–109.

Peters, N.L., 1989. Snipping the thread of life. Antimuscarinic side effects of medications in the elderly. *Archives of Internal Medicine* 149:2414–2420.

Petrohelos, M.A., 1974. Chloroquine-induced ocular toxicity. *Annals of Ophthalmology* 6:615–618.

Phillips, C.I., Clayton, R.M., Cuthbert, J., et al., 1996. Human cataract risk factors: significance of abstention from, and high consumption of, ethanol (U-curve) and nonsignificance of smoking. *Ophthalmic Research* 28:237–247.

Pickrell, L., and Purvin, V., 1987. Ischemic optic neuropathy secondary to intracarotid infusion of BCNU. *Journal of Clinical Neuro Ophthalmology* 7:87–91.

Polak, B.C.P., Leys, M., and van Lith, G.H.M., 1985. Blue–yellow colour vision changes are early symptoms of ethambutol oculotoxicity. *Ophthalmologica* 191:223–226.

Postel, E.A., Assalian, A., and Epstein, D.L., 1996. Drug-induced transient myopia and angle-closure glaucoma associated with supraciliary choroidal effusion. *American Journal of Ophthalmology* 122:110–112.

Potts, A.M., 1962. The concentration of phenothiazines in the eye of experimental animals. *Investigative Ophthalmology* 1:522–530.

Pridmore, S., Powell, G., and Wise, G., 1996. Photophobia and lithium. *Australian/New Zealand Journal of Psychiatry* 30:287–289.

Prin, R.F., DeLong, S.L., Cole, J.O., et al., 1970. Ocular changes occurring with prolonged high dose chlorpromazine therapy. *Archives of General Psychiatry* 23:464–468.

Radnot, M., and Follmann, P., 1973. Ocular side effects of oral contraceptives. *Annals of Clinical Research* 5:197–204.

Ramsey, M.S., and Fine, B.S., 1972. Chloroquine toxicity in the human eye. Histopathologic observations by electron microscopy. *American Journal of Ophthalmology* 73:229–235.

Rasmussen, K., Kirk, L., and Faurbye, A., 1976. Deposits in the lens and cornea of the eye during long-term chlorpromazine medication. *Acta Psychiatry Scandinavia* 53:1–6.

Reifler, D.M., Verdier, D.D., Davy, C.L., et al., 1987. Multiple chalazia and rosacea in a patient treated with amiodarone. *American Journal of Ophthalmology* 103:594–595.

Rennie, I.G., and Smerdon, D.L., 1985. The effect of a once-daily oral dose of nadolol on intraocular pressure in normal volunteers. *American Journal of Ophthalmology* 100:445–447.

Rietbrock, N., and Alken, R.G., 1980. Color vision deficiencies: a common sign of intoxication in chronically digoxin-treated patients. *Journal of Cardiovascular Pharmacology* 2:93–99.

Roberts, S.M., 1974. A review of the papers on the ocular toxicity of ethambutol hydrochloride (Myambutol), an anti-tuberculosis drug. *American Journal of Optometry and Physiological Optometry* 51:987–992.

Robertson, D.M., Hollenhorst, R.W., and Callahan, J.A., 1966. Ocular manifestations of digitalis toxicity. Discussion and report of three cases of central scotomas. *Archives of Ophthalmology* 76:640–645.

Robertson, D.M., Hollenhorst, R.W., and Callahan, J.A., 1966. Receptor function and digitalis therapy. *Archives of Ophthalmology* 76:852–857.

Rooklin, A.R., Lampert, S.I., Jaeger, E.A., et al., 1979. Posterior subcapsular cataracts in steroid-requiring asthmatic children. *Journal of Allergy Clinics and Immunology* 63:383–386.

Rosenberg, M.L., 1983. Reversible downbeat nystagmus secondary to excessive alcohol intake. *Journal of Clinical Neuro Ophthalmology* 11:315–319.

Rosenthal, A.R., Kolb, H., Bergsma, D., et al., 1978. Chloroquine retinopathy in the rhesus monkey. *Investigative Ophthalmology and Visual Science* 17:1158–1175.

Ruben, M., 1966. Contact lenses and oral contraceptives. *British Medical Journal* 1:1110.

Rubin, M.L., and Thomas, W.C., 1970. Diplopia and loss of accommodation due to chloroquine. *Arthritis and Rheumatology* 13:75–82.

Ruskiewicz, J.P., 1983. Birth control linked to vein occlusion. *Review of Optometry* 120:58–60.

Russo, P.A., and Chaglasian, M.A., 1994. Toxic optic neuropathy associated with ethambutol: implications for current therapy. *Journal of the American Optometry Association* 65:332–338.

Rynes, R.I., Krohel, G., Falbo, A., et al., 1979. Ophthalmologic safety of long-term hydroxychloroquine treatment. *Arthritis and Rheumatology* 22:832–836.

Sabroe, R.A., Archer, C.B., Harlow, D., et al., 1996. Minocycline-induced discolouration of the sclerae. *British Journal of Dermatology* 135:314–316.

Salazar-Bookaman, M.M., Wainer, I., and Patil, P.N., 1994. Relevance of drug–melanin interactions to ocular pharmacology and toxicology. *Journal of Ocular Pharmacology* 10:217–239.

Salmon, J.F., Carmichael, T.R., and Welsh, N.H., 1987. Use of contrast sensitivity measurement in the detection of subclinical ethambutol toxic optic neuropathy. *British Journal of Ophthalmology* 71:192–196.

Schenker, J.G., Ivry, M., and Oliver, M., 1972. The effect of oral contraceptives on microcirculation. *Obstetrics and Gynecology* 39:909–916.

Scott, D., 1977. Another beta blocker causing eye problems. *British Medical Journal* 2:1221.

Shearer, R.V., and Dubois, E.L., 1967. Ocular changes induced by long-term hydroxychloroquine (Plaquenil) therapy. *American Journal of Ophthalmology* 64:245–252.

Shingleton, B.J., Bienfang, D.C., Albert, D.M., et al., 1982. Ocular toxicity associated with high-dose carmustine. *Archives of Ophthalmology* 100:1766–1772.

Siddall, J.R., 1965. The ocular toxic findings with prolonged and high dosage chlorpromazine intake. *Archives of Ophthalmology* 74:460–464.

Siddall, J.R., 1968. Ocular complications related to phenothiazines. *Diseases of the Nervous System* 29:10–13.

Silman, A., and Shipley, M., 1997. Ophthalmological monitoring for hydroxychloroquine toxicity: a scientific review of available data. *British Journal of Rheumatology* 36:599–601.

Skalka, H.W., and Prchal, J.T., 1980. Effect of corticosteroids on cataract formation. *Archives of Ophthalmology* 98:1773–1777.

Smith, M.S., and Kreiger, A., 1970. Visual loss associated with oral contraceptives. *American Journal of Ophthalmology* 69:874–876.

Smith, S.E., Smith, S.A., Reynolds, F., et al., 1979. Ocular and cardiovascular effects of local and systemic pindolol. *British Journal of Ophthalmology* 63:63–66.

Spaeth, G.L., Rodrigues, M.M., and Weinreb, S., 1977. Steroid-induced glaucoma. A. Persistent elevation of intraocular pressure. B. Histopathological aspects. *Transactions of the American Ophthalmology Society* 75:353–381.

Spaide, R.F., Diamond, G., D'Amico, R.A., et al., 1987. Ocular findings in cystic fibrosis. *American Journal of Ophthalmology* 103:204–210.

Stern, R.S., Parrish, J.A., and Fitzpatrick, T.B., 1985. Ocular findings in patients treated with PUVA. *Journal of Investigative Dermatology* 85:269.

Stowe, G.C., Zakov, Z.N., and Albert, D.M., 1978. Central retinal vascular occlusion associated with oral contraceptives. *American Journal of Ophthalmology* 86:798–801.

Sykowski, P., 1949. Digitoxin intoxication resulting in retrobulbar optic neuritis. *American Journal of Ophthalmology* 32:572–574.

Taylor, H.R., 1980. The environment and the lens. *British Journal of Ophthalmology* 64:303–310.

Tekell, J.L., Silva, J.A., Maas, J.A., et al., 1996. Thioridazine-induced retinopathy. *American Journal of Psychiatry* 153:1234–1235.

Terrell, W.L., Haik, K.G., and Haik, G.M., 1988. Hydroxychloroquine sulfate and retinopathy. *Southern Medical Journal* 81:1327–1328.

Thaler, J.S., 1979. The effect of multiple psychotropic drugs on the accommodation of prepresbyopes. *American Journal of Optometry and Physiological Optometry* 56:259–261.

Thaler, J.S., 1982. Effects of benztropine mesylate (Cogentin) on accommodation in normal volunteers. *American Journal of Optometry and Physiological Optometry* 59:918–919.

Thaler, J.S., Curinga, R., and Kiracofe, G., 1985. Relation of graded ocular anterior chamber pigmentation to phenothiazine intake in schizophrenics. Quantification procedures. *American Journal of Optometry and Physiological Optometry* 62:600–604.

Tierney, D.W., 1988. Ocular chrysiasis. *Journal of the American Optometry Association* 59:960–962.

Tiffany, D.V., 1986. Optometric expert testimony. Foundation for the horizontal gaze nystagmus test. *Journal of the American Optometry Association* 57:705–708.

Tilden, M.E., Rosenbaum, J.T., and Fraunfelder, F.T., 1990. Systemic sulfonamides as a cause of bilateral, anterior uveitis. *Archives of Ophthalmology* 109:67–69.

Tobin, D.R., Krohel, G.B., and Rymes, R.I., 1982. Hydroxychloroquine. Seven-year experience. *Archives of Ophthalmology* 100:81–83.

Trusiewicz, D., 1975. Farnsworth 100-Hue test in the diagnosis of ethambutol-induced damage to optic nerve. *Ophthalmologica* 171:425–431.

Tse, D.T., and Ober, R.R., 1980. Talc retinopathy. *American Journal of Ophthalmology* 90:624–640.

Ubels, J.L., and MacRae, S.M., 1984. Vitamin A is present as retinol in tears of humans and rabbits. *Current Eye Research* 3:815–817.

Urban, R.C., and Cotlier, E., 1986. Corticosteroid-induced cataracts. *Survey of Ophthalmology* 31:102–110.

Van Dijk, B.W., and Spekreijse, H., 1983. Ethambutol changes the color coding of carp retinal ganglion cells reversibly. *Investigative Ophthalmology and Visual Science* 24:128–133.

Varga, M., 1976. Recent experiences of the ophthalmologic complications of oral contraceptives. *Annals of Ophthalmology* 8:925–934.

Walker, G.F., 1961. Blindness during streptomycin and chloramphenicol therapy. *British Journal of Ophthalmology* 45:555–559.

Watson, W.T.A, Shuckett, E.P., Becker, A.B., et al., 1994. Effect of nebulized ipratropium bromide on intraocular pressures in children. *Chest* 105:1439–1441.

Weidle, E.G., 1987. Lenticular chrysiasis in oral chrysotherapy. *American Journal of Ophthalmology* 103:240–241.

Weleber, R.G., Denman, S.T., Hanifin, J.M., et al., 1986. Abnormal retinal function associated with isotretinoin therapy for acne. *Archives of Ophthalmology* 104:831–837.

Weleber, R.G., and Shults, W.T., 1981. Digoxin retinal toxicity. Clinical and electrophysiologic evaluation of cone dysfunction syndrome. *Archives of Ophthalmology* 99:1568–1572.

Werblin, T.P., and Peiffer, R.L., 1987. Persistent hemorrhage after extracapsular surgery associated with excessive aspirin ingestion. *American Journal of Ophthalmology* 105:426.

Wetterholm, D.H., and Winter, F.C., 1964. Histopathology of chloroquine retinal toxicity. *Archives of Ophthalmology* 71:116–121.

Wettrell, K., and Pandolfi, M., 1975. Effect of oral administration of various beta-blocking agents on the intraocular pressure in healthy volunteers. *Experimental Eye Research* 21:451–456.

Williams, D.P., Troost, B.T., and Rogers, J., 1988. Lithium-induced downbeat nystagmus. *Archives of Neurology* 45:1022–1023.

Wilson, D.M., Martin, J.H.S., and Niall, J.F., 1973. Raised intraocular tension in renal transplant recipients. *Medical Journal of Australia* 32:482–484.

Wilson, G., and Mitchell, R., 1983. The effect of alcohol on the visual and ocular motor systems. *Australian Journal of Ophthalmology* 11:315–319.

Wirz-Justice, A., Remé, C., Prunte, A., et al., 1997. Lithium decreases retinal sensitivity, but this is not cumulative with years of treatment. *Biological Psychiatry* 41:743–746.

Wood, J.R., 1977. Ocular complications of oral contraceptives. *Ophthalmology Seminars* 2:371–402.

Woung, L.-C., Jou, J.-R., and Liaw, S.-L., 1995. Visual function in recovered ethambutol optic neuropathy. *Journal of Ocular Pharmacology and Therapeutics* 11:411–419.

Yablonski, M.E., Zimmerman, T.J., Waltman, S.R., and Becker, B., 1978. A fluorophotometric study of the effect of topical timolol on aqueous humor dynamics. *Experimental Eye Research* 27:135–142.

Yasuhara, T., Nishida, K., Uchida, K., et al., 1996. Corneal endothelial changes in schizophrenic patients with long-term administration of major tranquilizers. *American Journal of Ophthalmology* 121:84–88.

Yiannikas, C., Walsh, J.C., and McLeod, J.G., 1983. Visual evoked potentials in the detection of subclinical optic toxic effects secondary to ethambutol. *Archives of Neurology* 40:645–648.

Yospaiboon, Y., Lawtiantong, T., and Chotibutr, S., 1984. Clinical observations of ocular quinine intoxication. *Japanese Journal of Ophthalmology* 28:409–415.

Ophthalmic Toxicology
Edited by George C. Y. Chiou
Copyright © 1999 Taylor & Francis

8

Ophthalmic Toxicity by Local Agents

George C. Y. Chiou

Institute of Ocular Pharmacology and Department of Medical Pharmacology and Toxicology, Texas A&M University College of Medicine, College Station, Texas USA

- Adrenergic Stimulants and Blockers
- Antiglaucoma Agents
- Miotics and Mydriatics
- Cholinesterase Inhibitors and Reactivators and Chemical Warfare Agents
- Autacoids and Antihistamines
- Cardiovascular Drugs
- Blood-Related Agents
- Vitamins
- Agents for Deficiency Anemias
- Sedatives, Hypnotics, and Tranquilizers
- Antidepressants and Antiparkinsonism Agents
- Local Anesthetics
- Analgesics
- Antirheumatic and Antigout Agents
- Agents for Respiratory Diseases
- Antispasmodics
- Gastrointestinal Agents
- Chemotherapeutic Agents
- Disinfectants
- Scabicides and Pediculicides
- Antineoplastic Agents
- Antiwart Agents
- Antimalarial Agents
- Anthelminthics and Amoebocides
- Adrenal Corticosteroids
- Dermatologic Agents
- Antiseptics
- Preservatives
- Dyes
- Ophthalmic Implants
- Antiperspirants

- **Counterirritants**
- **Chelating Agents**
- **Decongestants**
- **Astringents**
- **Surfactants**
- **Cosmetics**
- **Insecticides**
- **Fishes and Jellyfish**
- **Toxins and Venoms**
- **Plants**
- **Gases**
- **Iodides**
- **Solvents**
- **Foreign Bodies**
- **Gun Powder**
- **Smog**
- **Pencils and Ink**
- **Tar**
- **Acids and Bases**
- **Enzymes**
- **Rare-Earth Salts**
- **Agents for Agricultural Use**
- **Substances for Commercial Use**
- **Substances for Medicinal Use**
- **Agents of Industrial Use**
- **Air Pollutants**
  - Irritation to the Eye
  - Measurements of Eye Irritation
  - Volcanic Eruption
  - Nitrogen Compounds
  - Sulfur Compounds
  - Photochemical Oxidants
  - Building Pollutants
  - Formaldehyde
  - Pyrolytic End Products
  - Occupational Hazards
  - Ammonia
  - Carbon Disulfide
  - Hydrogen Sulfide
  - Ethylene Oxide
  - Cyanide
  - Hydrogen Fluoride
  - *n*-Hexane
  - Toluene Diisocyanate
  - Formaldehyde
- **References**

Ever since the methods of chemical synthesis were invented, tens of thousands of new chemicals have been introduced into the world every year. A large portion of these compounds are reported to be irritating to the eyes. Obviously, it is not possible to cover all these agents in this chapter. Only a very small portion of these agents will be mentioned here by giving some representative chemicals in each class of agents, based on their uses.

ADRENERGIC STIMULANTS AND BLOCKERS

Adrenergic drugs may be either direct acting or indirect acting. Direct-acting adrenergics break down into alpha-adrenergics, such as **phenylephrine** (which is discussed more in mydriatics), and beta-adrenergics, such as **isoprenaline.** Direct-acting adrenergics have the side effects of decreased intraocular pressure (IOP) and allergy and irritation of the eye of sensitized individuals. There are also adrenergics which are not specific for either alpha- or beta-adrenergic sites: **bamethan** (discussed under glaucoma tests) and **epinephrine** (discussed under antiglaucoma drugs). Other direct-acting adrenergics are **methoxamine** and **norepinephrine** (Fraunfelder, 1982; Fraunfelder and Scafidi, 1978; Haddad et al., 1970; McReynolds et al., 1956).

Indirect acting adrenergics produce a variety of side effects which tend to vary with the drug. **Amphetamine** falls within this class; it has the side effects of mydriasis and retraction of the upper lid. **Ephedrine** has many side effects, including conjunctival vasoconstriction, decreased vision, allergic reactions of the eyelids or conjunctiva of sensitized individuals, conjunctivitis, irritation (with the further symptoms of lacrimation, rebound hyperemia, and photophobia), mydriasis, and aqueous "floaters" (bits of pigment debris). Another indirect adrenergic is **naphazoline.** This drug has the side effects of mydriasis and punctate epithelial keratitis. **Norepinephrine** may cause a decrease in the IOP, and **methoxamine** may cause widening of the palpebral fissure (Fraunfelder, 1982; Mitchell, 1957; Drance and Ross, 1970; Hull, 1975; Gilman et al., 1980; Pollack and Rossi, 1975).

There are many dopaminergic drugs which act on the central nervous system, but the only one used on the eyes is **dopamine.** Ten percent eye drops of **dopamine** produce mydriasis; however, they do not affect accommodation (Grant, 1986).

Adrenergic blockers may be either direct acting or indirect acting. The direct-acting blockers also are divided into alpha-adrenergic blocking agents, beta-adrenergic blocking agents, and nonspecific agents. The most prominent alpha-adrenergic blocking agent is **moxisylyte.** This drug has side effects that depend on the dosage. A 0.1% solution causes brief miosis. A 5% solution produces transient ptosis, hyperemia of the conjunctiva, and reduces IOP in glaucoma (side effects are not always objectionable). The primary beta-adrenergic blocking agent is **betadine.** This agent has the side effects of ptosis, miosis, and hyperemia of the conjunctiva, and it decreases IOP. Nonspecific adrenergic blockers include **practolol, propranolol** and **oxprenolol.** These drugs have the side effect of decreased IOP. **Oxprenolol** causes punctate keratitis and miosis. **Propranolol** also causes miosis; it also can cause decreased corneal reflex, conjunctival hyperemia and irritation (Fraunfelder,

1982; Cote and Drance, 1968; Felix et al., 1973; Rahi, 1976; Bucci, 1975; Holt and Waddington, 1975; Lewis et al., 1976).

Indirect-acting adrenergic blockers include **guanethidine** and **bretylium,** which are discussed under antiglaucoma agents (Wills, 1970).

ANTIGLAUCOMA AGENTS

One test for open-angle glaucoma is the use of **tolazoline,** an alpha-adrenergic blocking agent. This drug has the side effect of increasing IOP when injected subconjunctivally. Another test for open-angle glaucoma uses the alpha- plus beta-adrenergic agent **bamethan.** This agent has the side effects of increased IOP and redness and swelling of the eye (Fraunfelder, 1982; Duke-Elder, 1972; Sugar and Santos, 1955; Walsh and Hoyt, 1969).

A large number of drugs of several classes are used to control glaucoma. Some of the most common are adrenergic drugs. **Epinephrine** (adrenaline) is an adrenergic agonist which has an extensive list of reported side effects: decreased vision, mydriasis, allergic reactions of the eyelids or conjunctiva of sensitized persons, blepharoconjunctivitis (follicular), vasoconstriction of the conjunctiva, poliosis and pemphigoid lesions of the eyelids and conjunctiva. It may produce hyperplasia of the sebaceous glands of the eyelids, or symptoms of irritation (lacrimation, rebound hyperemia, photophobia, ocular pain, and ocular burning sensations). There may be adrenochrome deposits in the conjunctiva, in the cornea, or in the nasolacrimal system, cystoid macular edema, punctate keratitis, corneal edema, narrowing or occlusion of lacrimal canaliculi, subconjunctival or retinal hemorrhages, loss of eyelashes or eyebrows, paradoxical pressure elevation in open-angle glaucoma, scotomas, aqueous floaters (pigment debris), periorbital edema, iritis, cysts, and, in infected individuals, reactivation of corneal herpes simplex. Some of these symptoms may be secondary to changes in blood circulation in the eye and surrounding tissues produced by the continuously elevated levels of epinephrine used to treat glaucoma. The prodrug of epinephrine, **dipivefrin (DPE),** has many fewer side effects, including irritation, erythema of the eyelids, conjunctivitis, decreased vision, and mydriasis (Fraunfelder, 1982; Drance and Ross, 1970; Kaback, 1976; Theodore and Leibowitz, 1979; Becker and Morton, 1966; Waltman, 1977).

The most common beta-adrenergic blocker for treatment of glaucoma is **L-timolol.** This drug has the reported side effects of irritation (with hyperemia, ocular pain, and burning sensations), allergic reactions and erythema of the eyelids or conjunctiva, blepharoconjunctivitis, urticaria, purpura of the conjunctiva, decreased vision, myopia, visual hallucinations, decreased corneal reflex, keratoconjunctivitis, and myasthenic neuromuscular blocking effect (paralysis of the extraocular muscles and ptosis) (Fraunfelder, 1980, 1982; Van Buskirk, 1980; Wilson et al., 1980).

Guanethidine and **bretylium** are antiadrenergic norepinephrine-releasing blockers. They act by blocking the release of endogenous norepinephrine. **Guanethidine** has the side effects of irritation (with hyperemia, photophobia, ocular pain, edema, and burning sensations), Horner's syndrome (with miosis, ptosis, and enophthalmos), mydriasis, decreased IOP, and punctate keratitis. **Bretylium** (10%–25%) causes some reduction of ocular pressure in glaucoma and slight ptosis, but no irritation or injury (Fraunfelder, 1982; Bonomi and Di Comite, 1967; Davidson, 1973).

Glycerin is an osmotic agent given for acute glaucoma. Its side effects include irritation (with lacrimation, hyperemia, ocular pain, and burning sensations) and subconjunctival hemorrhages (Fraunfelder, 1982; American Medical Association, 1980, 365–366, 403; Hovland, 1971; Virno, 1963).

Direct-acting cholinomimetics include **carbachol** and **methacholine.** These agents have the side effects of allergic reactions and hyperemia of the eyelids or conjunctiva of sensitized individuals, blepharoclonus, and myopia. **Carbachol** can produce miosis, decreased vision, accommodative spasms, follicular conjunctivitis, ocular pain, retinal detachment, and, after intracameral injection, corneal edema. **Methacholine** can produce Adie's pupil (myosis), lacrimation, and even blood tears. Another drug in this family is **bethanechol.** It has the side effects of severe itching, burning, and tearing of the eyes (Fraunfelder, 1982; Gilman et al., 1980; Grant, 1986; Havener, 1978; Ellis, 1977; Fraunfelder, 1979; Vaughn et al., 1978).

MIOTICS AND MYDRIATICS

There are two main classes of miotics in general use: (1) cholinergic agents (cholinergic agonists), such as **aceclidine, carbachol, acetylcholine, methacholine,** and **pilocarpine;** and (2) anticholinesterases, such as **demecarium, echothiophate, isoflurophate (DFP), neostigmine, physostigmine, paraoxon,** and **nibufin.** General side effects of miotics include miosis, accommodative spasm, decreased vision, irritation of the eyes, decreased intraocular pressure (IOP), decreased anterior chamber depth, cataract, and even retinal detachment (of diseased retinas) (Grant, 1986; Hockwin and Swanson, 1976; Axelsohn and Holmberg, 1973; Axelsohn, 1986; Muller et al., 1956; Lebensohn, 1977; PDR, 1988, p. 1334).

One example of a cholinergic miotic is **pilocarpine.** Its side effects include an initial increase in IOP after administration, allergic reactions and hyperemia of the eyelids or conjunctiva of certain sensitive individuals, follicular conjunctivitis (after long-term use), transient myopia, and punctate keratitis. Other side effects can include blepharoclonus, increased axial lens diameter, decreased scleral rigidity, and, sometimes, retinal detachment or problems with color vision (dyschromatopsia) (Fraunfelder, 1982; Grant, 1986; Hockwin and Swanson, 1976).

An example of an anticholinesterase miotic is **isoflurophate (DFP).** This miotic may produce allergic reactions of the eyelids or conjunctiva in sensitive individuals, follicular conjunctivitis, edema of the eyelids or conjunctiva, pemphigoid lesion and depigmentation of the eyelids or conjunctiva, blepharoclonus, and iris or ciliary body cysts. Other side effects can include iritis, myopia, an initial increase in IOP, decreased scleral rigidity, occlusion of lacrimal canaliculi, or vitreous hemorrhages. Individuals who have had a surgical implant of a filtering bleb to control IOP may find the filtration decreased. **Nibufin** is another common anticholinesterase. Its side effects include increased tear production and changes in the b-wave of the elec-troretinogram (ERG) (Fraunfelder, 1982; Grant, 1986; PDR, 1988, p. 1334).

Mydriatics fall into two classes: anticholinergic drugs and adrenergic drugs. Examples of the anticholinergic mydriatics include **amprotropine, atropine, cyclopentolate, tropicamide, hemicholinium, eucatropine, homatropine,** and **scopolamine.** Adrenergic mydriatics include **hydroxyamphetamine, phenylephrine, pholedrine,** and **epinephrine. Epinephrine** and its side effects are presented under antiglaucoma drugs. Anticholinergic mydriatics have the general side effects of cycloplegia and decreased vision. They produce mydriasis, which may precipitate narrow-angle glaucoma, and they may increase intraocular pressure (with the exception of hemicholinium). Some drugs have more specific side effects. An example is **cyclopentolate,** which may produce irritation (with hyperemia, photophobia, ocular pain, and burning sensations), decrease or paralysis of accommodation, allergic reactions of the eyelids or conjunctiva in sensitized individuals, blepharoconjunctivitis, visual hallucinations, synechiae, keratitis, and shallow anterior chamber (Fraunfelder, 1982; Gilman et al., 1980; Havener, 1978; Awan, 1976; Ostler, 1975; Simcoe, 1962; German and Siddiqui, 1970).

CHOLINESTERASE INHIBITORS AND REACTIVATORS AND CHEMICAL WARFARE AGENTS

Edrophonium is a drug used to diagnose myasthenia gravis and which has a number of ocular side effects. These include photophobia, allergic reactions of the eyelids or conjunctiva, conjunctivitis, iritis, iris cysts, a decreased depth of the anterior chamber, vitreous hemorrhages, and cataracts (Fraunfelder, 1982; Gilman et al.,1980; PDR, 1988, p. 1334).

Diphenylchloroarsine, diphenylcyanoarsine, and **hexachloroethane** are three chemical warfare agents which have the side effects of ocular irritation and lacrimation. **Hexachloroethane** can cause blepharospasm, photophobia, and reddening of the conjunctiva. **Diphenylcyanoarsine** may cause necrosis of the corneal epithelium (Mann et al., 1948; Maumenee and Scholz, 1948; National Toxicity Program Working Group, 1989b; Hochmeister and Vycudilik, 1989). **Sarin** is a nerve gas with ocular side effects. This toxic agent can produce miosis and spasm of accommodation for viewing near objects (Maumenee and Scholz, 1948; Hochmeister and Vycudilik, 1989).

Pralidoxime is the cholinesterase reactivator most associated with ocular toxicity. This drug has the side effects of irritation (with hyperemia and burning sensations), subconjunctival hemorrhages, and iritis. It reverses miosis and accommodative spasms (Fraunfelder, 1982; Jager and Stagg, 1958; Byron and Posner, 1964).

AUTACOIDS AND ANTIHISTAMINES

Autacoids are mediators of inflammatory responses; most can occur endogenously. Autacoids of interest in ocular toxicity include **bradykinin, prostaglandins, pro-**

tamine, and **serotonin.** When **bradykinin** was injected into the vitreous of rabbits, it produced hyalitis and subcapsular changes in the lens (Grant, 1986; Haddad and Winchester, 1990; Spada et al., 1988).

There are many kinds of endogenous and exogenous **prostaglandins.** In the eye, a **prostaglandin** from the iris, known as **irin,** is a local mediator of a specific reaction to irritation of the eyes. This reaction is characterized by vasodilation in the iris, leakage of protein from the blood to the aqueous humor (breakdown of the blood–aqueous barrier), miosis, and a rise in intraocular pressure lasting one to two hours (Haddad and Winchester, 1990; Fleisher, 1988; Campochiaro and Sen, 1989).

When **protamine** was injected into the cornea of rabbits, it produced an immediate chalk-white opacity, apparently caused by the precipitation of acid mucopolysaccharides (Haddad and Winchester, 1990). **Serotonin** produces less severe side effects, including slight miosis and a slight reduction in intraocular pressure (Grant, 1986).

Antihistamines of interest for their ocular side effects include **antazoline, diphenhydramine, mepyramine,** and **prophenpyridamine.** Side effects of antihistamines include an atropine-like action characterized by slight dilation of the pupils and impairment of accommodation for far vision. **Mepyramine** and **antazoline** may cause rapid clouding of the corneal epithelium, local anesthesia, and transitory swelling of the cornea. High concentrations of **antazoline** can cause temporary keratitis epithelialis (Fraunfelder, 1982; Gilman et al., 1980; Wyngaarden and Seevers, 1951; Dukes, 1980).

CARDIOVASCULAR DRUGS

Cardiovascular drugs with ocular side effects include **digoxin, erythrophleum alkaloids, gitalin, ouabain,** and **squill.** All these drugs decrease intraocular pressure, and all except **ouabain** produce corneal edema. **Digoxin** may produce wrinkling of Descemet's membrane, **erythrophleum alkaloids** may produce chemosis; and intravitreal injection of **ouabain** may cause loss of vision (Fraunfelder, 1982; Grant, 1986; American Medical Association, 1980, pp. 365–366, 403; PDR, 1988, p. 1334; Robertson et al., 1966; Weleber and Shults, 1981). A 9.7% solution of **potassium thiocyanate** can cause loosening of the corneal epithelium (Grant, 1986).

Amyl nitrite is an agent for treatment of angina pectoris. Ocular side effects include stinging and transient lacrimation. There may be slight superficial injury of the eye or severe corneal damage (Fraunfelder, 1982; Grant, 1986; Cristini and Pagliarani, 1953; Robertson and Steves, 1977).

Several classes of drugs are used as vasodilators; the side effects depend on the individual drug. **Acetylcholine** has the side effects of lacrimation, miosis, and clouding of the aqueous humor. **Isoxsuprine** has the side effects of increased intraocular pressure, edema, and hyperemia of episcleral tissues. **Nicodan-percutan** has the side effects of loss of corneal epithelium, clouding of the corneal stroma, corneal opacity, and vascularization and wrinkling of Descemet's membrane (Fraunfelder, 1982; Grant, 1986).

BLOOD-RELATED AGENTS

The usual plasma expanders are **dextran** and **dextran sulfate.** These agents may cause clouding of the vitreous. **Dextran sulfate** has severe side effects of severe irritation, intraocular hemorrhage, and distention of the globe. **Dextran** may produce phthisis bulbi (Fraunfelder, 1982; Blake and Cassidy, 1979; Fothergill and Heaney, 1976).

The ocular side effects of anticoagulants depend on the agent given. **Citric acid** has the side effects in some patients of a severe conjunctival reaction, with corneal ulceration or severe, dense opacification of the cornea. **Heparin** has different side effects. Subconjunctival injection of **heparin** may cause subconjunctival or periocular hemorrhages, subconjunctival scarring, chemosis, and decreased intraocular pressure. Intracameral injection of **heparin** may cause corneal edema and opacification, conjunctival chemosis, hyperemia of the iris, and a transient increase in intraocular pressure. Three percent eye drops of **heparin** may affect the corneal epithelium (Fraunfelder, 1982; Gilman et al., 1980; PDR, 1988, p. 1334; Aronson and Elliott, 1972).

Phenylhydrazine is a hemolytic which was injected intravitreally. It caused inflammation of the eye, chorioretinitis, and degeneration of the retina (Grant, 1986). **Saponins** are hemolytic agents also. Topical contact of **saponins** with the eye causes irritation, tearing, pain, photophobia, chemosis, and hyperemia. There may be conjunctivitis, damage to the corneal epithelium, keratitis, corneal ulceration, and corneal leukoma (Chiou and Chuang, 1989; Chiou et al., 1989).

Choline is an agent in this class. Its ocular side effects include inflammation and hemorrhages in the conjunctiva and superficial corneal opacities with edema (PDR, 1988, p. 1334; Merchant, 1988).

VITAMINS

Some vitamins [**menadione (vitamin K) and vitamin A**] have ocular side effects. **Vitamin K** may have the effects of discomfort of the eye, conjunctival congestion, and moderate injury to the eye. **Vitamin A** may produce blepharoconjunctivitis and loss of hair from the lids (Fraunfelder, 1982; Grant, 1986; Oliver and Havener, 1958; Turtz and Turtz, 1960).

AGENTS FOR DEFICIENCY ANEMIAS

A number of agents are used to treat deficiency anemias. Many of the agents with ocular side effects are iron compounds: **ferrocholinate, ferrous fumarate, ferrous gluconate, ferrous succinate, ferrous sulfate, iron dextran, iron sorbitex,** and **polysaccharide-iron complex.** These agents have the side effects of irritation (with hyperemia and photophobia), yellow-brown discoloration or deposits in the eyelids, conjunctiva, cornea, and sclera. There may be hypopyon and ulceration of the eyelids, conjunctiva, and cornea (Fraunfelder, 1982; Grant, 1986; Dukes, 1980; Chisholm, 1950).

SEDATIVES, HYPNOTICS, AND TRANQUILIZERS

Some agents classified as sedatives or hypnotics have ocular side effects. **Chlorobutanol** has the side effects of irritation (foreign body sensation) and keratitis epithelialis (BIBRA Working Group, 1989, (a); Tripathi and Tripathi, 1989). **Alcohol (ethanol)** has the side effects of irritation (with ocular pain, hyperemia, edema, lacrimation, and burning sensation), keratitis, paralysis of the extraocular muscles, nystagmus, ptosis, corneal ulceration or necrosis, corneal opacities, and decreased vision (Fraunfelder, 1982; Grant, 1986; Adams and Brown, 1975; Gramberg-Danielsen, 1965; Olurin and Osuntokun, 1978).

Reserpine is a tranquilizer with the side effects of decreased intraocular pressure and hyperemia of the conjunctiva (Fraunfelder, 1982; Kaplan and Pilger, 1957; Raymond, 1963).

ANTIDEPRESSANTS AND ANTIPARKINSONISM AGENTS

Protriptyline is an antidepressant with a mydriatic side effect. It also may cause corneal opacities of unknown composition (Fraunfelder, 1982; Davidson, 1973).

Antiparkinsonism agents include **L-Dopa (levodopa)** and **trihexyphenidyl.** These drugs may produce mydriasis and irritation; **trihexyphenidyl** may have an anesthetic action. **Amantadine** may cause decreased vision (Fraunfelder, 1982; Grant, 1986; Spiers, 1969).

LOCAL ANESTHETICS

Local anesthetics may be used for local ophthalmic use, or the eyes may be exposed unintentionally. Local anesthetics include **benoxinate, bulacaine, bupivacaine, cocaine, cornecaine, dibucaine, dyslonine, lidocaine, phenacaine, piperocaine, proparacaine, procaine,** and **tetracaine.** These drugs produce a variety of ocular side effects. All can produce irritation, with lacrimation, hyperemia, ocular pain, or burning sensations. There may be allergic reactions of the eyelids or conjunctiva in sensitized individuals, or blepharoconjunctivitis. There may be punctate keratitis, a gray, ground-glass appearance of the cornea, corneal edema, corneal softening, erosions, sloughing, filaments, ulceration, vascularization, or scarring. Corneal wound healing may be delayed. **Bupivacaine, lidocaine,** and **procaine** may produce decreased vision, paresis or paralysis of the extraocular muscles, or a decrease in intraocular pressure. Other reported side effects include a decrease in the blink reflex, subconjunctival hemorrhages, hypopyon, or iritis. Cocaine can cause conjunctival vasoconstriction; it also may induce mydriasis, paralysis of accommodation, or even visual hallucinations (Fraunfelder, 1982; Grant, 1986; American Hospital Formulary Service, 1974; Burns and Gipson, 1978; Fraunfelder et al., 1979; Siegel, 1978).

ANALGESICS

Analgesics fall into two main classes: narcotic analgesics and antipyretic analgesics. Narcotic analgesics include **meperidine** and **morphine**. **Meperidine** has the side effects of blepharitis and nonspecific conjunctivitis. **Morphine** has the side effects of miosis and, possibly, increased intraocular pressure (Fraunfelder, 1982; Grant, 1986).

Antipyretic analgesics include **aspirin, sodium salicylate, ethylmorphine, ethylmorpholine,** and **trichloroethylene. Aspirin** and **sodium salicylate** have the side effects of conjunctival edema or scarring and of keratitis, with or without ulceration. **Ethylmorphine** has the side effects of conjunctival vasodilation and edema, and may either increase or decrease intraocular pressure. **Ethylmorpholine** may produce corneal epithelium injury, hazy cornea, blurring of vision, and colored halos around lights. **Trichloroethylene** may cause chemical burns of the lids, conjunctiva, and cornea. There may be smarting pain and injuries to the corneal epithelium or disturbances of vision (Fraunfelder, 1982; Grant, 1986; Dukes, 1980; Ros et al., 1976; Gorn, 1979; Smith, 1966; Vernon and Ferguson, 1969).

ANTIRHEUMATIC AND ANTIGOUT AGENTS

Antirheumatic agents include **aurothioglucose, aurothioglycanide, gold (Au), gold sodium thiomalate (sodium aurothiomalate),** and **gold thiosulfate (sodium aurothiosulfate).** These agents have the ocular side effects of irritation, corneal clouding, and iritis (Fraunfelder, 1982; Walsh and Hoyt, 1969; American Medical Association, 1980, pp. 365–366, 403; Gibbons, 1979; Roberts and Wolter, 1956).

Colchicine is an antigout agent with the ocular side effects of decreased vision, conjunctival hyperemia, corneal clouding, vascularization of the cornea, and opacification of the cornea (Fraunfelder, 1982; Walsh and Hoyt, 1969; Estable, 1948).

AGENTS FOR RESPIRATORY DISEASES

Polyoxyethylene dodecanol (Laurithyl) is an agent for the treatment of respiratory diseases. Reported ocular side effects include irritation and corneal damage (Anonymous, 1988a).

ANTISPASMODICS

Antispasmodics include a large number of agents of differing classes of drugs: **adiphenine, ambutonium, anisotropine, belladonna clidenium, dicyclomine, dephemanil, glycopyrrolate, hexocylium, isopropamide, mepenzolate, methantheline, methixene, methylatropine, oxyphencyclamine, oxyphenonium, pipenzolate, piperidolate, poldine, propantheline,** and **tridihexethyl. Atropine** and

LOCAL AGENTS

homatropine (German and Siddiqui, 1970) are also used as antispasmodics; they are discussed with the mydriatics.

Side effects vary with the drug in question. Many antispasmodics produce mydriasis (which may, in turn, precipitate narrow-angle glaucoma), a decrease or paralysis of accommodation or irritation (with hyperemia, edema, and photophobia). **Belladonna** may produce decreased vision or follicular blepharoconjunctivitis. **Oxyphenonium** may produce nonspecific conjunctivitis. Both **belladonna** and **oxyphenonium** may induce allergic reactions of the eyelids or conjunctiva; they also may increase intraocular pressure, decrease lacrimation, or cause micropsia and brawny scleritis (Fraunfelder, 1982; Gilman et al., 1980; American Medical Association, 1980, pp. 365–366, 403; Havener, 1978; Dukes, 1980; Lazenby et al., 1970; German and Siddiqui, 1970).

GASTROINTESTINAL AGENTS

The ocular effects of cathartics depend on the specific agent. **Gamboge** that comes in contact with the eye can produce purulent keratitis (Grant, 1986). **Mercurous chloride** will cause slight transient redness and swelling of the eye, inflammation or scarring of the conjunctiva. When soluble iodides or soluble bromides were given systemically at the same time that mercurous chloride was applied to the eye of experimental animals, they produced edema of the lids, hyperemia of the eye, tearing and mucoid or purulent discharge, erosions of the corneal epithelium, and clouding of the cornea (Grant, 1986; Haddad and Winchester, 1990; EPA Working Group, 1984). **Croton oil** is very toxic to the eyes, causing severe keratoconjunctivitis with pain, swelling, and purulent discharge. When croton oil is injected intracamerally, it causes violent iritis and necrosis of the cornea. When injected into the vitreous, it causes devastating endophthalmitis (Mazzanti et al., 1987, Hull, 1988; Willis et al., 1988).

Bile and **bilirubin** are toxic when they come into contact with the eyes. **Bile** causes corneal epithelial injury, corneal opacity, cataract, degeneration of the retina, and choroid and hypertrophy of the iris and ciliary process. **Bilirubin** causes severe loss of vision, intraocular hemorrhages, loss of the electroretinogram (ERG), and yellow staining of the retina (Grant, 1986).

CHEMOTHERAPEUTIC AGENTS

Copper sulfate is an antitrachoma agent. Its side effects include temporary inflammation and purulent reaction, discoloration of the cornea, local necrosis, and corneal opacity symblepharon (Thirumalaikolundusubramanian et al., 1984).

Antibacterials include several classes of agents of diverse chemical structure. Antibiotics are drugs derived from natural sources. Penicillin antibiotics include **amoxicillin, ampicillin, carbenicillin, cloxacillin, dicloxacillin, hetacillin, methicillin, nafcillin, oxacillin, benzathine penicillin G, hydrabamine penicillin V, potassium penicillin G, potassium penicillin V, potassium phenethicillin,** and **procaine** penicillin G. Polypeptide antibiotics include **bacitracin, colistimethate, colistin, polymyxin B,** and **capreomycin.** Cephalosporins include **cefazolin, cephalexin, cephaloglycin, cephaloridine, cephalothin,** and **cephradine.** Chloramphenicol is a bacteriostatic antibiotic. Bacteriostatic derivatives of polycyclic naphthalene carboxamide include **chlortetracycline, demeclocycline, doxycline, methacycline, minocycline, oxytetracycline,** and **tetracycline.** Aminoglycosidic antibiotics include **framycetin, neomycin, gentamicin, kanamycin,** and **streptomycin.** Other antibiotics include **clindamycin, erythromycin, lincomycin,** and **vancomycin** (Fraunfelder, 1982; Gilman et al., 1980; Grant, 1986; Walsh and Hoyt, 1969; American Medical Association, 1980, pp. 365–366, 403; Ellis, 1977; PDR, 1988, p. 1334; Dukes, 1980; Crews, 1977; Cole et al., 1957; Lamda et al., 1968; Krejci and Brettschneider, 1978; Lund, 1968; Edwards, 1963; Francois and Mortiers, 1976).

Sulfa drugs are synthetic compounds (in contrast to antibiotics, which are natural compounds) with antibacterial action. Sulfonamides include **sulfacetamide, sulfachlorpyridazine, sulfacytine, sulfadiazine, sulfadimethoxine, sulfamerazine, sulfameter, sulfamethazine, sulfamethizole, sulfamethoxazole, sulfamethoxypyridazine, sulfanilamide, sulfaphenazole, sulfapyridine, sulfasalazine, sulfathiazole,** and **sulfisoxazole.**

Side effects depend somewhat on the class of antibacterial agents (Haviland and Long, 1940; Boettner et al., 1974). All of the antibiotics may produce irritation, allergic reactions and/or edema of the eyelids or conjunctiva in sensitized individuals, and overgrowth of nonsusceptible organisms. After intracameral injection, they produce uveitis, corneal edema, and lens damage (with the exceptions of the cephalosporins).

Other side effects depend on the specific antibiotic. **Cloxacillin** may produce corneal opacities. **Nafcillin** may produce conjunctival necrosis. Polypeptides can produce blepharoconjunctivitis, urticaria, and keratitis. Cephalosporins can produce urticaria. **Chloramphenicol** can produce depigmentation and optic neuritis. **Lincomycin** can produce subconjunctival hemorrhages, and **erythromycin** may produce mydriasis. Retrobulbar injection of **clindamycin** can cause optic neuritis and optic atrophy. **Framycetin** and **neomycin** may cause urticaria, erythema, and follicular conjunctivitis. **Gentamycin** may also cause follicular conjunctivitis. **Synermycin,** after intracameral injection, may cause intense inflammation involving, principally, the uveal tissues. **Sparsomysin** may cause the retinal pigment to gather together in coarse clumps and produce disturbance of vision and ring scotomas. **Pleomycin,** after topical application of a 0.1% solution, causes corneal opacity (Grant, 1986; Zylic et al., 1989). Sulfonamides cause follicular conjunctivitis, deposits, and delayed corneal wound healing. Some of the sulfonamides, particularly **sulfadiazine, sulfanilamide, sulfapyridine,** and **sulfathiazole,** cause acute myopia and shallowing of the anterior chamber (Fraunfelder, 1982; Haviland and Long, 1940; Boettner et al., 1974).

Silver-containing antibacterial agents include **colloidal silver, silver nitrate,** and **silver protein.** These agents have the side effects of silver deposits in the cornea, conjunctiva, eyelids, lens, and lacrimal sac. They produce irritation with hyperemia, photophobia, ocular pain, and edema. There may be allergic reactions and edema of the eyelids or conjunctiva in sensitized individuals, or conjunctivitis and symblepharon. **Silver nitrate,** at caustic concentrations, can cause scarring or opacities of any ocular structure. There may be decreased vision and problems with color vision: objects will appear to have a yellow tinge (Fraunfelder, 1982; Goldstein, 1971; Grayson and Pieroni, 1970; Rosen, 1950).

Other antibacterial agents may have ocular side effects. **Ethylhydrocupreine** may cause corneal anesthesia and clouding of the corneal epithelium. **Hydragaphene** may cause irritation, and **1-(5-nitro-2-furfunylideneamin) guanidine** may cause depigmentation of the eyelashes and the skin of the eyelids (Grant, 1986; Boettner et al., 1974).

There are a variety of fungicide agents: **amphotericin B, chloranil, Nemagon, dodine, drazoxolon, ferban, 2-heptadecyl-2-imidazoline, methyl mercury compounds, mylone, nystatin, propionic acid, sulfur dust, tetrachlorophenol, tomatine, trichlorophenol, triphenyltin hydroxide, undecylenic acid,** and **zinc dimethyldithiocarbamate.** The side effects depend on the agent. **Methyl mercury compounds, sulfur dust,** and **undecylenic acid** can cause irritation and keratitis. **Mylone** can cause loss of the corneal epithelium. **Chloranil** can cause corneal necrosis. **Methyl mercury compounds** can cause vascularization of the cornea or conjunctivitis. **Triphenyltin hydroxide** can cause opacity of the cornea. **Amphotericin B** and **nystatin** can cause allergic reactions of the eyelids or conjunctiva, and treatment may lead to overgrowth of nonsusceptible organisms; **amphotericin B** and **undecylenic acid** can cause conjunctivitis. **Amphotericin B** also may cause edema of the conjunctiva (as may **tomatine**), corneal ulceration, necrosis, nodules or yellow discoloration, or may produce uveitis (Fraunfelder, 1982; Grant, 1986; Gilman et al., 1980; American Medical Association, 1980, pp. 365–366, 403; Havener, 1978; Ellis, 1977; PDR, 1988, p. 1334; Dukes, 1980).

Some antiviral agents have ocular side effects; the effects depend on the agent. *p*-**fluorophenylalanine** may cause delayed regeneration of the corneal epithelium. **Cytarabine** may cause ocular pain, iritis, and corneal opacities and ulceration. **Idoxuridine (IDU), trifluridine (F3T),** and **vidarabine** have similar side effects. They produce irritation, with lacrimation, hyperemia, photophobia, and ocular pain. There may be superficial punctate keratitis, corneal filaments, delayed wound healing, erosions or indolent ulceration, stromal opacities, and superficial vascularization. There may be allergic reactions and hyperemia of the eyelids or conjunctiva in sensitized individuals. There may be follicular conjunctivitis, conjunctival punctate staining, and conjunctival scarring. There may be narrowing or occlusion of the lacrimal punctum and ptosis (Fraunfelder, 1982; Grant, 1986; Havener, 1978; Elliott and Schut, 1965; Itoi, 1975).

Neoarsphenamine is an antisyphilis drug with the side effects of corneal edema and opacity. **Oxophenarsine,** injected into the corneal stroma, causes moderate to moderately severe injury to the cornea (Doukan, 1990).

DISINFECTANTS

Disinfectants with ocular toxicity include **cresols, propiolactone, propylene oxide, Savlon, triethylene glycol,** and **xylenol.** All produce ocular irritation. **Cresols, propiolactone, savlon,** and **triethylene glycol** produce corneal haziness or opacity. **Cresols** also may produce conjunctival and lid reactions. **Savlon** also may produce corneal edema, hyphemia, and wrinkling of Descemet's membrane. **Xylenol** causes severe and, presumably, permanent injury to the eye. **Propylene oxide** is moderately injurious to the eye. **Propiolactone** may cause miosis (Jones, 1990; Meylan et al., 1986; Hayka et al., 1990; Von Berg, 1988; Khurana et al., 1989; Anonymous, 1988g; Kanerva et al., 1989).

SCABICIDES AND PEDICULICIDES

Lindane is the most common drug used to kill mites and lice. It has the side effects of irritation, conjunctivitis, and hyperemia (Grant, 1986; Haddad and Winchester, 1990).

ANTINEOPLASTIC AGENTS

There are several classes of antineoplastic agents, and the side effects vary somewhat from group to group. **Cyclophosphamide** and **thiotepa** are alkylating agents. **Cyclophosphamide** may cause damage to the cornea. **Thiotepa** causes irritation, allergic reactions in sensitized individuals, poliosis, and depigmentation of the eyelids or conjunctiva. There may be delayed corneal wound healing, keratitis, corneal edema, occlusion of the lacrimal punctum, or corneal ulceration (Fraunfelder, 1982; Grant, 1986; Berkow et al., 1969; Olander et al., 1978).

   Fluorouracil is an antimetabolite. It may cause irritation, allergic reactions, hyperpigmentation, photosensitivity, and subconjunctival hemorrhages of the eyelids or conjunctiva. After intradermal eyelid injection, there may be periorbital edema and cicatricial ectropion (PDR, 1988, p. 1334; Christoophidis, 1979).

   Chromomycin A3 and **mitomycin C** are antibiotics with antineoplastic effects. **Chromomycin A3** destroys the retina when injected into the vitreous. **Mitomycin C** may cause blepharoconjunctivitis, uveitis, scleral degeneration, increased intraocular pressure, prolapse of the iris, and destruction of the retina (Grant, 1986; Van Dyk, 1976).

   Vinblastine and **vincristine sulfate** are vinca alkaloids. **Vinblastine** causes irritation, with lacrimation, hyperemia, and photophobia. It may cause keratitis, superficial gray opacities of the cornea, blepharospasm, decreased vision, and astigmatism. **Vincristine sulfate** causes degeneration of the retina after injection into the vitreous (Albert et al., 1967; Green, 1975; McLendon and Bron, 1978; Sanderson et al., 1976).

   Other antineoplastic agents have different specific ocular side effects. **Actinomycin D** may cause a severe intraocular reaction of both the anterior and posterior segments of the eye, with opacification of the lens and cornea. **Alloxan** can cause severe injury to the eye. There may be corneal edema, opacity, and vascularization, or glaucoma may develop. **Methotrexate** can cause irritation, such as foreign body sensation, tearing, and blurring of vision. There may be defects of the epithelium, wrinkling of Descemet's membrane, and hyperemia of the conjunctiva. **Triaziquone** may produce local pain or a violent local reaction, with extensive necrosis of the conjunctiva, and glaucoma (Grant, 1986; PDR, 1988, p. 1334; Herse, 1990; Loprinzi et al., 1990).

ANTIWART AGENTS

Chelidonium majus and **podophyllin** are antiwart agents with toxic effects to the eyes. They cause irritation, with burning, epiphora, and blepharospasm. There can be keratoconjunctivitis and iritis. **Chelidonium majus** can cause hypopyon. **Podophyllin** causes conjunctival hyperemia, loss of corneal epithelium, and deposits in the back of the cornea (Grant, 1986; PDR, 1988, p. 1334; Holdright and Jahanqiri, 1990; Miller, 1985; Beutner and van Krogh, 1990).

ANTIMALARIAL AGENTS

Modern antimalarial agents include **amodiaquine, chloroquine, hydroxychloroquine, mepacrine,** and **quinoline.** All except **quinoline** can cause corneal deposits. **Mepacrine** may cause conjunctival deposits or corneal haziness and edema. **Quinoline** can cause moderately severe injury to the eyes (Grant, 1986; Fraunfelder, 1982; Bernstein, 1967; Burns, 1966; Lal and Gupta, 1974).

ANTHELMINTHICS AND AMOEBOCIDES

Quinacrine is used in the treatment of tapeworm infestations. Also, it is used in prophylaxis against worm infections and for the treatment of malaria. It has the side effects of producing blue haloes around lights, edema of the eyelids, conjunctiva, or cornea, and yellow discoloration of the eyes. There may be irritation, with lacrimation and ocular pain (Fraunfelder, 1982; Chamberlain and Boles, 1946; Ferrara, 1943).

Piperazine is used in the treatment of oxyuriasis and ascariasis. It is very toxic when applied topically to the eyes; a drop of 10% solution causes very severe injury to rabbit eyes within 24 hours (Grant, 1986; Walsh and Hoyt, 1969; American Medical Association, 1980, pp. 365–366, 403).

Emetine and **ipecac** are used in the treatment of acute amebic dysentery, amebic hepatitis, and amebic abscesses. They have the side effects of irritation, with lacrimation, hyperemia, and photophobia. There may be allergic reactions of the eyelids or conjunctiva in sensitized individuals, conjunctivitis, or keratitis. **Emetine** causes conjunctival edema, blepharospasm, corneal ulceration, corneal opacities, and iritis. **Ipecac** causes miosis (Fraunfelder, 1982; Grant, 1986; Duke-Elder, 1972; Lasky, 1950).

ADRENAL CORTICOSTEROIDS

There are a variety of adrenal corticosteroids and preparations: **adrenal cortex injection, aldosterone, betamethasone, cortisone, desoxycorticosterone, dexamethasone, fludrocortisone, fluorometholone, fluprednisolone, hydrocortisone, midrysone, meprednisone, methylprednisolone, paramethasone, prednisolone, prednisone,** and **triamcinolone.** These agents produce a great variety of ocular side effects. There may be increased intraocular pressure, decreased resistance to infection, delayed healing of corneal or scleral wounds, mydriasis, or glaucoma. There may be ptosis, posterior subcapsular cataracts, or decreased vision. The drugs may enhance the lytic action of collagenase. There may be a changing of visual fields, with scotomas, constriction, an enlarged blind spot, or glaucoma field defect. There may be problems with color vision, such as dyschromatopsia or colored haloes around lights. Sensitized people may have allergic reactions to these drugs. There may be persistent erythema, telangiectasis of the eyelids or conjunctiva, or eyelid or conjunctiva depigmentation, poliosis, or scarring. There may be fat atrophy and skin atrophy of the eyelids. Some patients develop paralysis of accommodation, punctate keratitis, irritation (with lacrimation, photophobia, ocular pain, or burning sensations), or anterior uveitis. The corneal or scleral thickness may change, initially increasing and then decreasing. There may be development of toxic amblyopia, optic atrophy, granulomas, or retinal embolic phenomenon. Adrenal corticosteroids may enhance facultative intraocular pathogens or cause development of retinal hemorrhages, retinal degeneration and detachment, or ascending optic atrophy. Adrenal corticosteroids may aggravate certain diseases, including scleromalacia perforans, corneal "melting" diseases, Behcet's disease, Eales' disease, or presumptive ocular toxoplasmosis (Fraunfelder, 1982; Grant, 1986; Armaly, 1963; Becker, 1964; David and Berkowitz, 1969; O'Connor, 1976).

DERMATOLOGIC AGENTS

Dermatologic agents with ocular side effects include **benzoyl peroxide, chrysarobin, dithranol, exolan, hexachlorophene, resorcinol,** and **salicylic acid.** All these agents may produce irritation with lacrimation, hyperemia, photophobia, and burning sensations; all except **dithranol** and **exolan** can produce conjunctivitis. **Chrysarobin** can cause allergic reactions of the eyelids or conjunctiva in sensitized persons, edema, or brown-violet discolorations. **Chrysarobin** and **hexachlorophene** can produce keratitis; **hexachlorophene** and **exolan** can produce corneal edema. **Resorcinol** can produce corneal vascularization, necrosis, and perforation. Treatment with **benzoyl peroxide** can lead to corneal opacity, and **exolan** can increase the intraocular pressure (Fraunfelder, 1982; Grant, 1986; Gilman et al., 1980; Duke-Elder,

1972; Dukes, 1980; Willetts, 1969; Andersen and Maibach, 1980; Lerman et al., 1980).

ANTISEPTICS

A variety of chemicals and compounds are used as antiseptics; their ocular side effects depend on the specific agent.

Local antiseptics include **brilliant green, chlorhexidine** (see **Savlon** in Disinfectants section), **gentian violet, hexylresorcinol, oxychlorosene, picric acid, silver proteinates,** and **mercuric chloride.**

All local antiseptics can produce ocular irritation (with the exception of **silver proteinates**). **Silver proteinates** can cause discoloration of the conjunctiva (Goldstein, 1971; Grayson and Pieroni, 1970; Rosen, 1950; Hanna et al., 1974). **Gentian violet** can produce dark purple staining of the cornea and conjunctiva, loss of corneal epithelium, and corneal stroma cloudiness. **Hexylresorcinol** can cause corneal edema or hyperemia of the iris. **Brilliant green** can produce keratitis and corneal opacity and, sometimes, hypopyon. **Mercuric chloride** can produce moderate to moderately severe corneal damage (graded from 22 to 75 on a scale of 0 to 100) (Fraunfelder, 1982; Grant, 1986; Hanna et al., 1974; Anonymous, 1983a; Groden et al., 1990; Gomez et al., 1988; Stevens et al., 1989).

Camphor is an antiseptic which can produce superficial keratitis with temporary loss of corneal epithelium (Anonymous, 1986f, p. 94; Committee on Drugs, 1978).

Cetrimonium bromide has the same side effects as **Savlon** (Khurana et al., 1989).

Creosote has the side effects of irritation (with burning sensations, itching, hyperemia, photophobia, and ocular discharge). It also is reported to be a carcinogen (Haddad and Winchester, 1990; Anonymous, 1989o; Liire, 1988).

n-**Hexanol** has the potential to cause severe eye injury (graded at 9 on a scale of 0 to 10) (Grant, 1986; Kennah et al., 1989).

Mercuric oxycyanide can produce the side effects of corneal edema, wrinkling of Descemet's membrane, hyperemia of the iris, cataract and posterior synechiae, disturbance of vision, and secondary glaucoma (Haddad and Winchester, 1990; Brownstein et al., 1989).

Methylene blue can produce irritation, with stinging and epiphora (Grant, 1986; Norn, 1967).

Phenol can produce corneal ulceration and opacity, chemotic, entropion, and scarring of the conjunctiva. Edema of the lids may develop, along with iritis and disturbance of vision (Mozingo et al., 1988; Baranowski-Dutkiewicz, 1981).

Zinc phenosulfonate may cause corneal necrosis and opacity (Anonymous, 1986a).

Mercuric oxide (yellow) may cause deposits of the pigment in the lids, conjunctiva, cornea, and lens. There may be blepharitis or conjunctivitis. Injection of **mercuric oxide** into the anterior chamber causes inflammation and purulent exudate (Haddad and Winchester, 1990; Hopkins, 1979; Johnstone, 1948).

PRESERVATIVES

Ophthalmic preservatives may belong to several categories; many are either quaternary ammonium agents or organomercurial agents. **Benzalkonium** is the most important quaternary ammonium agent. It has the side effects of irritation (with lacrimation, hyperemia, photophobia, and edema), punctate keratitis, grey corneal epithelial haze, pseudomembrane formation, decreased corneal epithelial microvilli, and cytotoxicity to the corneal epithelial cells. It also is suggested that it may cause delayed corneal wound healing (Fraunfelder, 1982; Gasset, 1977).

Organomercurials include **mercuric oxide, nitromersol, phenylmercuric acetate, phenylmercuric nitrate,** and **thimerosal.** These compounds have the side effects of allergic reactions in sensitized individuals, erythema, edema, and hyperemia of the eyelids or conjunctivitis. They may produce blepharoconjunctivitis. **Mercuric oxide** may produce bluish-gray mercury deposits on the eyelids, conjunctiva, and cornea; **mercuric oxide** and **phenylmercuric acetate** or **nitrate** also may leave deposits on the lens. **Thimerosal** can produce cytotoxicity of the corneal epithelial cells (Fraunfelder, 1982; Grant, 1986; Theodore, 1953; Willetts, 1969; Collin, 1986).

Chlorobutanol is another preservative. It has the side effect of cytotoxicity to corneal epithelial cells. Phenylmercuric salts include **dinaphylmethane disulfonate** and the **phenylmercuric** salts of acetate, chloride, nitrate, and oleate. These compounds have the side effect of mercurialentis (Grant, 1986; Collin, 1986).

DYES

Ophthalmic dyes frequently are used for ocular diagnostic tests. Commonly used dyes are **alcian blue, fluorescein, rose bengal,** and **trypan blue.** These dyes have the side effects of staining mucus, connective tissue, ocular fluids, and degenerated epithelial cells. They will produce irritation (with ocular pain and burning sensations) and blue, yellow-orange, or red discolorations of the eyelids or conjunctiva. **Fluorescein** may produce problems with color vision (objects will have a yellow tinge) (Fraunfelder, 1982; Grant, 1986).

Normally, the ocular side effects due to these ophthalmic dyes are rare and transient. However, if the corneal epithelium is not intact, the topical application of **alcian blue** may cause long-term, or even permanent, stromal deposits of the dye (Fraunfelder, 1982; Grant, 1986).

Methylene blue is a dye used during ocular surgery as a tissue marker. It has the side effects of producing a burning sensation, and it stains corneal nerves (Grant, 1986; Havener, 1978; Norn, 1967).

Nonophthalmic dyes normally are not placed deliberately in the eye, though some ophthalmic dyes also have nonophthalmic uses. They are a class of potentially toxic compounds that may accidentally contaminate the eye. The list of nonophthalmic dyes is fairly long: **acridine red, acridine yellow, acriflavine, alkali violet, amethyst violet, alisolin concentrate, auramine, Bindschedler's green,**

Bismarck green, brilliant cresyl blue, brilliant firnblau, brilliant green, brilliant phoaphin 5G, brilliant victoria blue RB, chrysoidine, clematin, coriphosphine, crystal violet, diamond fuchsin, 2,3-dichlorophenolindophenol, echtblau 2B, ethyl violet, basic fuchsin, gentian violet, homacridine yellow, indelible pencils, indigo, indoin, Janus black, Janus green B, malachite green, Mendola blue, mepacrine, methyl green, methyl rosaniline, methyl violet, methylene blue, methylene green, new blue R, new fuchsin, night blue, pararosaniline, patent phosphin G, phenosafranin, p-phenylenediamine, phloxine B, phosphine, prune pure, rhodamine B, rhodamine 6G, rhodamine S, safranin O, setocyanin, setoglaucin, spirit blue, thiazin blue, thionin, toluidine blue, Victoria blue R, Victoria pure blue BO, Dupont FDL 316, Victoria R.B., and violet 4RN.

All of these dyes have the potential to produce injury to the eye. **Bindschedler's green** and **phloxine B** may produce opacification and vascularization of the cornea. **Brilliant green** may produce destructive keratitis with hypopyon. **Janus green B** may produce corneal edema and damage to the epithelium, and **2,3-dichlorophenolindophenol** may produce histologic and metabolic disturbances of the retina (Fraunfelder, 1982; Grant, 1986; Haddad and Winchester, 1990; Anonymous, 1986f, pp. 590–591, 180; Anonymous, 1989a).

OPHTHALMIC IMPLANTS

Flaxseeds sometimes have been placed in the conjunctival sac as a form of home remedy. **Flaxseeds** may produce erythema, edema, and a local gray mucoid discharge. Corneal edema and abrasions inferior to the conjunctival sac also have been observed (Grant, 1986).

Ivalov is used as an implant in orbits after enucleation of the eyes they contain. This procedure may produce a foreign body type of cellular reaction, like rejection of a foreign substance (Grant, 1986).

Silicone has been used for implants; **silicone** implants increase postoperative infections and glaucomatous reactions. Liquid **silicone** applied topically causes a burning sensation. Liquid **silicone** used intraocularly can produce cataracts and endothelial damage with corneal edema or vascularization (Fraunfelder, 1982; Armaly, 1962; Setula et al., 1989; Rosengren, 1969).

Polygenline is used as a substitute for the vitreous humor in patients being treated for retinal detachment. Signs of inflammation with clouding of the vitreous have been noted in rabbits who received intravitreal injection of **polygenline** at concentrations of 7% or greater (Grant, 1986).

ANTIPERSPIRANTS

Antiperspirants contain compounds such as **aluminum chloride,** employed in the form of liquids, powders, sprays, and sticks. Contamination of the eyes with antiperspirants can cause transient irritation, ocular pain, blepharospasm, transient epithelial damage, and persistent faint nebula in the corneal stroma (Grant, 1986; Haddad and Winchester, 1990; De Groot et al., 1988a).

COUNTERIRRITANTS

Drugs used as counterirritants include **allylisothiocyanate, arnica, veratrine,** and **2-naphthol.** All of these agents can produce irritation and lacrimation. **Veratrine** can induce irritation of the conjunctiva; **arnica** can produce edema of the lids or hyperemia of the conjunctiva. **Allylisothiocyanate** can cause keratitis, and **2-naphthol** causes cataracts, white, yellow-white, or pigmented spots and edema in the retina, and disturbance of vision (Grant, 1986; Passreiter et al., 1988; Anonymous, 1989b; Wells et al., 1989).

CHELATING AGENTS

A number of chelating agents are used clinically. **Deferoxamine** is used in the treatment of ocular siderosis and hematogenous pigment of the cornea. It has the side effects of causing allergic reactions in sensitized individuals and hyperemia of the eyelids or the conjunctiva. When a $5-\mu g$ sample of **deferoxamine** was injected intravitreally, it caused widespread hemorrhagic necrosis, particularly affecting the rods and cones of the retina and extinguishing the ERG. When $200-\mu g$ of **deferoxamine** was injected intravitreally, there was congestion of the uvea and exudative detachment of the choroid and retina (Fraunfelder, 1982; Gilman et al., 1980; Grant, 1986; PDR, 1988, p. 1334).

Dimercaprol is used in the treatment of arsenic, gold, or mercury poisoning. It has the side effect of irritation, with lacrimation, photophobia, burning sensations, and blepharospasm. There may be severe iritis, corneal infiltration, corneal vascularization, and permanent scarring (Fraunfelder, 1982; Grant, 1986; Scherling and Blondis, 1945; Petersen et al., 1990).

Edetate (EDTA) has the side effects of a mild stinging sensation, localized faint opacity of the cornea, and hyperemia of the iris and the conjunctiva (Petersen et al., 1990).

DECONGESTANTS

Decongestants with ocular side effects include **naphazoline** and **tetrahydrozoline.** These agents can cause conjunctival vasoconstriction, irritation, lacrimation, reactive hyperemia, and burning sensations. There may be punctate keratitis, decreased vision, or mydriasis which, in turn, may precipitate narrow-angle glaucoma. There may be allergic reactions of the eyelid or conjunctiva in sensitized individuals or increases in pigment granules in the anterior chamber. **Naphazoline** may produce conjunctivitis; **tetrahydrozoline** may cause blepharoconjunctivitis or a decrease in intraocular pressure (Fraunfelder, 1982; Gilman et al., 1980; Grant, 1986; American Medical Association, 1980, 365–366, 403; PDR, 1988, p. 1334).

ASTRINGENTS

Alum has been employed topically as an astringent and styptic and in the treatment of trachoma. It can cause corneal incrustation and turbidity (Grant, 1986).

Potassium permanganate can cause a hardened, eroded lesion of the eye, swelling of the lids and conjunctiva, subconjunctival hemorrhages, turbidity, and brown discoloration of the cornea (Grant, 1986).

Tannic acid has been employed topically as an astringent and hemostatic. It has the side effects of a slight or mild reaction, discoloration, and, sometimes, corneal injury (Grant, 1986).

Lead acetate can cause irritation, opacity, and lead encrustation of the cornea and conjunctiva (Grant, 1986; Trocme et al., 1988; Reuhl et al., 1989; Niebroj and Grszczynska, 1989).

SURFACTANTS

Surfactants fall into three classes: cationic surfactants, anionic surfactants, and nonionic surfactants. Cationic surfactants include **benzalkonium, benzethonium, cetrimonium (CTAB), cetylpyridinium, decyltrimethylammonium, dodecyl-trimethylammonium, Emcol E607, Emulsol 607, 607M, G271, hexadecyl-trimethylammonium, Isothan Q15,** and **tetradecyltrimethylammonium.** All of these agents can cause irritation and injury to the eyes; **benzalkonium** can cause degeneration of the iris or chorioretinitis (Grant, 1986; Tripathi and Tripathi, 1989; Barney et al., 1988; Kahn et al., 1990; Lemp and Zimmerman, 1988).

Anionic surfactants include **Aerosol OS, Aerosol OT, alkyl sodium sulfate series** from **octyl** to **octadecyl, Armour #600 KOP soap, dodecyl sodium sulfate, Duponol ME, Duponol WAT, Eutsufon, Igepon AP, Ivory soap, Lissapol N, Naconol NRSF, Santomerse D, sodium lauryl sulfate, Duponol C, Tergitol-4, Tergitol-07, Tergitol-08, triethanolamine lauryl sulfate (Drene), Triton W30, Triton X30, Ultrawet 30DS,** and **Ultrawet 60L.**

All anionic surfactants cause irritation, discomfort, and potential injury to the eyes. There may be hyperemia of the conjunctiva, edema of the corneal epithelium, and temporary clouding of the cornea (Grant, 1986; Haddad and Winchester, 1990; Martin et al., 1962; Kennah et al., 1989; Anonymous, 1983b, 1985a).

Nonionic surfactants include **Brij-30, G1690, G2132, G3721, Laurithyl,** and **Triton X155.** Side effects include irritation, with ocular pain and photophobia, loss of the corneal epithelium, and corneal opacity (Grant, 1986; Haddad and Winchester, 1990; Martin et al., 1962; Kennah et al., 1989; Booman et al., 1988).

COSMETICS

Cosmetics usually are not single substances but are mixtures of substances, both natural and synthetic. **Eye cosmetics** contain numerous inert oily or waxy substances and coloring materials, such as **lecithin, cholesterin, cocoa butter, paraffin, di-ethylene glycol stearate, triethanolamine, stearic acid, carbon black, iron oxide,** and other inorganic pigments. Contamination of the eye with **eye cosmetics** can produce pigmentation of the palpebral conjunctiva, slight irregularities of the surface of the conjunctiva, mild burning or foreign-body sensations, and tearing (Grant, 1986; Haddad and Winchester, 1990; Gosselin et al., 1976; CTFA, 1976; Kirk and Othmer, 1980; Anonymous, 1986b, 1988b, 1989b, 1983d; Heine and Laubstein, 1990).

Hair cosmetics include a variety of preparations for a variety of purposes, none of which should bring them in contact with the eyes (Heine and Laubstein, 1990). Hair dyes may be either *p*-**phenylenediamine-type hair dyes** or **henna** or **2,4-diaminophenol.** *p*-**Phenylenediamine** derived dyes can cause irritation, with burning sensations, ocular pain, tearing, redness, swelling, and edema of the lids. There also may be edema and hyperemia of the conjunctiva. There may be loss of the corneal epithelium and corneal ulceration. Dyes also may produce iritis, iridocyclitis, exophthalmos, lost vision, or retrobulbar neuritis with central scotoma (Haddad and Winchester, 1990; Nigam and Saxena, 1988; Gouche, 1989; Matsunaga et al., 1988; Tosti et al., 1988).

Henna is a natural compound. It may have the side effects of swelling of the lids, tearing, discharge, and severe pain (Haddad and Winchester, 1990; Nigam and Saxena, 1988; Gouche, 1989; Natow, 1986; Bracher et al., 1987–1988; Pruett et al., 1987).

2,4-Diaminophenol may cause dark brown staining of the corneal stroma or permanent corneal opacification and vascularization (Grant, 1986).

Hair sprays and **lacquers** may produce ocular irritation, a transient stinging sensation, or a temporary fine keratitis epithelialis (Heine and Laubstein, 1990; Bracher et al., 1987–1988; Pruett et al., 1987).

Hair tonics that contact the eye may cause stinging and burning sensations, ocular pain, swelling, and redness of the lids (Grant, 1986).

Hair-waving preparations, such as **thioglycolates,** generally produce keratitis. They also may produce irritation, burning sensations, conjunctival inflammation, corneal epithelial erosion, turbidity of the cornea, mydriasis, cycloplegia, loss of convergence, and disturbance of vision (Grant, 1986).

Skin lotions, such as **Parabens** and **Triacetin,** can cause eye irritation. **Parabens** causes redness and swelling of the eyelids. **Triacetin** causes ocular pain and much redness of the conjunctiva (Grant, 1986; DeGroot et al., 1988b).

Nail hardener may cause allergic reactions of the eye and conjunctiva in sensitized individuals. **Nail polish** and **nail polish remover** can cause temporary solvent burns, swelling and vesiculization of the lids, and itching (Grant, 1986; Haddad and Winchester, 1990).

Lip Magik is a cosmetic preparation that should be mentioned, because it can cause discomfort and blurred vision, hyperemia, and chemosis of the conjunctiva (De Groot et al., 1988b).

Some common cosmetic ingredients can cause ocular side effects. **Isopropyl alcohol** and **hexylene glycol** both can cause irritation and mild transitory injury (graded 4 on a scale of 1 to 10), and **2-cyanoacrylic acid methyl ester**, an ingredient in glue, can cause irritation, haze of the cornea, inflammation of the eye, and blurred vision (Golubovic and Parunovic, 1990; Koo et al., 1989; Kinnunen and Hannuksela, 1989; Anonymous, 1986f, pp. 309, 337; Anonymous, 1986h, 1989e, 1984, 1985b; De Respinis, 1990; Siegal and Zaidman, 1989).

INSECTICIDES

A variety of compounds used as insecticides have unpleasant or dangerous effects on accidental topical contact with the eyes. These insecticides include *bis*(**tri-*n*-butyltin**) **oxide, mixtures of carbaryl** and **dimethoate, copper acetoardenite, Delna, Derris, 1,1-dichloro-1-nitroethane, Deet, HETP, hexachloroeyelopentadiene, irsbornyl thiocyanoacetate, lead arsenate, malathione, methyl isothiocyanate, naphthalene, nicotine, parathione, phenothiazine, pyrethrum, trichloroacetonitrile, tetraethylpyrophosphate (TEPP),** and **trichlorobenzene.** All of these compounds can produce irritation and ocular pain (**nicotine, parathion, trichlorobenzene**), photophobia (**phenothiazine**), or lacrimation (**1,1-dichloro-1-nitroethane, Deet, trichloroacetonitrile**). The eyelids or conjunctiva often are affected by topical contamination; there may be edema (**Deet, malathione,** or **pyrethrum**), hyperemia (**malathione** or **pyrethrum**), conjunctivitis (after **Delna** or **Deet**), injury (after **lead arsenate**), reaction (**nicotine**), or swelling of the lids (after a mixture of **carbaryl** and **dimethoate**). **Phenothiazine** and **pyrethrum** may cause corneal edema; corneal clouding or opacity may be induced by *bis*(**tri-*n*-butyltin)oxide, Deet, methyl isothiocyanate,** or **nicotine.** There may be corneal ulceration, vascularization and scarring, hemorrhages of the iris, or hypopyon after exposure to *bis*(**tri-*n*-butyltin) oxide.** There may be corneal epithelium injury after **Deet** or **methyl isothiocyanate,** a corneal haze or serious injury to the eye after **pyrethrum** exposure, corneal infiltration after **nicotine,** or keratitis epithelialis after a mixture of **carbaryl** and **dimethoate.** Miosis may be induced by **HETP, parathione,** or **tetraethylpyrophosphate** or **trichlorfon. Parathione** and **tetraethylpyrophosphate** may cause disturbed vision (Gilman et al., 1980; Grant, 1986; Haddad and Winchester, 1990; Arena, 1970; Hayes, 1975; Pullicino and Aquilina, 1989; Moster et al., 1987; Hata et al., 1986; Francis, 1986; EPA/OTS, 1987; Kennedy, 1986; Coyes et al., 1986; Anonymous, 1981b, 1982b, 1985f, 1986d; Ubels et al., 1987; Anand et al., 1987; Whorton and Obrinsky, 1983; Olson, 1983; Kelly, 1981).

FISHES AND JELLYFISH

Some kinds of **fish** are actually toxic; most of them can produce gases when decomposing which are toxic to the eyes. **Trimethylamine** is a gas released during the putrefaction of fish. **Eel blood** is especially irritating. **Jellyfish** and other coelenterates possess stinging cells which can inject anything they contact with toxins. Decomposing fish evolve gases which have induced bilateral keratitis epithelialis in fishermen.

Eel blood can produce a burning sensation and purulent discharge of the eyes, photophobia, inflammation and chemosis of the conjunctiva, keratitis, and swelling of the lids. **Jellyfish** can produce irritation, ocular pain and blepharospasm, photophobia, swelling of the lids, and injury to the corneal epithelium. **Trimethylamine** can cause hemorrhagic conjunctivitis, loss of corneal epithelium, corneal edema, opacity, and vascularization (Grant, 1986; Haddad and Winchester, 1990; Anonymous, 1986f, p. 607; McCormick and Davis, 1988; Rapoza et al., 1986).

TOXINS AND VENOMS

Moths flying into the eyes may cause irritation (Preisova et al., 1988). **Caterpillar hairs** of many species are really spines containing a toxin. If spines enter the eye, they can cause irritation, conjunctivitis, keratitis, uveitis, and necrosis (Verin and Comte, 1987; Martin et al., 1986; Marti-Huguet et al., 1987). **Cantharides** can cause conjunctivitis, keratitis, iritis, edema of the skin, a fibrinous exudate, hyperemia, and necrosis of the eyes (Rivand et al., 1990). **Bee stings** cause ocular pain, photophobia, clouding and swelling of the cornea, corneal infiltration and vascularization, keratitis, conjunctivitis, iritis, hypopyon, cataract, abscess of the lens, and, more rarely, glaucoma. There may be optic atrophy or optic neuritis (Surkova and Semonov, 1989; Agrawal, 1985). **Tarantula hairs** also can irritate the eye (Llered et al., 1988).

Skunks spray anything that threatens them with a powerful irritant and may aim for the eyes. Spray from a **skunk** causes irritation, conjunctivitis, and, sometimes, corneal opacity and vascularization (Grant, 1986; Haddad and Winchester, 1990).

Diphtheria toxin is topically toxic to the eyes, causing hyperemia and edema of the conjunctiva and opacification of the cornea (Grant, 1986).

Spider venoms can cause ocular irritation, with swelling of the lids, conjunctival edema, and subconjunctival hemorrhages (Adams, 1989).

Toad poisons are produced in the toad's skin and may contact the eyes if a toad is handled and then the eyes touched. **Toad poisons** can cause irritation, swelling of the lids, hyperemia of the conjunctiva, conjunctivitis, corneal and conjunctival anesthesia, paresis of the eye muscles, ptosis and corneal clouding, keratitis, iritis, mydriasis, decreased IOP, and central retinal edema (Grant, 1986; Van Tittelboom et al., 1988).

Wasp stings can cause swelling of the lids, ocular pain, and bullous keratitis (Kam et al., 1989; see Bee stings also).

Tetanus toxin is a neurotoxin. The effect of **tetanus toxin** on the iris has been shown to resemble postganglionic parasympathectomy (Grant, 1986).

PLANTS

A great variety of plants can cause irritation or changes in the eyelids, conjunctiva, or cornea. Some of the species include *Actaea rubra*, *Agrostemma* **seed**, *Araroba*, **burdock burs, capsaicin, carrageenan, cashew nut shell oil, castor beans, chestnut shell, crownflower,** *Dieffenbachia* **plants,** *Ecballia elaterium*, *Euphorbia*, **wild** fig, *Hura crepitans*, *Hyacinth* bulbs, **Jequirity bean, manchineel, mesquite thorn, morel,** *Mucuna pruriens,* **mustard oil, onion, pepper, peppermint oil, pig weed, poison ivy and related species of** *Rhus,* **primula,** *Pyracanthus* **extract, ricin, snuff, tea,** and **teakwood,** as well as **tobacco smoke** and **wood dust.**

All of these plants and plant-derived substances can cause irritation, ocular pain, lacrimation, burning, photophobia, tearing, blurring of vision, blepharospasm, and itching (Grant, 1986). Other effects depend somewhat on the agent. **Capsaicin** causes abnormal permeability of the blood vessels of the conjunctiva (Waldrep and Crosson, 1988; Agrawal et al., 1985; Szallasi and Blumberg, 1989). Edema or swelling of the eyelids or conjunctiva can be produced by **burdock burs** (Grant, 1986; Biger and Abulafia, 1986), **cashew nut shell oil** (Reginella et al., 1989; Geller, 1989), **crownflower** (Vighetto et al., 1990), *Ecballium elaterium* (Yesilada et al., 1988), *Euphorbia* (Grant, 1986), **manchineel** (Grant, 1986; Mozherenko, 1985), **pepper** (Grant, 1986), **poison ivy** (Baer, 1990), **primula** (Grant, 1986), **tobacco smoke** (Sibony et al., 1988; Kjaergaard and Pedersen, 1989), or **wood dust** (Vedal et al., 1986; Hansen et al., 1990; Hinds, 1988). Conjunctivitis can be induced by **cashew nut shell oil, castor beans** (de Zotte et al., 1988), *Ecballium elaterium,* *Euphorbia,* **wild fig** (Grant, 1986), *Hura crepitans* (Grant, 1986; Mozherenko, 1985), *Mucuna* pruriens (Leads from the MMWR, 1986), **mustard oil** (Grant, 1986), **Pyracanthus extract** (Subiza et al., 1990), **ricin** (de Zotte et al., 1988), **snuff,** or **tea** (Grant, 1986). Hyperemia of the conjunctiva can be produced by contact with *Euphorbia,* **manchineel, primula** (Epstein, 1990), or **wood dust** (Anonymous, 1986f, pp. 635–636). Chemosis can be induced by *Euphorbia,* **mustard oil** (Grant, 1986), or **manchineel** (Mozherenko, 1985). Conjunctival necrosis or ulcer can be produced by **chestnut shell** or **jequirity bean** (Grant, 1986). **Teakwood** can cause dermatitis in the lids (Anonymous, 1986f, pp. 635–636). Damage of the corneal epithelium can be produced by **crownflower, morel,** or **peppermint oil** (Grant, 1986). **Wild fig** and **burdock burs** can cause corneal ulcers; **burdock burs** also cause scarring and erosion of the cornea and corneal edema, as does **crownflower.** Corneal clouding or opacity may be produced by **burdock burs, carrageenan** [BIBRA Working Group, 1987, (a)], *Ecballium elaterium,* **wild fig, jequirity beans,** or **mustard oil** (Grant, 1986). **Burdock burs** and **carrageenan** can cause corneal vascularization. Keratitis can be produced by *Euphorbia,* **peppermint oil,** or *Rhizoma galanoa* (Grant, 1986). Corneal infiltration can be induced by **jequirity beans** or **peppermint oil.** Keratitis epithelialis can be induced by **mustard oil, primula** (Epstein, 1990), or **wood dust. Peppermint oil** can cause deposits on the cornea or release of pigment into the anterior chamber (Grant, 1986). Keratoconjunctivitis can be induced by *Agrostemma* **seed** (Grant, 1986), **manchineel** (Mozherenko, 1985), or **morel** (Grant, 1986). **Castor beans** can produce symblepharon (de Zotte et al., 1988), while **jequirity bean** and **burdock burs** can produce inflammation of the anterior chamber (Grant, 1986). **Carrageenan** can cause an acute rise in intraocular pressure, and **crownflower** (Grant, 1986) can cause a wrinkling of Descemet's membrane. Iritis may be produced by *Euphorbia,* **jequirity bean, mustard oil, primula,** *Pyracanthus* **extract,** or *Rhizoma galanga* (Hinds, 1988; Subiza et al., 1990; Vache and Bodnur, 1988; Epstein, 1990; Anonymous, 1986f, pp. 635–636; Sussman and Dorian, 1990; Dugan et al., 1989; Oji, 1990; Critchfield et al., 1988; Brooks et al., 1986).

Some other plants also are known to cause ocular problems. *Aloe* **barbs** cause uveitis. *Acacia* **extract** (Hansen et al., 1990) can cause non-necrotizing inflammation, and *Acacia* **thorn** (Vaishya, 1990) can cause iridocyclitis. **Belladonna** causes blurring of the vision and impairment of accommodation for near objects, with pupil dilation, shallow anterior chamber, and increased intraocular pressure (Fraunfelder, 1982; Brooks et al., 1986).

Datura cornigera can cause mydriasis and cycloplegia (Dugan et al., 1989). *Laminaria* **digitata** can induce glaucoma (Brooks et al., 1986).

GASES

Many substances are used in tear gases: **bromoacetone, bromomethyl ethyl ketone, bromoxylene, chloroacetone, chloroaceophenone, *o*-chloroenzylidene malononitrile, dichloroformoxime, ethyl bromoacetate, alpha-iodotoluene, pelargonic acid morpholide, trichloroethane, trichloromethane sulfonyl chloride,** and **trichloromethanediol.** All tear gases can produce irritation, lacrimation, and smarting of the eyes.

Chloroacetophenone can produce blepharospasm, and ***o*-chlorobenzylidene malononitrile** can produce burning and pain. Corneal opacity can be induced by **bromoacetone, chloroacetone, chloroacetophenone,** or **ethyl bromoacetate.** Corneal necrosis or ulceration can be induced by **bromoacetone, bromomethyl ethyl ketone,** or **chloroacetophenone.** Corneal edema can be produced by **ethyl bromoacetate;** this substance and **bromomethyl ethyl ketone** can produce corneal scarring. **Dichloroformoxime** may even produce blindness (Folb and Talmud, 1989; Fuchs and in der Wiesche, 1990; Leenutaphong and Goerz, 1989; Petersen et al., 1989; Goh, 1987; Mauchee et al., 1986; Sargent et al., 1986; Jarkman et al., 1985).

War gases include **allyl alcohol, alpha-bromobenzylcyanide, chlorine, chloropicrin, cyanogen chloride, ethylarsine dichloride, lewisite, methyl arisine dichloride, mustard gas, nitrogen mustard, nitrosamines, phenarsazine chloride, phenylcarbylamine, phosgene, sulfuryl chloride, tetrachlorosilane, thiodiglycol,** and **xylyl bromides** (Grant, 1986; Goldman and Dacre, 1989; Pierard and Dowlati, 1989). All of these agents can produce irritation. Many are lacrimatory: **allyl alcohol, chlorine, chloropicrin, cyanogen chloride, ethylarsine dichloride, lewisite, methyl arisine dichloride, mustard gas, nitrogen mustard, phenarsazine chloride, phenylcarbylamine, sulfuryl chloride,** and **xylyl bromides.** Many produce ocular pain (**allyl alcohol, chloropicrin, lewisite, thiodiglycol**), blepharospasm (**chlorine, cyanogen chloride, lewisite, mustard gas, nitrogen mustard, phenylcarbylamine,** and **phosgene**), or photophobia and burning sensations (**allyl alcohol, chlorine, cyanogen chloride, mustard gas, nitrogen mustard,** and **phenylcarbylamine**). There may be edema and hyperemia of the eyelids and conjunctiva (**allyl alcohol, cyanogen chloride, mustard gas, phosgene,** or **dithioglycol**) or conjunctivitis (**cyanogen chloride**). Many cause corneal clouding or opacity (**allyl alcohol, mustard gas, nitrogen mustard, phenylcarbylamine,** or **phosgene**), corneal edema (**allyl alcohol, alpha-bromobenzylcyanide, mustard gas,** and **nitrogen mustard**), or corneal necrosis or ulceration (**ethylarsine dichloride, lewisite, methyl arisine dichloride, mustard gas, nitrogen mustard, phenarsazine chloride, phenylcarbamine, phosgene,** or **sulfuryl chloride**). There may be keratitis (**allyl alcohol, ethyl isothiocyanate, mustard gas,** or **nitrogen mustard**). Other symptoms of exposure may be uveitis from **nitrosamines,** injury of the iris from **nitrogen mustard** or **nitrosamines,** or lens damage from **nitrogen mustard.**

Nerve gas has been dealt with elsewhere; **sarin** can produce miosis and spasm of accommodation for near objects.

Other gases of interest in ocular toxicology include **arsine, carbon dioxide, carboxide, chlorine dioxide, chlorine monofluoride, chlorine oxide, chlorine trifluoride, cyanogen, dichlorodifluoromethane (F-12, Freon F-12), ethylamine, fluorine, formaldehyde, germanium tetrafluoride, hydrogen chloride gas, hydrogen selenide,** and **nitrosyl chloride** (Bake et al., 1988; Anonymous, 1986f, p. 118; Zeitling et al., 1989; Stahlbom et al., 1991; Akesson et al., 1986; Ding 1989; Weber et al., 1988; Krootila et al., 1986; Alderman and Bergin, 1986; Bellander and Hagmar, 1982; Abhyankar et al., 1989). All these gases can cause irritation. **Formaldehyde** can cause lacrimation and photophobia, corneal vascularization, chemosis, and iritis. There may be swelling of the lids after exposure to **formaldehyde** and **arsine.** Corneal edema may follow exposure to **chlorine dioxide, chlorine monofluoride, F-12,** or **formaldehyde.** Some gases cause corneal ulcer or erosion: **chlorine trifluoride, ethylamine, formaldehyde,** and **hydrogen chloride gas;** the latter two gases also may cause corneal clouding or opacity. **Chlorine dioxide** and **formaldehyde** can cause cataract; **chlorine dioxide** also may cause pupil dilation and paralysis of obduction (Dreyfors et al., 1989; Luck and Kaye, 1989; Rabinovitch et al., 1989).

Sodium chloroacetate is a chemical defoliant. Contact with the eyes causes temporary corneal clouding and ulceration (Scarborough et al., 1989).

IODIDES

Iodides have, on topical contact, the effects of lacrimation, edema of the eyelids, conjunctival hyperemia, keratoconjunctivitis, hypopyon, hemorrhagic iritis, and vitreous opacities (Grant, 1986; Anonymous, 1986f, p. 399; Fiore, 1989).

SOLVENTS

A great variety of substances and preparations are used as solvents. The effects of topical exposure of the eyes to solvents depends on the nature of the solvent. Some solvents only produce irritation of the eyes; these include **benzyl acetate, *n*-butyl formate, *n*-butyl methyl ketone, ethyl benzene, isoamyl alcohol, isopropyl** acetate, methyl cyclohexanol, methyl cyclohexanone, methyl formate, methyl isobutyl ketone, 2,5-tetrahydrofurandimethanol, and tetrahydronaphthalene.

Other solvents produce irritation and slight to severe injuries to the eyes. Slight injury is produced by contact with dichloroethyl ether, N, N-dimethylacetamide, dimethyl phthalate, dioxane, epichlorohydrin, 2-ethoxyethanol, or isophorone (ECETOC Working Group, 1989). Moderate injury follows contact with n-butanol, cyclohexanol, cyclohexanone, diacetone alcohol, dimethylaniline, ethyl formate, isobutyl alcohol, methyl acetate, methyl propyl ketone, npropyl alcohol, or pyridine. Severe injury follows exposure to ethylenediamine, ethyl chloroacetate, or bisphenol A. Other solvents with toxic properties on the eyes include acetone, amyl acetate, amyl alcohol, benzyl alcohol, 2-butoxyethanol, butyl acetate, p-tertiary-butyltoluene, diacetin, 1,2-dichloroethane (Anonymous, 1986f, p. 594), diethyleneglycol monoethyl ether, N, N-dimethylformamide, dimethylsulfoxide (DMSO), ethyl alcohol, ethyl acetate, ethyl ethyl ketone, glycerol, methanol, methyl cellosolve, morpholine, nitroparaffins, phosphorus oxychloride, alpha-picoline, sulfolane, tetrachloroethylene, toluene, turpentine, and xylene (Anonymous, 1986f, pp. 637–638).

All these solvents, except benzyl alcohol, cause irritation. Burning, stinging sensations, lacrimation, ocular pain, blurring of vision, blepharospasm, and conjunctival injury follow exposure to acetone or sulfolane. Many solvents cause hyperemia of the conjunctiva: amyl acetate, amyl alcohol, butyl acetate, 2-butoxyethanol, diacetin, 1,2-dichloroethane, ethyl alcohol, methyl cellosolve, methanol, methyl ethyl ketone, toluene, turpentine, and xylene. Chemosis or swelling follows exposure to 2-butoxyethanol, p-tertiary butyltoluene, or methyl cellosolve. DMSO and glycerol cause dilation of blood vessels in the eye. Ethyl alcohol and morpholine can cause necrosis or ulceration. Diethylene glycol monoethyl ether causes conjunctivitis. Amyl alcohol and phosphorus oxychloride cause corneal injury; many agents cause corneal epithelial injury and edema: acetone, amyl acetate, 1,2-dichloroethane, DMSO, ethyl acetate, ethyl alcohol, tetrachloroethylene, toluene, turpentine, and xylene. Several agents cause corneal edema (acetone, benzyl alcohol, ethyl alcohol, glycerol, and methyl ethyl ketone) or corneal opacity (acetone, 2-butoxyethanol, diethylene glycol monoethyl ether, ethyl alcohol, methyl ethyl ketone, morpholine, or turpentine). Benzyl alcohol and xylene cause corneal keratopathy. Toluene, isobutyl alcohol, and n-butanol can cause vacuolar keratitis. Benzyl alcohol, 1,2-dichloroethane, ethyl alcohol, and glycerol can cause endothelial injury; ethyl alcohol also produces corneal infiltration and vascularization. Acetone can cause cataract, and diethylene glycol monoethyl ether can cause iritis. Nitroparaffins can cause mydriasis, and alpha-picoline can cause diplopia. Toluene causes dilation of the pupil and impairment of pupillary reaction to light. Glycerol may cause retinal edema, and amyl acetate can cause retrobulbar neuritis. Turpentine, injected intracamerally, causes fibrinopurulent inflammation and, injected subconjunctivally, causes phthisis bulbi (ECETOC Working Group, 1985, 1986, 1989; Anonymous, 1986f, pp. 637–638, 631, 630, 601–602, 594, 572, 501, 500, 440, 537, 516, 507, 242–244, 237, 233, 221, 206, 203, 199, 186, 178, 171, 159,

156, 151, 408, 402, 401, 397, 395, 391, 378–379, 372, 367, 386, 18, 9, 6–7, 366, 361, 339, 337, 336, 330, 329, 305–308, 280, 259, 83, 76, 73, 29; Anonymous, 1985b, 1987d, 1988c,d,e,m, 1989c,h,f,g; BIBRA Working Group, 1988(a); NIOSH Working Group, 1976, 1978; National Toxicity Program Working Group, 1989a,b; EPA Working Group, 1982; Illing et al., 1987; WHO Working Group, 1987, 1985, 1984a,b; Reutter, 1989; Ansell and Fowler, 1988; Ballantyne and Myers, 1987, Lundberg, 1987; Haley, 1987; O'Donoghue, 1985; Von Burg, 1982).

FOREIGN BODIES

The ocular side effects of foreign bodies in the eye depend on the nature of the foreign body; some substances produce specific reactions of the eye. **Glass, lead metal foreign bodies, peat dust,** and **plastics** cause irritation and can cause injury mechanically (Macewen, 1989; Schein et al., 1983). **Copper metal foreign bodies** and **alloys of brass, bronze,** or **aluminum containing copper** also can cause purulent inflammation, fibrinous iritis, changes of the vitreous and retina, widespread inflammatory and degenerative changes, pigment migration, or macular injury. There may be development of cataract, chalcosis, and glaucoma (Micovic et al., 1990; Good and Gross, 1988).

Iron and **iron compounds** cause siderosis on various ocular tissues. There may be discolorations of ocular tissues. The pupil may become larger or smaller (mydriasis or miosis), and there may be poor reaction to light. Cataract, retinal degeneration, disturbance of vision, or glaucoma may develop (Good and Gross, 1988; Sneed and Weingeist, 1990; Zagorski et al., 1989).

The materials packed in a golf ball may include **sodium hydroxide, barium sulfate,** and **zinc sulfide.** These materials may be corrosive; they may produce deposits in conjunctival and palpebral tissues and macrophage reaction (Grant, 1986).

Common dusting powders are **starch powder** and **talc. Talc** can cause conjunctival inflammation and symblepharon. Injected into the anterior chamber, it produces pseudohypopyon (Grant, 1986). **Starch powder** has been associated with petechial hemorrhages in the retina; injected into the anterior chamber, **starch powder** produces granulomatous reactions and transitory leukocytic and fibrinous exudate (Adams et al., 1990; Kanai et al., 1989; Karcioglu et al., 1988).

GUN POWDER

Gun powder can produce corneal injury, with coagulation of the epithelium and stippling of the epithelium with black particles (Grant, 1986).

Mercury fulminate is a detonator, a powerful explosive. Exposure to **mercury fulminate** may produce conjunctival irritation and itching erythema and swelling of the eyelids (Grant, 1986; Haddad and Winchester, 1990).

SMOG

Smog contains **nitro-olefins, peroxyacetyl nitrate, peroxybenzoyl nitrate, ozone, aldehydes,** and **organic peroxides.** These compounds cause irritation, lacrimation, conjunctival hyperemia, and whitening of the corneal epithelium. **Nitro-olefins** can cause inflammation of the conjunctiva and lids and dilation of superficial blood vessels (Grant, 1986).

PENCILS AND INK

Indelible pencils and **colored pencils** cause injury that depends on the location of the foreign material and its content of cationic dye. Injury from a pencil may cause permanent corneal opacification, ulceration of the conjunctiva, panophthalmis, or necrosis (Grant, 1986).

Hectograph ink can cause burning sensations if it contacts the eyes (Grant, 1986).

TAR

Tar and carbon come in several forms. **Charcoal** has the side effects of irritation, discoloration, and inflammation of the anterior segment of the eye, and can cause fine particles to become embedded in the cornea and conjunctiva. **Coal tar** can cause reddening and squamous eczema of the lid margins, erosions of the corneal epithelium, superficial changes in the corneal stroma, conjunctivitis, discoloration of the cornea, and epithelioma of the lid margin. **Pitch** can cause irritation, chemosis, ulceration and infiltration of the cornea, hypopyon, staining of the cornea and conjunctival discoloration, and deformities of the lids (Liire, 1988; NIOSH Working Group, 1978; Thomson, 1989; BIBRA Working Group, 1986, (a); Anonymous, 1989j; Algvere et al., 1988).

ACIDS AND BASES

Some acids produce specific ocular injury. **Acetic acid** causes irritation, lacrimation, photophobia, swelling of the lids, corneal edema, anesthesia, epithelial injury, and opacity. There may be conjunctival hyperemia, iritis, or a small pupil fixed by posterior synechiae (BIBRA Working Group, 1987, (b); Anonymous, 1986f, p. 4). **Chrysophanic acid** can cause ocular inflammation (Grant, 1986).

Chromic acid can cause corneal infiltration, vascularization, opacification, and ulceration. There may be brown staining of the eye and keratitis. It may also cause occlusion of the central retinal vein (NIOSH Working Group, 1973).

Citraconic acid can cause slight transient injury of the eye (Grant, 1986).

Diphenylarsenic acid can cause tearing, swelling of the lids, and conjunctival hyperemia (Grant, 1986).

Formic acid causes corneal opacity, loss of the endothelium, infiltration and vascularization, and swelling of the epithelium and stroma. There may be hypopyon, iritis and opacity (Grant, 1986). **Mesaconic acid** causes moderate acid-type injury (Grant, 1986).

Pimelic acid causes moderate irritation, swelling of the lids, and corneal opacity (Passi et al., 1989).

Alkalies include **ammonium hydroxide (ammonia), calcium hydroxide (lime), diethylethanolamine, diethylenetriamine, diisopropylamine, 3-dimethylamino-propylamine, sodium hydroxide (lye), tetraethylammonium hydroxide,** and **tetramethylammonium hydroxide.** All alkalies are highly toxic to the eyes, causing irritation, corneal opacification, sloughing of the epithelium, edema, necrosis, infiltration, ulceration perforation, vascularization, scarring, regeneration of the epithelium and endothelium, and loss of corneal mucoid. There may be iritis, followed by disappearance of iritis, cataract, glaucoma, ischemic necrosis, edema of the conjunctiva and limbal region of the sclera, symblepharon, or staphyloma (Hopkins, 1979; Ormerod et al., 1989; Chung, 1988; Mattax and McCulley, 1988; Anonymous, 1979, Anonymous, 1986f, pp. 28, 204; 1988i; WHO Working Group, 1986; Millen et al., 1989; Wrong, 1988; BIBRA Working Group, 1988, (b); 1989, (b); Kriteriegruppen for Hygieniskagransvarden, 1983; Chung, 1990).

Other substances classified as alkalies are **neurine** and **putrescine. Neurine** causes hemorrhagic conjunctivitis and corneal edema with opacities. **Putrescine** causes mucoid discharge and a slight reaction of the eyes (Grant, 1986).

Ethanolamine and **ethanolamine oleate** are sclerosing agents. **Ethanolamine** causes injury similar to that caused by ammonia. Subconjunctival injection of **ethanolamine oleate** causes a severe local reaction (Grant, 1986; BIBRA Working Group, 1989, (b)).

Substances classified as amines include **aliphatic amines, 2-chloroethylamines, cyclic amines, 2-aminoethoxyethanol,** and *N***-aminoethylmorpholine.** These amines cause severe injury to the eyes. Contact with the eyes causes irritation, burning sensations, photophobia, destruction of the corneal epithelium, edema of the corneal epithelium, and keratitis (Grant, 1986; Anonymous, 1987c; Sutton, 1963; Warren and Selchan, 1988; Albrecht and Stephenson, 1988; Deschamps et al., 1988).

ENZYMES

Hyaluronidase is an enzyme used as a spreading agent. It can cause redness and irritation of the eyes, myopia, astigmatism, iritis, and glaucoma; it causes changes in the trabecular meshwork (Grant, 1986).

A number of proteolytic enzymes can have toxic effects on the eyes. **Chymotrypsin** can cause corneal edema, uveitis, scleritis, or an increase in the IOP; it lyses zonular fibers, causing forward displacement of the lens. **Fibrinolysin** can cause disturbance of the endothelium. **Ficin** can be injurious to the eye. **Protease** can cause corneal edema and severe exudative and fibrinous reactions. **Streptokinase** can cause iritis or retinitis. **Trypsin** can cause burning sensations of the eyes, loss of epithelium, destruction of the burning cornea, chorioretinitis, retinal degeneration, or cataract. **Urokinase** can cause irritation, clouding of the cornea, uveitis, increased or decreased IOP, hypopyon, or chemosis (Grant, 1986; Fernandex-Durango et al., 1990; Shearer, 1989; Gondorowa et al., 1990).

RARE-EARTH SALTS

Commonly encountered rare-earth salts include **dysprosium chloride, erbium chloride, gadolinium chloride, praseodymium chloride, samarium chloride, scandium chloride,** and **terbium chloride.** These salts all can cause irritation and redness and edema of the conjunctiva. Many produce conjunctival ulcers (**erbium chloride, dysprosium chloride, scandium chloride,** and **terbium chloride**) or corneal opacity and vascularization (**praseodymium chloride, samarium chloride, scandium chloride,** and **terbium chloride**). **Praseodymium chloride** also produces conjunctival hyperemia and corneal leucoma, and **terbium chloride** causes hyperemia of the iris (Grant, 1986; Ji and Cui, 1988; Wald, 1990; London, 1988).

Other rare-earth salts that cause irritation and conjunctival ulceration are **holmium chloride, thulium chloride, ytterbium chloride,** and **neodymium chloride** (Wald, 1990).

AGENTS FOR AGRICULTURAL USE

Blasticidin-s is an antimicrobial agent used in agriculture. Accidental topical contamination can produce conjunctivitis, keratitis, or hyperemia of the iris (Grant, 1986; Yamashita et al., 1987).

Herbicides (weed killers) include **isocil, 4(2-methyl-4-chlorophenoxy) bubric acid, Natrin, monochloroacetic acid,** and **pentachlorophenol.** Herbicides can cause ocular irritation. **Monochloroacetic acid** can cause corneal epithelial injury. **Natrin** may cause severe damage to the eyes, and **pentachlorophenol** is suspected of causing retrobulbar neuritis (Grant, 1986; Haddad and Winchester, 1990; Vale et al., 1987; Kennedy, 1987).

Other herbicides include **barban, *N*, *N*-diallyl-2-chloroacetamide (CDAA), 2,6-*di-tert*-bubl-*p*-tolylmethylcarbamate (Azak), butofen, dinitro-*o*-cresol (DNOC), diquat, endothal, paraquat,** and *s*-**propyl bublethylthiocarbamate** (Grant, 1986; Scarborough et al., 1989; Hoffer and Taitelman, 1989; Hart, 1987). All of these chemicals can cause irritation. **Diquat** can cause hyperemia of the conjunctiva. **Paraquat** can cause loss of the conjunctival epithelium or loss of the corneal epithelium and corneal scarring (Vale et al., 1987; Hart, 1987). **Butofen** can cause damage to the cornea, while **CDAA** can cause serious damage to the whole eye.

Fertilizers include **ammonia, cyanamide, basic slag, superphosphate, sodium nitrate,** and **urea.** All can cause irritation and are caustic to the eyes. Urea may cause loosening of the epithelium from the stroma or a slow decrease in electrical resistance of the cornea. ***Ammonia*** (Anonymous, 1986f, p. 28; Anonymous, 1979; WHO

Working Group, 1986; Millen et al., 1989; Wrong, 1988) has many topical effects, including irritation, stinging and pain, tearing, and blepharospasm. Rarely, there is keratitis epithelialis. There may be fine, band-shaped corneal clouding, corneal endothelial damage, or corneal stroma edema. There may be iritis or lens damage; severe **ammonia** burns develop all the serious complications caused by strong alkalies in general (Fraunfelder, 1982; Grant, 1986; Havener, 1978; Haddad and Winchester, 1990; Anonymous, 1981a; American Hospital Formulary Service, 1976; Hughes, 1946a,b; Stanley, 1965; Ebert et al., 1990; Wrong, 1988; Douglas and Coe, 1987; Brands, 1987).

Sodium nitrate may cause irritation, with tearing, blepharitis, conjunctival hyperemia, and conjunctivitis. There may be corneal infiltration, superficial corneal clouding, or clouding of the lens (Haddad and Winchester, 1990; Ji and Cui, 1988; Mozingo et al., 1988). **Calcium superphosphate** may cause irritation and corneal burns or even superficial necrosis of the cornea (Grant, 1986).

Soil fumigants include **sodium *N*-methyl-dithiocarbamate** and the so-called **DD mixture.** They can cause ocular irritation (Nesterova, 1988; Van Joost and de Jong, 1988).

Arsenic trioxide is used in agriculture. It can cause the effects of irritation, itching, burning, lacrimation, and photophobia. There may be conjunctivitis, hyperemia, chemosis, or edema of the lids after topical contamination. Corneal injury and opacity may develop. When placed in the anterior chamber, **arsenic trioxide** produces a local necrotizing action (Anonymous, 1987b, 1985e, 1986g; Stern and Knapp, 1986).

SUBSTANCES FOR COMMERCIAL USE

A number of substances are used as bleaches: **chlorinated lime, hypochlorites, hypochlorite and ammonia mixtures; potassium persulfate, sodium hypochlorite,** and **sulfur dioxide.**

All bleaches could cause irritation, with a smarting, burning, or stinging sensation, pain, and lacrimation. All but **potassium persulfate** cause hyperemia of the conjunctiva. **Hypochlorite** and **ammonia mixtures, sodium hypochlorite,** and **sulfur dioxide** can cause keratitis; **sulfur dioxide** also can cause conjunctivitis, corneal opacity and vascularization, and disturbance of vision. **Chlorinated lime** can cause caustic lime burns to the eye (Grant, 1986; Haddad and Winchester, 1990; Pashley et al., 1985; Jessen, 1989).

Cleaning agents include **nitrogen trichloride** and mixtures of compounds used as **oven cleaners.** These preparations can cause irritation and damage to the corneal epithelium and conjunctiva. **"Drano"** is a drain cleaner; in granular, solid form, it consists mainly of sodium hydroxide and can cause devastating damage to the eye (Grant, 1986; Vigoli et al., 1985; Barbee et al., 1983).

Ozone, sodium hydroxide, and **sulfamic acid** are industrial cleaners. All three are irritating (McDonnell et al., 1983; Rowes et al., 1983; Ng et al., 1985); **sulfamic acid** may cause swelling of the lids and blepharospasm and also may cause moderate conjunctivitis, edema, and keratitis (Anonymous, 1982a, 1985c). **Sodium hydroxide** causes erosion of the conjunctiva, devastating injuries of the eye, and increased IOP (Grant, 1986; Haddad and Winchester, 1990; McDonnell et al., 1983; Anonymous, 1987h; Nelson and Kopietz, 1987; Flynn et al., 1984; Moon and Robertson, 1983; Chung and Fagerholm, 1987).

Shampoos may contain **pyrinate, chirimoya** or **cherimoya seeds, "Duponol WAT,"** or **selenium sulfide.** Topical side effects of shampoos can include ocular pain (after **pyrinate** or **chirimoya** or **cherimoya seeds**), irritation, or superficial keratitis (**selenium sulfide**). There may be mild injury to the cornea ("**duponol WAT**"), erosion of the epithelium (from **chirimoya** or **cherimoya seeds**), or loss of the corneal epithelium (**pyrinate**) (Grant, 1986; Haddad and Winchester, 1990; DeGroot et al., 1988a; Morgan et al., 1987; Freeberg et al., 1986; Peer and Ben Ezra, 1988; Clarke, 1986; Del Palacio-Hernanz et al., 1987).

Glues for gluing wood contain a urea–formaldehyde resin. This resin can cause photophobia, blepharospasm, and corneal disturbance (Grant, 1986; Haddad and Winchester, 1990; De Respinis, 1990; Carlson and Wilhelmus, 1987; EPA/OTS, 1983; 1986; Haley, 1987).

Gold is sometimes toxic in industrial settings. Metallic **gold dust** can cause atrophic changes in the retina when introduced into the corneal stroma. **Gold chloride** can cause slight irritation, brown stains of the eye, iritis, nebula, or leukoma with vascularization. **Gold cyanide** induces corneal clouding and severe iritis. **Gold sodium thiosulfate** has been injected into the anterior chamber and has been found to cause injury to the endothelium, corneal edema, and vascularization (Grant, 1986; Haddad and Winchester, 1990; McGuiness and Beaumont, 1985; Fowler, 1987; American Medical Association, 1980, pp. 104–106, 1092; Grubb et al., 1986; McCormick et al., 1985).

Ethylene oxide is used as a fumigant for foodstuffs and medical devices. It can produce irritation, with soreness and a foreign-body sensation in the eye, tearing, conjunctivitis, or keratitis (Estrig et al., 1987).

Matches ignite with a release of irritating oxides. They may cause allergic blepharitis and conjunctivitis (Grant, 1986).

Chemicals used in photography include **hydroquinone, lithium hydroxide,** and **trisodium phosphate.** These chemicals can produce irritation, photophobia, lacrimation, corneal injury, ulceration, or corneal opacification and vascularization. Chronic injury from **hydroquinone** can arise with discoloration, hypesthesia, distortion of the cornea, brownish staining in the cornea and conjunctiva, scarring of the corneal epithelium, corneal flattening, and stigmatism or disturbance of vision (Grant, 1986; BIBRA Working Group, 1986, (b); NIOSH Working Group, 1978).

Depilatories are intended to remove hair and cause breakdown of beta-keratin. They are thus corrosive and cause injuries to the cornea resembling severe calcium hydroxide burns (Grant, 1986; Haddad and Winchester, 1990).

Ethylene glycol is used in antifreeze. Exposure to the vapor or spray causes ocular irritation, edema of the lids, and corneal opacity. When it is splashed into the eyes, there is discomfort with a temporary conjunctival reaction. After intracameral injection, iritis and corneal opacity develop (Haddad and Winchester, 1990; Ballantyne and Myers, 1987; BIBRA Working Group, 1988, (c); Anonymous, 1986f, p. 253).

p-Dichlorobenzene is used to protect clothing against moths. This agent can cause irritation, ocular pain, or cataracts (Haddad and Winchester, 1990; Siegel and Watson, 1986; Anonymous, 1986f, p. 179).

Sodium hexametaphosphate is the principal ingredient in water softeners. Side effects of topical contact with this compound include chemosis and hemorrhages in the conjunctiva and nictitating membrane (of species with a nictitating membrane), corneal edema, and hyperemia of the iris (Grant, 1986).

Many kinds of detergents are used in industry; many of them have been dealt with in the section on Surfactants. Other detergent agents are carbon tetra- chloride, polyethyleneglycol ethers, soaps, enzyme–detergent combinations, or "pHisoHex." Soap can cause stinging pain, conjunctival hyperemia and damage of the corneal epithelium. Polyethyleneglycol ethers can produce inflammation, corneal hypesthesia, corneal edema, ulceration, vascularization, and keratitis epithe- lialis. "pHisoHex" also can cause corneal edema, and enzyme–detergent combi- nations can cause transient conjunctivitis. Carbon tetrachloride can cause reduc- tion of central visual acuity and visual field abnormalities (Grant, 1986; Haddad and Winchester, 1990; DeGroot et al., 1988a; Freeberg et al., 1986; Shapkin-Gunko et al., 1989; Martin et al., 1962).

Fire-extinguisher fluids may contain carbon tetrachloride, methyl bromide, chlorobromomethane, or tetrachloroethylene. These compounds may cause su- perficial injury to the eye. Chlorobromomethane, in particular, causes severe burn- ing sensations, photophobia, hyperemia, and edema of the conjunctiva and lids; there may be transient corneal epithelial injury (Haddad and Winchester, 1990; Hezemans- Boer et al., 1988; Anonymous, 1986f, pp. 125–126; Illing et al., 1987; WHO Work- ing Group, 1984b; Miller, 1982; Wirtschafter, 1933; Smith, 1950).

Acriflavine is a germicide with the side effects of irritation and of corneal injury, opacity, and vascularization (Ng and Goh, 1989).

Sodium chloride is used in many industrial situations and also is used as a topical agent to reduce corneal edema. Side effects include hyperemia and a transitory rise in the IOP (Fraunfelder, 1982; Grant, 1986; Walsh and Hoyt, 1969; Huang et al., 1989; Kruger et al., 1990). Solutions of sodium chloride that are used as topical os- motic agents may produce irritation, hyperemia, ocular pain and burning sensations, corneal dehydration, subconjunctival hemorrhages, or increases in IOP (Fassihi and Naidoo, 1989).

Antimony trichloride is highly corrosive. Topical effects include strong irritation and destruction of the cornea and conjunctiva (Grant, 1986; Haddad and Winchester, 1990).

SUBSTANCES FOR MEDICINAL USE

Ammonium chloride can cause hyperemia of the iris or hemorrhages of the iris. It may induce a salt cataract, increase in the intraocular pressure, or fibrin in the anterior chamber with corneal edema (WHO Working Group, 1986; Anonymous, 1986f, p. 21).

Ointments which contact the eye may cause interference with corneal wound healing. There may be intraocular penetration of ointment bases and oils. Water-soluble or greaseless ointment bases may cause keratitis (Anonymous, 1986e).

Paraffin may cause considerable tissue reaction. There may be loss of vision following an embolus of **paraffin** reaching the retinal arteries. When paraffin is put into the anterior chamber, it causes slight inflammatory reactions and clouding of the cornea (Grant, 1986; Willis et al., 1988).

Radiopaque x-ray media are used in orbitography. One procedure involves retrobulbar injection of a mixture of 25% sodium diatrizoate and 1% lidocaine. This procedure has caused rapidly reduced vision, dilation of the pupil, weakness of abduction, and nystagmus (Finger et al., 1990). In another case, an unidentified **radiopaque medium** caused pain, edema, diplopia, and severe granulomatous reaction when injected along the floor of the orbit (Grant, 1986).

Orbital injection of **diodone** causes edema of the lids and transient loss of vision (Grant, 1986). **Amylopectin sulfate** and **polyethylene sulfonic acid** were injected into the eye in a study of experimental retinal detachment. **Amylopectin** caused iritis and contraction of vitreous strands and retinal adhesions. **Polyethylene sulfonic acid** caused uveitis, vitreous opacities, partial liquifaction and formation of strands, detachment of the retina, cataract, dislocation of the lens, band keratopathy, and superficial calcification of the cornea (Grant, 1986; Refojo, 1988).

Tattooing of the cornea may cause uveitis (Grant, 1986).

Gastric juice contaminating the eyes can cause corneal ulceration (Grant, 1986).

Hemoglobin, injected into the vitreous, caused damage of the rods; the so-called AU visual cells disappeared (Schuchereba et al., 1990).

Catechol, in solid form, causes burns of the eye (Anonymous, 1986f, p. 112).

AGENTS OF INDUSTRIAL USE

Workers with aircraft and missiles have the potential danger of ocular contamination with some unusual agents. **Dural** causes irritation, conjunctivitis, and blepharitis. Propellants may be ocular toxins. **Pentaborane** produces miosis. **Tetranitromethane** produces irritation, and **methylhydrazine** causes corneal edema, swelling, and injury of the corneal epithelium (Grant, 1986; Anonymous, 1986f, p. 459; Anonymous, 1989f; Yarbrough et al., 1985–1986).

Workers in building and masonry can come into contact with **calcium hydroxide** (slaked lime) and **calcium oxide** (quicklime). These agents have caustic effects resembling lime burns (Logai et al., 1989; O'Grady, 1989; BIBRA Working Group, 1988, (b); Anonymous, 1986f, p. 92).

The chemical industry brings workers into proximity with a number of toxic chemicals. Methylating agents include **dimethyl sulfate, methyl bromide, methyl chloride,** and **methyl iodide.** All these agents produce irritation, and all except **methyl chloride** produce lacrimation. **Dimethyl sulfate** produces pain and photophobia, corneal opacity, and necrosis and edema of the lids. Conjunctival hyperemia is reported after exposure to **dimethyl sulfate** and **methyl chloride**. **Methyl bromide** and **methyl chloride** can produce blurring of vision and diplopia. **Methyl bromide** can produce retinal hemorrhage; **methyl chloride** can produce ptosis (Wang et al., 1988; Anger et al., 1986; Hezemans-Boer et al., 1988; Anonymous,1986f, pp. 380–381, 399).

Agents used in routine organic synthesis can be toxic. The nature of the injury depends on the agent. **Acetonitrile** causes damage like acetone. **Diketene** and **thionyl chloride** cause irritation. **Methylamine** causes irritation, hemorrhages in the conjunctiva, corneal opacity, and edema. **Red phosphorus** is sometimes used in organic synthesis; when injected into the anterior chamber, it produces hypopyon and dilation of blood vessels of the iris. **Potassium metal** produces severe ocular injuries (Grant, 1986; Anonymous, 1986f, pp. 373, 572; Sharir et al., 1987; Kiteriegruppen for Hygieniskagransvarden, 1983).

Other agents commonly used in chemical manufacture are **acetic anhydride, acetyl chloride, allyl chloride, barium hydroxide, boron tribromide, chlorosulfonic acid, cyanic acid, cyclododecatriene, ethylenimine, mercuric iodide, phosphorus trichloride, piperidine,** and **triethylamine** (Albrecht and Stephenson, 1988). All cause irritation; many cause severe damage to the eyes (**acetyl chloride, barium hydroxide, chlorosulfonic acid,** and **triethylamine**). **Acetic anhydride** causes burning sensations and photophobia and edema of the eyelids or conjunctiva. **Acetic anhydride, cyanic acid,** and **ethyleneimine** can produce lacrimation. **Chlorosulfonic acid** causes swelling of the lids. **Cyclododecatriene, ethylenimine,** and **phosphorus trichloride** can produce conjunctivitis; **cyclododecatriene** can also cause dermatitis of the lids. **Acetic anhydride** and **chlorosulfonic acid** can cause corneal edema; **ethylenimine** can cause keratitis. Many agents (**acetic anhydride, barium hydroxide, boron tribromide, phosphorus trichloride,** and **piperidine**) can cause clouding or opacity of the cornea; **boron tribromide** also causes corneal hypesthesia, scarring, and vascularization. **Acetic anhydride, boron tribromide,** and **triethylamine** all can cause erosions to the eye; when injected into the anterior chamber they produce damage to the eye, purulent exudate and inflammation (Grant, 1986; BIBRA Working group, 1987, (c); Anonymous, 1986f, pp. 5, 486; Anonymous, 1988j).

Many substances are used as catalysts in industrial synthesis. Common catalysts with ocular toxic properties include **aluminum alkyls, antimony pentachloride, *t*-butyl hydroperoxide, cyclohexanone peroxide, diacetyl peroxide, *N*-methyl morpholine, osmium tetroxide,** various **organic peroxides, phosphorus pentachloride, silver(II)oxide, tetramethylbutanediamine, triethylenediamine,** and **vanadium pentoxide** (Grant, 1986; Anonymous, 1986f, p. 485; Shichi, 1990; Albrecht and Stephenson, 1988).

Antimony pentachloride can cause severe injury to the eyes. **Cyclohexanone peroxide** can cause moderately severe corneal injury with superficial opacity and associated conjunctival inflammation. ***t*-Butyl hydroperoxide** and ***N*-methyl morpholine** can cause moderate injury of the eyes; ***N*-methyl morpholine** can also cause sloughing of the epithelium, corneal haze, or conjunctival hyperemia. **Osmium tetroxide** can cause keratitis epithelialis or blurring of vision by fixing corneal proteins. **Diacetyl peroxide** (Albrecht and Stephenson, 1988), **tetramethylbutanediamine,** and **triethylenediamine** can all cause corneal damage, irritation, lacrimation, burning sensations, ocular pain, and photophobia. Corneal epithelial edema can be produced by *N*-**methyl morpholine, osmium tetroxide, tetramethylbutanediamine,** or **triethylenediamine; tetramethylbutanediamine** also can cause mydriasis and cycloplegia. **Vanadium pentoxide** can cause conjunctivitis (Grant, 1986).

Calcium chloride and **phosphorus peroxide** are used as drying and dehydrating agents. They can cause irritation on topical exposure. **Calcium chloride** can produce superficial injuries to the eye and miosis (BIBRA Working Group, 1989, (c); Hightower and Farnum, 1985; Krootila et al., 1986; Singh et al., 1985–1986); **phosphorus peroxide** is more dangerous, causing burns to the lids, conjunctiva, and cornea and leaving blue-white opacities (Grant, 1986; Albrecht and Stephenson, 1988).

Many chemicals are used in the manufacture of dyes, including **acrylamide, anthraquinone, aniline, benzene, barium chloride,** *bis*-**(chloromethyl) anthracene, benzoyl chloride, 2,4-dinitrophenol (DNP), lactic acid, manganese compounds, nitric acid,** *m*-**nitroaniline, nitronaphthalene, oxalic acid,** *p*-**phenylenediamine, phthalic anhydride, quinones, sodium hydrosulfite, titanium tetrachloride,** and *o*-**toluidine.** All these agents can produce ocular irritation; other side effects depend on the agent. **Anthraquinone** can produce inflammation, and injuries to the eyes can follow exposure to **benzoyl chloride, 2,4-dinitrophenol,** *o*-**toluidine,** or **titanium tetrachloride.** *bis* **(Chloromethyl) anthracene** can induce blepharospasm and, like *p*-**phenylenediamine,** may produce conjunctival hyperemia. Conjunctival edema may follow exposure to *p*-**phenylenediamine** or **sodium hydrosulfite.** Conjunctivitis may be induced by *p*-**phenylenediamine** and **phthalic anhydride. Nitric acid** can produce necrosis of the eyelids or conjunctiva, and sometimes symblepharon. **Quinones** and *m*-**nitroaniline** can stain the conjunctiva. Superficial corneal injury can follow exposure to **acrylamide;** there also may be vitreous opacities. Corneal opacity and clouding can be produced by *bis***(chloromethyl) anthracene,** *m*-**nitroaniline, oxalic acid,** *p*-**phenylenediamine,** or **nitric acid. Lactic acid** can cause corneal epithelial coagulation and, sometimes, corneal necrosis, perforation, and vascularization or hypopyon; **nitronaphthalene** can cause keratitis. Corneal ulceration can be produced by *p*-**phenylenediamine,** and corneal opacification and vascularization can be produced by **manganese compounds. Acrylamide, barium chloride,** and *p*-**phenylenediamine** can produce iritis or iridocyclitis. **Phthalic anhydride** can produce exophthalmos or proptosis. Cataract can follow exposure to **acrylamide, lactic acid,** or **nitronaphthalene** (Takahasi et al., 1988; BIBRA Working Group, 1990; BIBRA Working Group, 1987, (d); Anonymous, 1985d, 1988f, 1989i,m, 1990a; Anonymous, 1986, pp. 387–388, 451, 487, 509, 244, 228; NIOSH Working Group, 1976, p. 78; BIBRA Working Group, 1989, (d); Venables, 1989; Anson, 1988; Ladefoged, 1982).

Agents used in the explosives industry include **nitrogen dioxide, sulfuric acid, sulfur trioxide, tetryl, trinitrobenzene, fulfuric acid,** and **trinitrotoluene (TNT).**

All these substances except **trinitrobenzene** can cause irritation. **Sulfuric acid** and **sulfur trioxide** can cause devastating damage to the eye. **Tetryl** can cause dermatitis of the eyelids and conjunctivitis or keratitis and iridocyclitis. **Nitrogen dioxide** can cause damage of the corneal epithelium and corneal opacity. **Sulfuric acid** and **trinitrotoluene** can induce cataract, and **fulfuric acid** can induce glaucoma. **Trinitrobenzene** can cause yellowing of the conjunctiva or sclera or optic neuritis and amblyopia. **Trinitrotoluene** can cause disturbance of vision, pupil dilation, blurring, and hyperemia of the optic nerve heads (Grant, 1986; Vevchenko and Vysochin, 1988; WHO Working Group, 1978; Anonymous, 1986f, p. 586).

Fuels are of many kinds; some of the fuels used in industry or in hobbies include **dimethylamineborane, dimethylhydrazine, fuel for model airplanes** (a mixture of methyl alcohol, nitromethane or nitropropane, and castor oil), **hydrazine, petroleum products,** and, at some places, **uranium compounds.** All can cause irritation. **Dimethylamineborane** and **petroleum products** cause hyperemia of the conjunctiva; **dimethylamineborane** and **fuel for model airplanes** can cause conjunctival edema. **Uranium compounds** are capable of producing moderately severe injury to the eyes and necrosis of the eyelids and conjunctiva; they also may produce perforating ulceration of the cornea. **Fuel for model airplanes** and **petroleum products** can cause injury to the corneal epithelium. **Petroleum products** can cause cataract and, after subconjunctival injection, they may cause chemosis and exophthalmos and corneal clouding (Grant, 1986; Anonymous, 1986f, pp. 210, 310; Anonymous, 1987g; 1989k).

The manufacture of lubricants involves some special compounds: **barium oxide, decyl alcohol,** and **silicone oil. Decyl alcohol** is slightly injurious to the eyes, but **barium oxide** causes severe alkali burns of the eyes (Anonymous, 1989n). **Silicone oil** causes corneal edema, vascularization and scarring, glaucoma, and cataract (Bennett and Abrams, 1990; Suzuki et al., 1990; Setula et al., 1989).

The manufacture of apparatus for laboratory use involves the use of some particular compounds: **platinum salts** and **polytetrafluoroethylene.** These substances cause irritation and lacrimation. **Platinum salts** cause burning sensations, photophobia, and conjunctival hyperemia. **Polytetrafluoroethylene** can cause etching of the cornea (Butcher et al., 1989; Adenis et al., 1989; Steinkogler, 1988; Johnson et al., 1989).

Some compounds encountered in the pharmaceutic industry include **bromal, *n*-butyl amine, dichloroethyl acetate** (Robert et al., 1988), **halazone, methyl cellulose, *o*-nitrobenzylchloride, phenothiazine, phosphoric acid, polysorbate 80, tartaric acid,** and **triethanolamine.** All these substances, except **methylcellulose** and **polysorbate 80,** cause irritation. Severe injury to the eyes can be induced by *n*-**butyl amine. Phosphoric acid** and **triethanolamine** can cause hyperemia of the conjunctiva. **Dichloroethyl acetate** can cause conjunctivitis and corneal ulceration. Corneal edema can be induced by **phosphoric acid, polysorbate 80,** and **triethanolamine. Triethanolamine** also can produce hyperemia of the iris. **Methyl cellulose** can produce iridocyclitis and increases in the IOP, and **phenothiazine** can cause corneal keratitis (Grant, 1986; Anonymous, 1983e, 1988k; Booman et al., 1988; EPA/OTS, 1989a).

Compounds used in the manufacture of plastics include **acrylic acid, acrylonitrile, dibutyl phthalate, dibutyl tin dichloride, ethyl acrylate, furfural, levulinic acid, methocryonitrile, methyl acrylate, polyvinyl chloride, toluene diisocyanates, tributyl phosphate,** and **vinyl acetate.** Side effects depend on the compound. **Vinyl acetate** can cause slight injury to the eyes; **methyl acetate** causes mild injury, while **acrylic acid** and **levulinic acid** cause severe injury to the eyes. **Methocryonitrile** and **toluene diisocyanates** cause irritation and blepharospasm; these compounds, as well as **methyl acrylate** and **dibutyl tin dichloride,** can cause lacrimation. **Furfural** and **toluene diisocyanates** can cause swelling of the eyelids or corneal edema. **Toluene diisocyanates** can cause conjunctivitis, keratitis, iridocyclitis, or glaucoma. **Dibutyl tin dichloride** can cause hyperemia of the conjunctiva, and **furfural** can cause hemorrhage of the conjunctiva. **Acrylonitrile** can cause transient disturbance of the cornea. **Ethyl acrylate** and **tributyl phosphate** can cause injury of the epithelium (Grant, 1986; EPA/OTS, 1989b; EPA Working Group, 1983; Anonymous, 1986f, pp. 280, 580–581, 591, 621; Anonymous, 1986i; BIBRA Working Group, 1987, (e); BIBRA Working Group, 1988, (d); Nielsen et al., 1989; Maki-Paakkanen and Norppa, 1988; BIBRA Working Group, 1987, (f)).

Gilsonite is a mineral hydrocarbon used in making roads and roofs and causes irritation (Keimig et al., 1987).

Arsenic trichloride is used in the ceramic industry. It can produce irritation, blepharospasm, photophobia, or lacrimation. There may be redness of the conjunctiva after exposure, corneal ulceration, and corneal opacity (Anonymous, 1980).

Lead chloride is used in the manufacture of white lead. It causes moderate purulent reactions and general inflammation of the eye (Grant, 1986).

Agents used in the manufacture of perfumes include **acetophenone** (BIBRA Working Group, 1987, (f)), **allyl bromide, menthol, methylal, methyl salicylate, 1-naphthol, octanol, oil of citronella, phenethyl alcohol,** and **propyl acetate. Oil of citronella** and **methyl salicylate** can cause slight eye injury; **acetophenone, menthol,** and **1-naphthol** can cause severe injury. **Octanol** can cause irritation and corneal epithelial injury, while **phenethyl alcohol** can cause clouding of the epithelium (Grant, 1986; BIBRA Working Group, 1986, (c); Anonymous, 1986f, pp. 371, 500; Anonymous, 1989b; ECETOC Working Group, 1987).

Industrial reducing agents include **calcium carbide** and **lithium hydride. Calcium carbide** causes injuries like lime burns. **Lithium hydride** causes irritation, inflammation, corneal opacity, and ulceration (Grant, 1986; Anonymous, 1986f, p. 349).

The manufacture of matches uses **white phosphorus** and **phosphorus sesquisulfide. White phosphorus** causes blepharospasm, photophobia, lacrimation, corneal opacity, interstitial vascularization, episcleritis, and inflammation of the eye. **Phosphorus sesquisulfide** causes irritation, blepharitis, and conjunctivitis (Grant, 1986; Mozingo et al., 1988).

Chemicals used in the manufacture of rubber include **chloroprene, cyclohexyl-amine, diethanolamine, dibenzathiazyl disulfide, diethylamine, 1,3-diethylthio-urea, dimethylamine, diphenyl guanidine, (MBTS), 1-mercaptobenzothiazole, methyl vinyl ketone, styrene, sulfur monochloride,** and **thiram. Cyclohex-ylamine** and **dimethylamine** can cause severe injury to the eye; **diethanolamine** causes moderate injury. **Sulfur monochloride** causes irritation and corrosion. **Diphenyl guanidine** causes conjunctival edema, while **styrene** causes hyperemia of the conjunctiva. **Dimethylamine** can cause hemorrhage of the conjunctiva or corneal edema and infiltration, and **1,3-diethylthiourea** can cause keratitis or oc-ular pain with photophobia and blurred vision. **Chloroprene** and **methyl vinyl ke-tone** can cause conjunctivitis; these agents, as well as **diethylamine** and **styrene,** can cause corneal epithelial injury. **Diphenyl guanidine** and **3-diethylthiourea** can cause punctate corneal epithelial defects, while **cyclohexylamine, diethylamine,** and **dimethylamine** can cause corneal opacity (BIBRA Working Group, 1986, (d); Anonymous, 1986f, pp. 161–162, 135, 197, 206, 410, 545, 573; BIBRA Working Group, 1988, (e); BIBRA Working Group, 1989, (e); Ogawa et al., 1989; Ken-nah et al., 1989; Fielder and Lowing, 1981; Dalvi, 1988; BIBRA Working Group, 1986, (e)).

The manufacture of soaps involves the use of **oleic acid, potassium carbonate, potassium hydroxide, sodium aluminate, sodium carbonate,** and **sodium silicate. Potassium hydroxide** and **sodium aluminate** cause injuries like alkali burns. **Oleic acid** causes inflammation, scarring, necrosis and vascularization of the eyes, and corneal abscess. **Potassium carbonate** induces ocular pain and slight transient op-tical irregularities of the epithelium. **Sodium carbonate** and **sodium silicate** cause damage of the corneal epithelium (Anonymous, 1986f, pp. 495, 409, 264; Anony-mous, 1987e,f; Babaian et al., 1989; Burns and Paterson, 1989; BIBRA Working Groups, 1988, (f)).

Thioglycolic acid is a reagent that causes ocular pain, conjunctival edema, hyper-emia, necrotic neovascularization, and corneal opacity (Anonymous, 1986f, p. 521).

Synthesis of resins involves the use of **diglycidylresorcinol, epon, maleic acid,** and **maleic anhydride.** These agents produce irritation. **Maleic anhydride** produces burning sensations in the eyes, while **maleic acid** causes conjunctival hyperemia and corneal edema, opacity, and vascularization (BIBRA Working Group, 1989, (f); Anonymous, 1986c; Anonymous, 1986f, p. 353; BIBRA Working Group, 1985; Dreyfors et al., 1989; Venables, 1989).

Manufacture of textiles, woolens, and cloth involves some special reagents. Man-ufacture of textiles involves **carbon disulfide, divinyl sulfone, glycolic acid, naph-thalenebutylsulfonate sodium,** and **thioformaldehyde. Divinyl sulfone** causes se-vere burns; **glycolic acid** causes irritation and moderately severe injury. **Carbon disulfide** causes keratitis epithelialis, retrobulbar neuritis, and disturbance of vision. Manufacture of woolens involves **ficin,** which induces injuries to the eyes. Manufac-ture of some kinds of cloth involves **urea–formaldehyde,** which causes irritation of the eye. Manufacture of nylon involves **1,6-hexanediamine,** which causes ocular irritation (Schwartz, 1989; Vale and Rycroft, 1988; Anonymous, 1989j, 1986j; Peters, 1986).

Nitrocellulose paint or **lacquer** can cause keratitis, cataract, and optic neuritis (Grant, 1986; Morgan et al., 1990).

Manufacture of glass requires **silica,** which causes inflammation of the eye, corneal edema, opacity and vascularization, necrosis of the retina, and atrophy of the choroid. Removing color from glass involves **sodium selenite,** which causes severe injury to the eyes (NIOSH Working Committee, 1977; Watanabe and Shearer, 1989; David et al., 1988).

Compounds used in soldering are **fluorides, zinc chloride,** and **zinc sulfate. Zinc chloride** causes pain and redness of the eye, and it can cause corneal ulcer, vascularization, and opacity. It also may cause iritis or acute angle-closure glaucoma. **Fluorides** are necrotic to the conjunctiva and cause inflammation of the eye or corneal edema. Both **fluorides** and **zinc chloride** can cause injury of the epithelium or hemorrhages of the iris. **Zinc chloride** and **zinc sulfate** can cause cataract (Grant, 1986; Anonymous, 1986f, pp. 514, 272–273; Anonymous, 1986k, 1988h; Ding, 1989).

Manufacture of batteries involves **lead sulfate** and **nickel metal.** When **lead sulfate** was placed in the anterior chamber, it produced a moderate purulent reaction and inflammation of the eye. **Nickel metal** can cause conjunctivitis and epiphora (Walsh and Hoyt, 1969; Cremers and Hofstee, 1989).

Allyl amines are used in the manufacture of mercurial diuretics. They cause severe ocular irritation (Grant, 1986).

Compounds used in the cotton industry include **aniline, pyridine, formaldehyde, nitrogen oxide, hydrochloric acid, sulfuric acid,** and **sodium hydroxide.** Some of these substances are discussed elsewhere in this chapter. All of them cause clouding of the corneal stroma, vitreous opacities, retinal arteriosclerosis, and myopia (Anonymous, 1986f, pp. 507, 276–277; Anonymous, 1988f; Dutertre-Catella et al., 1989; Fielder, 1981; Burns and Paterson, 1989).

Fiberglass dust can cause irritation of the conjunctiva and cornea (Emmett, 1983; NIOSH Working Committee, 1977).

Strontium hydroxide is used in the refining of sugar. It causes serious burns to the eyes like other strong alkalies (Grant, 1986).

Hydrofluoric acid (HF) is used in the cleaning of cast iron, copper, and brass, and in etching glass. It causes irritation, ocular pain, conjunctival hyperemia, loss of the epithelium from the cornea and conjunctiva, and edema of the lid, conjunctiva, and cornea (Caravata, 1988; Flood, 1988).

Yttrium chloride is a rare-earth metal salt used in the preparation of pure metal. It can cause corneal opacity and corneal vascularization (Anonymous, 1986f, p. 641; London, 1989).

Indium trichloride is used in electroplating; it causes irritation (Anonymous, 1986f, p. 322).

Copper cyanide plating bath is used in the electroplating of copper and can cause alkali burns (Mozingo et al., 1988).

Some chemicals and substances used in the automotive industry are ocular toxins. **Brake fluid** is composed of alcohols, glycols, and a lubricant, such as castor oil. Topical contamination causes severe smarting and burning sensations and injury of the corneal epithelium (Grant, 1986).

Tetraethyl lead is a gasoline additive. It can cause slight mydriasis, photophobia, smarting sensations, blepharospasms, and contractions of the visual field (Grant, 1986).

Cobalt compounds are used to make metal alloys. These compounds can cause corneal injury, corneal opacification and vascularization, and uveitis (BIBRA Working Group, 1988, (g); Anonymous, 1990b).

The manufacture of mirrors involves the use of **mercury metal (liquid)** or of **silver metal, silver ammonium compounds,** or **silver nitrate. Liquid mercury metal** causes corneal opacity, band keratopathy, purulent reactions, local abscesses, detachment of the retina, and shrinkage and atrophy of the eye. **Silver nitrate** can cause argyria and edema of the conjunctiva and lids, symblepharon, or cataract. **Silver ammonium compounds** and **silver nitrate** can cause corneal opacity and scarring, while exposure to **silver metal** can cause retinal atrophy (Merigan, 1989; Anonymous, 1986f, pp. 529–531; Pifers et al., 1989).

Makare is used in cabinet making. Exposure to **makare** causes ocular irritation with lacrimation and swelling of the eyelids (Grant, 1986).

Pinha is a substance employed in the preparation of an alcoholic tincture used in repelling lice. It can induce the side effects of edema and erosions of the corneal epithelium, chemosis of the conjunctiva, and dermatitis of the lids (Grant, 1986).

The synthesis of polymers can involve the use of **methyl polymers** and **diepoxybutane. Methyl polymers** can cause ocular irritation. **Diepoxybutane** can cause severe injury, with loosening and sloughing of the epithelium, and opacification of the corneal stroma with scarring and vascularization (Grant, 1986; Illing and Shillaker, 1985; Anonymous, 1971).

Bicycloheptadiene dibromide is an alkylating agent. It can cause conjunctivitis and hemorrhage in the fundus (Grant, 1986).

Difluoro is an intermediate in the chemical manufacture of **sarin. Difluoro** can cause irritation and opacity (see War Gases).

There are a number of miscellaneous compounds used in manufacturing which can be ocular toxins. **Nitrosomethyl urethane** is used in the synthesis of diazomethane (Anonymous, 1986f, p. 173). It can produce irritation, hyperemia, blepharospasm, chemosis, and loss of the corneal epithelium or edema of the corneal epithelium. There may be keratitis, epithelialis, and blurring of vision after exposure. **Sulfosalicylic acid** is used in the precipitation of proteins. It can cause hazing of the cornea and hyperemia of the iris. **Tetraethoxysilane** is used as a waterproofing agent. It can cause ocular irritation and opacities of the cornea; **1,3-butadiene** and **1,4-butynediol** can cause irritation. **Copper chloride** can cause severe injury to the cornea with permanent opacification. **Iodine monobromide** can cause corrosion of the eye. **Methyl *n*-butyl ketone** causes moderate irritation (Anonymous, 1986f, p. 173). **Tantalum fluoride** causes burns of the cornea (Anonymous, 1986f,

p. 554). **Mortar, plaster,** and **Portland cement** cause injuries like a lime burn (Grant, 1986; Mozingo, 1988; Illing and Shillaker, 1985; Clark et al., 1989; BIBRA Working Group, 1981, (g); Fielder and Lowing, 1981; Parke et al., 1988; Yu et al., 1990).

AIR POLLUTANTS

Air pollutants are gaseous particles which, when added to the air, cause adverse effects on humans. Air pollutants are subdivided into outdoor and indoor pollutants. Outdoor air pollutants include, but are not limited to, carbon monoxide, nitrogen oxides, sulfur oxides, hydrocarbons, ozone, and particulate matter, whereas indoor air pollutants include formaldehyde, acrolein, hydrocarbons, and biological organisms (Godish, 1985). Where the indoor air is polluted by second-hand smoke, the air will contain more than 4,000 chemicals, many of which are potentially deadly, including at least 43 known compounds that cause cancer. These harmful agents include cadmium, ammonia, benzene, acetone, formaldehyde, and thousands of other toxic gases and airborne particles. Particles represent both solid and liquid phases which disperse in the air as a suspension. The smog produced by gas condensation and concomitant photochemical reactions can reduce visibility and cause eye irritation.

Irritation to the Eye

Although eye irritation is the most frequently reported toxic symptom associated with exposure of humans to air pollution, this ophthalmic effect is largely overlooked (Wilson, 1974). Eye irritants in the atmosphere can be formed by the interaction of hydrocarbons with sulfur oxides and nitrogen oxides. Smogs can be divided into two systems, synthetic and natural. Synthetic smog systems include formaldehyde, peroxybenzol nitrate (PB_2N) (Heuss and Glasson, 1968), peroxyacetyl nitrate (PAN), and acrolein. These synthetic smog materials are produced from automobile exhaust, olefin–nitrogen oxide mixtures, or by ultraviolet irradiation of aromatic hydrocarbons and nitrogen oxides. Natural smog could come from volcanic eruption, photochemical reactions, and the like. Most studies are limited to synthetic smog materials, however.

Measurements of Eye Irritation

Tearing is the most common sign of eye irritation. Tears are secreted from lacrimal glands and from accessory glands. Tears from lacrimal glands contain lysozyme, whereas tears from accessory glands, the goblet cells of the conjunctiva, do not contain lysozyme (McEwen and Goodner, 1969). Tears are unique fluids which contain a specific tear protein (STP) that does not correspond to any protein in the serum (Bonavida, et al., 1969). Although the role of STP is not clear, there is an interesting relationship between STP and lysozyme: a decrease in lysozyme concentration with an increase in STP. Changes in lysozyme concentration are presently used as a biomarker of eye irritation. Dose–response relationship measurements have been attempted to relate the degree of eye irritation with the concentration of smog. In general, more accurate results are obtained with synthetic smog than with natural smog.

Intense efforts have been made to determine the degree of eye irritation objectively. Because of small tear sample size, capillary electrophoresis has to be used to analyze its chemical contents, particularly the lysozyme. Another approach to the measurement of eye irritation is the use of electrophysiological measurement of neuronal responses subsequent to stimulation of sensory receptors in the cornea (Tower, 1940). Electrodes can be attached to the long ciliary nerves (Lele and Weddell, 1959) or trigeminal nerve complex (Mosso and Kruger, 1972, 1973) to detect the chemical stimulation of the cornea.

Determination of lysozymes and pH values of tears coupled with sensitive detectors, such as laser-induced fluorescent detectors, may provide a reasonable approach to establish a more precise relationship between the concentration of the irritants and the degree of eye irritation produced.

Clinical symptoms of eye irritation include foreign-body sensation, hyperemia, chemosis of conjunctiva, tearing, and dry sensation of the eye (Heuss and Glasson, 1968). Of all these air pollutants, PAN was found to be 200-fold more irritating to the eye than formaldehyde (Heuss and Glasson, 1968), whereas ozone was found not to be an important eye irritant (Schuck and Doyle, 1959; Hamming et al., 1967). Because of limited air exchange, outdoor pollutants can be concentrated in the indoor environment. Further, some buildings contain toxic air pollutants sufficient to cause adverse effects on humans. These effects are called *sick building syndrome*. Eye irritation is the first physical sign and symptom to be noted in this syndrome (Nero, 1988). The eye irritation includes watery eyes, burning sensation, stinging eyes, foreign-body sensation, and rubbing and itching of the eyes.

Volcanic Eruption

Six weeks after the volcanic eruption of Mt. St. Helens, it was found that 4–8% of the urban population in the high air fallout area complained of eye irritation (Fraunfelder et al., 1983). The ocular problems included foreign-body sensation, hyperemia, and irritative conjunctivitis. Individuals who wore contact lenses or who had dry-eye syndrome were bothered the most by the volcanic ash exposure. Wearers of hard contact lenses had more problems than wearers of soft contact lenses. The ocular symptoms usually subsided in one to two days after leaving the ash environment. The volcanic ash caused hyperproduction and secretion of mucus. However, the toxic effect of the volcanic pollutants was less than expected, possibly due to the small size of the particulate matter. Also, the ash was chemically inert and contained only 4–6% of free silica (Klopfer, 1989).

Particulate matter refers to small particles with diameters in the range 0.005–500 μm. The smallest particles are fumes (0.03–0.3 μm) and smoke (0.05–1.00 μm). Mists (0.5–3 μm) are liquid particulates formed by vapor condensation, whereas sprays (710 μm) are liquid formed by atomization of another liquid (Klopfer, 1989). The largest particles are dust (>100 μm), which are solids formed by mechanical processes, including coal and ash cement. Usually, the larger the particle the more irritating it is to the eye.

Carbon monoxide (CO) is the major air pollutant in the atmosphere exerting toxic effects on the eye. In heavy, slow traffic, it results in 30 ppm of CO in the air to develop a level of 5% carboxyhemoglobin, and to decrease the sensitivity to light, particularly at night (Halperin et al., 1959). At 500 ppm of CO, retinal hemorrhage and papilledema occur. CO intoxication can also produce ocular neuropathy, including cortical blindness (Grimsdale, 1934), visual field reduction (Fink, 1951), nystagmus, optic neuritis, optic atrophy, and pupillary abnormality (Bilchik and Muller-Bergh, 1971). In addition to carboxyhemoglobin formation by CO decreasing the oxygen-carrying capacity of the blood, CO also binds to visual receptors in the central and/or peripheral visual system to exert its toxicological effects.

Ischemic retinopathy is another manifestation of CO intoxication (Bilchik and Muller-Bergh, 1971). Retinal venous congestion, hyperemia of papilla, and fine retinal hemorrhage might occur occasionally.

Nitrogen Compounds

Nitrogen compounds include N_2O, NO, and $NO_2 \cdot N_2O$ and NO are colorless, odorless, and tasteless gases that produce little irritation to the eye. Their major adverse effects on the eye come from their oxidation, as they are involved in various photochemical reactions with hydrocarbons, ozones, and formaldehyde. NO_2 is yellowish to reddish in color and has a rather pungent, irritating property. It is produced by the oxidation of NO, particularly on a sunny day, and is quite irritating to the eye. The resident time of NO and NO_2 in the atmosphere is approximately 3–4 days.

Sulfur Compounds

Most of the sulfur compounds which pollute the air are sulfur oxides, particularly SO_2, which attains sufficient concentrations to produce adverse effects in humans. SO_2 is a colorless gas but produces an unpleasant taste and odor in concentrations of 0.3–1.0 ppm. At concentrations higher than 3 ppm, it has a pungent odor and is quite irritating to the eye. SO_2 undergoes further oxidation in the air to sulfate ($SO_4 =$). SO_2 is effectively removed from the atmosphere by natural processes. Since it is highly soluble in water, it can be effectively removed during rain.

Photochemical Oxidants

Organic nitrites are formed by photochemical reactions involving a series of hydrocarbons and NO_x (NO and NO_2 together). Organic nitrite compounds include peroxyacyl nitrate (PAN), peroxypropionyl nitrate (PPN), and peroxybutery nitrate (PBN).

Among these, PAN is the most important pollutant as it can cause eye irritation. Hydrocarbons which can enter into photochemical oxidation include aliphatic hydrocarbons, olefins, and polyunsaturated hydrocarbons. They are precursors to form aromatic hydrocarbons, such as benzopyrene, benzene, and so on.

Photochemical oxidants refer to chemicals that can be oxidized easily, not by oxygen directly, but by chemical reactions with NO_x, oxygen, and sunlight. They include O_3, NO_2, PAN, and related compounds. These reactions can raise the concentration of primary pollutants, such as formaldehyde, olefins, and various organic formaldehydes.

Building Pollutants

Building pollutants contribute primarily to indoor pollution. Formaldehyde is a common material used in wall paneling and pressed wood insulation. Xylene and toluene are solvents associated with paint products. Cyclopentadine is a carpet adhesive which primarily causes eye irritation. Dimethyl acetamide is used in plastic office dividers and is a potent irritant. Methacrylate and methanol are present in signature machines and duplicators. Ozone is produced by photocopying machines.

Formaldehyde

As mentioned previously, formaldehyde is widely used in building materials. It is also widely used in industry as various chemical products. Formaldehyde is very irritating to the eyes. Approximately 10% of the U.S. population may be hypersensitive to the irritating effect of formaldehyde, particularly in the eyes. The main source of this chemical in the indoor environment is its use as a urea–formaldehyde foam insulation. Formaldehyde is slowly liberated from the urea–formaldehyde foam as it degrades. The formaldehyde liberation is directly proportional to the temperature and humidity of the building. As the temperature and humidity increase, the formaldehyde concentration also will increase.

Pyrolytic End Products

Burning wood, charcoal, straw, dung, kerosene, and petroleum products with open fire in a room during wintertime contribute greatly to indoor air pollution; gas stoves release carbon monoxide, various nitrogen oxides, formaldehyde analogs, and hydrocarbon particles that irritate the eyes. The other indoor pollutant of greatest concern is tobacco smoke. Acrolein and formaldehyde released in the air can cause eye irritation in smoke-filled rooms. It should be understood that the adverse health effects of pyrolytic end products are present not only in the eye but also in other systems, such as the pulmonary, cardiovascular, and central nervous systems.

Occupational Hazards

Occupationally related disease of the eye was first noted by Ramazzini (1964). He described in detail in his book of occupational medicine that a noxious gas (H_2S) caused toxic injuries to the eyes of workers who worked in the sewer systems. These workers developed red, inflamed eyes and complained of a burning sensation. The prognosis of these workers was rather poor, as they ultimately lost their eyesight. Hydrogen sulfide can be present in relatively high concentrations in septic pools, sewers, and underground passages. This gas is quite toxic, and its irritant properties can cause severe conjunctivitis and keratitis (Ramazzini, 1964). Two of the classic texts on occupationally related diseases and injuries to the eye were written by Minton (1949) and, later, by Grant (1986).

The occurrence of eye injuries caused by hazardous chemicals in the workplace is rather common and widespread. Damage to the eye can result from local topical injuries or from systemic absorption of these chemicals. These effects on the eye may occur either immediately or insidiously. An extensive list of chemicals that have injurious effects on the eye has been compiled by Grant (1986) and Anger and Johnson (1985). In this chapter, only a few of the most commonly encountered chemicals are mentioned as examples.

Ammonia

Inadvertent release of ammonia gas from accidents or agricultural and industrial equipment is a frequent, unfortunate occurrence today. Ammonia is a colorless gas that has a characteristic pungent odor. It is quite hygroscopic in that it combines with water to form ammonium hydroxide. The severity of the damage to the eye is attributed to the dissociation of ammonium hydroxide into the hydroxyl ion. The eye is especially sensitive to these caustic burns of a strong base. Such injuries are usually associated with an increase in intraocular pressure (Highman, 1969) and the destruction of tissues. The clinical course after exposure to ammonia is similar to that seen in individuals with acute angle-closure glaucoma associated with corneal edema and a semidilated fixed pupil. To minimize the damage of the eye, a prompt, vigorous ocular irrigation with water is essential. Topical steroid cream and antibiotics should be given prophylactically. Even a vigorous and timely treatment may not prevent the fatal destruction of cornea resulting in blindness when the exposure to ammonia is severe (Birken et al., 1981).

The characteristic pungent order of ammonia is readily detectable by the smell well below the toxic level. Ammonia odor usually can be detected at 30 ppm, whereas the eye irritation occurs at 50 ppm (Rom, 1983).

Carbon Disulfide

Carbon disulfide is a volatile, colorless, flammable liquid with an ethereal odor. Its technical grade, however, has a rather unpleasant odor because of contamination by other sulfides. According to the National Institute of Occupational Safety and Health (NIOSH), over 20,000 workers in the United States are exposed to carbon disulfide annually (NIOSH, 1977).

The effects of carbon disulfide on the ocular system have been reviewed (NIOSH Working Group, 1984). It causes retinal hemorrhages or microaneurysms (Goto and Hottar, 1967; Goto et al., 1971). The frequency of microaneurysms was found to be directly related to the extent of carbon disulfide exposure. Ophthalmodynamography has been used as a diagnostic test for detecting early signs of carbon disulfide–induced cerebral involvement (Maugeri and Cavalleia, 1966). Grant indicated that the peripheral and central signs and symptoms were quite varied. In severe, chronic poisoning, retrobulbar neuritis occurred which resulted in visual disturbances, including central scotoma, decreased visual acuity, and impaired color discrimination of red and green (Grant, 1986).

Hydrogen Sulfide

Hydrogen sulfide is a highly toxic gas widely used in various industrial processes. It is also found in natural gas, volcanoes, certain natural spring waters, sewers, sewer treatment plants, wells, and caissons.

Hydrogen sulfide is a rapidly acting poison with an extremely high knockdown potency. It is colorless, heavier than air, and has a well-recognized odor of rotten egg. Although this gas can be easily detected at very low concentrations, people should not rely on the olfactory system to detect this gas, as olfactory fatigue occurs rapidly at 100–150 ppm. This fatigue leads to the impression that the hydrogen sulfide gas is diminishing in concentration, whereas it may be actually increasing (Rom, 1983).

At concentrations of 200 ppm, H_2S causes pain in the eye, visual blurring, and superficial corneal turbidity (Environmental Protection Agency, 1986). At lower concentrations, the unpleasant odor of H_2S is detected first, a few hours before ocular symptoms develop. A gradual onset of ocular symptoms includes scratchy, irritating, tearing, and burning sensations. Slit-lamp biomicroscopic examination reveals only a conjunctival hyperemia and keratitis. More exposure can lead to increased burning, discomfort, photophobia, and color halos. As the exposure becomes more severe, the corneal surface may become lusterless and eroded from death and loss of epithelial cells.

Ethylene Oxide

Ethylene oxide is a reactive compound that is used extensively for sterilization, particularly in hospitals and pharmaceutical firms. Therefore, it becomes an increasing concern of workers in hospitals and pharmaceutical firms as they are routinely exposed to high levels of ethylene oxide. There appears to be a correlation between ethylene oxide exposure and cataract formation (Jay et al., 1982).

This reactive gas is colorless and has a characteristic ethereal odor. It is a potent alkylating agent acting directly on nucleophils, such as -OH, -SH, $-NH_2$ and -COOH groups of purines, pyrimidino, and amino acids. This reaction may be the basis of the mutagenicity and carcinogenicity of ethylene oxides (Ehrenberg et al., 1974). It also binds to histidine moiety in hemoglobin.

Exposure to high concentrations of ethylene oxide results in irritation lacrimation, conjunctival inflammation, and clouding of the cornea.

Cyanide

Cyanide is widely used in industry and is present in many poisonous plants. Its acute toxic effects on vision include mydriasis, blindness, and damage of optic nerve and retina (Grant, 1986). In experimental animals, marked central retinal edema, lesions in the retina and the optic nerve, degeneration in the optic nerve, optic chiasma, and changes in the electroretinogram have been reported.

Chronic cyanide exposures such as tobacco smoking (Smith and Duckett, 1965) and cassava ingestion, result in optic neuropathies (Wilson, 1967), optic neuritis (Osuntokun, 1968), and tobacco amblyopia (Darby and Wilson, 1967).

Hydrogen Fluoride

Hydrogen fluoride in aqueous solution is called hydrofluoric acid, which is widely used in the etching of silica products, in the production of semiconductors, and in many other industries. Hydrofluoric acid is extremely irritating to the mucous membrane, conjunctiva, and skin. It causes irritation to the eye at concentrations as low as 5 ppm. Hydrogen fluoride's presence in industrial air can cause conjunctival hyperemia in the palpebral fissure, although corneal disturbances are rare (Grant, 1986). With direct contact of hydrofluoric solution in the eye, there is an immediate coagulation and sloughing of corneal epithelium with moderate conjunctival inflammation developing. Further, chemosis and corneal opacity can develop.

n-Hexane

n-Hexane is an organic solvent widely used in industry. Its ocular toxicity includes blurred vision, polyneuropathy, optic atrophy, and retrobulbar neuritis. In experimental animals, visual loss, abnormal pupillary reflexes, and nystagmus have been noted (Spencer and Schaumberg, 1977; Schaumberg and Spencer, 1976). The most important aspect of n-hexane ocular toxicity is the development of retinal toxicity and macular damage which causes color discrimination defects (Mergler et al., 1987). Furthermore, n-hexane exposure is related to the diminution of foveal reflex and incipiency of lens opacification.

Toluene Diisocyanate

Toluene diisocyanate is a reactive chemical that is used in the production of polyurethane foam. Its toxicity to the eye includes decreased visual acuity, red, irritated eyes, blurred vision, mild edema of corneal epithelium, and conjunctival inflection (Luckenback and Kielar, 1980).

Formaldehyde

Formaldehyde is an intermediate that is used widely in many occupations (NIOSH, 1981). Exposure to formaldehyde at concentrations as low as 0.05 ppm results in detectable eye irritation. Lacrimation occurs at concentrations of 20 ppm in the air. An accidental splash of 40% formalin solution in the eye causes immediate pain, but the eye appears uninjured for the first few hours. During the next 12 hr, however, all the areas of the cornea will show damage and edema, and the interior segment will develop degeneration, opacification, photophobia, swelling of the lid, and chemosis.

REFERENCES

Abhyankar, A., Bhambure, N., Kamath, N.N., et al. 1989. Six month follow-up of fourteen victims with short-term exposure to chlorine gas. *Journal of the Society of Occupational Medicine* 39:131–132.

Adams, A.J., and Brown, B. 1975. Alcohol prolongs time course of glare recovery. *Nature* 257:481.

Adams, H.A., Hossemer, V., Jacobi, K.W., and Kempelmann, G. 1990. Plasma level of lidocaine and adrenaline in local anesthesia with addition of colloid in eye surgery. *Fortschritte der Ophthalmologie* 87:209–213.

Adams, M.E. 1989. Structure and pharmacology of spider venoms. In *FEDRIP Database*, National Technical Information Service (NTIS).

Adenis, J.P., Leboutet, M.J., Salomon, J.L., Duprat, F., and Loubet, R. 1989. Experimental and clinical study of conjunctival–scleral tolerance of PTFE (Goretex) suture compared to polygalactine (Vicryl). *Ophtalmologie* 3:231–232.

Agrawal, R.C., Sarode, A.V., Lalitha, V.S., and Bhide, S.V. 1985. Chili extract treatment and induction of eye lesion in hamsters. *Toxicology Letter* 28:1–7.

Agrawal, R.K. 1985. Traumatic cataract following bee sting. *Indian Journal of Ophthalmology* 33:59–60.

Akesson, B., Bengtsson, M., and Floren, I. 1986. Visual disturbances after industrial triethylamine exposure. *International Archives of Occupational Environmental Health* 57:297–302.

Albert, D.M., Wong, V.G., and Henderson, E.S. 1967. Ocular complications of vincristine therapy. *Archives of Ophthalmology* 78:709.

Albrecht, W.N., and Stephenson, R.L. 1988. Health hazards of tertiary amine catalysts. *Scandinavian Journal of Work Environmental Health* 14:209–219.

Alderman, L.C., and Bergin, J.J. 1986. Hydrogen selenide poisoning: an illustrative case with review of the literature. *Archives of Environmental Health* 41:354–358.

Algvere, P., Wallow, I.H., and Martini, B. 1988. The development of vitreous membranes and retinal detachment induced by intravitreal carbon microparticles. *Graefes Archives of Clinical Experimental Ophthalmology* 226:471–478.

American Hospital Formulary Service. 1974. *American Hospital Formulary Service*, vol. 2, pp. 72–100. Washington, DC: American Society of Hospital Pharmacists.

American Hospital Formulary Service. 1976. *American Hospital Formulary Service*, vol. 2, p. 28. Washington, DC: American Society of Hospital Pharmacists.

American Medical Association. 1980. *American Medical Association Drug Evaluations*, 4th ed. New York: John Wiley.

Anand, M., Gapal, K., Mehrotra, S., Chandra, S.V., Ray, P.K., and Paul, A.K. 1987. Ocular toxicity of organochlorinated pesticides in rabbits. *Journal of Toxicology and Cutaneous Ocular Toxicology* 6:161–171.

Andersen, K.E., and Maibach, H.I. 1980. Allergic reaction to drugs used topically. *Clinical Toxicology* 16:415.

Anger, W.K., and Johnson, B.L. 1985. Chemicals affecting behavior. In *Neurotoxicology of Industrial and Commercial Chemicals*, ed. J.L. O'Donoghue, pp. 51–148. Boca Raton, FL: CRC Press.

Anger, W.K., Moody, L., Burg, J., et al. 1986. Neurobehavioral evaluation of soil and structural fumigation using methyl bromide and sulfuryl fluoride. *Neurotoxicology* 7:137–156.

Anonymous. 1971. Diepoxybutane *IARC Monographs on the Evaluation of the Carcinogenic Risk of Chemicals to Humans* 11:115–123.

Anonymous. 1979. Ammonia. In *Medical and Biological Effects of Environmental Pollutants*, p. 354. National Research Council.

Anonymous. 1980. Arsenic and arsenic compounds. *IARC Monographs on the Evaluation of the Carcinogenic Risk of Chemicals to Humans* 23:39–141.

Anonymous. 1981a. Calcium cyanamide. *Cahiers de Medecine Interprofessionnelle* 21:43.

Anonymous. 1981b. Chemical hazard information profile draft report. Diethyl phosphorochlorothioate. CAS No. 2524-04-1. Washington, DC: EPA, Office of Toxic Substances.

Anonymous. 1982a. Sulfamic acid. *Cahiers de Medecine Interprofessionnelle* 22:11.

Anonymous. 1982b. Information profiles on potential occupational hazards: phthalates. Center for Chemical Hazard Assessment, SCRTR 82-520. Syracuse: Syracuse Research Corp.

Anonymous. 1983a. Final report on the safety assessment of sodium borate and boric acid. *Journal of the American College of Toxicology* 2:87–125.

Anonymous. 1983b. Final report on the safety assessment of sodium lauryl sulfate and ammonium lauryl sulfate. *Journal of the American College of Toxicology* 2:127–181.

Anonymous. 1983c. Final report on the safety assessment of PEG-2, -6, -8, -12, -20, -32, -40, -50, -100, and -150 stearates. *Journal of the American College of Toxicology* 2:17–34.

Anonymous. 1983d. Final report on the safety assessment of vinyl acetate/cotonic acid copolymer. *Journal of the American College of Toxicology* 2:125–140.

Anonymous. 1983e. Final report on the safety assessment of triethanolamine, diethanolamine and monoethanolamine. *Journal of the American College of Toxicology* 2:183–235.

Anonymous. 1984. Final report on the safety assessment of dioctyl adipate and diisopropyl adipate. *Journal of the American College of Toxicology* 3:101–130.

Anonymous. 1985a. Final report on the safety assessment of benzethonium chloride and methylbenzethonium chloride. *Journal of the American College of Toxicology* 4:65–106.

Anonymous. 1985b. Final report on the safety assessment of butylene glycol, hexylene glycol, ethoxydiglycol and dipropylene glycol. *Journal of the American College of Toxicology* 4:223–248.

Anonymous. 1985c. Sulfamic acid. Cahiers de notes documentaires. *Securité et Hygiene du Travail 3rd Qtr.* 120:393–396.

Anonymous. 1985d. Final report on the safety assessment of 2-nitro-*p*-phenylenediamine and 4-nitro-*o*-phenylenediamine. *Journal of the American College of Toxicology* 4:161–202.

Anonymous. 1985e. Arsenous oxide. In *EPA Chemical Profiles*. Washington, DC: EPA.

Anonymous. 1985f. Paris green. In *EPA Chemical Profiles*. Washington, DC: EPA.

Anonymous. 1986a. Final report on the safety assessment of zinc phenolsulfonate. *Journal of the American College of Toxicology* 5:373–390.

Anonymous. 1986b. Final report on the safety assessment of hydroquinone and pyrocatechol. *Journal of the American College of Toxicology* 5:123–165.

Anonymous. 1986c. Final report on the safety assessment of toluenesulfonamide/formaldehyde resin. *Journal of the American College of Toxicology* 5:471–490.

Anonymous. 1986d. Final report on the safety assessment of drometrizole. *Journal of the American College of Toxicology* 5:455–470.

Anonymous. 1986e. Final report on the safety assessment of hydroquinone and pyrocatechol. *Journal of the American College of Toxicology* 5:123–165.

Anonymous. 1986f. *Documentation of the Threshold Limit Values of Biological Exposure Indices*, 5th ed. American Confederation Government of Individual Hygienists.

Anonymous. 1986g. *Arsenic and Its Compounds (Except Arsine)*. Toronto: Industrial Accident Prevention Association.

Anonymous. 1986h. Final report on the safety assessment of toluenesulfonamide/formaldehyde resin. *Journal of the American College of Toxicology* 5:471–490.

Anonymous. 1986i. Methyl acrylate. *IARC Monographs on the Evaluation of the Carcinogenic Risks of Chemicals to Humans* 39:99–112.

Anonymous. 1986j. Vinylidene chloride. *IARC Monographs on the Evaluation of the Carcinogenic Risk of Chemicals to Humans* 39:195–226.

Anonymous. 1986k. *Zinc Chloride*. Calcutta: Indian Chemical Manufacturers Association, India Exchange Place.

Anonymous. 1987a. Eye safety: irritants, exposure effects, and protective devices. *Government Reports, Announcements and Index, Jan 1976–May 1987*.

Anonymous. 1987b. Arsenic trioxide. In *Arbetarskyddsnamnden*. Stockholm.

Anonymous. 1987c. Diaminotoluenes. In *Environmental Health Criteria 74* Geneva: World Health Organization, International Programme on Chemical Safety, (IPCS).

Anonymous. 1987d. Final report on the safety assessment of *n*-butyl alcohol. *Journal of the American College of Toxicology* 6:403–424.

Anonymous. 1987e. Final report on the safety assessment of oleic acid, lauric acid, palmatic acid, myristic acid and stearic acid. *Journal of the American College of Toxicology* 6:321–401.

Anonymous. 1987f. Final report on the safety assessment of sodium sesquicarbonate, sodium bicarbonate, and sodium carbonate. *Journal of the American College of Toxicology* 6:121–138.

Anonymous. 1987g. Hydrazine. *Environmental Health Criteria*, p. 68. Geneva: WHO.

Anonymous. 1987h. *Sodium hydroxide*. Hamilton, Ontario: Canadian Centre for Occupational Health and Safety.

Anonymous. 1988a. Final report on the safety assessment of stearate-2,-4,-6,-7,-10,-11,-13,-15 and -20. *Journal of the American College of Toxicology* 7:881–910.

Anonymous. 1988b. Final report on the safety assessment of 2,3-naphthalenediol. *Journal of the American College of Toxicology* 7:353–357.

Anonymous. 1988c. Final report on the safety assessment of methylene chloride. *Journal of the American College of Toxicology* 7:741–835.

Anonymous. 1988d. Final report on the safety assessment of amyl acetate and isoamyl acetate. *Journal of the American College of Toxicology* 7:705-719.

Anonymous. 1988e. 3-methylbutanol-1. *Toxikologische Bewertungen* 95:1–17.

Anonymous. 1988f. *Aniline*. Chicago: National Safety Council.

Anonymous. 1988g. *Cresols, All Isomers*. U.S. Department of Health and Human Services. Cincinnati: Public Health Service, Center for Disease Control.

Anonymous. 1988h. *Inorganic Fluorides*. Chicago: National Safety Council.

Anonymous. 1988i. Nine toxicity studies on diisopropylamine with cover letter. EPA/OTS Doc #89-880000108.

Anonymous. 1988j. Occupational safety and health guidelines for chemical hazards. Division of Standard Development and Technology Transfer, OHHS (NIOSH) Publ. #89-104 Suppl. 12-OHG. Cincinnati: National Institute of Occupational Safety and Health.

Anonymous. 1988k. *Phosphoric Acid*. Paris: Institut National de Recherche et de Securité.

Anonymous. 1988m. *Trichlorofluoromethane*. Paris: Institut National de Recherche et de Securité.

Anonymous. 1989a. Final report on the safety assessment of 4-amino-2-hydroxytoluene. *Journal of the American College of Toxicology* 8:569–578.

Anonymous. 1989b. Final report on the safety assessment of 1-naphthol. *Journal of the American College of Toxicology* 8:749–768.

Anonymous. 1989c. Final report on the safety assessment of morpholine. *Journal of the American College of Toxicology* 8:707–748.

Anonymous. 1989d. Final report on the safety assessment of 4-amino-2-hydroxytoluene. *Journal of the American College of Toxicology* 8:569–588.

Anonymous. 1989e. Final report on the safety assessment of ethyl acetate and butyl acetate. *Journal of the American College of Toxicology* 8:681–705.

Anonymous. 1989f. Consensus report for nitromethane and tetranitromethane. *Arbete Och Halsa* 32:55–63.

Anonymous. 1989g. Consensus report for diacetone alcohol. *Arbete Och Halsa* 32:26–33.

Anonymous. 1989h. 1,1,2,2-tetrachlorethane. *Beratergremium fuer umweltrelevante Altstoffe (BUA)* 29:1–83.

Anonymous. 1989i. *Benzene*. Hamilton, Ontario: Canadian Centre for Occupational Health and Safety.

Anonymous. 1989j. Eye safety: irritants, exposure effects and protective devices Jan. 1976–June 1989. (Citations from the Energy Department Base.) *Government Reports, Announcements and Index*, Issue 16.

Anonymous. 1989k. *Hydrazine Hydrate and Aqueous Solutions*. Paris: Institut National de Recherche et de Securité.

Anonymous. 1989m. Soluble barium compounds (as barium). *Noticias de Seguridad* 51:insert 4.

Anonymous. 1989n. *Soluble Barium Compounds (as Barium)*. Paris: Institut National de Recherche et de Securité.

Anonymous. 1989o. Consensus report for creosote. *Arbete Och Halsa* 32:18–25.

Anonymous. 1990a. *Aniline*. Commission of the European Communities. International Programme on Chemical Safety (IPCS). Geneva: World Health Organization.

Anonymous. 1990b. Toxicity of cobalt. *Government Reports, Announcements and Index*, Issue 05.

Ansell, J.M., and Fowler, J.A. 1988. The acute oral toxicity and primary ocular and dermal irritation of selected n-alkyl-2-pyrrolidones. *Food and Chemical Toxicology* 25:475–479.

Anson, S.W. 1988. Mechanisms of chemically induced photosensitivity. In *Crisp Data Base*. Washington, DC: National Institutes of Health.

Arena, J.M. 1970. *Poisoning: Toxicology, Symptoms, Treatment*, 2nd ed. Springfield, IL: Charles C. Thomas.

Armaly, M.F. 1962. Ocular tolerance to silicones. *Archives of Ophthalmology* 68:390.

Armaly, M.F. 1963. Effect of corticosteroids on intraocular pressure and fluid dynamics I. Effect of dexamethasone in the normal eye. *Archives of Ophthalmology* 70:482.

Aronson, S.B., and Elliott, J.H. 1972. *Ocular Inflammation*, pp. 91–92. St. Louis: C.V. Mosby.

Awan, K.J. 1976. Adverse systemic reactions of topical cyclopentolate hydrochloride. *Annals of Ophthalmology* 8:695.

Axelsohn, U. 1986. Glaucoma, miotic therapy and cataract. *Acta Ophthalmologica* 46:83–105.

Axelsohn, U., and Holmberg, A. 1973. The frequency of cataract after miotic therapy. *Acta Ophthalmologica* 44:421–429.

Babaian, Ea., Nazerotian, R.A., and Khachatrian, R.R. 1989. Toxicological characteristics and hygienic standardization on the levels of sodium hydrocarbonate and potassium carbonate in the air of the work place. *Gigiena Truda i Professionalnye Zabolevaniia (Moskva)* 5:30–32.

Baer, R.L. 1990. Poison ivy dermatitis. *Cutis* 46:34–36.

Bake, M. Ia., Rusakova, N.E., and Emke, I.A. 1988. Gas-chromatographic analysis of carboxide in the air of the work area. *Gigiena Truda i Professionalnye Zabolevaniia (Moskva)* 9:46–47.

Ballantyne, B., and Myers, R.C. 1987. The comparative acute toxicity and primary irritancy of the monohexyl ethers of ethylene and diethylene glycol. *Veterinary and Human Toxicology* 29:361–366.

Baranowski-Dutkiewicz, B. 1981. Skin absorption of phenol from aqueous solutions in men. *International Archives of Occupational Environmental Health* 49:99.

Barbee, S.J., Thackara, J.W., and Rinehart, W.E. 1983. Acute inhalation toxicology of nitrogen trichloride. *American Industrial Hygiene Association Journal (Fairfax VA)* 44:145–146.

Barney, N.P., Kleinman, R.E., Trocme, S.D., Block, K.J., and Allansmith, M.R. 1988. Attenuation of rat conjunctival response by repeated haptan application. *Current Eye Research* 7:843–848.

Becker, B. 1964. The side effects of corticosteroids. *Investigative Ophthalmology* 3:492.

Becker, B., and Morton, W.R. 1966. Topical epinephrine in glaucoma suspects. *American Journal of Ophthalmology* 62:272.

Bellander, T., and Hagmar, L. 1982. Kriteriengruppen-for-hygieniska-gansvarden. Morfolin. *Arbete Och Halsa* 32:1–32.

Bennett, S.R., and Abrams, G.W. 1990. Band keratopathy from emulsified silicone oil. *Archives of Ophthalmology* 108:1387.

Berkow, J.W., Gills, J.P., and Wise, J.B. 1969. Depigmentation of eyelids after topically administered thiotepa. *Archives of Ophthalmology* 82:415.

Bernstein, H.N. 1967. Chloroquine ocular toxicity. *Survey of Ophthalmology* 12:415.

Beutner, K.R., and van Krogh, G. 1990. Current status of podophyllotoxin for the treatment of genital warts. *Seminars in Dermatology (Philadelphia PA)* 9:148–151.

BIBRA Working Group. 1985. Maleic acid. In *Toxicity Profile*. British Industrial Biology Research Association.

BIBRA Working Group. 1986. (a) Carbon black. (b) Hydroquinone. (c) Menthol. (d) Cyclohexylamine. (e) 2-Mercaptobenzothiazol and its sodium salt. In *Toxicity Profile*. British Industrial Biology Research Association.

BIBRA Working Group. 1987. (a) Carrageenan. (b) Acetic acid and its common salt. (c) Acetic anhydride. (d) Methyl cyclopentadienyl manganese tricarbonyl. (e) Dibutyl phthalate. (f) Acetophenone. In *Toxicity Profile*. British Industrial Biology Research Association.

BIBRA Working Group. 1988. (a) Methyl n-amyl ketone. (b) Calcium hydroxide. (c) Ethylene glycol. (d) Ethyl acrylate. (e) Diethanolamine. (f) Methyl silicate. (g) Cobalt naphthenate. In *Toxicity Profile*. British Industrial Biology Research Association.

BIBRA Working Group. 1989. (a) Chlorobutanol. (b) Ethanolamine. (c) Calcium chloride. (d) N,N'-diphenyl-para-phenylenediamine. (e) Diethylamine and its hydrochloride. (f) 1,2-dihydro-2,2,4-trimethylquinoline (monomer and polymer). (g) Alpha-methylstyrene. In *Toxicity Profile*. British Industrial Biology Research Association.

BIBRA Working Group. 1990. Lactic acid. In *Toxicity Profile*. British Industrial Biology Research Association.

Biger, Y., and Abulafia, C. 1986. Eye injuries due to cactus thorns. *Harefuah* 110:611–612.

Bilchik, R.C., and Muller-Bergh, H.A. 1971. Ischemic retinopathy due to carbon monoxide poisoning. *Archives of Ophthalmology* 86:142–144.

Birken, G.A., Fabri, P.J., and Carey, L.C. 1981. Acute ammonia intoxication complicating multiple trauma. *Journal of Trauma* 33:820–822.

Blake, J., and Cassidy, H. 1979. Ocular hypersensitivity to dextran. *Irish Journal of Medical Science* 148:249.

Boettner, E.A., Fralick, F.B., and Wolter, J.R. 1974. Conjunctival concretions of sulfadiazine. *Archives of Ophthalmology* 92:446.

Bonavida, B., Sapse, T., and Sercarz E. 1969. Specific tear albumin: a unique lachrymal protein absent from serum and other secretions. *Nature* 221:375–376.

Bonomi, L., and Di Comite, P. 1967. Outflow facility after guanethidine sulfate administration. *Archives of Ophthalmology* 78:337.

Booman, K.A., Cascieri, T.M., Demetrulias, J., et al. 1988. In vitro methods for estimating eye irritancy of cleaning products phase I: preliminary assessment. *Journal of Toxicology and Cutaneous Ocular Toxicology* 7:173–185.

Bracher, M., Faller, C., Spengler, J., and Reinhardt, C.A. 1987–1988. Comparison of in vitro cell toxicity with an in vivo eye irritation. *Molecular Toxicology* 1:561–570.

Brands, A. 1987. Asphyxiant gases. In *Handbook of Toxicology*, eds. Haley, T.J. and Berndt, W.O., pp. 472–503. New York: Hemisphere Publishing.

Brooks, A.M., West, R.H., and Gillies, W.E. 1986. The risks of precipitating acute angle-closure glaucoma with the clinical use of mydriatic agents. *Medical Journal of Australia* 145:34–36.

Brownstein, S., Liszaner, A.D., and Jackson, W.B. 1989. Ocular complications of a topical methylene blue–vasoconstrictor–anesthetic preparation. *Canadian Journal of Ophthalmology* 24:317–324.

Bucci, M.G. 1975. Topical administration of oxprenolol (beta blocking agent) in the therapy of glaucoma. Preliminary note. *Bulletin Oculist* 54:235.

Burns, F.R., and Paterson, C.A. 1989. Prompt irrigation of chemical eye injuries may avert severe damage. *Occupational Health Safety* 58:33–36.

Burns, R.P. 1966. Delayed onset of chloroquine retinopathy. *New England Journal of Medicine* 275:693.

Burns, R.P., and Gipson, I. 1978. Toxic effects of local anesthetics. *Journal of the American Medical Association* 240:347.

Butcher, B. T., Bernstein, I.L., and Schwartz, J.H. 1989. Guidelines for the clinical evaluation of occupational asthma due to small molecular weight chemicals. *Journal of Allergy and Clinical Immunology* 84:834–838.

Byron, H.M., and Posner, H. 1964. Clinical evaluation of Protopam. *American Journal of Ophthalmology* 57:409.

Campochiaro, P.A., and Sen, H.A. 1989. Adenosine and its agonists cause retinal vasodilation and hemorrhages. Implication for ischemic retinopathies. *Archives of Ophthalmology* 107:412–416.

Caravata, E.M. 1988. Acute hydrofluoric acid exposure. *American Journal of Emergency Medicine* 6:143–150.

Carlson, A.N., and Wilhelmus, K.R. 1987. Giant papillary conjunctivitis associated with cyanoacrylate glue. *American Journal of Ophthalmology* 104:437–438.

Chamberlain, W.P., and Boles, D.J. 1946. Edema of the cornea precipitated by quinacrine (Atabrine). *Archives of Ophthalmology* 35:120.

Chiou, G.C.Y., and Chuang, C.Y. 1989. Improvement of systemic absorption of insulin through eyes with absorption enhancers. *Journal of Pharmaceutical Science* 78:815–818.

Chiou, G.C.Y., Chuang, C.Y., and Chang, M.S. 1989. Systemic delivery of insulin through eyes to lower the glucose concentration. *Journal of Ocular Pharmacology* 5:81–91.

Chisholm, J.F. 1950. Iron pigmentation of the palpebral conjunctiva. *American Journal of Ophthalmology* 3:1108.

Christoophidis, N. 1979. Ocular side effects with 5-fluorouracil. *Australian/New Zealand Journal of Medicine* 9:143.

Chung, J.H. 1988. Experimental corneal alkali wound healing. *Acta Ophthalmologica* 66(suppl.) 187:5–35.

Chung, J.H. 1990. Healing of rabbit corneal alkali wounds in vitro. *Cornea* 9:36–40.

Chung, J.H., and Fagerholm, P. 1987. Endothelial healing in rabbit corneal alkali wounds. *Acta Ophthalmologica (Copenhagen)* 65:648-656.

Clark, C.R., Ferguson, P.W., Katchen, M.A., Dennis, M.W., and Craig, B.K. 1989. Comparative toxicity of shale and petroleum-derived distillates. *Toxicology and Industrial Health* 5:1005–1016.

Clarke, J.S. 1986. Corneal abrasions following the use of A-200 pyrinate shampoo. *Pediatric Emergency Care* 2:65.

Cole, J.G., Cole, H.G., and Janoff, L.A. 1957. A toxic ocular manifestation of chloramphenicol therapy. *American Journal of Ophthalmology* 44:18.

Collin, H.B. 1986. Ultrastructural changes to corneal stromal cells due to ophthalmic preservatives. *Acta Ophthalmologica (Copenhagen)* 64:72–78.

Committee on drugs. 1978. Camphor—who needs it? *Pediatrics* 62:404.

Cote, G., and Drance, S.M. 1968. The effect of propranolol on human intraocular pressure. *Canadian Journal of Ophthalmology* 3:207.

Coyes, M.J., Barnett, P.G., Midtling, J.E., et al. 1986. Clinical confirmation of organophosphate poisoning of agricultural workers. *American Journal of Industrial Medicine* 10:399–409.

Cremers, P.M., and Hofstee, A.W. 1989. Dangers of batteries. *Journal of Toxicology and Clinical Experiments* 9:11–19.

Crews, S.J. 1977. Ocular adverse reaction to drugs. *Practitioner* 219:72.

Cristini, G., and Pagliarani, N. 1953. Amyl nitrate test in primary glaucoma. *British Journal of Ophthalmology* 37:741.

Critchfield, J.W., Calendra, A.J., Nesburn, A.B., and Kenney, M.C. 1988. Keratoconus I. Biochemical studies. *Experimental Eye Research* 46:953–963.

CTFA, 1976. *CTFA Cosmetic Ingredient Dictionary*, 2nd ed. Washington, DC: Cosmetic, Toiletry and Fragrance Association.

Dalvi, R.R. 1988. Toxicity of thiram (tetramethylthiuram disulfide). A review. *Veterinary and Human Toxicology* 30:480–482.

Darby, P.W., and Wilson, J. 1967. Cyanide smoking and tobacco amblyopia. *British Journal of Ophthalmology* 51(5):336–338.

David, D.S., and Berkowitz, J.S. 1969. Ocular effects of topical and systemic corticosteroids. *The Lancet* 2:149.

David, L.L., Takemoto, L.J., Anderson, L.S., and Shearer, T.R. 1988. Proteolytic changes in main intrinsic polypeptide (MIP26) from membranes in selenite cataract. *Current Eye Research* 7:411–417.

Davidson, S.I. 1973. Reports of ocular adverse reactions. *Transactions of the Ophthalmology Society United Kingdom* 93:495.

De Groot, A.C., Beverdam, E.G., Ayong, C.T., Coenraads, P.J., and Nater, J.P. 1988a. The role of contact allergy in the spectrum of adverse effects caused by cosmetics and toiletries. *Contact Dermatitis* 19:195–201.

De Groot, A.C., Bruynzeel, D.P., Bos, J.D., Van der Meeren, H.L., Van Joost, T., Jagtman, B.A., and Weyland, J.W. 1988b. The allergens in cosmetics. *Archives of Dermatology* 124:1525–1529.

Del Palacio-Hernanz, A., Delgado Vincente, S., Menendez Kamos, F., and Rodriguez-Noriega-Belanstegai, A. 1987. Randomized comparative clinical trial of itraconazole and selenium sulfide shampoo for the treatment of pityriasis versicolor. *Reviews of Infectious Disorders* 9(suppl. 1):S121–S127.

De Respinis, P.A. 1990. Cyanoacrylate nail glue mistaken for eye drops. *Journal of the American Medical Association* 263:2301.

Deschamps, D., Garnier, R., Savoye, J., Chabaux, C.H., Fethymiou, M.L., and Fournier, E. 1988. Allergic and irritant contact dermatitis from diethyl-beta-chloroethylamine. *Contact Dermatitis* 18:103–105.

de Zotte, R., Patussi, V., Fiorito, A., and Larese, F. 1988. Sensitization to green coffee beans (GCB) and castor bean (CB) allergens among dock workers. *International Archives of Occupational and Environmental Health (Berlin)* 61:7–12.

Ding, Y.P. 1989. Chronic effect of fluorine in the eye. *Chung Hua I Hsueh Tsa Chih* 69:695–697.

Douglas, R.B., and Coe, J.E. 1987. The relative sensitivity of the human eye and lung to irritating gases. *Annals of Occupational Hygiene* 31:265–267.

Doukan, G. 1990. Venerologie d'antefois. *Revue du Praticien (Paris)* 40:1689–1690.

Drance, S.M., and Ross, R.A. 1970. The ocular effects of epinephrine. *Survey of Ophthalmology* 14:330.

Dreyfors, J.M., Jones, S.B., and Sayed, Y. 1989. Hexamethylene tetramine: a review. *American Industrial Hygiene Assocation Journal* 50:579–585.

Dugan, G.M., Gumbmann, M.R., and Friedman, M. 1989. Toxicological evaluation of jimson weed (*Datura stramonium*) seed. *Food and Chemical Toxicology* 27:501–510.

Duke-Elder, S. 1972. *Systems of Ophthalmology*, vol. 14, part 2, pp. 1046, 1187. St. Louis: C.V. Mosby.

Dukes, M.N.G., ed. 1980. *Meyler's Side Effects of Drugs*, vol. 9, pp. 365–368. Amsterdam: Excerpta Medica.

Dutertre-Catella, H., Phu-Lich, N., Huyen, V.N., Olivier, L., Truhaut, R., and Claude, J.C. 1989. Eye and skin irritation induced by picolines. *Archives of Toxicology* (Suppl. 13):428–432.

Ebert, E., Leist, K.H., and Mayer, D. 1990. Summary of safety evaluation toxicity studies of glufosinate ammonium. *Food and Chemical Toxicology* 28:339–349.

ECETOC Working Group. 1985. Xylenes. *ECETOC Joint Assessment of Commodity Chemicals* 6:1–59.

ECETOC Working Group. 1986. Ethylbenzene. *ECETOC Joint Assessment of Commodity Chemicals* 7:1–39.

ECETOC Working Group. 1987. Methyl isobutyl ketone. *ECETOC Joint Assessment of Commodity Chemicals* 8:29.

ECETOC Working Group. 1989. Isophorone. *ECETOC Joint Assessment of Commodity Chemicals* 10:1–55.

Edwards, T.S. 1963. Transcient myopia due to tetracycline. *Journal of the American Medical Association* 186:69.

Ehrenberg, L., Hiesche, K.D., Osterman-Golkar, S., et al. 1974. Evaluation of genetic risks of alkylating agents: tissue doses in the mouse from air contaminated with ethylene oxide. *Mutation Research* 24:83–91.

Elliott, G.A., and Schut, A.L. 1965. Studies with cytarabine HCl (CA) in normal eyes of man, monkey and rabbit. *American Journal of Ophthalmology* 60:1074.

Ellis, P.P. 1977. *Ocular Therapeutics and Pharmacology*, 5th ed., pp. 16, 47, 50, 187. St. Louis: C.V. Mosby.

Emmett, E.A. 1983. Occupational skin disease. *Journal of Allergies and Clinical Immunology* 72:649–656.

Environmental Protection Agency. 1986 Health assessment document for hydrogen sulfide. Report number EPA/600/8-86/026A. Washington, DC: Office of Health and Environmental Assessment.

EPA/OTS. 1983. Report on eye irritation in rabbits using Elmer's plastic resin cascamite glue. EPA/OTS Doc. #878213874.

EPA/OTS. 1986. Rabbit eye irritation test with liquid urea–formaldehyde resin. EPA/OTS Doc. #868600010.

EPA/OTS. 1987. Acute toxicological properties of Dursban 24E insecticide. EPA/OTS Doc. #86-870002320.

EPA/OTS. 1989a. Rabbit eye irritation after introduction of approximately 10 mg of solid or 0.1 mg of liquid into the conjunctival sac, with cover letter dated 060789. EPA/OTS Doc #86-890000314.

EPA/OTS. 1989b. Acute oral LD50 and subacute feeding (28 days) in albino rats and acute dermal LD50, primary skin irritation and acute eye irritation in albino rabbits, with attached cover sheets and letter. EPA/OTS Doc #86-890000524S.

EPA Working Group. 1982. An exposure and risk assessment for trichloroethanes. EPA-440/4–85-018.

EPA Working Group. 1983. Health assessment document for acrylonitrile. Final report. EPA-600-8-82007F.

EPA Working Group. 1984. Mercury health effects update. In *Health Issue Reassessment*. Document EPA-600/8-84-019F. Washington, DC: Environmental Protection Agency.

Epstein, E. 1990. Primula contact dermatitis: an easily overlooked diagnosis. *Cutis* 45:411–416.

Estable, J.J. 1948. The ocular effect of several irritant drugs applied directly to the conjunctiva. *American Journal of Ophthalmology* 31:837.

Estrig, W.J., Cavalieri, S.A., Wald, P., Becker, C.E., Jones, J.R., and Cone, J.E. 1987. Evidence of neurologic dysfunction related to long-term ethylene oxide exposure. *Archives of Neurology* 44:1283–1286.

Fassihi, A.R., and Naidoo, N. T. 1989. Irritation associated with tear-replacement ophthalmic drops: a pharmaceutical and subjective investigation. *South African Medical Journal* 75:233–235.

Felix, R.H., I've, F.A., and Dahl, M.G.C. 1973. Cutaneous and ocular reactions to practolol. *British Medical Journal* 2:452.

Fernandex-Durango, R., Trivino, A., Ramirez, J.M., et al. 1990. Immunoreactive atrial natriuretic factor in aqueous humor: its concentration is increased with high intraocular pressure in rabbit eyes. *Vision Research* 30:1305–1310.

Ferrara, A. 1943. Optic neuritis from high doses of Atebrin. *Rassegna Italian Ophthalmology* 12:123.

Fielder, R.J. 1981. Formaldehyde. *HSE Toxic Review* 2:1–18.

Fielder, R.J., and Lowing, R. 1981. Styrene. *HSE Toxic Review* 1:1–42.

Finger, P. T., Ho, T.K., Fastenberg, D.M., Hyman, R.A., Stroh, E.M., Packer, S., and Perry, H.D. 1990. Intraocular radiation blocking. *Investigative Ophthalmology and Visual Science* 31:1724–1730.

Fink, A.I. 1951. Carbon monoxide asphyxia with visual sequelae. *American Journal of Ophthalmology* 34:1024–1027.

Fiore, P.M. 1989. Drug-induced ocular sensitization. *Internal Ophthalmology Clinic* 29:147–150.

Fleisher, L.N. 1988. Effects of inhibitors of arachidonic acid metabolism on endotoxin-induced ocular inflammation. *Current Eye Research* 7:321–327.

Flood, S. 1988. Hydrofluoric acid burns. *American Family Physician* 37:175–182.

Flynn, W.J., Manger, T.F., and Hill, R.M. 1984. Corneal burns: a quantitative comparison of acid and base. *Acta Ophthalmologica (Copenhagen)* 62:542–548.

Folb, P.I., and Talmud, J. 1989. Tear gas—its toxicology and suggestions for management of its acute effects in man. *South African Journal of Medicine* 46:295.

Fothergill, R., and Heaney, G.A. 1976. Reactions to dextran. *British Journal of Medicine* 2:11502.

Fowler, J.F., Jr. 1987. Selection of patch test materials for gold allergy. *Contact Dermatitis* 17:23–25.

Francis, B.M. 1986. Teratogenicity of bifenox and nitrofen in rodents. *Journal of Environmental Science Health Bulletin* 21:303–317.

Francois, J., and Mortiers, P. 1976. The injurious effects of locally and generally applied antibiotics on the eye. *Tijdschrift Voor Sociale Geneeskunde (Assen)* 32:139.

Fraunfelder, F. T. 1979. Corneal edema after use of carbachol. *Archives of Ophthalmology* 97:975.

Fraunfelder, F. T. 1980. Interim report: National Registry of Possible Drug-Induced Ocular Side Effects. *Ophthalmology* 87:87.

Fraunfelder, F. T. 1982. *Drug-Induced Ocular Side Effects and Drug Interactions*, 2nd ed., pp. 364–372. Philadelphia: Lea and Febiger.

Fraunfelder, F. T., and Scafidi, A.F. 1978. Possible adverse effects from topical ocular 10% phenylephrine. *American Journal of Ophthalmology* 85:447.

Fraunfelder, F. T., Kalina, R.E., Buist, A.S., Berstein, R.S., and Johnson, D.S. 1983. Ocular effects following the volcanic eruptions of Mount St. Helens. *Archives of Ophthalmology* 101:373–378.

Fraunfelder, F. T., Sharp, J.D., and Silver, B.E. 1979. Possible adverse effects from topical anesthetics. *Documenta Ophthalmologica* 18:341.

Freeberg, F.E., Nixon, G.A., Reer, P.J., Weaver, J.E., Bruce, R.D., Griffith, J.F., and Sanders, L.W., 3rd. 1986. Human and rabbit eye responses to chemical insult. *Fundamentals of Applied Toxicology* 7:626–634.

Fuchs, T., and in der Wiesche, M. 1990. Contact allergies to CN and CS ("tear gas") in participants in demonstrations. *Zeitschrift fur Hautkrankheiten (Berlin)* 65:288–292,295.

Gasset, A.R. 1977. Benzalkonium chloride toxicity to the human cornea. *American Journal of Ophthalmology* 84:169.

Geller, M. 1989. Poison ivy, mangoes, cashews and dermatitis. *Annals of Internal Medicine* 110:1036–1037.

German, E., and Siddiqui, N. 1970. Atropine toxicity from eye drops. *New England Journal of Medicine* 282:689.

Gibbons, R.B. 1979. Complications of chrysotherapy. A review of recent studies. *Archives of Internal Medicine* 139:343.

Gilman, A.G., Goodman, L.S., and Gilman, A., eds. 1980. *The Pharmacological Basis of Therapeutics*, 6th ed., pp. 151–153, 164–166. New York: Macmillan.

Godish, T. 1985. *Air Quality* Chelsea, MI: Lewis Publishers.

Goh, C.L. 1987. Allergic contact dermatitis to mace tear gas. *Australian Journal of Dermatology* 28:115–116.

Goldman, M., and Dacre, J.C. 1989. Lewisite: its chemistry, toxicology and biological effects. *Reviews of Environmental Contamination Toxicology* 110:75–115.

Goldstein, J.H. 1971. Effects of drugs on cornea, conjunctiva and lids. *International Ophthalmology Clinic* 11:13.

Golubovic, S., and Parunovic, A. 1990. Cyanoacrylate glue in the treatment of corneal ulcerations. *Fortschritte der Ophthalmologie (Berlin)* 87:378–381.

Gomez, J. T., Robinson, N.M., Osato, M.S., and Wilhelmus, K.R. 1988. Comparison of acridine orange and gram stains in bacterial keratitis. *American Journal of Ophthalmology* 106:735–737.

Gondorowa, R.A., Bordjugowa, G.G., Choroschilowa-Maselewa, I.P., Tschesnokowa, N.B., Ilatowskaja, L.W., and Sosulina, N.E. 1990. Treatment of eye burns with a polyvalent proteolytic inhibitor. *Klinische Monatsblatter fur Augenheilkunde (Stuttgart)* 197:1–5.

Good, P., and Gross, K. 1988. Electrophysiology and metallosis: support for an oxidative (free radical) mechanism in the human eye. *Ophthalmalogica* 196:204–209.

Gorn, R.A. 1979. The detrimental effect of aspirin on hyphema rebleed. *Annals of Ophthalmology* 11:351.

Gosselin, R.E., Hodge, H.D., Smith, R.P., and Gleson, M.N. 1976. *Clinical Toxicology of Commercial Products*, 4th ed. Baltimore: Williams and Wilkins.

Goto, S., and Hottar, R. 1967. The medical and hygiene of carbon disulfide poisoning in Japan. In *Toxicology of Carbon Disulfide*, eds. Briber, H. and Teisinger, J., pp. 219–230. Amsterdam: Excerpta Medica Foundation.

Goto, S., Hottar, R., and Sugimoto, K. 1971. Studies on chronic carbon disulfide poisoning patho-genesis of renal microaneurysm due to carbon disulfide with special reference to a subclinical defect of carbo-hydrate metabolism. *Internationales Archiv fur Arbeitsmedizin (Berlin)* 28:151–156.

Gouche, R. 1989. Hazards of henna. *Anesthesia Analgesic* 69:416–417.

Gramberg-Danielsen, B. 1965. Ophthalmological findings after the use of alcohol. *Zentralblatt Verkehrs Medizin* 11:129.

Grant, W.M. 1986. *Toxicology of the Eye*, 3rd ed. Springfield, IL: Charles C. Thomas.

Grayson, M., and Pieroni, D. 1970. Severe silver nitrate injury to the eye. *American Journal of Ophthalmology* 70:227.

Green, W.R. 1975. Retinal and optic nerve atrophy induced by intravitreous vincristine in the primate. *Transactions of the American Ophthalmology Society* 73:389.

Grimsdale, H. 1934. A case of gas poisoning with unusual ophthalmological complications. *British Journal of Ophthalmology* 18:443–446.

Groden, L.R., Rodnite, J., Brinser, J.H., and Genvert, G.I. 1990. Acridine orange and gram stains in infectious keratitis. *Cornea* 9:122–124.

Grubb, B.R., Matthews, D.O., and Bentley, P.J. 1986. Ocular chrysiasis: accumulation of gold in the rabbit eye. *Current Eye Research* 5:891–893.

Haddad, L.M., and Winchester, J.F. 1990. *Clinical Management of Poisoning and Drug Overdose*, vol. 130, pp. 315–316. Philadelphia: W.B. Saunders.

Haddad, N.J., Moyer, N.J., and Riley, F.C. 1970. Mydriatic effect of phenylephrine hydrochloride. *American Journal of Ophthalmology* 70:729.

Haley, T.J. 1987. Solvents and chemical intermediates. In *Handbook of Toxicology*, eds. T.J. Haley and W.O. Berndt, pp. 504–554. New York: Hemisphere Publishing.

Halperin, M.N., McFarland, R.A., and Niven, J. 1959. The time course of effects of carbon monoxide on visual thresholds. *Journal of Physiology* 86:142–144.

Hamming, W.J., MacBeth, W.G., and Chass, R.L. 1967. The photochemical air pollution syndrome. *Archives of Environmental Health* 14:137–149.

Hanna, C., Fraunfelder, F. T., and Sanchez, J. 1974. Ultrastructural study of argyrosis of the cornea and conjunctiva. *Archives of Ophthalmology* 92:18.

Hansen, B.M., Brahn, G., and Tilsley, D.A. 1990. Contact allergy to Australian blackwood (*Acacia melanoxylum* R. Br.). Isolation and identification of new hydroxyflavin sensitizers. *Contact Dermatitis* 23:33–39.

Hart, T.B. 1987. Paraquat—a review of safety in agricultural and horticultural use. *Human Toxicology* 6:13–18.

Hata, S., Bernstein, E., and Davis, L.E. 1986. Atypical ocular bobbing in acute organophosphate poisoning. *Archives of Neurology* 43:185–186.

Havener, W.H. 1978. *Ocular Pharmacology*, 4th ed., pp. 263–264. St. Louis: C.V. Mosby.

Haviland, J.W., and Long, P.H. 1940. Skin and ocular reactions to sulfathiazole therapy. *Bulletin Johns Hopkins Hospital* 66:263.

Hayes, W.J. 1975. *Toxicology of Pesticides*. Baltimore: Williams and Wilkins.

Hayka, B.J., Zhu, L., Sens, D., Tapert, M.J., and Crouch, R.K. 1990. Cytolysis of corneal epithelial cells by hydrogen peroxide. *Experimental Eye Research* 50:11–16.

Heine, A., and Laubstein, B. 1990. Contact dermatitis from cyclohexanone-formaldehyde resin (L2 resin) in a hair lacquer spray. *Contact Dermatitis* 22:108.

Herse, P.R. 1990. Diurnal and long-term variations in corneal thickness in the normal and alloxan-induced diabetic rabbit. *Current Eye Research* 9:451–457.

Heuss, J.M., and Glasson, A. 1968. Hydrocarbon reactivity and eye irritation. *Environmental Science Technology* 2:1109–1116.

Hezemans-Boer, M., Toonstra, J., Meulenbelt, J., Zwavaling, J.H., Sangster, B., and van Vloten, W.A. 1988. Skin lesions due to exposure to methyl bromide. *Archives of Dermatology* 124:917-921.

Highman, V.N. 1969. Early rise in intraocular pressure after ammonia burns. *British Medical Journal* 2:259–260.

Hightower, K.R., and Farnum, R. 1985. Calcium induces opacities in cultured human lenses. *Experimental Eye Research* 41:565-568.

Hinds, W.C. 1988. Basis for particle size-selecting sampling for wood dust. *Applied Industrial Hygiene* 3:67–72.

Hochmeister, M., and Vycudilik, W. 1989. Morpho-toxicological findings following war gas effect (S-Last). *Beitrage zur Gerichtlichen Medizin (Vienna)* 47:533–538.

Hockwin, O., and Swanson, A. 1976. Comments on the influence of miotics on the lens. *Annals of Ophthalmology* 8:895–896.

Hoffer, E., and Taitelman, U. 1989. Exposure to paraquat through skin absorption: clinical and laboratory observations of accidental splashing on healthy skin of agricultural workers. *Human Toxicology* 8:483–485.

Holdright, D.R., and Jahanqiri, M. 1990. Accidental poisoning with podophyllin. *Human Experimental Toxicology* 9:51–56.

Holt, P.J.A., and Waddington, E. 1975. Oculocutaneous reaction to oxprenolol. *British Medical Journal* 2:539.

Hopkins, J. 1979. Hexachlorophene: more bad news than good. *Food Cosmetic Toxicology* 17:410.

Hovland, K.R. 1971. Effects of drugs on aqueous humor dynamics. *International Ophthalmology Clinics (Boston MA)* 11:99.

Huang, A.J., Belldegrun, R., Hanninen, L., Kenyon, K.R., Tseng, S.C., and Refojo, M.F. 1989. Effects of hypertonic solutions on conjunctival epithelium and mucin-like glycoprotein discharge. *Cornea* 8:15–20.

Hughes, W.F., Jr. 1946a. Alkali burns to the eye I. Review of literature and summary of present knowledge. *Archives of Ophthalmology* 35:423.

Hughes, W.F., Jr. 1946b. Alkali burns to the eye II. Clinical and pathological course. *Archives of Ophthalmology* 36:189.

Hull, D.S. 1975. Effect of norepinephrine on the corneal epithelium. *American Journal of Ophthalmology* 79:245.

Hull, D.S. 1988. Drugs, pathological conditions and corneal epithelium (rabbits). In *Crisp Database*. Washington, DC: National Institutes of Health.

Illing, H.P.A., and Shillaker, R.O. 1985. 1,3-butadiene and related compounds. *HSE Toxic Review* 11:1–34.

Illing, H.P.A., Mariscotti, S.P., and Smith, A.M. 1987. Tetrachloroethylene (tetrachloroethane, perchloroethylene). *HSE Toxic Review* 17:1–81.

Itoi, M. 1975. Teratogenicities of ophthalmic drugs I. Antiviral ophthalmic drugs. *Archives of Ophthalmology* 93:46.

Jager, B.V., and Stagg, G.N. 1958. Toxicity of diacetyl monoxime and of pyridine-2-aldoxime methiodide in man. *Bulletin Johns Hopkins Hospital* 102:203.

Jarkman, S., Skoog, K.D., and Nilsson, S.E. 1985. The c-wave, the electroretinogram and the standing potential of the eye as highly sensitive measures of effects of low doses of trichloroethylene, methyl chloroform and halothane. *Documenta Ophthalmologica* 60:375–382.

Jay, W.M., Swift, T.R., and Hull, D.S. 1982. Possible relationship of ethylene oxide to cataract formation. *American Journal of Ophthalmology* 93:727–732.

Jessen, H.J. 1989. Improving the quality of bathing water by oxygen releasing substances. *Zeitschrift fur die Gesamte Hygiene und ihre Grenzgebiete (Berlin)* 35:376–380.

Ji, Y.J., and Cui, M.Z. 1988. Toxicological studies on safety of rare earths used in agriculture. *Biomedical Environmental Science* 1:270–276.

Johnson, R.N., Flynn, H.W., Jr., Parel, J.M., and Portugal, L.M. 1989. Transient hypopyon with marked anterior chamber fibrin following pars plana vitrectomy and silicone oil injection. *Archives of Ophthalmology* 107:683–686.

Johnstone, R.T. 1948. *Occupational Medicine and Industrial Hygiene*, p. 216. St Louis: C.V. Mosby.

Jones, R.D. 1990. Xylene/amitraz: a pharmacological review and profile. *Veterinary and Human Toxicology* 32:446–448.

Kaback, M.B. 1976. The effects of dipivalyl epinephrine on the eye. *American Journal of Ophthalmology* 81:768.

Kahn, M., Barney, N.P., Briggs, R.M., Block, K.J., and Allansmith, M.R. 1990. Penetrating the conjunctival barrier. The role of molecular weight. *Investigative Ophthalmology and Visual Science* 31:258–261.

Kam, J., Waron, M., Barishak, Y.R., Schachner, E., and Ishay, J.S. 1989. Intraocular pressure in cats is lowered by drops of hornet venom. *Comparative Biochemistry and Physiology [C]* 92:329–331.

Kanai, A., Alba, R.M., Takano, T., et al. 1989. The effect on the cornea of alpha cyclodextrin vehicle for cyclosporin eye drops. *Transplant Proceedings* 21:3150–3152.

Kanerva, L., Estlander, T., and Jolanki, R. 1989. Allergic contact dermatitis from dental composite resins due to aromatic epoxy actylates and aliphatic acrylates. *Contact Dermatitis* 20:201–211.

Kaplan, M.R., and Pilger, I.S. 1957. The effect of rauwolfia serpentina derivatives on intraocular pressure. *American Journal of Ophthalmology* 43:550.

Karcioglu, Z.A., Aran, A.J., Holmes, D.L., Kapiciglu, Z., and Lopez, J. 1988. Inflammation due to surgical glove powders in the rabbit eye. *Archives of Ophthalmology* 106:808–811.

Keimig, D.G., Castellan, R.M., Kullman, D.G., and Kinsley, K.B. 1987. Respiratory health status of gilsonite workers. *American Journal of Industrial Medicine* 11:287–296.

Kelly, T.E. 1981. Evaluation of effects of a tick dip on dog's eyes. *Journal of the American Veterinary Medical Association* 178:64–65.

Kennah, H.E., Albulesen, D., Hignet, S., and Barrow, C.S. 1989. A critical evaluation of predicting ocular irritancy potential from an in vitro cytotoxicity assay. *Fundamental Applications in Toxicology* 12:281–290.

Kennah, H.E., Hignet, S., Laux, P.E., Dorko, J.D., and Barrow, C.S. 1989. An objective procedure for quantitating eye irritation based upon changes in corneal thickness. *Fundamental and Applied Toxicology* 12:258–268.

Kennedy, G.L., Jr. 1986. Acute toxicity studies with oxamyl. *Fundamental Applied Toxicology* 6:423–429.

Kennedy, G.L., Jr. 1987. Acute and environmental toxicity studies with hexazinone. *Fundamental and Applied Toxicology* 4:603–611.

Khurana, A.K., Ahluwalic, B.K., and Scod, S. 1989. Savlon keratopathy, a clinical profile. *Acta Ophthalmologica (Copenhagen)* 67:465–466.

Kinnunen, T., and Hannuksela, M. 1989. Skin reactions to hexylene glycol. *Contact Dermatitis* 21:154–158.

Kirk, R.E., and Othmer, D.F., eds. 1980. *Encyclopedia of Chemical Technology*, vol. 12, 3rd ed. New York: John Wiley.

Kjaergaard, S.K., and Pedersen, D.F. 1989. Dust exposure, eye redness, eye cytology and mucous membrane irritation in a tobacco industry. *International Archives of Occupational and Environmental Health* 61:519–525.

Klopfer, J. 1989. Effects of environmental air pollution on the eye. *Journal of Clinical Review.* 60:773–778.

Koo, D., Bourier, B., Wesley, M., Courtwright, P., and Reingold, A. 1989. Epidemic keratoconjunctivitis in a university medical center ophthalmology clinic; need for re-evaluation of the design and disinfection of instruments. *Infectious Control Hospital Epidemiology* 10:547–552.

Krejci, L., and Brettschneider, I. 1978. Yellow-brown cornea: a complication of topical use of tetracycline. *Ophthalmic Research* 10:131.

Kriteriegruppen for Hygieniskagransvarden. 1983. Consensus report for some aliphatic amines. *Arbete Och Halsa* 36:19–34.

Krootila, K., Uusitalo, H., Lehtosalo, J.I., and Palkama, A. 1986. Effect of topical chemical irritation on the blood–aqueous barrier of the rat eye. *Ophthalmic Research* 18:248–252.

Kruger, R.A., Higgins, J., Rashford, S., Fitzgerald, B., and Land, R. 1990. Emergency eye care. *Australian Family Physician* 19:934–938.

Ladefoged, O. 1982. Industribensin. *Arbete Och Halsa* 21:1–54.

Lal, S., and Gupta, A.K. 1974. Lenticular deposits associated with chloroquine keratopathy. *Indian Journal of Ophthalmology* 22:34.

Lamda, P.A., Sood, N.N., and Moorthy, S.S. 1968. Retinopathy due to chloramphenicol. *Scott Medical Journal* 13:166.

Lasky, M.A. 1950. Corneal response to emetine hydrochloride. *Archives of Ophthalmology* 44:47.

Lazenby, G.W., Reed, J.W., and Grant, W.M. 1970. Anticholinergic medication in open-angle glaucoma. Long term tests. *Archives of Ophthalmology* 84:719.

Leads from the MMWR. 1986. Mucana pruriens–associated pruritus, New Jersey. *Journal of the American Medical Association* 255:313.

Lebensohn, J.E. 1977. Spectacular adverse reactions from pilocarpine. *American Journal of Ophthalmology* 83:281.

Leenutaphong, V., and Goerz, G. 1989. Allergic contact dermatitis from chloroacetophenone (tear gas). *Contact Dermatitis* 20:316.

Lele, P.P., and Weddell, G. 1959. Sensory nerves of the cornea and cutaneous sensibility. *Experimental Neurology* 1:334–359.

Lemp, M.A., and Zimmerman, L.E. 1988. Toxic endothelial degeneration in ocular surface disease treated with topical medications containing benzalkonium chloride. *American Journal of Ophthalmology* 105:670–673.

Lerman, S., Megaw, J., and Willis, I. 1980. Potential ocular complications from PUVA therapy and their prevention. *Journal of Investigative Dermatology* 74:197.

Lewis, B.S., Setzen, M., and Kokoris, N. 1976. Ocular reaction to oxprenolol. A case report. *South African Medical Journal* 50:482.

Liire, J. 1988. Creosote. Nordiske-expertgruppen for gransvardesdocumentation. *Arbete Och Halsa* 33:7–51.

Llered, R.W., Spaulding, A.G., Sanitato, J.J., and Wander, A.H. 1988. Ophthalmia nodosa caused by tarantula hairs. *Ophthalmology* 95:166–169.

Logai, J.M., Guseva, O.G., and Kalvinsh, I.Ia. 1989. The use of lysomotropic preparations in treating some experimental chemical burns. *Oftalmologicheskii Zhurnal (Odessa)* 8:497–500.

London, J.E. 1988. Toxicological study of gadolinium nitrate. *Government Reports, Announcements and Index*, Issue 23.

London, J.E. 1989. Preliminary toxicological study of yttrium barium copper oxide. *Government Reports, Announcements and Index*, Issue 10.

Loprinzi, C.L., Love, R.R., Garrity, J.A., and Ames, M.M. 1990. Cyclophosphamide, methotrexate and 5-fluorouracil (CMF) induced ocular toxicity. *Cancer Investigation* 8:459–465.

Luck, J., and Kaye, S.B. 1989. An unrecognized form of hydrogen sulfide keratoconjunctivitis. *British Journal of Industrial Medicine* 46:748–749.

Luckenback, M., and Kielar, R. 1980. Toxic corneal epithelial edema from exposure to high atmosphere concentration of toluene diisocyanate. *American Journal of Ophthalmology* 90:682–686.

Lund, M.H. 1968. Colistin sulfate ophthalmic in the treatment of ocular infections. *Archives of Ophthalmology* 81:4.

Lundberg, I. 1987. Methylene chloride. *Arbete Och Halsa* 40:75–120.

Macewen, C.J. 1989. Eye injuries: a prospective survey of 5,671 cases. *British Journal of Ophthalmology* 73:888–894.

Maki-Paakkanen, J., and Norppa, H. 1988. Vinyl acetate. *Arbete Och Halsa* 33:77–113.

Mann, I., Pirie, A., and Pullinger, B.D. 1948. An experimental and clinical study of the reaction of the anterior segment of the eye to chemical injury, with special reference to chemical warfare agents. *British Journal of Ophthalmology (Suppl.)* 13:1.

Marti-Huguet, T., Pujol, O., Cabiro, I., Oteyza, J.A., Roca, G., and Marsa, J. 1987. Endophthalmos caused by intravitreal caterpillar hairs. Treatment by direct photocoagulation with argon lasar. *Journal of French Ophthalmology* 10:559–564.

Martin, G., Draize, J.H., and Kelley, E.A. 1962. Local anesthesia in eye mucosa produced by surfactants in cosmetic formulations. *Proceedings of the Scientific Section of Toilet Goods Association* 37:2.

Martin, X., Uffer, S., and Gaillond, C. 1986. Ophthalmia nodosa and the oculoglandular syndrome of Parinand. *British Journal of Ophthalmology* 70:536–542.

Matsunaga, K., Hosokawa, K., Suzuki, M., Arima, Y., and Hayakawa, R. 1988. Occupational allergic contact dermatitis in beauticians. *Contact Dermatitis* 18:94–96.

Mattax, J.B., and McCulley, J.P. 1988. Corneal surgery following alkali burns. *International Ophthalmology Clinics* 28:76–82.

Mauchee, O.M., Strengel, R., and Schopf, E. 1986. Chloroacetophenone allergy. *Hautarzt* 37:392–401.

Maugeri, U., and Cavalleia, V.L. 1966. Ophthalmodynamography in occupational carbon disulfide poisoning. *Medical Lav* 57:730–740 (Italian).

Maumenee, A.E., and Scholz, R.O. 1948. The histopathology of the ocular lesions produced by the sulfur and nitrogen mustards. *Bulletin Johns Hopkins Hospital* 82:121.

Mazzanti, G., Bolle, P., Martinoli, L., Piccinelli, D., Gagurina, E., Animati, F., and Mugne, Y. 1987. Croton acrostachys, a plant used in traditional medicine: purgative and inflammatory activity. *Journal of Ethnopharmacology* 19:213–219.

McCormick, D.P., and Davis, A.L. 1988. Injuries in sailboard enthusiasts. *British Journal of Sports Medicine* 22:95–97.

McCormick, S.A., DiBartolomeo, A.G., Raju, V.K., and Schwab, I.R. 1985. Ocular chrysiasis. *Ophthalmology* 92:1432–1435.

McDonnell, F., Horstman, D.H., Hazucha, M.J., Seal, E., Jr., Haak, E., Salaam, S.A., and House, D.E. 1983. Pulmonary response during exposure to low concentrations of ozone. *Advanced Medicine Environmental Toxicology* 5:139–144.

McEwen, W.K., and Goodner, E.K. 1969. Secretion of tears and blinking. In *The Eye*, vol. 3, ed., H. Davson, pp. 27–38. New York: Academic Press.

McGuiness, R., and Beaumont, P. 1985. Gold dust retinopathy after the ingestion of canthaxanthine to produce skin-bronzing. *Medical Journal of Australia* 143:622–623.

McLendon, B.F., and Bron, A.L. 1978. Corneal toxicity from vinblastine solution. *British Journal of Ophthalmology* 62:97.

McReynolds, W.U., Havener, W.H., and Henderson, J.W. 1956. Hazards of the use of sympathomimetic drugs in ophthalmology. *Archives of Ophthalmology* 56:176.

Merchant, J.A. 1988. Epidemiological assessment of laboratory animal allergy. In *Crisp Database*. Washington, DC: National Institutes of Health.

Mergler, D., Blain, L., and Lagace, J.P. 1987. Solvent related colour vision loss: an indication of neural damage. *Archives of Occupational Environmental Health* 59:313–321.

Merigan, W.H. 1989. Visual indices of neurotoxicity. In *Crisp Database*. Washington, DC: National Institutes of Health.

Meylan, W., Papa, L., De Rose, C.T., and Stura, J.F. 1986. Chemical of current interest: propylene oxide: health and environmental effects profile. *Toxicology and Industrial Health (Princeton NJ)* 2:219–260.

Micovic, V., Milenkovic, S., and Opric, M. 1990. Acute aseptic panophthalmitis caused by a copper foreign body. *Fortschritte der Ophthalmologie (Berlin)* 87:362–363.

Millen, T.P., Kucan, J.O., and Smoot, E.C., 3rd. 1989. Anhydrous ammonia injuries. *Journal of Burn Care Rehabilitation* 10:448–453.

Miller, N.R. 1982. *Walsh and Hoyt's Clinical Neuro-Ophthalmology*, 4th ed. Baltimore: Williams and Wilkins.

Miller, R.A. 1985. Podophyllin. *International Journal of Dermatology* 24:491–498.

Minton, J. 1949. *Occupational Eye Diseases and Injuries*, pp. 39–110. New York: Grune and Stratton.

Mitchell, D.W.A. 1957. The effect of ephedrine instillation on intraocular pressure. *British Journal of Physiology and Ophthalmology* 14:38.

Moon, M.E., and Robertson, J.F. 1983. Retrospective study of alkali burns of the eye. *Australian Journal of Ophthalmology* 11:281–286.

Morgan, E.W., Hiatt, G.F., and Korte, D.W. 1990. Primary ocular irritation potential of Ball Powder (trade name) in male rabbits. *Government Reports, Announcements and Index*, Issue 01.

Morgan, R.L., Sorenson, S.S., and Castles, T.R. 1987. Prediction of ocular irritation by corneal pachymetry. *Food and Chemical Toxicology* 25:609–613.

Mosso, J.A., and Kruger, L. 1972. Spinal trigeminal neurons excited by noxious and thermal stimuli. *Brain Research* 38:206–210.

Mosso, J.A., and Kruger, L. 1973. Receptor categories represented in spinal trigeminal nucleus caudalis. *Journal of Neurophysiology* 26:472–488.

Moster, M.F., Winklerova, S., and Nemecek, R. 1987. The toxic effect of organophosphorus compounds on the rabbit eye I. Ultrastructural changes in the cornea. *Ceskoslovenska Oftalmologie (Praha)* 43:354–365.

Mozherenko, V.P. 1985. Plants in the treatment of eye disease. *Meditsinskaia Sestra (Moskva)* 44:53–54.

Mozingo, D.W., Smith, A.A., McManus, W.F., Pruitt, B.A., Jr., and Mason, A.D., Jr. 1988. Chemical burns. *Journal of Trauma* 28:142–147, 642–647.

Müller, H.K., Kleifeld, O., Hockwin, O., and Dardenne, U. 1956. Der Einfluss von Pilocarpin und Mintacol auf den Stoffwechsel der Linse. *Bericht uber die Zusammenkunft der Deutschen Ophthalmologischen Gesellschaft (Munchen)* 60:115–118.

National Institute of Occupational Safety and Health. 1981. *Formaldehyde: Evidence of Carcinogenicity*. U.S. Department of Health and Human Services, Current Intelligence Bulletin 34. Washington, DC: U.S. Government Printing Office.

National Institute of Occupational Safety and Health. 1977. *Occupational Exposure to Carbon Disulfide.* Publication Number 77–156. Washington DC: Department of Health, Education and Welfare.

National Toxicity Program Working Group. 1989a. Toxicology and carcinogenesis studies of benzyl alcohol in F344/N rats and B6C3F1 mice (gavage studies). *National Toxicology Program Technical Report Series* 343:1–158.

National Toxicity Program Working Group. 1989b. Toxicology and carcinogenesis studies of hexachloroethane in F344/N rats (gavage study). *National Toxicology Program Technical Report Series* 361:120.

Natow, A.J. 1986. Henna. *Cutis* 38:21.

Nelson, J.D., and Kopietz, L.A. 1987. Chemical injuries to the eyes. Emergency, intermediate, and long-term care. *Postgraduate Medicine* 81:62–75.

Nero, A.V., Jr. 1988. Controlling indoor air pollution. *Scientific American* 258:42–48.

Nesterova, M.F. 1988. Evaluation of soil fumigants from the standpoint of nutrition. *Gigiena i Sanitariia (Moskva)* 6:83-84.

Ng, S.K., and Goh, C.L. 1989. Contact allergy to sodium hypochlorite in Insol. *Contact Dermatitis* 21:281.

Ng, T.P., Tsin, T.W., and O' Kelly, F.J. 1985. An outbreak of illness after occupational exposure to ozone and acid chlorides. *British Journal of Industrial Medicine* 42:686–690.

Niebroj, T., and Grszczynska, M. 1989. Reaction of Langerhans cells of the corneal epithelium to topically applied lead. *Klinika Oczna (Warszawa)* 91:54.

Nielsen, J., Fahraens, C., Bensryd, I., Akesson, B., Welinder, H., Linden, K., and Skerfving, S. 1989. Small airways function in workers processing polyvinyl chloride. *Internal Archives of Occupational and Environmental Health* 61:427–430.

Nigam, P.K., and Saxena, A.K. 1988. Allergic contact dermatitis to henna. *Contact Dermatitis* 18:55–56.

NIOSH Working Committee. 1977. Occupational exposure to fibrous glass. In *Criteria for a Recommended Standard*, pp. 77–152. National Institute of Occupational Safety and Health.

NIOSH Working Group. 1973. Occupational exposure to chromic acid. HSM 73–11021, p. 83. National Institute of Occupational Safety and Health.

NIOSH Working Group. 1976. *Criteria for a Recommended Standard*, pp. 76–184. National Institute of Occupational Safety and Health.

NIOSH Working Group. 1978. *Criteria for a Recommended Standard*, pp. 78–213. National Institute of Occupational Safety and Health.

NIOSH Working Group. 1984. Health effects of occupational exposure to CS_2. TIC #00135185, Chap. 7, pp. 1–15. National Institute of Occupational Safety and Health.

Norn, M.S. 1967. Methylene blue (methylthionine) vital staining of the cornea and conjunctiva. *Acta Ophthalmologica* 45:347.

O'Connor, G.R. 1976. Periocular corticosteroid injections: uses and abuses. *Eye Ear Nose Throat and Mouth* 55:83.

O'Donoghue, J.L. 1985. Alkanes, alcohols, ketones and ethylene oxide. In *Neurotoxicity of Industrial and Commercial Chemicals*, vol. I, ed. J.F. O' Donoghue, pp. 61–97. Boca Raton, FL: CRC Press.

O'Grady, T.C. 1989. Mass eye casualties at sea. *Military Medicine* 154:596–598.

Ogawa, Y., Kamata, E., Suzuki, S., et al. 1989. Toxicity of 2-mercaptobenzothiazole in mice. *Eisei Shikenjo Hokoku* 107:44–50.

Oji, E.O. 1990. Clinical and pathological effects on the rabbit's eye of some plant-derived ophthalmic swabs. *Annals of the Roal College of Surgeons England* 72:340–343.

Olander, K., Haik, K.G., and Haik, G.M. 1978. Management of pterygia. Should thiotepa be used? *Annals of Ophthalmology* 10:853.

Oliver, K.T., and Havener, W.H. 1958. Eye manifestations of chronic vitamin A intoxication. *Archives of Ophthalmology* 60:19.

Olson, R.J. 1983. Occupational eye disorders. *Environmental and Occupational Medicine* 367–372.

Olurin, O., and Osuntokun, O. 1978. Complications of retrobulbar alcohol injections. *Annals of Ophthalmology* 10:474.

Ormerod, L.D., Abelson, M.B., and Kenyon, K.R. 1989. Standard models of corneal injury using alkali-immersed filter discs. *Investigative Ophthalmology and Visual Science* 30:2148–2153.

Ostler, H.B. 1975. Cycloplegics and mydriatics. Tolerance, habituation and addiction after topical administration. *Archives of Ophthalmology* 93:432.

Osuntokun, B.O. 1968. An ataxic neuropathy in Nigeria. *Brain* 91(part II):215–248.

Parke, A., Bhattacherjee, P., Palmer, R.M., and Lazarus, N.R. 1988. Characterization and quantification of copper sulfate–induced vascularization of the rabbit cornea. *American Journal of Pathology* 138:123–128.

Pashley, E.L., Birdsong, N.L., Bowman, K., and Pashley, D.H. 1985. Cytotoxic effects of NaOCl on vital tissue. *Journal of Endodontics* 11:525–528.

Passi, S., Picardo, M., Mingrone, G., Breathnach, A.S., and Nazzaro-Porro, M. 1989. Azelaic acid—biochemistry and metabolism. *Acta Dermato-Venereologica. Supplementum (Oslo)* 143:8–13.

Passreiter, C.M., Florack, M., Willhua, G., and Goertz, G. 1988. Allergic contact dermatitis caused by Asteraceae. Identification of an 8,9-epoxythymol-diester as the contact allergen of *Arnica sachalinensis*. *Dermatosen in Beruf und Umwelt. Occupational and Environmental Dermatoses (Aulendorf)* 36:79–82.

PDR. 1988. Physician's Desk Reference, 42nd ed. Oradell, NJ: Edward R. Barnhart.

Peer, J., and Ben Ezra, D. 1988. Corneal damage following the use of the pediculocide A 200 pyrinate. *Archives of Ophthalmology* 106:106–107.

Peters, A.C. 1986. Toxicity tests of 1,6-hexanediamine (rats, mice). NIH proposal.

Petersen, K.K., Schroder, H.M., and Eiskjaer, S.P. 1989. CS tear gas spray as an injurious agent. Clinical aspects. *Ugeskrift for Laeger (Copenhagen)* 151:1388–1389.

Petersen, P.E., Evans, R.B., Johnstone, M.A., and Henderson, W.R., Jr. 1990. Evaluation of ocular hypersensitivity to dipivalyl epinephrine by component eye-drop testing. *Journal of Allergy Clinical Immunology* 85:954–958.

Pierard, G.E., and Dowlati, A. 1989. The deleterious effects of vesicant war gases. *Review Medicine Liège* 44:133–137.

Pifers, J.W., Friedlander, B.R., Kintz, R.J., and Stockdale, D.K. 1989. Absence of toxic effects in silver reclamation workers. *Scandinavian Journal of Work Environmental Health* 15:210–221.

Pollack, I.P., and Rossi, H. 1975. Norepinephrine in the treatment of ocular hypertension and glaucoma. *Archives of Ophthalmology* 93:173.

Preisova, J., Riebel, O., Ulkova, E., Prokes, B., and Hnilicka, B. 1988. Moth fragments as intraocular foreign bodies. *Klinische Monatsblatter fur Augenheilkunde (Stuttgart)* 192:30–32.

Pruett, R.C., Weiter, J.J., and Goldstein, R.B. 1987. Myopic cracks, angioid streaks and traumatic tears in Bruch's membrane. *American Journal of Ophthalmology* 103:537–543.

Pullicino, P., and Aquilina, J. 1989. Opso clonus in organophosphate poisoning. *Archives of Neurology* 46:704-705.

Rabinovitch, S., Greyson, N.D., Weiser, W., and Hoffstein, V. 1989. Clinical and laboratory features of acute sulfur dioxide inhalation poisoning: two-year follow-up. *American Journal of Respiratory Disorders* 139:556–558.

Rahi, A.H.S. 1976. Pathology of practolol-induced ocular toxicity. *British Journal of Ophthalmology* 60:312.

Ramazzini, B. 1964. Diseases of workers. (Translated by W.C. Wright.) From *De Morbis Artificum Diatriba, 1713*. New York: Hafner.

Rapoza, P.A., West, S.K., Newland, H.S., and Taylor, H.R. 1986. Ocular jellyfish stings in Chesapeake Bay watermen. *American Journal of Ophthalmology* 102:536–537.

Raymond, L.F. 1963. Ocular pathology in reserpine sensitivity. Report of two cases. *Journal of the Medical Society of New Jersey* 60:417.

Refojo, M.F. 1988. Synthetic hydrophylic polymers for eye surgery (rabbits). In *Crisp Database*. Washington, DC: National Institutes of Health.

Reginella, R.F., Fairfield, J.C., and Marks, J.G., Jr. 1989. Hyposensitization to poison ivy after working in a cashew nut shell oil processing factory. *Contact Dermatitis* 20:274–279.

Reuhl, K.R., Rice, D.C., Gilbert, S.G., and Hallett, J. 1989. Effects of chronic development lead exposure on monkey neuroanatomy—visual system. *Toxicology and Applied Pharmacology* 99:501–509.

Reutter, S. 1989. Trichloroethane: a summary of the toxicological data. *Government Reports Announcements and Index*, Issue 18.

Rivand, C., Gerault, A., Frau, E., and Faye, M. 1990. Eye injuries caused by vesicatory insects. *Journal of French Ophthalmology* 13:47–50.

Robert, Y., Gloor, B., Wachsmuth, E.D., and Herbst, M. 1988. Evaluation of the tolerance of the intraocular injection of hydroxypropyl methyl cellulose in animal experiments. *Klinische Monatsblatter fur Augenheilkunde (Stuttgart)* 192:337–339.

Roberts, W.H., and Wolter, J.R. 1956. Ocular chrysiasis. *Archives of Ophthalmology* 56:48.

Robertson, D., and Steves, R.M. 1977. Nitrates and glaucoma. *Journal of the American Medical Association* 237:117.

Robertson, D.M., Hollenhorst, R.W., and Callahan, J.A. 1966. Ocular manifestations of digitalis toxicity. *Archives of Ophthalmology* 76:640.

Rom, W.N. 1983. *Environmental and Occupational Medicine*, pp. 225–276. Boston: Little, Brown.

Ros, A.M., Juhlin, L., and Michaelsson, G. 1976. A follow-up study of patient with recurrent urticaria and hypersensitivity to aspirin, benzoates, and azo dyes. *British Journal of Dermatology* 95:19.

Rosen, E. 1950. Argyrolentis. *American Journal of Ophthalmology* 33:797.

Rosengren, B. 1969. Silicone injection into the vitreous in hopeless cases of retinal detachment. *Acta Ophthalmologica* 47:757.

Rowes, M.D., Nowak, K.M., and Moskowitz, P.D. 1983. Health effects of oxidants. *Environmental International* 9:515–528.

Sanderson, P.A., Kuwabara, T., and Cogan, D.G. 1976. Optic neuropathy presumably caused by vincristine therapy. *American Journal of Ophthalmology* 81:146.

Sargent, E.V., Kirk, G.D., and Hite, M. 1986. Hazard evaluation of monochloroacetone. *American Industrial Hygiene Association Journal* 47:375–378.

Scarborough, M.E., Ames, R.G., Lipsett, M.J., and Jackson, R.J. 1989. Acute health effects of community exposure to cotton defoliants. *Archives of Environmental Health* 44:351–360.

Schaumberg, H.H., and Spencer, P.S. 1976. Degeneration in central and peripheral nervous system produced by pure *n*-hexane: an experimental study. *Brain* 99:183.

Schein, D.D., Hibberd, P.L., Shingleton, B.J., et al. 1983. The spectrum and burden of ocular injury. *Ophthalmology* 95:300–305.

Scherling, S.S., and Blondis, R.R. 1945. The effect of chemical warfare agents on the human eye. *Military Surgery* 96:70.

Schuchereba, S. T., Clifford, C.B., Vargas, J.A., Bunch, D., and Bowman, P.D. 1990. Morphological alterations in rat retina after hypervolemic infusion of cross-linked hemoglobin. *Biometer Artificial Cells and Artificial Organs* 18:299–307.

Schuck, E.A., and Doyle, G.J. 1959. Photooxidation of hydrocarbons in mixtures containing oxides of nitrogen and sulfur dioxide. *Air Pollution Foundation Report*. (San Marino, CA) 29:104–112.

Schwartz, C.S. 1989. Toxicity of advanced composite matrix materials. *Applied Industrial Hygiene* Special issue:23–28.

Setula, K., Ruusuvaara, P., Punnonen, E., and Laatikainen, L. 1989. Changes in corneal endothelium after treatment of retinal detachment with intraocular silicone oil. *Acta Ophthalmologica (Copenhagen)* 67:37–43.

Shapkin-Gunko, V.A., Leus, N.F., and Drozhzhina, G.I. 1989. Characteristics of the development of cataract models against a background of poisoning. *Oftalmologicheskii Zhurnal (Odessa)* 2:116–119.

Sharir, M., Chen, V., and Blumenthal, M. 1987. Red phosphorus as a cause of corneal injury. A case report. *Ophthalmologica* 194:204–208.

Shearer, T.R. 1989. Calcium activated proteases in cataract formation. In *Crisp Database*. Washington, DC: National Institutes of Health.

Shichi, H. 1990. Glutathione-dependent detoxification of peroxides in bovine ciliary body. *Experimental Eye Research* 50:813–818.

Sibony, P.A., Evinger, C., and Manning, K.A. 1988. The effects of tobacco smoking on smooth pursuit eye movements. *Annals of Neurology* 23:238–241.

Siegal, J.E., and Zaidman, G.W. 1989. Surgical removal of cyanoacrylate adhesive after accidental instillation in the anterior chamber. *Ophthalmic Surgery* 20:179–181.

Siegel, E., and Watson, S. 1986. Mothball toxicity. *Pediatric Clinics of North America* 33:369–374.

Siegel, R.K. 1978. Cocaine hallucinations. *American Journal of Psychiatry* 135:309.

Simcoe, C.W. 1962. Cyclopentolate (Cyclogyl) toxicity. *Archives of Ophthalmology* 67:406.

Singh, G., Bohnke, M., Vom Domarus, D., Draeger, J., Linstrom, R.L., and Doughman, D.J. 1985–1986. Vital staining of corneal epithelium. *Cornea* 4:80-91.

Smith, A.D.M., and Duckett, S. 1965. Cyanide, vitamin B_{12}, experimental demyelination and tobacco amblyopia. *British Journal of Experimental Pathology* 46:615–622.

Smith, A.R. 1950. Optic atrophy following inhalation of carbon tetrachloride. *Archives Industrial Hygiene* 1:348.

Smith, G.F. 1966. Trichloroethylene: a review. *British Journal of Industrial Medicine* 23:249.

Sneed, S.R., and Weingeist, T.A. 1990. Management of siderosis bulbi due to a retained iron-containing intraocular foreign body. *Ophthalmology* 97:375–379.

Spada, C.S., Woodward, D.F., Hawley, S.B., Nieves, A.L., Williams, L.S., and Feldman, B.J. 1988. Synergistic effects of LTB4 and LTD4 on leucocyte emigration into the guinea pig conjunctiva. *American Journal of Pathology* 130:354–368.

Spencer, P.S., and Schaumberg, H.H. 1977. Neurotoxic properties of certain allophatic hexacarbons. *Proceedings of the Royal Society of Medicine* 70:37–39.

Spiers, A.S.D. 1969. Mydriatic response to sympathomimetic amines in patients treated with L-dopa. *The Lancet* 2:1301.

Stahlbom, B., Lundh, T., Floren, I., and Akesson, B. 1991. Visual disturbances in man as a result of experimental and occupational exposure to dimethylethylamine. *British Journal of Industrial Medicine* 48:26–29.

Stanley, J. 1965. Strong alkali burns to the eye. *New England Journal of Medicine* 273:1265.

Steinkogler, F.J. 1988. Polytetrafluoroethylene in enucleation surgery. *Fortschritte der Ophthalmologie (Berlin)* 85:321–322.

Stern, G.A., and Knapp, A. 1986. Iatrogenic peripheral corneal disease. *International Ophthalmology Clinic* 26:77–89.

Stevens, E., Ectors, M., and Cornil, A. 1989. Case of acute poisoning by mercuric oxycyanide. *Acta Clinica Belgica (Bruxelles)* 44:116–122.

Subiza, J., Subiza, J.L., Alonso, M., Hinojosa, M., Garcia, R., Jerez, M., and Subiza, E. 1990. Allergic conjunctivitis to chamomile tea. *Annals of Allergy* 65:127–132.

Sugar, S., and Santos, R. 1955. The priscoline provocation test. *American Journal of Ophthalmology* 40:510.

Surkova, V.K., and Semonov, E.N. 1989. Eye injury caused by bee sting. *Vestnik Oftalmologii (Moskva)* 105:71–72.

Sussman, G.L., and Dorian, W. 1990. Psyllium anaphylaxis. *Allergy Proceedings* 11:241–242.

Sutton, W.L. 1963. Aliphatic and alicyclic amines. In *Industrial Hygiene and Toxicology*, vol. 2, 2nd ed., eds. D.W. Fassett, and D.D. Iris, pp. 2037–3067. New York: Wiley Interscience.

Suzuki, M., Okada, T., Takeuchi, S., Ishii, Y., Yamashita, H., and Hori, S. 1990. The effect of silicone oil on the ocular tissues. *Nippon Ganka Gakkai Zasshi* 94:160–166.

Szallasi, A., and Blumberg, P.M. 1989. Resiniferatoxin, a phorbol-related diterpene, acts as an ultrapotent analog of capsaicin, the irritant constituent of red pepper. *Neuroscience* 30:515–520.

Takahasi, W.K., Saito, T.R., Amao, H., Kosaka, T., Obata, M., Umeda, M., and Shirazu, Y. 1988. Acute reversible cataract due to nitro compounds in Japanese quail *Cornutix cornutix japonica*. *Jikken Dobutsu* 37:239–243.

Theodore, F.H. 1953. Drug sensitivities and irritations to the conjunctiva. *Journal of the American Medical Association* 151:25.

Theodore, J., and Leibowitz, H.M. 1979. External ocular toxicity of dipivalyl epinephrine. *American Journal of Ophthalmology* 88:1013.

Thirumalaikolundusubramanian, P., Chandramohen, M., and Johnson, E.S. 1984. Copper sulphate poisoning. *Journal of the Indian Medical Association* 82:6.

Thomson, S.A. 1989. Toxicology of carbon fibers. *Applied Industrial Hygiene* Special issue:29–33.

Tosti, A., Melino, M., and Bardazzi, F. 1988. Contact dermatitis due to glyceryl monothioglycolate. *Contact Dermatitis* 19:71–72.

Tower, S. 1940. Unit for sensory reception in cornea. *Journal of Neurophysiology* 3:486–500.

Tripathi, B.J., and Tripathi, R.C. 1989. Cytotoxic effects of benzalconium chloride and chlorbutanol on human corneal epithelial cells in vitro. *Lens Eye Toxicity Research* 6:395–403.

Trocme, S.D., Bonini, S., Barney, N.P., Block, K.J., and Allansmith, M.R. 1988. Late-phase reaction to topically induced ocular anaphylaxis in the rat. *Current Eye Research* 7:437–443.

Turtz, C.A., and Turtz, A.L. 1960. Vitamin-A intoxication. *American Journal of Ophthalmology* 50:165.

Ubels, J.L., Eddhauser, H.F., Nemioff, B.J., Meyer, L.A., and Dicherson, C.L. 1987. Ocular miotic and irritative effects of aerosol and topically applied dichlorvos and propoxur insecticides on rabbit and monkey eyes. *Journal of Toxicology and Cutaneous Ocular Toxicology* 6:61–77.

Vache, J., and Bodnur, M. 1988. Dieffenbachia and the eye. *Ceskoslovenska Oftalmologie (Praha)* 44:453–455.

Vaishya, R. 1990. A thorny problem: the diagnosis and treatment of acacia thorn injuries. *Injury* 21:99–100.

Vale, J.A., Meredith, T.J., and Buckley, B.M. 1987. Paraquat poisoning: clinical features and immediate general management. *Human Toxicology* 6:41–47.

Vale, P. T., and Rycroft, R.J.G. 1988. Occupational irritant contact dermatitis from fibreboard containing urea-formaldehyde resin. *Contact Dermatitis* 19:62.

Van Buskirk, E.M. 1980. Adverse reactions from timolol administration. *Ophthalmology* 87:447.

Van Dyk, J.J. 1976. Adriamycin in the treatment of cancer. *South African Medical Journal* 50:61.

Van Joost, T., and de Jong, G. 1988. Sensitization to DD soil fumigant during manufacture. *Contact Dermatitis* 18:307–308.

Van Tittelboom, T., Kuhn, D., and Strauven, A. 1988. Eye injuries from toad poison. *Journal of Toxicology and Clinical Experiments* 8:95–99.

Vaughn, E.D., Hull, D.S., and Green, K. 1978. Effect of intraocular miotics on corneal endothelium. *Archives of Ophthalmology* 96:1897.

Vedal, S., Chan Yeung, M., Enarson, D., Fera, T., MacLean, L., Tse, K.S., and Langille, R. 1986. Symptoms and pulmonary function in western red cedar workers related to duration of employment and dust exposure. *Archives of Environmental Health* 41:179–183.

Venables, K.M. 1989. Low molecular weight chemicals, hypersensitivity and direct toxicity. The acid anhydrides. *British Journal Industrial Medicine* 46:222–232.

Verin, P., and Comte, P. 1987. Emergency treatment of the projection of caterpillar hairs into the cornea. *Bulletin of the Society of French Ophthalmology* 87:403–404.

Vernon, R.J., and Ferguson, R.K. 1969. Effects of trichloroethylene on visual motor performance. *Archives Environmental Health* 18:894.

Vevchenko, M.S., and Vysochin, V.I. 1988. Detection of occupational trinitrotoluene cataract. *Vrachebnoe Delo (Kiev)* 2:108–109.

Vighetto, A., Grochowicki, M., and Juillet-Reitz, M. 1990. A rare cause of accidental pharmacologic mydriasis. *Presse Medicale (Paris)* 19:219.

Vigoli, J., Whitehead, B., and Marcus, S.M. 1985. Oven-cleaner pads: new risk for corrosive injury. *American Journal of Emergency Medicine* 3:412–414.

Virno, M. 1963. Oral glycerol in ophthalmology. *American Journal of Ophthalmology* 55:1133.

Von Berg, R. 1988. Toxicology update. *Journal of Applied Toxicology* 8:145–148.

Von Burg, R. 1982. Toxicology updates. Xylene. *Journal of Applied Toxicology* 2:269–271.

Wald, P.H. 1990. Review of the literature on the toxicity of rare-earth metals as it pertains to the engineering demonstration surrogate test. Revision 1. *Government Reports, Announcements and Index*, Issue 17.

Waldrep, J.C., and Crosson, C.E. 1988. Induction of keratouveitis by capsaicin. *Current Eye Research* 7:1173–1182.

Walsh, F.B., and Hoyt, W.F. 1969. *Clinical Neuro-Ophthalmology*, vol. 1, 3rd ed., pp. 447. Baltimore: Williams and Wilkins.

Waltman, S.R. 1977. Corneal endothelial changes with long-term topical epinephrine therapy. *Archives of Ophthalmology* 95:1357.

Wang, Y., Xia, J., and Wang, Q.W. 1988. Clinical report on 62 cases of acute dimethyl sulfate intoxication. *American Journal of Industrial Medicine* 13:455–467.

Warren, D.W., Jr., and Selchan, D.F. 1988. An industrial hygiene appraisal of triethylamine and dimethylethylamine exposure limits in the foundry industry. *American Industrial Hygiene Association Journal* 49:630–634.

Watanabe, H., and Shearer, T.R. 1989. Lens crysallins in aqueous and vitreous humor in selenite overdose cataract. *Current Eye Research* 8:979–986.

Weber, R., Budmiger, H., and Siegenthaler, W. 1988. Chronic formaldehyde exposure—a misunderstood disease? *Schweizerische Medizinische Wochenschrift. Journal Suisse de Medecine (Basel)* 118:457–461.

Weleber, R.B., and Shults, W.T. 1981. Digoxin retinal toxicity. Clinical and electrophysiologic evaluation of a cone dysfunction syndrome. *Archives of Ophthalmology* 99:1568.

Wells, P.G., Wilson, B., and Lubek, B.M. 1989. In vivo murine studies on the biochemical mechanism of naphthalene cataractogenesis. *Toxicology and Applied Pharmacology* 99:466–473.

WHO Working Group. 1978. Photochemical oxidants. *Environmental Health Criteria* 7:1–110.

WHO Working Group. 1984a. Trichloroethylene. *Environmental Health Criteria*, 50:1–133.

WHO Working Group. 1984b. Tetrachloroethylene. *Environmental Health Criteria* 31:1–48.

WHO Working Group. 1985. Toluene. *Environmental Health Criteria* 52:1–146.

WHO Working Group. 1986. Ammonia. *Environmental Health Criteria* 54:1–210.

WHO Working Group. 1987. *tert*-Butanol. *Environmental Health Criteria* 65:67–92.

Whorton, M.D., and Obrinsky, D.L. 1983. Persistence of symptoms after mild to moderate acute organophosphate poisoning among 19 farm field workers. *Journal of Toxicology and Environmental Health* 11:347–354.

Willetts, G.S. 1969. Ocular side-effects of drugs. *British Journal of Ophthalmology* 53:252.

Willis, C.M., Stephens, C.J.M., and Wilkinson, J.D. 1988. Experimentally-induced irritant contact dermatitis. Determination of optimum irritant concentrations. *Contact Dermatitis* 18:20–24.

Wills, J.H. 1970. Toxicity of anticholinesterases and treatment of poisoning. In *Anticholinesterase Agents, International Encyclopedia of Pharmacology and Therapeutics*, ed. Karacaman, A.G., p. 355. Oxford: Pergamon Press.

Wilson, J. 1967. Leber's hereditary optic atrophy—a possible disorder of cyanide detoxication. *Excerpta Medica International Congress Series* 154:70–73.

Wilson, K.W. 1974. Survey of eye irritation and lachrymation in relation to air pollution. Report proposed for the NY Coordination Research Council, Inc., pp. 1–45. Copley International Corporation.

Wilson, R.P., Spaeth, G.L., and Poryzees, E. 1980. The place of timolol in the practice of ophthalmology. *Ophthalmology* 87:451.

Wirtschafter, Z.T. 1933. Toxic amblyopia and accompanying physiological disturbances in carbon tetrachloride intoxication. *American Journal of Public Health* 23:1035.

Wrong, O. 1988. Ammonia burns to the eye. *British Medical Journal of Clinical Research* 296:1263.

Wyngaarden, V.B., and Seevers, M.H. 1951. Toxic effects of antihistamine drugs. *Journal of the American Medical Association* 145:277.

Yamashita, M., Nakamura, K., Naito, H., et al. 1987. Acute blasticidin-s poisoning. *Veterinary and Human Toxicology* 29:8–11.

Yarbrough, B.E., Garrettson, L.K., Zolet, D.I., Cooper, K.R., Kellaher, A.B., and Steele, M.H. 1985–1986. Severe central nervous system damage and profound acidosis in persons exposed to pentoborane. *Journal of Toxicology and Clinical Toxicology* 23:519–536.

Yesilada, E., Tanaka, S., Sezik, E., and Tabata, M. 1988. Isolation of an anti-inflammatory principle from the fruit juice of *Ecballium elaterium*. *Journal of National Produce* 51:504–508.

Yu, H.S., Pastor, S.A., Lam, K.W., and Yee, R.W. 1990. Ascorbate-enhanced copper toxicity on bovine corneal endothelial cells in vitro. *Current Eye Research* 9:177–182.

Zagorski, Z., Palae, O., Grabowski, J., Lang, G.K., and Naumann, G.O. 1989. Comparative studies in chronic ocular chalcosis. *Klinika Oczna (Warszawa)* 91:73–75.

Zeitling, G.L., Hobin, K., Platt, J., and Woitkoski, N. 1989. Accumulation of carbon dioxide during eye surgery. *Journal of Clinical Anesthesia* 1:262–267.

Zylic, Z., De Grip, W.J., Wagener, D.J., Van Rennes, H., Van der Kleijn, E., Van den Brock, L.A., and Ottenheijm, H.D. 1989. Studies on retinotoxic potential of a novel antitumor antibiotic—sparsomycin—in rats. *Anticancer Research* 9:923–927.

Ophthalmic Toxicology
Edited by George C. Y. Chiou
Copyright © 1999 Taylor & Francis

9

Treatment of Chemical Ocular Injury

Linda C. Epner

*Department of Ophthalmology, Cullen Eye Institute, Baylor College of Medicine,
Houston, Texas, USA*

- **General Principles**
- **Experimental Animal Treatment Models**
  - Use of Trapidil and Hydrocortisone for Treatment of Corneal Neovascularization
  - Paracentesis and Anterior Chamber Irrigation With Phosphate Buffer
  - Treatment of Hydrofluoric Acid Burns
  - Evaluation of Hypertonic Saline and Glucose on Alkali Corneal Burns
  - Ascorbic Acid for Corneal Burns
  - Investigational Use of Tissue Adhesive for Corneal Perforations
  - Medroxyprogesterone for Prevention of Alkali-Burn Perforations
  - Epidermal Growth Factor in Alkali Corneal Reepithelialization
  - Conservative Management of Symblephara
  - Platelet Activating Factor Antagonism
  - Corticosteroid Use on Ulceration in Alkali Burns
- **Surgical Treatment**
  - Conjunctiva
  - Cornea
  - Corneal Perforation
- **References**

GENERAL PRINCIPLES

Immediate and copious irrigation of the injured eye with a bland irrigating solution is the key element in the treatment of any chemical injury to the eye. Begin irrigation on-site within seconds after the injury and continue en route to, and at, the emergency facility (Pfister and Koski, 1982; Pfister, 1983; Campochiaro et al., 1990). To begin irrigation, the eyelids should be spread open with a lid retractor (Desmarres), or even with the fingertips if a retractor is not available, and flooded with a bland solution, such as water or Ringer's intravenous fluid (Nelson and Kopietz, 1987; Burns and Paterson, 1989). Remove any goggles, glasses, or contact lenses that may interfere with irrigation (Pyramid Films Corp., 1981). The victim should be asked to roll the eyes in all directions to improve irrigation of ocular surfaces, including conjunctival cul-de-sacs. The eyes should be examined carefully, including sweeping of the conjunctival fornices, to remove any foreign particles, such as solid chemicals that, if retained, will continue to leak chemicals into the eyes despite irrigation. Any foreign particles may be gently lifted off the conjunctiva of the cornea with a clean tissue or cotton-tip applicator. Alternatively, foreign particles, once identified, may be irrigated off the ocular surface as well.

Irrigation after arrival at the medical facility should be continued using suspended bags of pH-balanced intravenous fluid connected by sterile tubing with or without a scleral contact lens on the injured eye. Continue irrigation for a minimum of one liter of irrigation fluid for a mild injury to several hours of irrigation for a severe alkali injury. Periodically, the pH of the conjunctival cul-de-sac should be checked with litmus paper, continuing irrigation until the pH is normal again. Alkalies cause deeper ocular damage and may remain deep in ocular tissue, acting as a reservoir of base. They can continue to produce ocular damage despite irrigation. Alkali injuries, therefore, require prolonged irrigation until the pH is normal and remains normal with repeated checks.

After irrigation, the eye should be examined at the slit-lamp with fluorescein stain to look for any epithelial defects and for the depth of the anterior chamber. Once it is determined that the patient will tolerate mydriasis without risk of angle closure, a strong cycloplegic agent, such as atropine 1%, should be started twice daily. Topical antibiotic eye drops also are indicated, four times a day, to prevent infection. If possible, an attempt should be made to measure the intraocular pressure. Secondary glaucoma, especially, develops in alkali burns due to collagen shrinkage. Acetazolamide (an oral carbonic anhydrase inhibitor) may be started to control intraocular pressure. In severe alkali burns, normalization of the pH of the aqueous by anterior chamber paracentesis with reformation with balanced salt solution or phosphate buffer may be useful, but this procedure is controversial (Pfister, 1983; Campochiaro et al., 1990; Deutsch and Feller, 1985).

The role of topical steroids also is controversial. They may be used safely during the first week after injury whether the corneal epithelium is intact or not. Beyond the first week, experimental data suggests that they may contribute to corneal ulceration, and even perforation, due to interference with new collagen synthesis, which is necessary in the reparative process (Donshik et al., 1978). If topical steroids are used at all, they should be discontinued after the first week until the corneal epithelium is again intact.

There is an outpouring of collagenase after chemical burns, which leads to corneal ulceration. Various collagenase inhibitors have been advocated in the treatment of alkali burns. These agents include acetylcysteine (Mucomyst 10% or 20%), cysteine, penicillamine 0.15 M, calcium ethylenediaminetetraacetic acid (EDTA), and medroxyprogesterone (Pfister et al., 1983; Deutsch and Feller, 1985; Newsome and Gross, 1977). Collagenase inhibitors act either reversibly or irreversibly to inhibit collagenase action or synthesis.

Ascorbate levels in the aqueous humor are normally 15–20 times the plasma level (Pfister and Koski, 1982). Alkali injuries cause a dramatic and prolonged drop in ascorbate levels (Levinson et al., 1976). Since ascorbate is necessary for fibroblast collagen synthesis and critical for postinjury corneal repair, it has been used to treat alkali burns (Pfister and Koski, 1982). Either topical 10% solution or high oral dosages (2 g four times a day) may be used to maintain high aqueous ascorbate levels to minimize ulceration.

Severe alkali injuries, in particular, may result in vision and even eye-threatening scarring. Symblepharon formation should be minimized by symblephara rings, scleral contact lenses, and lysis of early conjunctival adhesions as they form. Once symblephara are fixed, however, surgical measures are required to release them. These include conjunctival autografts if a normal conjunctiva is available and buccal mucosal grafts if it is not (Thoft, 1982; Paton and Milauskas, 1970).

Often, despite very aggressive treatment of alkali and other chemical burns to the eye, severe scarring of the cornea, eyelids, and intraocular tissues occurs. Any rehabilitative surgery, such as penetrating keratoplasties, lid repairs, and so on, should be delayed for as long as possible, preferably for at least 1 year postinjury (Pfister and Koski, 1982). This allows inflammation to clear and improves the success rate of rehabilitative surgery (Panda et al., 1984; Abel et al., 1975; Dohlman et al., 1967; Tragakis et al., 1974). Other issues that must be addressed in a timely fashion include continued treatment of any glaucoma and any formed cataracts. Keratoprosthesis is reserved for the most difficult of cases where lid function cannot be restored and penetrating keratoplasties have failed (Kozarsky et al., 1987; Polack and Heimke, 1980).

EXPERIMENTAL ANIMAL TREATMENT MODELS

Use of Trapidil and Hydrocortisone for Treatment of Corneal Neovascularization

Benelli et al. studied the effect of trapidil, a medication used clinically to treat ischemic heart disease, on corneal neovascularization. They noted a similar degree of antiangiogenic effect by trapidil or hydroxycortisone-21-phosphate when topically applied four times a day to silver nitrate- or potassium nitrate-injured rat cornea. When used together, topical trapidil and hydrocortisone produced a marked decrease in corneal neovascularization (Benelli et al., 1995).

Paracentesis and Anterior Chamber Irrigation With Phosphate Buffer

Bennett et al. (1978) designed an experimental model using albino rabbits to determine the effect of phosphate buffer irrigation of the anterior chamber in alkali-burned corneas in rabbits. Alkali burns were produced by using one drop of 0.5 N NaOH placed on an 8-mm filter paper disk that was applied to the rabbit cornea for 40 sec.

The rabbits were divided into five experimental groups. Groups 1 and 2 served as controls, receiving either corneal burns with no irrigation (group 2) or phosphate irrigation with no burn (group 1). Groups 3, 4, and 5 all received corneal burns, but phosphate buffer irrigation was instituted at varying times: immediate treatment, 15 min later, and 30 min later. After 6 weeks, eyes were examined clinically and histologically to determine the amount of corneal opacification and cataract formation. Burned corneas not receiving buffer irrigation uniformly developed extensive corneal vascularization and cataract formation. In contrast, burned corneas receiving phosphate buffer irrigation within 15 min developed less corneal vascularization and cataract formation. All eyes developed cataracts if buffer irrigation occurred at 30 min. Control eyes were unaffected by buffer irrigation, either clinically or histologically. This study suggests that early paracentesis and normalization of aqueous pH with phosphate buffer in alkali-burned corneas may decrease the degree of injury to the eye.

Treatment of Hydrofluoric Acid Burns

Hydrofluoric (HF) acid is used commonly in a variety of industrial settings. Eye injuries involving HF acid result in more serious damage compared with other acids, due to the ability of the fluoride ion to penetrate and cause liquefactive necrosis. McCulley et al. (1983) investigated the benefit of various irrigation solutions and topical ointments in treating HF corneal burns in rabbits. Some of the irrigating solutions investigated included $MgCl_2$, NaCl, lanthanum chloride ($LaCl_3$), 0.2% hyamine, and zephiran. Magnesium oxide or $MgSO_4$ topical petrolatum ointments also were tried. Many of the above proved unsuitable for treatment due to toxicity in normal rabbit eyes. The study revealed that the best treatment for HF burns remains immediate irrigation with water, isotonic saline (NaCl), or $MgCl_2$. Repetitive irrigation was found to be less effective than single irrigation with increased risk of corneal ulceration. Since water and isotonic saline are the most immediately available irrigation solutions at the time of injury, they remain the gold standard for treatment of HF and other acid ocular burns.

Evaluation of Hypertonic Saline and Glucose on Alkali Corneal Burns

Alkali burns to the cornea produce edema, which is thought to be a precondition for revascularization (Singh and Foster, 1987). An inadequate glucose supply to the cornea also is implicated in stromal ulceration (Pfister et al., 1971). These observations prompted evaluation of hypertonic saline and glucose ointment on rabbit corneal burns by Korey et al. (1977). Corneal burns were produced by applying 0.5 N NaOH-soaked filter paper for 30 sec with the rabbit under general anesthesia, followed by 60-sec lavage with distilled water. The rabbits were divided into three groups and treated with either vehicle, 40% glucose, or 5% NaCl ophthalmic ointment. Eyes were examined at 3 weeks and 6 weeks, both clinically and histologically, for corneal neovascularization, corneal ulceration, lenticular clouding, and red reflex. The results of this study demonstrate that treatment of corneal alkali burns with hypertonic glucose and saline ointments in rabbits resulted in much less corneal ulceration and neovascularization. Notably, there was no difference between hypertonic glucose and saline in the degree of corneal ulceration, and corneal clarity was better with hypertonic NaCl. Histologically, NaCl-treated rabbit eyes demonstrated more endothelium regeneration.

Ascorbic Acid for Corneal Burns

Levinson et al. (1976) found that ascorbate levels in the aqueous dramatically drop after alkali injury to rabbit cornea. They hypothesized that treating alkali-burned eyes with topical or subconjunctival injections of ascorbate to normalize aqueous ascorbate levels may help corneal healing. In their studies (Levinson et al., 1976; Pfister and Paterson, 1977; Pfister et al., 1978), New Zealand rabbits were anesthetized with pentobarbital sodium. Uniformly sized corneal burns were produced by filling a 6- or 12-mm lucite well with 1 N NaOH placed on the proptosed cornea. The NaOH was pipetted out after 20 sec, and the lucite well and cornea were rinsed with saline for 5 sec. Control rabbits received no treatment, while the remainder of the rabbits received daily injections of ascorbate either subcutaneously or topically. The researchers discovered that ascorbate-treated rabbits were less likely to develop descemetoceles and corneal perforation. Their findings have been confirmed by others (Nirankari et al., 1981; Petroutsos and Pouliquen, 1984). Ascorbate's mechanism of action remains unclear. It is known that ascorbate is necessary for new collagen synthesis, but it also may act to inhibit collagenase activity (Nirankari et al., 1981). Others feel it works as a superoxide radical scavenging agent (Petroutsos and Pouliquen, 1984).

Investigational Use of Tissue Adhesive for Corneal Perforations

Descemetocele formation leading to corneal perforation is a formidable treatment challenge. CHC tissue adhesive (carbohexoxymethyl 2-cyanoacrylate monomer) produced by Ethicon has been used on an investigative basis for treatment of corneal perforations. Investigators at the Wilmer Institute have been studying its use since 1974 (Hirst et al., 1982). The glue is applied under microscopic control with topical anesthetic. After meticulously drying the perforation site, the anterior chamber is partially reformed with a small air bubble at the perforation site. A small drop of the tissue adhesive is then placed at the perforation site. After the glue has dried, it can be covered with a bandage-style soft contact lens, or a more definitive surgery may be performed once the anterior chamber is fully reformed. The tissue adhesive can be left in place for up to a year if it does not dislodge spontaneously sooner. It may be removed easily, if necessary, with a pair of sterile, fine-toothed forceps. Investigators at Wilmer have found in a retrospective study that the incidence of enucleation after corneal perforation had decreased from 19% to 6% since initiation of tissue adhesive treatment, and 29% compared with 19% of the patients achieved visual acuities 20/200 or better (Hirst et al., 1982).

Medroxyprogesterone for Prevention of Alkali-Burn Perforations

Newsome and Gross (1977) examined the effects of a known collagenase synthesis inhibitor, medroxyprogesterone, on collagenase activity in alkali-burned rabbit cornea. Albino rabbits were anesthetized with intravenous sodium pentobarbital, and uniformly sized alkali burns were induced by 1 N NaOH-soaked gauze disks. Rabbits were separated into control and treatment groups. Treated rabbits were further subdivided by mode of medroxyprogesterone administration: (a) topical drops consisting of 0.5% suspension of medroxyprogesterone in 1% methylcellulose daily or twice daily, (b) subconjunctival depot injections of 10 mg Depo-Provera repeated at weekly intervals, and (c) 200-mg intramuscular injections of Depo-Provera into the hind leg of rabbits at 7- to 8-day intervals.

All three modes of administration were effective in preventing corneal perforation. Only 4 out of 85 untreated corneas healed, compared with 51 out of 87 treated corneas that reepithelialized without perforation. There was a three- to four-fold decrease in collagenolytic activity in the treated animals compared with the controls. The rates of corneal ulceration were similar; approximately one-quarter in each group ulcerated but did not perforate. Of note, far fewer medroxyprogesterone-treated animals developed corneal perforation (8 out of 87) compared with a greater than 50% perforation rate in untreated corneas (49 out of 85 eyes). Further studies are necessary to delineate minimum effective dosages that may be as effective as the large doses used in this study.

Epidermal Growth Factor in Alkali Corneal Reepithelialization

Treatment of poorly reepithelializing corneas and recurrent corneal erosions is a major therapeutic challenge in alkali-burned corneas. Currently available treatment modalities, including bandage contact lenses, ascorbate, topical corticosteroids, and so on, often fail. Epidermal growth factor (EGF) is a polypeptide known to stimulate corneal epithelial cell proliferation. It is isolated from mouse submaxillary glands. EGF was studied in a double-masked fashion to evaluate its effect on corneal reepithelialization in alkali-burned rabbit corneas (Singh and Foster, 1987). Rabbits were anesthetized with intravenous sodium pentobarbital and topical 0.5% proparacaine eye drops. Ten-millimeter circular corneal alkali burns were produced by placing 1 N NaOH-soaked 10-mm-diameter Whatman filter paper disks on central corneas for 1 min. Eyes were rinsed with distilled water, and methylene blue (0.5%) was used to confirm the area of epithelial loss. Mouse EGF eye drops were produced by suspending 0.05 μg/ml EGF in phosphate buffer saline. Rabbits were randomly assigned to three treatment groups. Groups A and B received EGF drops or placebo drops four times a day, beginning 16 hr after the alkali injury; then drops were reversed, and those receiving placebo drops received EGF, and vice versa, beginning on day 6 after the alkali injury. Group C served as control, receiving no treatment drops at all. The results showed increased corneal epithelial wound healing in eyes receiving EGF. When EGF drops were discontinued, the corneal epithelium broke down again centrally. Those rabbits receiving placebo drops initially showed incomplete reepithelialization; however, once EGF was started, the wound closed completely. Histopathological studies revealed poorly adherent epithelium growing over no basement membrane and alkali-burned cornea stroma. The authors conclude that, although EGF enhances epithelial growth in alkali-burned rabbit corneas, it has no effect on adherence of the epithelium to its underlying damaged stroma and, thus, has no effect in preventing the well-known complication of recurrent erosions. The authors suggest that a combination of EGF and other factors that may enhance epithelial attachment to underlying stroma may prove to be helpful therapeutic modalities in the future (Singh and Foster, 1987).

Conservative Management of Symblephara

One of the most difficult complications of alkali burns is shortening of the conjunctival fornices from scarring and the formation of adhesions between raw deepithelialized conjunctival surfaces (symblephara). Since treatment of extensive, formed symblephara is quite difficult, many different techniques have been tried to prevent their formation in the first place. Treatment modalities include symblephara rings, a scleral conformer fitted to prevent shortening of conjunctival fornices, or scleral contact lens. Other modalities that have been tried with limited success include plastic wrap and eggshell membrane lining of conjunctival fornices (Croll and Croll, 1952). A standard prophylactic treatment is daily sweeping of conjunctival fornices to lyse any forming symblepharon with a glass rod (Belin and Hannush, 1987).

Platelet Activating Factor Antagonism

In addition to prostaglandins (PGs) and leukotrienes (LTs), platelet activating factor (PAF) is considered to be involved in the inflammatory reaction. It follows that PAF antagonists could be used as anti-inflammatory agents after alkali burns (Bazan et al., 1987). PAF stimulates release of arachidonic acid and production of hydroxyeicosatetraenoic acid (HETE). In this study, a PAF antagonist, BN 52021, was applied topically to NaOH-burned corneas of New Zealand white rabbits in which 6 μl of labeled arachidonic acid were injected into the anterior chamber. The PAF antagonist was applied according to three experimental designs varying the spacing and frequency of drops. Postmortem analysis of corneal buttons were analyzed to measure levels of PGs and HETEs. Results showed that the PAF antagonist significantly inhibited production of radiolabeled cyclooxygenase and lipoxygenase products (HETEs) after alkali injury, especially when applied in an uninterrupted manner during the immediate postinjury period every 30 min, for a total of nine times. No effect was noted, however, in the amount of protein content in aqueous humor with PAF antagonist.

Corticosteroid Use on Ulceration in Alkali Burns

A study was done by Donshik et al. (1978) to evaluate the effect of topical corticosteroid drops on ulcerated alkali-burned corneas. The study was performed on albino rabbits. The results show that topical steroids given during postinjury weeks 2 and 3 resulted in increased severity of corneal ulcerations. The mechanism for this still is unclear, but may be related to inhibition of new collagen synthesis, rather than steroid enhancement of collagenase enzyme activity. Generally, if topical steroids are to be used at all after severe alkali corneal ulceration, they should be used only during the immediate postinjury period, days 1 through 6, then discontinued until the cornea is intact again. If, at any time during steroid use, corneal melting begins, steroids should be discontinued immediately.

SURGICAL TREATMENT

"Conjunctival transdifferentiation" is the process by which normal corneal epithelium replacement occurs via migration and differentiation of conjunctival limbal stem cells in a centripetal manner. In severe chemical corneal injuries in which limbal stem cells are entirely destroyed, normal corneal reepithelialization is impossible. This leads to the well-known postinjury complications: (a) recurrent corneal erosions, (b) recurrent epithelial defects, (c) corneal stromal neovascularization, (d) persistent inflammation, and (e) corneal stromal thinning and even perforation and blindness (Kenyon and Tseng, 1989).

Surgical transplantation of conjunctiva and cornea are frequently done to relieve symptoms of eye injury for therapeutic or cosmetic benefit. Details of surgical techniques are not covered here. Readers are encouraged to consult the original literature or surgical texts if interested.

Conjunctiva

Autologous Limbal Stem Cell Conjunctival Transplantation

Unilateral chemical injuries in which there is severe conjunctival scarring may benefit from autologous conjunctival transplantation from the normal fellow eye. The scarred abnormal conjunctiva is dissected free, and the normal graft conjunctiva is then sutured in place either as a single doughnut-shaped graft or as multiple, smaller islands of conjunctiva.

Kenyon and Tseng performed limbal stem cell autografts from normal eyes to injured eyes to reestablish a normal stem cell population, leading to stable corneal reepithelialization. They performed stem cell autografts on 26 consecutive patients with corneal injury (including 20 patients with chemical corneal injuries) with a mean follow-up time of 18 months. Key features of their surgical technique include the following: (a) sharing of remaining healthy basal stem cells between injured and healthy eyes (only half of the donor stem cells were transplanted, leaving a healthy population of stem cells to maintain the donor corneal integrity); (b) gentle debridement of recipient corneal stromal vascularization and clearing of limbus to bare sclera at recipient site; (c) donor site conjunctiva marked focally with light cautery to mark proper orientation of graft; (d) thin dissection of donor conjunctiva, avoiding Tenon's tissue; (e) excision of two arcuate grafts, measuring ~3 mm × 11 mm, extending 4 clock hours and separated by 180°. Each graft extended 0.5 mm onto clear cornea and 2 mm onto bulbar conjunctiva; (f) grafts sutured with 10-0 nylon on corneal border and 8-0 vicryl on conjunctival border; and (g) donor site closed with two 8-0 vicryl sutures or left bare sclera for reepithelialization (Kenyon and Tseng, 1989).

The majority of patients (17/26) gained improved visual acuity with no intraoperative or postoperative complications, such as corneal perforations. There was rapid, permanent healing of corneal epithelial defect and a decrease in corneal stromal neovascularization, resulting in improved cosmesis with decreased photophobia. The donor eye was unharmed as some stem cells were preserved (Kenyon and Tseng, 1989).

Stem cell limbal autograft may be used as a viable treatment option in patients with both acute and chronic chemical corneal injury as well as in patients with corneal injury secondary to other etiologies (Kenyon and Tseng, 1989).

Conjunctival Flap

A Gunderson conjunctival flap is another technique that has been used in eyes with nonhealing epithelium and poor visual potential. A variation on the Gunderson technique has been described by Paton and Milauskas (1970). The keys to a successful flap include (a) no buttonholes, (b) an absence of traction from the flap base, and (c) thinness of the flap. It is important to remove Tenon's capsule from the undersurface of the dissected flap prior to securing on the cornea. The free margin of the flap is sutured to the episclera and the eye patched for 12–24 hr postoperatively. Most patients experience pain relief. Vision is limited by density of the central corneal scar and the thickness of the conjunctival flap.

Cornea

Pressure Patch

Mild contact thermal burns to the cornea, such as those from curling irons, may cause opacification of the corneal epithelium. Conservative management of such injuries includes topical cycloplegia, antibiotic eye drops, and pressure patching of the injured eye with a soft sterile eye pad over the closed eyelid. The injured cornea usually reepithelializes within 24–72 hr, depending on the size of the epithelial defect (Bloom et al., 1986).

Therapeutic Contact Lenses

Hydrophilic contact lenses can be used in patients with delayed healing of corneal and conjunctival injuries after chemical or thermal burns (Leibowitz and Berrospi, 1975; Bechara et al., 1987). Any necrotic tissue from the injured site should be gently debrided prior to placement of the bandage contact lens. These lenses allow regeneration of the epithelium and patient comfort. Hydrophilic contact lenses also have been used as a mode of therapy for descemetoceles. The cornea in a descemetocele is reduced in the involved area to only Descemet's membrane with no overlying stroma or epithelium.

Keratoplasty

Keratoplasty has been used as a surgical treatment for a variety of ocular conditions. It may be used in the late treatment of alkali burns, although the prognosis is not as favorable as penetrating keratoplasties performed for other ocular disorders, such as keratoconus or corneal stromal dystrophies. Postcorneal transplants performed after severe chemical injuries may be complicated by poor wound healing, severe dry eye, recurrent epithelial breakdown, and glaucoma. These complications can be minimized by pre-and postoperative glaucoma control, preservation of donor epithelium, and control of postoperative inflammation (Belin and Hannush, 1987).

Corneal Perforation

Corneal Perforation Repair

When a full-thickness corneal defect occurs, it may be repaired by several techniques. A peripheral corneal perforation away from the visual axis may be repaired with a scleral or corneal patch graft (Larsson, 1948). As sclera is opaque, this technique is not suitable for corneal defects that are within the visual axis. Donor corneal tissue may be used as a lamellar patch graft (Dohlman et al., 1967; Tragakis et al., 1974) for central perforations. Sutures should be placed away from the visual axis, and deep corneal bites should be used to avoid "cheese-wiring" of sutures through edematous corneal tissue. In some cases, very tiny corneal perforations may seal themselves spontaneously. Techniques used to plug a perforation include bandage soft contact lenses, autogenous Tenon's capsule, and cyanoacrylate adhesive glue. Cyanoacrylate adhesives provide a relatively simple means of closing a corneal perforation that is small (< 2 mm) or temporizing until penetrating keratoplasty may be performed with a formed anterior chamber. Since the polymerized adhesive leaves an irregular surface, a bandage contact lens should be placed over the site after placing the glue plug. The glue plug usually dislodges spontaneously within several weeks or is removed at the time of the corneal transplant (Mandelbaum and Udell, 1987).

Keratoprosthesis

When ocular scarring is so severe that penetrating keratoplasty techniques have failed, prosthokeratoplasty may be considered as a last resort. Keratoprosthesis may provide a limited amount of sight in the end stages of severe scarring disorders, such as cicatricial pemphigoid, erythema multiforme (Stevens–Johnson syndrome), and severe chemical burns. Various types of keratoprostheses have been tried with limited success. Polack and Heimke (1980) designed a two-piece ceramic kerato-prosthesis. It consists of an aluminum oxide, 10-mm-long optical cylinder, and an 8.5-mm-diameter retaining disk with 12 suture holes and a central 3-mm opening (Kozarsky et al., 1987). Complications of keratoprostheses include infection, extrusion of implant, glaucoma, and retinal detachment (Cardona and DeVoe, 1977).

REFERENCES

Abel, R., Jr., Binder, P.S., Polack, F.M., and Kaufman, H.E. 1975. The results of penetrating keratoplasty after chemical burns. *Transactions of the American Academy of Ophthalmology* 79:584–595.

Bazan, H.E.P., Braquet, P., Peddy, S.T.K., and Bazan, N.G. 1987. Inhibition of the alkali burn-induced lipoxygenation of arachidonic acid in the rabbit cornea by a PAF antagonist. *Journal of Ocular Pharmacology* 3:357–365.

Bechara, S.J., Kara-Jose, N., and Pettinati, A.H. 1987. Therapeutic use of contact lenses in alkali burns of the cornea. *Cornea* 6:117–121.

Belin, M.W., and Hannush, S.B. 1987. Mucous membrane abnormalities. In *Surgical Intervention in Corneal and External Diseases*, ed. R.I. Abbot, pp. 159–176. Orlando, FL: Grune & Stratton.

Benelli, U., Lepri, A., Nardi, M., Danesi, R., and Del Tacca, M. 1995. Trapidil inhibits endothelial cell proliferational angiogenesis in the chicken chorioallantoic membrane and in the rat cornea. *Journal of Ocular Pharmacology and Therapeutics* 11:157–166.

Bennett, T.O., Peyman, G.A., and Rutgard, J. 1978. Intracameral phosphate buffer in alkali burns. *Canadian Journal of Ophthalmology* 13:93–95.

Bloom, S.M., Gittinger, J.W., Jr., and Kazarian, E.L. 1986. Management of corneal thermal burns. *American Journal of Ophthalmology* 102:536.

Burns, F.R., and Paterson, C.A. 1989. Prompt irrigation of chemical eye injuries may avert severe damage. *Occupational Health and Safety* 58:33–36.

Campochiaro, P.A., Fogle, J.A., and Spyker, D.A. 1990. Chemical and drug injury to the eye. In *Chemical Management of Poisoning and Drug Overdoses*, eds. L.M. Haddad and J.F. Winchester, pp. 370–378. Philadelphia: W.B. Saunders.

Cardona, H., and DeVoe, A.G. 1977. Prosthokeratoplasty. *Transactions of the American Academy of Ophthalmology and Otolaryngology* 83:272–275.

Croll, M., and Croll, L.J. 1952. Egg membrane for chemical injuries of eye, new adjuvant treatment. *American Journal of Ophthalmology* 35:1585–1586.

Deutsch, T.A., and Feller, D.B. 1985. *Paton and Goldberg's Management of Ocular Injuries*, 2nd ed., pp. 93–100. Philadelphia: W.B. Saunders.

Dohlman, C.H., Boruchoff, S.A., and Sullivan, G.L. 1967. A technique for the repair of perforated corneal ulcer. *Archives of Ophthalmology (Chicago)* 77:519–525.

Donshik, P.C., Berman, M.B., Dohlman, C.H., Gage, J., and Rose, J. 1978. Effect of topical corticosteroids on ulceration in alkali-burned corneas. *Archives of Ophthalmology* 96:2117–2120.

Hirst, L.W., Smiddy, W.E., and Stark, W.J. 1982. Corneal perforations, changing methods of treatment 1960–1980. *Ophthalmology (Rochester)* 89:630–635.

Kenyon, K.R., and Tseng, S.C.G. 1989. Limbal autograft transplantation for ocular surface disorders. *Ophthalmology* 96:709–723.

Korey, M., Peyman, G.A., and Berkowitz, R. 1977. The effect of hypertonic ointments on corneal alkali burns. *Annals of Ophthalmology* 9:1383–1387.

Kozarsky, A.M., Knight, S.H., and Waring, G.O., 3rd. 1987. Clinical results with a ceramic keratoprosthesis placed through the eyelid. *Ophthalmology* 94:904–911.

Larsson, S. 1948. Treatment of perforated corneal ulcer by autoplastic scleral transplantation. *British Journal of Ophthalmology* 32:54–57.

Leibowitz, H.M., and Berrospi, A.R. 1975. Initial treatment of descemetocele with hydrophilic contact lenses. *Annals of Ophthalmology* 1975:1161–1166.

Levinson, R.A., Paterson, C.A., and Pfister, R.R. 1976. Ascorbic acid prevents corneal ulceration and perforation following experimental alkali burns. *Investigative Ophthalmology* 15:986–993.

Mandelbaum, S., and Udell, I.J. 1987. Noninfected corneal perforations. In *Surgical Intervention in Corneal and External Diseases*, ed. R.L. Abbott, pp. 87–106. Orlando, FL: Grune & Stratton.

McCulley, J.P., Whiting, D.W., Pettit, M.G., and Lauber, S.E. 1983. Hydrofluoric acid burns of the eye. *Journal of Occupational Medicine* 25:447–450.

Nelson, J.D., and Kopietz, L.A. 1987. Chemical injuries to the eye. Emergency, intermediate and long-term care. *Postgraduate Medicine* 81:62–66,69–71,75.

Newsome, N.A., and Gross, J. 1977. Prevention of medroxyprogesterone of perforation in the alkali-burned rabbit cornea: inhibition of collagenolytic activity. *Investigative Ophthalmology and Visual Science* 16:21–31.

Nirankari, V.S., Varma, S.D., Lakhanpal, V., and Richards, R.D. 1981. Superoxide radical scavenging agents in treatment of alkali burns. An experimental study. *Archives of Ophthalmology* 99:886–887.

Panda, A., Mohan, M., Gupta, H.K., and Chawdhary, S. 1984. Keratoplasty in alkali burned corneas. *Indian Journal of Ophthalmology* 32:441–446.

Paton, D., and Milauskas, A.T. 1970. Indications, surgical technique and results of thin conjunctival flaps on the cornea: a review of 122 consecutive cases. *International Ophthalmology Clinics* 10:329–345.

Petroutsos, G., and Pouliquen, Y. 1984. Effect of ascorbic acid on ulceration in alkali-burned corneas. *Ophthalmic Research* 16:185–189.

Pfister, R.R. 1983. Chemical injuries of the eye. *Ophthalmology (Rochester)* 90:1246–1253.

Pfister, R.R., Friend, J., and Dohlman, C.H. 1971. The anterior segments of rabbits after alkali burns: metabolic and histologic alterations. 1971. *Archives of Ophthalmology* 86:189–193.

Pfister, R.R., and Koski, J. 1982. Alkali burns of the eye: pathophysiology and treatment. *Southern Medical Journal* 75:417–422.

Pfister, R.R., and Paterson, C.A. 1977. Additional clinical and morphological observations on the favorable effect of ascorbate on experimental ocular alkali burns. *Investigative Ophthalmology and Visual Science* 16:478–487.

Pfister, R.R., Paterson, C.A., and Hayes, S.A. 1978. Topical ascorbate decreases the incidence of corneal ulceration after experimental alkali burns. *Investigative Ophthalmology and Visual Science* 17:1019–1024.

Polack, F.M., and Heimke, G. 1980. Ceramic keratoprostheses. *Ophthalmology (Rochester)* 87:693–698.

Pyramid Films Corp. 1981. Preserving eyesight through quick response. *Occupational Health and Safety* 50:70–73.

Singh, G., and Foster, C.S. 1987. Epidermal growth factor in alkali-burned corneal epithelial healing. *American Journal of Ophthalmology* 103:802–807.

Thoft, R.A. 1982. Indications for conjunctival transplantation. *Ophthalmology (Rochester)* 89:335–339.

Tragakis, M.P., Rosen, J., and Brown, S.I. 1974. Transplantation of the perforated cornea. *American Journal of Ophthalmology* 78:518–522.

Index

Milton Keynes UK
Ingram Content Group UK Ltd.
UKHW021822071024
449327UK00021B/1394